The Anatomy of Melancholy

What It Is, With All The Kinds, Causes, Symptomes, Prognostics, And Several Cures Of It. In Three Partitions, With Their Several Sections, Members and Subsections, Philosophically, Medicinally, Historically Opened and Cut Up (Volume I)

Democritus Junior

Alpha Editions

This Edition Published in 2020

ISBN: 9789354211591

Design and Setting By
Alpha Editions
www.alphaedis.com
Email – info@alphaedis.com

As per information held with us this book is in Public Domain.
This book is a reproduction of an important historical work. Alpha Editions
uses the best technology to reproduce historical work in the same manner
it was first published to preserve its original nature. Any marks or number
seen are left intentionally to preserve its true form.

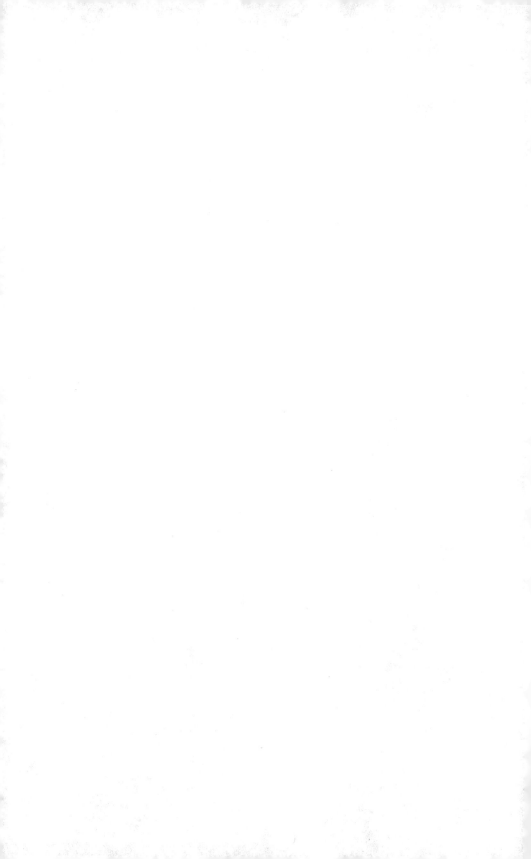

HONORATISSIMO DOMINO,

NON MINVS VIRTVTE SVA,

QUAM GENERIS SPLENDORE,

ILLVSTRISSIMO,

GEORGIO BERKLEIO

MILITI DE BALNEO,

BARONI DE BERKLEY, MOUBREY, SEGRAVE,

D. DE BRUSE,

DOMINO SVO MULTIS NOMINIBUS OBSERVANDO,

HANC SUAM

MELANCHOLIÆ ANATOMEN,

JAM SEXTO REVISAM,

D. D.

DEMOCRITUS Junior.

ADVERTISEMENT.

THE work now restored to public notice has had an ex-
traordinary fate. At the time of its original publication it
obtained a great celebrity, which continued more than half a
century. During that period few books were more read, or
more deservedly applauded. It was the delight of the learned,
the solace of the indolent, and the refuge of the uninformed.
It past through at least eight editions, by which the bookseller,
as WOOD *records, got an estate; and, notwithstanding the ob-*
jections sometimes opposed against it, of a quaint style, and too
great an accumulation of authorities, the fascination of its wit,
fancy, and sterling sense, have borne down all censures, and
extorted praise from the first writers in the English language.
The great JOHNSON *has praised it in the warmest terms, and*
the ludicrous STERNE *has interwoven many parts of it into his*
own popular performance. MILTON *did not disdain to build*
two of his finest poems on it; and a host of inferior writers have
embellished their works with beauties not their own, culled from
a performance which they had not the justice even to mention.
Change of times, and the frivolity of fashion, suspended in some
degree, that fame which had lasted near a century; and the suc-
ceeding generation affected indifference towards an author, who
at length was only looked into by the plunderers of literature,
the poachers in obscure volumes. The plagiarisms of Tristram
Shandy, *so successfully brought to light by* DR. FERRIAR, *at*
length drew the attention of the public towards a writer, who,
though then little known, might without impeachment of modesty
lay claim to every mark of respect; and inquiry proved, beyond
a doubt, that the calls of justice had been little attended to by
others, as well as the facetious Yorick. WOOD *observed, more*
than a century ago, that several authors had unmercifully
stolen matter from BURTON *without any acknowledgement.*
The time, however, at length arrived, when the merits of the
"Anatomy of Melancholy" were to receive their due praise.
The book was again sought for and read, and again it became

ADVERTISEMENT.

an applauded performance. Its excellencies once more stood confest, in the increased price which every copy offered for sale produced; and the increased demand pointed out the necessity of a new edition. This is now presented to the public in a manner not disgraceful to the memory of the author; and the undertakers of it rely with confidence, that so valuable a repository of amusement and information will continue to hold the rank it has been restored to, firmly supported by its own merit, and safe from the influence and blight of any future caprices of fashion.

The Argument of the Frontispiece [1].

TEN distinct Squares here seen apart,
Are joyn'd in one by Cutter's art.

1. Old Democritus under a tree,
Sits on a stone with book on knee;
About him hang there many features
Of cats, dogs, and such like creatures,
Of which he makes anatomy,
The seat of black choler to see.
Over his head appears the skie,
And Saturn Lord of melancholy.

2. To the left a landscape of Jealousie,
Presents itself unto thine eye.
A kingfisher, a swan, an hern,
Two fighting-cocks you may discern,
Two roaring bulls each other hie,
T' assault concerning venery.
Symboles are these; I say no more,
Conceive the rest by that's afore.

3. The next of solitariness,
A portraiture doth well express,
By sleeping dog, cat; buck and doe,
Hares, conies in the desart go;
Bats, owls the shady bowers over,
In melancholy darkness hover.
Mark well: If't be not as't should be,
Blame the bad Cutter, and not me.

4. I' th' under column there doth stand
Inamorato with folded hand;
Down hangs his head, terse and polite,
Some dittie sure he doth indite.
His lute and books about him lie,
As symptomes of his vanity.
If this do not enough disclose,
To paint him, take thyself by th' nose.

5. Hypochondriacus leans on his arm,
Winde in his side doth him much harm,
And troubles him full sore, God knows,
Much pain he hath and many woes.
About him pots and glasses lie,
Newly brought from's Apothecary.
This Saturn's aspects signifie,
You see them portraid in the skie.

6. Beneath them kneeling on his knee,
A superstitious man you see:
He fasts, prays, on his idol fixt,
Tormented hope and feare betwixt;
For hell perhaps he takes more pain,
Then thou dost heaven itself to gain.
Alas poor soule, I pitie thee,
What stars incline thee so to be?

7. But see the madman rage downright
With furious looks, a ghastly sight!
Naked in chains bound doth he lie
And roars amain he knows not why!
Observe him; for as in a glass,
Thine angry portraiture it was.
His picture keep still in thy presence;
'Twixt him and thee there's no difference.

8. 9. Borage and hellebor fill two scenes,
Soveraign plants to purge the veins
Of melancholy, and chear the heart
Of those black fumes which make it smart;
To clear the brain of misty fogs,
Which dull our senses, and soule clogs.
The best medicine that ere God made
For this malady, if well assaid.

10. Now last of all to fill a place,
Presented is the Author's face;
And in that habit which he wears,
His image to the world appears,
His minde no art can well express,
That by his writings you may guess.
It was not pride, nor yet vain glory,
(Though others do it commonly)
Made him do this: if you must know,
The Printer would needs have it so.
Then do not frown or scoffe at it,
Deride not, or detract a whit,
For surely as thou dost by him,
He will do the same again.
Then look upon't, behold and see,
As thou lik'st it, so it likes thee.
And I for it will stand in view,
Thine to command, Reader, adiew.

[1] These verses refer to the old folio Frontispiece, which was divided into ten compartments that are here severally explained. Though it was impossible to reduce that Frontispiece to an octavo size for this edition, the lines are too curious to be lost.

The Author's Abstract of Melancholy, Διαλογικῶς.

WHEN I go musing all alone,
Thinking of divers things fore-
known,
When I build castles in the ayr,
Void of sorrow and void of feare,
Pleasing myself with phantasms
sweet,
Methinks the time runs very fleet.
  All my joyes to this are folly,
    Naught so sweet as melancholy.
When I go walking all alone,
Recounting what I have ill done,
My thoughts on me then tyrannize,
Feare and sorrow me surprise,
Whether I tarry still or go,
Methinks the time moves very slow.
  All my griefs to this are jolly,
    Naught so sad as melancholy.
When to myself I act and smile,
With pleasing thoughts the time
beguile,
By a brook side or wood so green,
Unheard, unsought for, or unseen,
A thousand pleasures do me bless,
And crown my soule with happiness.
  All my joyes besides are folly,
    None so sweet as melancholy.
When I lie, sit, or walk alone,
I sigh, I grieve, making great
mone,
In a dark grove, or irksome den,
With discontents and Furies then,
A thousand miseries at once
Mine heavy heart and soule en-
sconce.
  All my griefs to this are jolly,
    None so sour as melancholy.
Me thinks I hear, me thinks I see,
Sweet musick, wondrous melodie,
Towns, palaces, and cities fine ;
Here now, then there ; the world is
mine.
Rare beauties, gallant ladies shine,
What e'er is lovely or divine.
  All other joyes to this are folly,
    None so sweet as melancholy.
Methinks I hear, methinks I see
Ghosts, goblins, fiends ; my phan-
tasie
Presents a thousand ugly shapes,
Headless bears, black men, and apes,
Doleful outcries, and fearful sights,
My sad and dismall soule affrights.
  All my griefs to this are jolly,
    None so damn'd as melancholy.

Me thinks I court, me thinks I kiss,
Me thinks I now embrace my
miss.
O blessed dayes, O sweet content,
In Paradise my time is spent.
Such thought may still my fancy
move,
So may I ever be in love.
  All my joyes to this are jolly,
    Naught so sweet as melancholy.
When I recount loves many frights,
My sighs and tears, my waking
nights,
My jealous fits ; O mine hard fate
I now repent, but 'tis too late.
No torment is so bad as love,
So bitter to my soule can prove,
  All my griefs to this are jolly,
    Naught so harsh as melancholy.
Friends and companions get you
gone,
'Tis my desire to be alone ;
Ne'er well but when my thoughts
and I
Do domineer in privacie.
No gemm, no treasure like to this,
'Tis my delight, my crown, my bliss,
  All my joyes to this are folly,
    Naught so sweet as melancholy.
'Tis my sole plague to be alone,
I am a beast, a monster grown,
I will no light nor company,
I finde it now my misery.
The scean is turn'd, my joyes are gone,
Feare, discontent, and sorrows come.
  All my griefs to this are jolly,
    Naught so fierce as melancholy.
I'll not change life with any King,
I ravisht am : can the world bring
More joy, then still to laugh and smile,
In pleasant toyes time to beguile ?
Do not, O do not trouble me,
So sweet content I feel and see.
  All my joyes to this are folly,
    None so divine as melancholy.
I'll change my state with any
wretch
Thou canst from gaole or dunghill
fetch :
My pain's past cure, another hell,
I may not in this torment dwell,
Now desperate I hate my life,
Lend me a halter or a knife ;
  All my griefs to this are jolly,
    Naught so damn'd as melancholy.

Democritus Junior ad Librum suum.

VADE liber, qualis, non ausim dicere, fœlix,
    Te nisi fœlicem fecerit alma dies.
Vade tamen quocunque lubet, quascunque per oras,
    Et Genium Domini fac imitere tui.
I blandas inter Charites, mystamque saluta
    Musarum quemvis, si tibi lector erit.
Rura colas, urbem, subeasve palatia regum,
    Submisse, placide, te sine dente geras.
Nobilis, aut si quis te forte inspexerit heros,
    Da te morigerum, perlegat usque lubet.
Est quod Nobilitas, est quod desideret heros,
    Gratior hæc forsan charta placere potest.
Si quis morosus Cato, tetricusque Senator
    Hunc etiam librum forte videre velit,
Sive magistratus, tum te reverenter habeto ;
    Sed nullus ; muscas non capiunt aquilæ.
Non vacat his tempus fugitivum impendere nugis,
    Nec tales cupio ; par mihi lector erit.
Si matrona gravis casu diverterit istuc,
    Illustris domina, aut te Comitissa legat :
Est quod displiceat, placeat quod forsitan illis,
    Ingerere his noli te modo, pande tamen.
At si virgo tuas dignabitur inclyta chartas
    Tangere, sive schedis hæreat illa tuis :
Da modo te facilem, et quædam folia esse memento
    Conveniant oculis quæ magis apta suis.
Si generosa ancilla tuos aut alma puella
    Visura est ludos, annue, pande lubens.
Dic, Utinam nunc ipse meus [1] (nam diligit istas)
    In præsens esset conspiciendus herus.
Ignotus notusve mihi de gente togatâ
    Sive aget in ludis, pulpita sive colet,
Sive in Lycæo, et nugas evolverit istas,
    Si quasdam mendas viderit inspiciens,
Da veniam auctori, dices ; nam plurima vellet
    Expungi, quæ jam displicuisse sciat.
Sive Melancholicus quisquam, seu blandus Amator,
    Aulicus aut Civis, seu bene comptus Eques
Huc appellat, age et tuto te crede legenti,
    Multa istic forsan non male nata leget.
Quod fugiat, caveat, quodque amplexabitur, ista
    Pagina fortassis promere multa potest.

[1] Hæc comice dicta, cave ne male capias.

xiv Democritus Junior ad Librum suum.

At si quis Medicus coram te sistet, amice
    Fac circumspecte, et te sine labe geras:
Inveniet namque ipse meis quoque plurima scriptis,
    Non leve subsidium quæ sibi forsan erunt.
Si quis Causidicus chartas impingat in istas,
    Nil mihi'vobiscum, pessima turba vale :
Sit nisi vir bonus, et juris sine fraude peritus ;
    Tum legat, et forsan doctior inde siet.
Si quis cordatus, facilis, lectorque benignus
    Huc oculos vertat, quæ velit ipse legat ;
Candidus ignoscet, metuas nil, pande libenter,
    Offensus mendis non erit ille tuis,
    Laudabit nonnulla.   Venit si Rhetor ineptus,
    Limata et tersa, et qui bene cocta petit,
Claude citus librum ; nulla hîc nisi ferrea verba,
    Offendent stomachum quæ minus apta suum.
At si quis non eximius de plebe poëta,
    Annue ; namque istic plurima ficta leget.
Nos sumus e numero, nullus mihi spirat Apollo,
    Grandiloquus Vates quilibet esse nequit.
Si Criticus Lector, tumidus Censorque molestus,
    Zoilus et Momus, si rabiosa cohors :
Ringe, freme, et noli tum pandere, turba malignis
    Si occurrat sannis invidiosa suis :
Fac fugias ; si nulla tibi sit copia eundi,
    Contemnes tacite, scommata quæque feres.
Frendeat, allatret, vacuas gannitibus auras
    Impleat, haud cures ; his placuisse nefas.
Verum age si forsan divertat purior hospes,
    Cuique sales, ludi, displiceantque joci,
Objiciatque tibi sordes, lascivaque : dices,
    Lasciva est Domino et Musa jocosa tuo,
Nec lasciva tamen, si pensitet omne; sed esto ;
    Sit lasciva licet pagina, vita proba est.
Barbarus, indoctusque rudis spectator in istam
    Si messem intrudat, fuste fugabis eum :
Fungum pelle procul (jubeo); nam quid mihi fungo ?
    Conveniunt stomacho non minus ista suo.
Sed nec pelle tamen : læto omnes accipe vultu,
    Quos, quas, vel quales, inde vel unde viros.
Gratus erit quicunque venit, gratissimus hospes
    Quisquis erit, facilis difficilisque mihi.
Nam si culpârit, quædam culpâsse juvabit ;
    Culpando faciet me meliora sequi.
Sed si laudârit, neque laudibus efferar ullis,
    Sit satis hisce malis opposuisse bonum.
Hæc sunt quæ nostro placuit mandare libello,
    Et quæ dimittens discere jussit Herus.

ACCOUNT OF THE AUTHOR.

ROBERT BURTON was the son of Ralph Burton, of an ancient and genteel family at Lindley, in Leicestershire, and was born there 8 February, 1576 [1]. He received the first rudiments of learning at the free school of Sutton Coldfield, in Warwickshire [2], from whence he was, at the age of seventeen, in the long vacation, 1593, sent to Brazen Nose College, in the condition of a commoner, where he made a considerable progress in logic and philosophy. In 1599 he was elected student of Christ-church, and, for form sake, was put under the tuition of Dr. John Bancroft, afterwards Bishop of Oxford. In 1614 he was admitted to the reading of the Sentences, and on the

[1] His elder brother was William Burton, the Leicestershire antiquary, born August 24, 1575, educated at Sutton Coldfield, admitted commoner, or gentleman commoner, of Brazen Nose college, 1591; at the Inner Temple, May 20, 1593; B. A. June 22, 1594; and afterwards a barrister and reporter in the court of Common Pleas. " But his natural genius," says Wood, " leading him to the studies of heraldry, genealogies, and antiquities, he became excellent in those obscure and intricate matters; and look upon him as a gentleman, was accounted, by all that knew him, to be the best of his time for those studies, as may appear by his description of Leicestershire." His weak constitution not permitting him to follow business, he retired into the country, and his greatest work, The Description of Leicestershire, was published in folio, 1622. He died at Falde, after suffering much in the civil war, April 6, 1645, and was buried in the parish church belonging thereto, called Hanbury.

[2] This is Wood's account. His will says, Nuneaton; but a passage in this work [vol. i. p. 517.] mentions Sutton Coldfield: probably, he may have been at both schools.

ACCOUNT OF THE AUTHOR.

29th of November, 1616, had the vicarage of St. Thomas, in the west suburb of Oxford, conferred on him by the dean and canons of Christ-church, which, with the rectory of Segrave in Leicestershire, given to him in the year 1636, by George Lord Berkeley, he kept, to use the words of the Oxford antiquary, with much ado to his dying day. He seems to have been first beneficed at Walsby, in Lincolnshire, through the munificence of his noble patroness, Frances, countess dowager of Exeter, but resigned the same, as he tells us, for some special reasons. At his vicarage he is remarked to have always given the sacrament in wafers. Wood's character of him is, that—" he was an exact mathematician, a curious calculator of nativities, a general read scholar, a thorough-paced philologist, and one that understood the surveying of lands well. As he was by many accounted a severe student, a devourer of authors, a melancholy and humorous person ; so by others, who knew him well, a person of great honesty, plain dealing and charity. I have heard some of the ancients of Christ-church often say, that his company was very merry, facete, and juvenile ; and no man in his time did surpass him for his ready and dextrous interlarding his common discourses among them with verses from the poets, or sentences from classic authors ; which being then all the fashion in the university, made his company the more acceptable." He appears to have been a universal reader of all kinds of books, and availed himself of his multifarious studies in a very extraordinary manner. From the information of Hearne, we learn, that John Rouse, the Bodleian librarian, furnished him with choice books for the prosecution of his work. The subject of his labour and amusement seems to have been adopted from the infirmities of his own habit and constitution. Mr. Granger says, " He composed this book with a view of relieving his own melancholy, but increased it to such a degree, that nothing could make him laugh, but going to the bridge-foot and hearing the ribaldry

ACCOUNT OF THE AUTHOR. xvii

of the bargemen, which rarely failed to throw him into a violent fit of laughter. Before he was overcome with this horrid disorder, he in the intervals of his vapours was esteemed one of the most facetious companions in the university."

His residence was chiefly at Oxford; where in his chamber in Christ-church College, he departed this life, at or very near the time which he had some years before foretold, from the calculation of his own nativity, and which, says Wood, "being exact, several of the students did not forbear to whisper among themselves, that rather than there should be a mistake in the calculation, he sent up his soul to heaven through a slip about his neck." Whether this suggestion is founded in truth, we have no other evidence than an obscure hint in the epitaph hereafter inserted, which was written by the author himself, a short time before his death. His body, with due solemnity, was buried near that of Dr. Robert Weston, in the north aisle which joins next to the choir of the cathedral of Christ-church, on the 27th of January 1639-40. Over his grave was soon after erected a comely monument, on the upper pillar of the said aisle, with his bust, painted to the life. On the right hand is the following calculation of his nativity:

VOL. I.   a

ACCOUNT OF THE AUTHOR.

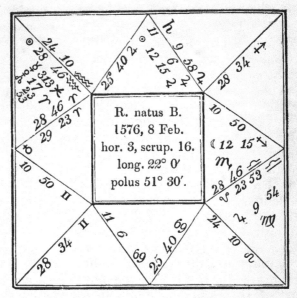

and under the bust, this inscription of his own com_
position.

> Paucis notus, paucioribus ignotus,
> Hîc jacet *Democritus* junior,
> Cui vitam dedit et mortem
> Melancholia.
> Ob. 8. Id. Jan. A.C. MDCXXXIX.

Arms:—Azure on a bend O. between three dogs
heads O. a crescent G.

A few months before his death, he made his will, of
which the following is a copy:

Extracted from the Registry of the Prerogative Court of Canterbury.

In Nomine Dei Amen. August 15th One thousand six hundred thirty nine because there be so many casualties to which our life is subject besides quarrelling and contention which happen to our Successors after our Death by reason of unsettled Estates I Robert Burton Student of Christchurch Oxon.

ACCOUNT OF THE AUTHOR. xix

though my means be but small have thought good by this my
last Will and Testament to dispose of that little which I have
and being at this present I thank God in perfect health of Bodie
and Mind and if this Testament be not so formal according to
the nice and strict terms of Law and other Circumstances peradventure required of which I am Ignorant I desire howsoever
this my Will may be accepted and stand good according to my
true Intent and meaning First I bequeath Animam Deo Corpus
Terræ whensoever it shall please God to call me I give my
Land in Higham which my good Father Ralphe Burton of
Lindly in the County of Leicester Esquire gave me by Deed of
Gift and that which I have annexed to that Farm by purchase
since now leased for thirty eight pounds per Ann. to mine Elder Brother William Burton of Lindly Esquire during his life
and after him to his Heirs I make my said Brother William
likewise mine Executor as well as paying such Annuities and
Legacies out of my Lands and Goods as are hereafter specified
I give to my nephew Cassibilan Burton twenty pounds Annuity
per Ann. out of my Land in Higham during his life to be paid at
two equall payments at our Lady Day in Lent and Michaelmas
or if he be not paid within fourteen Days after the said Feasts
to distrain on any part of the Ground on or any of my Lands
of Inheritance Item I give to my Sister Katherine Jackson during her life eight pounds per Ann. Annuity to be paid at the
two Feasts equally as above said or else to distrain on the Ground
if she be not paid after fourteen days at Lindly as the other
some is out of the said Land Item I give to my Servant John
Upton the Annuity of Forty Shillings out of my said Farme
during his life (if till then my Servant) to be paid on Michaelmas
day in Lindley each year or else after fourteen days to distrain
Now for my goods I thus dispose them First I give an Cth
pounds to Christ Church in Oxford where I have so long lived
to buy five pounds Lands per Ann. to be yearly bestowed on
Books for the Library Item I give an hundredth pound to the
University Library of Oxford to be bestowed to purchase five
pound Land per Ann. to be paid out Yearly on Books as Mrs.
Brooks formerly gave an hundred pounds to buy Land to the
same purpose and the Rent to the same use I give to my Brother George Burton twenty pounds and my watch I give to
my brother Ralph Burton five pounds Item I give to the Parish
of Seagrave in Leicestershire where I am now Rector ten
pounds to be given to certain Feoffees to the perpetual good
of the said *Parish Oxon* * Item I give to my Niece Eugenia
Burton One hundredth pounds Item I give to my Nephew
Richard Burton now Prisoner in London an hundredth pound

---

* So in the Register.

a 2

XX ACCOUNT OF THE AUTHOR.

to redeem him Item I give to the Poor of Higham Forty Shillings where my land is to the poor of Nuneaton where I was once a Grammar Scholar three pound to my Cousin Purfey of Wadlake [Wadley] my Cousin Purfey of Calcott my Cousin Hales of Coventry my Nephew Bradshaw of Orton twenty shillings a piece for a small remembrance to Mr. Whitehall Rector of Cherkby myne own Chamber Fellow twenty shillings I desire my Brother George and my Cousin Purfey of Calcott to be the Overseers of this part of my Will I give moreover five pounds to make a small Monument for my Mother where she is buried in London to my Brother Jackson forty shillings to my Servant John Upton forty shillings besides his former Annuity if he be my servant till I dye if he be till then my Servant *—ROBERT BURTON—Charles Russell Witness— John Pepper Witness.

An Appendix to this my Will if I die in Oxford or whilst I am of Christ Church and with good Mr. Paynes August the Fifteenth 1639.

I give to Mr. Doctor Fell Dean of Christ Church Forty Shillings to the Eight Canons twenty Shillings a piece as a small remembrance to the poor of St. Thomas Parish Twenty Shillings to Brasenose Library five pounds to Mr. Rowse of Oriel Colledge twenty shillings to Mr. Heywood xxs. to Doctor Metcalfe xxs. to Mr. Sherley xxs. If I have any Books the University Library hath not let them take them If I have any Books our own Library hath not let them take them I give to Mrs. Fell all my English Books of Husbandry one excepted   to her Daughter Mrs. Catherine Fell my Six pieces of Silver Plate and six Silver spoons to Mrs. Iles my Gerards Harball To Mrs. Morris my Country Farme Translated out of French 4. and all my English Physick Books to Mr. Whistler the Recorder of Oxford I give twenty Shillings to all my fellow Students M^rs of Arts a Book in fol. or two a piece as Master Morris Treasurer or Mr. Dean shall appoint whom I request to be the Overseer of this Appendix and give him for his pains Atlas Geografer and Ortelius Theatrum Mond' I give to John Fell the Deans Son Student my Mathematical Instruments except my two Crosse Staves which I give to my Lord of Donnol if he be then of the House To Thomas Iles Doctor Iles his Son Student Soluntch on Paurrhelia and Lucians Works in 4 Tomes If any books be left let my Executors dispose of them with all such Books as are written with my own hands and half my Melancholy Copy for Crips hath the other half To Mr. Jones Chaplain and Chanter my Surveying Books

* So in the Register.

ACCOUNT OF THE AUTHOR.   xxi

and Instruments To the Servants of the House Forty Shillings
ROBERT BURTON — Charles Russell Witness — John
Pepper Witness—This Will was shewed to me by the Testator
and acknowledged by him some few days before his death to
be his last Will Ita Testor John Morris S Th D Prebendari'.
Eccl Chri' Oxon. Feb. 3. 1639.

  Probatum fuit Testamentum suprascriptum, &c. 11°
  1640 Juramento Willmi Burton Fris' et Executoris
  cui &c. de bene et fideliter administrand' &c. coram
  Mag'ris Nathanaele Stephens Rectore Eccl. de
  Drayton, et Edwardo Farmer, clericis, vigore com-
  missionis, &c.

' The only work our author executed, was that now
reprinted, which probably was the principal employment of his life. Dr. Ferriar says, it was originally
published in the year 1617 ; but this is evidently a mistake [1]; the first edition was that printed in 4to. 1621 ;
a copy of which is at present in the collection of JOHN
NICHOLS, ESQ. the indefatigable illustrator of the *History of Leicestershire;* to whom, and to ISAAC REED,
ESQ. of Staple Inn, this account is greatly indebted for
its accuracy. The other impressions of it were in 1624,
1628, 1632, 1638, 1651-2, 1660, and 1676, which last,
in the title-page, is called the eighth edition.

The copy from which the present is re-printed, is
that of 1651-2 ; at the conclusion of which is the following address.

"TO THE READER.

" Be pleased to know (Courteous Reader) that since the last
Impression of this Book, the ingenuous Author of it is deceased,
leaving a Copy of it exactly corrected, with several considerable Additions by his own hand; this Copy he committed to my
care and custody, with directions to have those Additions inserted in the next Edition; which in order to his command,
and the Publicke Good, is faithfully performed in this last Impression."   *H. C.*
        (*i. e. HENRY CRIPPS.*)

[1] Originating, perhaps, in a note, p. 448, 6th edit. (vol. ii. p. 212 of the present)
in which a book is quoted as having been "printed at Paris 1624, *seven* years after
Burton's First Edition." As, however, the editions after that of 1621 are regularly
marked in succession, to the 8th, printed in 1676, there seems very little reason
to doubt that, in the note above alluded to, either 1624 has been a misprint for
1628, or *seven* years for *three* years. The numerous typographical errata in other
parts of the work strongly aid this latter supposition.

xxii ACCOUNT OF THE AUTHOR.

The following testimonies of various authors, will serve to show the estimation in which this work has been held.

"The ANATOMY OF MELANCHOLY, wherein the author hath piled up variety of much excellent learning. Scarce any book of philology in our land hath, in so short a time, passed so many editions." *Fuller's Worthies*, fol. 16.

" 'Tis a book so full of variety of reading, that gentlemen who have lost their time, and are put to a push for invention, may furnish themselves with matter for common or scholastical discourse and writing."
Wood's Athenæ Oxonienses, vol. i. p. 628. 2d edit.

"If you never saw BURTON UPON MELANCHOLY, printed 1676, I pray look into it, and read the ninth page of his preface, " Democritus to the Reader." There is something there which touches the point we are upon ; but I mention the author to you, as the pleasantest, the most learned, and the most full of sterling sense. The wits of Queen Anne's reign, and the beginning of George the Ist. were not a little beholden to him."
Archbishop Herring's Letters, 12mo. 1777. p. 149.

"BURTON'S ANATOMY OF MELANCHOLY, he (Dr. Johnson) said, was the only book that ever took him out of bed two hours sooner than he wished to rise."
Boswell's Life of Johnson, vol. i. p. 580. 8vo. edit.

"BURTON'S ANATOMY OF MELANCHOLY is a valuable book," said Dr. Johnson. "It is, perhaps, overloaded with quotation ; but there is great spirit and great power in what Burton says when he writes from his own mind."
Ibid. vol. ii. p. 325.

"It will be no detraction from the powers of Milton's original genius and invention, to remark, that he seems to have borrowed the subject of *L'Allegro* and *Il Penseroso*, together with some particular thoughts, expressions, and rhymes, more especially the idea of a contrast between these two dispositions, from a forgotten poem prefixed to the first edition of BURTON's ANATOMIE OF MELANCHOLY, entitled, 'The Author's Abstract of Melancholy; or, A Dialogue between Pleasure and Pain.' Here Pain is Melancholy. It was written, as I conjecture, about the year 1600. I will make no apology for abstracting and citing as much of this poem as will be sufficient

ACCOUNT OF THE AUTHOR. xxiii

to prove, to a discerning reader, how far it had taken possession of Milton's mind. The measure will appear to be the
same; and that our author was at least an attentive reader of
Burton's book, may be already concluded from the traces of
resemblance which I have incidentally noticed in passing
through the *L'Allegro* and *Il Penseroso*."

After extracting the lines, Mr. Warton adds, " as to the
very elaborate work to which these visionary verses are no un-
suitable introduction, the writer's variety of learning, his quotations from scarce and curious books, his pedantry sparkling
with rude wit and shapeless elegance, miscellaneous matter,
intermixture of agreeable tales and illustrations, and, perhaps
above all, the singularities of his feelings, cloathed in an un-
common quaintness of style, have contributed to render it,
even to modern readers, a valuable repository of amusement
and information." *Warton's Milton*, 2d edit. p. 94.

"The ANATOMY OF MELANCHOLY is a book which has been
universally read and admired. This work is, for the most part,
what the author himself styles it, " a cento;" but it is a very
ingenious one. His quotations, which abound in every page,
are pertinent; but if he had made more use of his invention
and less of his common-place book, his work would perhaps
have been more valuable than it is. He is generally free from
the affected language and ridiculous metaphors which disgrace
most of the books of his time."
Granger's Biographical History.

" BURTON'S ANATOMY OF MELANCHOLY, a book once the
favourite of the learned and the witty, and a source of sur-
reptitious learning, though written on a regular plan, consists chiefly of quotations: the author has honestly termed
it a cento. He collects, under every division, the opinions of
a multitude of writers, without regard to chronological order,
and has too often the modesty to decline the interposition of
his own sentiments. Indeed the bulk of his materials generally overwhelms him. In the course of his folio he has con-
trived to treat a great variety of topics, that seem very loosely
connected with the general subject, and, like *Bayle*, when he
starts a favourite train of quotations, he does not scruple to let
digression outrun the principal question. Thus, from the doctrines of religion to military discipline, from inland navigation
to the morality of dancing schools, every thing is discussed and
determined." *Ferriar's Illustrations of Sterne*, p. 58.

" The archness which Burton displays occasionally, and his
indulgence of playful digressions from the most serious discus-

xxiv   ACCOUNT OF THE AUTHOR.

sions, often give his style an air of familiar conversation, notwithstanding the laborious collections which supply his text.
He was capable of writing excellent poetry, but he seems to
have cultivated this talent too little.   The English verses prefixed to his book, which possess beautiful imagery, and great
sweetness of versification, have been frequently published.
His Latin elegiac verses addressed to his book, shew a very
agreeable turn for raillery."   *Ibid.* p. 58.

" When the force of the subject opens his own vein of prose,
we discover valuable sense and brilliant expression.   Such is his
account of the first feelings of melancholy persons, written probably from his own experience."   (See vol. i. 126, 127. of the
present edition.)   *Ibid.* p. 60.

" During a pedantic age like that in which Burton's production appeared, it must have been eminently serviceable to
writers of many descriptions.   Hence the unlearned might
furnish themselves with appropriate scraps of Greek and Latin,
whilst men of letters would find their enquiries shortened, by
knowing where they might look for what both ancients and
moderns have advanced on the subject of human passions.   I
confess my inability to point out any other English author who
has so largely dealt in apt and original quotations."
             Manuscript note of the late George Steevens, Esq. to
             his copy of THE ANATOMY OF MELANCHOLY.

DEMOCRITUS JUNIOR

TO THE READER.

GENTLE reader, I presume thou wilt be very inquisitive to know what antick or personate actor this is, that so insolently intrudes, upon this common theatre, to the worlds view, arrogating another man's name, whence he is, why he doth it, and what he hath to say. Although, [1] as he said, *Primum si noluero, non respondebo : quis coacturus est?* (I am a free man born, and may chuse whether I will tell : who can compel me ?) if I be urged, I will as readily reply as that Egyptian in [2] Plutarch, when a curious fellow would needs know what he had in his basket, *Quum vides velatam, quid inquiris in rem absconditam?* It was therefore covered, because he should not know what was in it. Seek not after that which is hid: if the contents please thee, [3] *and be for thy use, suppose* the man in the moon, *or whom thou wilt, to be the author:* I would not willingly be known. Yet, in some sort to give thee satisfaction, which is more than I need, I will show a reason, both of this usurped name, title, and subject. And first of the name of Democritus ; lest any man, by reason of it, should be deceived, expecting a pasquil, a satyre, some ridiculous treatise (as I myself should have done), some prodigious tenent, or paradox of the earths motion, of infinite worlds, *in infinito vacuo, ex fortuitâ atomorum collisione,* in an infinite waste, so caused by an accidental collision of motes in the sun, all which Democritus held, Epicurus and their master Leucippus of old maintained, and are lately revived by Copernicus, Brunus and some others. Besides, it hath been always

---

[1] Seneca, in Ludo in mortem Claudii Cæsaris.   [2] Lib. de Curiositate.
    [3] Modo hæc tibi usui sint, quemvis auctorem fingito. Wecker.

VOL. I.   B

DEMOCRITUS TO THE READER.

an ordinary custom, as [1] Gellius observes, *for later writers and impostors, to broach many absurd and insolent fictions, under the name of so noble a philosopher as* Democritus, *to get themselves credit, and by that means the more to be respected* as artificers usually do, *novo qui marmori ascribunt Praxitelem suo.* 'Tis not so with me.

> [2] Non hic Centauros, non Gorgonas, Harpyiasque,
> Invenies: hominem pagina nostra sapit.

> No Centaurs here, or Gorgons, look to find:
> My subject is of man and humane kind.

Thou thy self art the subject of my discourse.

> [3] Quidquid agunt homines, votum, timor, ira, voluptas,
> Gaudia, discursus, nostri farrago libelli.

> Whate'er men do, vows, fears, in ire, in sport,
> Joys, wandrings, are the summ of my report.

My intent is no otherwise to use his name, than Mercurius Gallobelgicus, Mercurius Britannicus, use the name of Mercurie, [4] Democritus Christianus, &c. although there be some other circumstances for which I have masked my self under this visard, and some peculiar respects, which I cannot so well express, until I have set down a brief character of this our Democritus, what he was, with an epitome of his life.

Democritus, as he is described by [5] Hippocrates, and [6] Laërtius, was a little wearish old man, very melancholy by nature, averse from company in his latter dayes, [7] and much given to solitariness, a famous philosopher in his age, [8] *coævus* with Socrates, wholly addicted to his studies at the last, and to a private life; writ many excellent works, a great divine, according to the divinity of those times, an expert physician, a politician, an excellent mathematician, as [9] Diacosmus and the rest of his works do witness. He was much delighted with the studies of husbandry, saith [10] Columella; and often I find him cited by [11] Constantinus and others treating of that subject. He knew the natures, differences of all beasts, plants, fishes, birds; and, as some say, could [12] understand the tunes and voices of them. In a word, he was *omnifariam doctus*, a general scholar, a great student; and, to the intent he might better contemplate, [13] I find it related by some, that he put out his

---

[1] Lib. 10. c. 12. Multa a male feriatis in Democriti nomine commenta data, nobilitatis, auctoritatisque ejus perfugio utentibus. [2] Martialis, lib. 10. epigr. 14. [3] Juv. Sat. 1. [4] Auth. Pet. Besseo. edit. Coloniæ 1616. [5] Hip. Epist. Damaget. [6] Laërt. lib. 9. [7] Hortulo sibi cellulam seligens, ibique seipsum includens, vixit solitarius. [8] Floruit Olympiade 80; 700 annis post Trojam. [9] Diacos. quod cunctis operibus facile excellit. Laërt. [10] Col. lib. 1. c. 1. [11] Const. lib. de agric. passim. [12] Volucrum voces et linguas intelligere se dicit Abderitanus. Ep. Hip. [13] Sabellicus, exempl. lib. 10. Oculis se privavit, ut melius contemplationi operam daret, sublimi vir ingenio, profundæ cogitationis, &c.

DEMOCRITUS TO THE READER.

eyes, and was in his old age voluntarily blind, yet saw more than all Greece besides, and [1] writ of every subject : *Nihil in toto opificio naturæ, de quo non scripsit :* a man of an excellent wit, profound conceit; and, to attain knowledge the better in his younger years, he travelled to Egypt and [2] Athens, to confer with learned men, [3] *admired of some, despised of others.* After a wandering life, he settled at Abdera, a town in Thrace, and was sent for thither to be their law-maker, recorder, or town-clerk, as some will; or as others, he was there bred and born. Howsoever it was, there he lived at last in a garden in the suburbs, wholly betaking himself to his studies and a private life, [4] *saving that sometimes he would walk down to the haven,* [5] *and laugh heartily at such variety of ridiculous objects, which there he saw.* Such a one was Democritus.

But, in the mean time, how doth this concern me, or upon what reference do I usurp his habit? I confess, indeed, that to compare my self unto him for ought I have yet said, were both impudency and arrogancy. I do not presume to make any parallel. *Antistat mihi millibus trecentis :* [6] *parvus sum ; nullus sum; altum nec spiro, nec spero.* Yet thus much I will say of my self, and that I hope without all suspicion of pride, or self-conceit, I have lived a silent, sedentary, solitary, private life, *mihi et Musis,* in the university, as long almost as Xenocrates in Athens, *ad senectam fere,* to learn wisdom as he did, penned up most part in my study: for I have been brought up a student in the most flourishing college of Europe, [7] *augustissimo collegio,* and can brag with [8] Jovius, almost, *in eâ luce domicilii Vaticani, totius orbis celeberrimi, per 37 annos multa opportunaque didici ;* for thirty years I have continued (having the use of as good [9] libraries as ever he had) a scholar, and would be therefore loth, either, by living as a drone, to be an unprofitable or unworthy member of so learned and noble a society, or to write that which should be any way dishonourable to such a royal and ample foundation. Something I have done : though by my profession a divine, yet *turbine raptus ingenii,* as [10] he said, out of a running wit, an unconstant, unsettled mind, I had a great desire (not able to attain to a superficial skill in any) to have some smattering in all, to be *aliquis in omnibus, nullus in singulis ;*

---

[1] Naturalia, moralia, mathematica, liberales disciplinas, artiumque omnium peritiam callebat.   [2] Veni Athenas; et nemo me novit.   [3] Idem contemptui et admirationi habitus.   [4] Solebat ad portam ambulare, et inde, &c. Hip. Ep. Dameg.   [5] Perpetuo risu pulmonem agitare solebat Democritus. Juv. Sat. 7.   [6] Non sum dignus præstare matellam. Mart.   [7] Christ Church in Oxford.   [8] Præfat. hist.   [9] Keeper of our college library lately revived by Otho Nicolson, Esquire.   [10] Scaliger.

B 2

DEMOCRITUS TO THE READER.

which [1] Plato commends, out of him [2] Lipsius approves and furthers, *as fit to be imprinted in all curious wits, not to be a slave of one science, or dwell altogether in one subject, as most do, but to rove abroad*, centum puer artium, *to have an oar in every mans boat, to* [3] *taste of every dish, and to sip of every cup;* which, saith [4] Montaigne, was well performed by Aristotle, and his learned countrey-man Adrian Turnebus. This roving humour (though not with like success) I have ever had, and, like a ranging spaniel, that barks at every bird he sees, leaving his game, I have followed all, saving that which I should, and may justly complain, and truly, *qui ubique est, nusquam est,* which [5] Gesner *did in modesty;* that I have read many books, but to little purpose, for want of good method, I have confusedly tumbled over divers authors in our libraries with small profit, for want of art, order, memory, judgement. I never travelled but in map or card, in which my unconfined thoughts have freely expatiated, as having ever been especially delighted with the study of cosmography. [6] Saturn was lord of my geniture, culminating, &c. and Mars principal significator of manners, in partile conjunction with mine ascendent; both fortunate in their houses, &c. I am not poor, I am not rich; *nihil est, nihil deest;* I have little, I want nothing: all my treasure is in Minerva's tower. Greater preferment as I could never get, so am I not in debt for it. I have a competency *(laus Deo)* from my noble and munificent patrons. Though I live still a collegiat student, as Democritus in his garden, and lead a monastique life, *ipse mihi theatrum,* sequestred from those tumults and troubles of the world, *et tanquam in speculâ positus* ([7] as he said), in some high place above you all, like *Stoicus sapiens, omnia sæcula præterita præsentiaque videns, uno velut intuitu,* I hear and see what is done abroad, how others [8] run, ride, turmoil, and macerate themselves in court and countrey. Far from those wrangling law-suits, *aulæ vanitatem, fori ambitionem, ridere mecum soleo:* I laugh at all, [9] *only secure, lest my suit go amiss, my ships perish,* corn and cattle miscarry, trade decay, *I have no wife nor children, good or bad, to provide for;* a meer spectator of other mens fortunes and adventures, and how they act their parts, which me thinks are diversly presented unto

---

[1] In Theæt. [2] Phil. Stoic. li. diff. 8. Dogma cupidis et curiosis ingeniis imprimendum, ut sit talis qui nulli rei serviat, aut exacte unum aliquid elaboret, alia negligens, ut artifices, &c. [3] Delibare gratum de quocunque cibo, et pitissare de quocunque dolio jucundum. [4] Essays, lib. 3. [5] Præfat. bibliothec. [6] Ambo fortes et fortunati. Mars idem magisterii dominus juxta primam Leovitii regulam. [7] Heinsius. [8] Calide ambientes, solicite litigantes, aut misere excidentes, voces, strepitum, contentiones, &c. [9] Cyp. ad Donat. Unice securus, ne excidam in foro, aut in mari Indico bonis eluam, de dote filiæ, patrimonio filii non sum solicitus.

DEMOCRITUS TO THE READER. 5

me, as from a common theatre or scene. I hear new news
every day: and those ordinary rumours of war, plagues, fires,
inundations, thefts, murders, massacres, meteors, comets,
spectrums, prodigies, apparitions, of towns taken, cities besieged in France, Germany, Turky, Persia, Poland, &c.
daily musters and preparations, and such like, which these
tempestuous times afford, battles fought, so many men slain,
monomachies, shipwracks, piracies, and sea-fights, peace,
leagues, stratagems, and fresh alarms—a vast confusion of
vows, wishes, actions, edicts, petitions, law-suits, pleas, laws,
proclamations, complaints, grievances—are daily brought to
our ears; new books every day, pamphlets, currantoes, stories,
whole catalogues of volumes of all sorts, new paradoxes,
opinions, schisms, heresies, controversies in philosophy, religion, &c. Now come tidings of weddings, maskings, mum-
meries, entertainments, jubiles, embassies, tilts and tourna-
ments, trophies, triumphs, revels, sports, playes; then again,
as in a new shifted scene, treasons, cheating tricks, rob-
beries, enormous villanies in all kinds, funerals, burials, death
of princes, new discoveries, expeditions; now comical, then
tragical matters. To day we hear of new lords and officers
created, to morrow of some great men deposed, and then
again of fresh honours conferred; one is let loose, another
imprisoned; one purchaseth, another breaketh; he thrives,
his neighbour turns bankrupt; now plenty, then again dearth
and famine; one runs, another rides, wrangles, laughs, weeps,
&c. Thus I daily hear, and such like, both private and publick news. Amidst the gallantry and misery of the world,
jollity, pride, perplexities and cares, simplicity and villany,
subtlety, knavery, candour and integrity, mutually mixt and
offering themselves, I rub on, *privus privatus:* as I have still
lived, so I now continue *statu quo prius,* left to a solitary life,
and mine own domestick discontents; saving that sometimes,
ne quid mentiar, as Diogenes went into the city and Democritus to the haven, to see fashions, I did for my recreation
now and then walk abroad, look into the world, and could
not chuse but make some little observation, *non tam sagax
observator, ac simplex recitator,* not, as they did, to scoff or
laugh at all, but with a mixt passion:

[1] Bilem, sæpe jocum vestri movere tumultus.

I did sometime laugh and scoff with Lucian, and satyrically
tax with Menippus, lament with Heraclitus, sometimes again
I was [2] *petulanti splene cachinno,* and then again, [3] *urere bilis
jecur,* I was much moved to see that abuse which I could
not amend: in which passion howsoever I may sympathize

[1] Hor.   [2] Per.   [3] Hor.

DEMOCRITUS TO THE READER.

with him or them, 'tis for no such respect I shroud my self under his name, but either, in an unknown habit, to assume a little more liberty and freedom of speech, or if you will needs know, for that reason and only respect which Hippocrates relates at large in his epistle to Damegetus, wherein he doth express, how, coming to visit him one day, he found *Democritus* in his garden at Abdera, in the suburbs, [1] under a shady bower, [2] with a book on his knees, busie at his study, sometime writing, sometime walking. The subject of his book was melancholy and madness: about him lay the carkasses of many several beasts, newly by him cut up and anatomized; not that he did contemn Gods creatures, as he told Hippocrates, but to find out the seat of this *atra bilis*, or melancholy, whence it proceeds, and how it is engendered in mens bodies, to the intent he might better cure it in himself, by his writings and observations [3] teach others how to prevent and avoid it. Which good intent of his Hippocrates highly commended, Democritus Junior is therefore bold to imitate, and, because he left it imperfect, and it is now lost, *quasi succenturiator Democriti*, to revive again, prosecute, and finish in this treatise.

You have had a reason of the name. If the title and inscription offend your gravity, were it a sufficient justification to accuse others, I could produce many sober treatises, even sermons themselves, which in their fronts carry more phantastical names. Howsoever, it is a kind of policy in these dayes, to prefix a phantastical title to a book which is to be sold: for as larks come down to a day-net, many vain readers will tarry and stand gazing, like silly passengers, at an antick picture in a painter's shop, that will not look at a judicious piece. And indeed, as [4] Scaliger observes, *nothing more invites a reader than an argument unlooked for, unthought of, and sells better than a scurrile pamphlet, tum maxime cum novitas excitat palatum.* Many men, saith [5] Gellius, *are very conceited in their inscriptions*, and able, (as [6] Pliny quotes out of Seneca) to make him loyter by the way, *that went in haste to fetch a mid-wife for his daughter, now ready to lye down.* For my part, I have honourable [7] precedents for this I have done: I will cite one for all, Anthonie Zara, Pap. Episc. his

---

[1] Secundum mœnia locus erat frondosis populis opacus, vitibusque sponte natis: tenuis prope aqua defluebat, placide murmurans, ubi sedile et domus Democriti conspiciebatur.   [2] Ipse composite considebat, super genua volumen habens, et utrinque alia patentia parata, dissectaque animalia cumulatim strata, quorum viscera rimabatur.   [3] Cum mundus extra se sit, et mente captus sit, et nesciat se languere, ut medelam adhibeat.   [4] Scaliger, Ep. ad Patisonem. Nihil magis lectorem invitat quam inopinatum argumentum; neque vendibilior merx est quam petulans liber.   [5] Lib. xx. c. 11. Miras sequuntur inscriptionum festivitates.   [6] Præfat. Nat. Hist. Patri obstetricem parturienti filiæ accersenti moram injicere possunt.   [7] Anatomy of Popery. Anatomy of Immortality. Angelus Salas, Anatomy of Antimony, &c.

DEMOCRITUS TO THE READER. 7

Anatomy of Wit, in four sections, members, subsections, &c. to be read in our libraries.

If any man except against the matter or manner of treating of this my subject, and will demand a reason of it, I can allege more than one. I write of melancholy, by being busie, to avoid melancholy. There is no greater cause of melancholy than idleness, *no better cure than business*, as [1]Rhasis holds: and howbeit, *stultus labor est ineptiarum*, to be busied in toyes is to small purpose, yet hear that divine Seneca, better *aliud agere quam nihil*, better do to no end, than nothing. 1 writ therefore, and busied my self in this playing labour, *otiosâque diligentiâ ut vitarem torporem feriandi*, with Vectius in Macrobius, *atque otium in utile verterem negotium;*

[2]—Simul et jucunda et idonea dicere vitæ,
Lectorem delectando simul atque monendo.

To this end I write, like them, saith Lucian, that *recite to trees, and declaim to pillars, for want of auditors;* as [3]Paulus Ægineta ingenuously confesseth, *not that any thing was unknown or omitted, but to exercise my self* (which course if some took, I think it would be good for their bodies, and much better for their souls); or peradventure, as others do, for fame, to shew myself *(Scire tuum nihil est, nisi te scire hoc sciat alter).* I might be of Thucydides opinion, [4]*to know a thing and not to express it, is all one as if he knew it not.* When I first took this task in hand, *et, quod ait* [5]*ille, impellente genio negotium suscepi,* this I aimed at [6]*vel ut lenirem animum scribendo,* to ease my mind by writing, for I had *gravidum cor, fœtum caput,* a kind of imposthume in my head, which 1 was very desirous to be unladen of, and could imagine no fitter evacuation than this. Besides, I might not well refrain; for, *ubi dolor, ibi digitus,* one must needs scratch where it itches. I was not a little offended with this malady, shall I say, my Mistris *melancholy,* my Egeria, or my *malus genius;* and for that cause, as he that is stung with a scorpion, I would expel, *clavum clavo,* [7]comfort one sorrow with another, idleness with idleness, *ut ex viperâ theriacum,* make an antidote out of that which was the prime cause of my disease. Or as he did, of whom [8]Felix Plater speaks, that though he had some of Aristophanes frogs in his belly, still crying *Brecc' ckex, coax, coax, oop, oop,* and for that cause studied physick seven years, and travelled

---

[1] Cont. l. 4. c. 9. Non est cura melior quam labor. [2] Hor. [3] Non quod de novo quid addere, aut a veteribus prætermissum, sed propriæ exercitationis caussâ. [4] Qui novit, neque id quod sentit exprimit, perinde est ac si nesciret. [5] Jovius, Præf. Hist. [6] Erasmus. [7] Otium otio, dolorem dolore, sum solatus. [8] Observat. l. 1.

8   DEMOCRITUS TO THE READER.

over most part of Europe, to ease himself; to do my self good,
I turned over such physicians as our libraries would afford, or
my [1] private friends impart, and have taken this pains. And
why not? Cardan professeth he writ his book *De consola-
tione* after his sons death, to comfort himself; so did Tully
write of the same subject with like intent after his daughters
departure, if it be his at least, or some impostors put out in
his name, which Lipsius probably suspects. Concerning my
self, I can peradventure affirm with Marius in Sallust, [2] *that
which others hear or read of, I felt and practised my self:
they get their knowledge by books, I mine by melancholizing:
experto crede Roberto.* Something I can speak out of experience, *ærumnabilis experientia me docuit;* and with her in
the poet, [3] *Haud ignara mali miseris succurrere disco.* I
would help others out of a fellow-feeling, and as that vertuous
lady did of old, [4] *being a leper her self, bestow all her portion
to build an hospital for lepers,* I will spend my time and knowledge, which are my greatest fortunes, for the common good
of all.

   Yea, but you will inferr, that this is [5] *actum agere,* an unnecessary work, *cramben bis coctam apponere,* the same again
and again in other words. To what purpose? [6] *Nothing is
omitted that may well be said:* so thought Lucian in the like
theam. How many excellent physicians have written just
volumes and elaborate tracts of this subject? no news here:
that which I have is stoln from others; [7] *dicitque mihi mea
pagina, fur es.* If that severe doom of [8] Synesius be true,
*it is a greater offence to steal dead mens labours, than their
cloaths,* what shall become of most writers? I hold up my
hand at the bar amongst others, and am guilty of felony in
this kind: *habes confitentem reum,* I am content to be pressed
with the rest. 'Tis most true, *tenet insanabile multos scribendi cacoëthes;* and [9] *there is no end of writing of books,* as
the wise man found of old, in this [10] scribling age especially,
wherein [11] the *number of books is without number,* (as a worthy
man saith) *presses be oppressed,* and out of an itching humour,
that every man hath to show himself, [12] desirous of fame
and honour, *(scribimus indocti doctique ——)* he will write
no matter what, and scrape together, it boots not whence.

---

[1] M. Joh. Rous, our Protobib. Oxon. Mr. Hopper, Mr. Guthridge, &c.   [2] Quæ
illi audire et legere solent, eorum partim vidi egomet, alia gessi: quæ illi literis,
ego militando didici. Nunc vos existimate, facta an dicta pluris sint.   [3] Dido,
Virg.   [4] Camden, Ipsa elephantiasi correpta elephantiasis hospitium construxit.
[5] Iliada post Homerum. -   [6] Nihil prætermissum quod a quovis dici possit.
[7] Martialis.   [8] Magis impium mortuorum lucubrationes quam vestes furari.
[9] Eccl. ult.   [10] Libros eunuchi gignunt, steriles pariunt.   [11] D. King,
præfat. lect. Jonas, the late right reverend lord bishop of London.   [12] Homines
famelici gloriæ ad ostentationem eruditionis undique congerunt. Buchananus.

DEMOCRITUS TO THE READER.

[1] *Bewitched with this desire of fame, etiam mediis in morbis,* to the disparagement of their health, and scarce able to hold a pen, they must say something, [2] *and get themselves a name,* saith Scaliger, *though it be to the down-fall and ruine of many others.* To be counted writers, *scriptores ut salutentur,* to be thought and held Polymathes and Polyhistors, *apud imperitum vulgus ob ventosæ nomen artis,* to get a paper kingdom: *nullâ spe quæstûs, sed amplâ famæ,* in this precipitate, ambitious age, *nunc ut est sæculum, inter immaturam eruditionem, ambitiosum et præceps* ('tis [3] Scaligers censure) and they that are scarce auditors, *vix auditores,* must be masters and teachers, before they be capable and fit hearers. They will rush into all learning, *togatam, armatam,* divine, humane authors, rake over all indexes and pamphlets for notes, as our merchants do strange havens for traffick, write great tomes, *cum non sint reverâ doctiores, sed loquaciores,* when as they are not thereby better scholars, but greater praters. They commonly pretend publick good: but, as [4] Gesner observes, 'tis pride and vanity that eggs them on; no news, or ought worthy of note, but the same in other terms. *Ne feriarentur fortasse typographi, vel ideo scribendum est aliquid ut se vixisse testentur.* As apothecaries, we make new mixtures every day, pour out of one vessel into another; and as those old Romans rob'd all the cities of the world, to set out their bad sited Rome, we skim off the cream of other mens wits, pick the choice flowers of their till'd gardens to set out our own sterile plots. *Castrant alios, ut libros suos, per se graciles, alieno adipe suffarciant* (so [5] Jovius inveighs); they lard their lean books with the fat of others works. *Ineruditi fures, &c.* (a fault that every writer finds, as I do now, and yet faulty themselves) [6] *Trium literarum homines,* all thieves; they pilfer out of old writers to stuff up their new comments, scrape Ennius dung-hills, and out of [7] Democritus pit, as I have done. By which means it comes to pass, [8] *that not only libraries and shops are full of our putid papers, but every close-stool and jakes: Scribunt carmina, quæ legunt cacantes;* they serve to put under pies, to [9] lap spice in, and keep roast-meat from burning. *With us in France,* saith [10] Scaliger, *every man hath liberty to write, but few ability.* [11] *Heretofore learning was graced by judicious scholars, but now*

---

[1] Effascinati etiam laudis amore, &c. Justus Baronius.   [2] Ex ruinis alienæ existimationis sibi gradum et famam struunt.   [3] Exercit. 288.   [4] Omnes sibi famam quærunt, et quovis modo in orbem spargi contendunt, ut novæ alicujus rei habeantur auctores. Præf. biblioth.   [5] Præf. hist.   [6] Plautus. [7] E Democriti puteo.   ·   [8] Non tam refertæ bibliothecæ quam cloacæ.   [9] Et quidquid chartis amicitur ineptis.   [10] Epist. ad Petas. In regno Franciæ omnibus scribendi datur libertas, paucis facultas.   [11] Olim literæ ob homines in pretio, nunc sordent ob homines.

10 DEMOCRITUS TO THE READER.

noble sciences are vilified by base and illiterate scriblers, that either write for vain-glory, need to get money, or as parasites to flatter and collogue with some great men: they put out [1]*burras, quisquiliasque, ineptiasque.* [2]*Amongst so many thousand authors you shall scarce find one, by reading of whom you shall be any whit better, but rather much worse, quibus inficitur potius, quam perficitur,* by which he is rather infected, than any way perfected.

—————————— [3] Qui talia legit,
Quid didicit tandem, quid scit, nisi somnia, nugas?

So that oftentimes it falls out (which Callimachus taxed of old) a great book is a great mischief. [4] Cardan finds fault with Frenchmen and Germans, for their scribling to no purpose: *non, inquit, ab edendo deterreo, modo novum aliquid inveniant:* he doth not bar them to write, so that it be some new invention of their own; but we weave the same web still, twist the same rope again and again: or, if it be a new invention, 'tis but some bauble or toy which idle fellows write, for as idle fellows to read: and who so cannot invent? [5]*He must have a barren wit, that in this scribling age can forge nothing.* [6]*Princes shew their armies, rich men vaunt their buildings, souldiers their manhood, and scholars vent their toyes;* they must read, they must hear, whether they will or no.

[7] Et quodcunque semel chartis illeverit, omnes
Gestiet a furno redeuntes scire lacuque,
Et pueros et anus——.

What once is said and writ, all men must know,
Old wives and children as they come and go.

What a company of poets hath this year brought out! as Pliny complains to Sosius Senecio. [8]*This* April, *every day some or other have recited.* What a catalogue of new books all this year, all this age (I say), have our Frank-furt marts, our domestick marts, brought out! twice a year, [9]*proferunt se nova ingenia et ostentant;* we stretch our wits out, and set them to sale: *magno conatu nihil agimus.* So that, which [10] Gesner much desires, if a speedy reformation be not had, by some princes edicts and grave supervisors, to restrain this liberty, it will run on *in infinitum. Quis tam avidus librorum helluo,*

[1] Ans. pac.   [2] Inter tot mille volumina vix unus a cujus lectione quis melior evadat, immo potius non pejor.   [3] Palingenius.   [4] Lib. 5. de sap.
[5] Sterile oportet esse ingenium quod in hoc scripturientum pruritu, &c.   [6] Cardan. præf. ad consol.   [7] Hor. ser. I. sat. 4.   [8] Epist. lib. 1. Magnum poëtarum proventum annus hic attulit: mense Aprili nullus fere dies quo non aliquis recitavit.   [9] Idem.   [10] Principibus et doctoribus deliberandum relinquo, ut arguantur auctorum furta, et millies repetita tollantur, et temere scribendi libido coërceatur, aliter in infinitum progressura.

2

DEMOCRITUS TO THE READER. 11

who can read them? As already, we shall have a vast chaos
and confusion of books: we are [1]oppressed with them; [2]our
eyes ake with reading, our fingers with turning. For my part,
I am one of the number; *nos numerus sumus :* I do not deny
it. I have only this of Macrobius to say for my self, *Omne
meum, nihil meum,* 'tis all mine, and none mine. As a good
house-wife, out of divers fleeces, weaves one piece of cloth, a
bee gathers wax and honey out of many flowers, and makes a
new bundle of all,

Floriferis ut apes in saltibus omnia libant,

I have laboriously [3]collected this cento out of divers writers,
and that *sine injuriâ :* I have wronged no authors, but given
every man his own; which [4]Hierom so much commends in
Nepotian; he stole not whole verses, pages, tracts, as some do
now a days, concealing their authors names; but still said this
was Cyprians, that Lactantius, that Hilarius, so said Minutius
Felix, so Victorinus, thus far Arnobius: I cite and quote
mine authors (which howsoever some illiterate scriblers account pedantical, as a cloke of ignorance, and opposite to their
affected fine stile, I must and will use) *sumpsi, non surripui ;*
and what Varro, lib. 6. de re rust. speaks of bees, *minime
maleficæ, nullius opus vellicantes faciunt deterius,* I can say of
my self. Whom have I injured? The matter is theirs most
part, and yet mine : *apparet unde sumptum sit* (which Seneca
approves) ; *aliud tamen, quam unde sumptum sit, apparet ;*
which nature doth with the aliment of our bodies, incorpo-
rate, digest, assimilate, I do *concoquere quod hausi,* dispose of
what I take: I make them pay tribute, to set out this my
Maceronicon: the method only is mine own: I must usurp
that of [5]*Wecker e Ter. nihil dictum quod non dictum prius :
methodus sola artificem ostendit :* we can say nothing but what
hath been said, the composition and method is ours only,
and shows a scholar. Oribasius, Aëtius, Avicenna, have all
out of Galen, but to their own method, *diverso stylo, non di-
versâ fide.* Our poets steal from Homer; he spews, saith
Ælian, they lick it up. Divines use Austins words *verbatim*
still, and our story-dressers do as much; he that comes last is
commonly best,

—— donec quid grandius ætas
Postera, sorsque ferat melior.——

[1] Onerabuntur ingenia, nemo legendis sufficit. [2] Libris obruimur: oculi
legendo, manus volitando dolent. Fam. Strada, Momo. Lucretius. [3] Quidquid ubique bene dictum facio meum, et illud nunc meis ad compendium, nunc
ad fidem et auctoritatem alienis, exprimo verbis: omnes auctores meos clientes
esse arbitror, &c. Sarisburiensis ad Polycrat. prol. [4] In Epitaph. Nep.
illud Cyp. hoc Lact. illud Hilar. est, ita Victorinus, in hunc modum loquutus est
Arnobius, &c. [5] Præf. Syntax. med.

12   DEMOCRITUS TO THE READER.

Though there were many giants of old in physick and philosophy, yet I say with [1]Didacus Stella, *A dwarf standing on
the shoulders of a giant, may see farther than a giant himself;*
I may likely add, alter, and see farther than my predecessors:
and it is no greater prejudice for me to indite after others,
than for Ælianus Montaltus, that famous physician, to write
de morbis capitis after Jason Pretensis, Heurnius, Hildesheim,
&c. Many horses to run in a race, one logician, one rheto-
rician, after another. Oppose then what thou wilt,

> Allatres licet usque nos et usque,
> Et gannitibus improbis lacessas;

I solve it thus. And for those other faults of barbarism,
[2]Dorick dialect, extemporanean style, tautologies, apish imitation, a rhapsody of rags gathered together from several
dung-hills, excrements of authors, toyes, and fopperies, confusedly tumbled out, without art, invention, judgment, wit,
learning, harsh, raw, rude, phantastical, absurd, insolent, in-
discreet, ill-composed, indigested, vain, scurrile, idle, dull
and dry; I confess all ('tis partly affected): thou canst not
think worse of me than I do of my self. 'Tis not worth the
reading, I yield it: I desire thee not to lose time in perusing
so vain a subject; I should be peradventure loth my self to
read him or thee so writing: 'tis not *operæ pretium.* All I
say, is this, that I have [3]precedents for it, which Isocrates
calls *perfugium iis qui peccant,* others as absurd, vain, idle,
illiterate, &c. *Nonnulli alii idem fecerunt,* others have done as
much, it may be more, and perhaps thou thy self: *Novimus
et qui te, &c.* we have all our faults; *scimus, et hanc veniam,
&c.* [4]thou censurest me, so have I done others, and may do
thee: *Cædimus, inque vicem, &c.* 'tis *lex talionis, quid pro quo.*
Go now censure, criticise, scoff and rail.

> [5]Nasutus sis usque licet, sis denique nasus,
>   Non potes in nugas dicere plura meas,
> Ipse ego quam dixi, &c.

> Wer'st thou all scoffs and flouts, a very Momus,
> Than we our selves, thou canst not say worse of us.

Thus, as when women scold, have I cryed whore first; and,
in some mens censures, I am afraid I have overshot my self.
Laudare se vani, vituperare stulti: as I do not arrogate, I
will not derogate. *Primus vestrum non sum, nec imus,* I am
none of the best, I am none of the meanest of you. As I

---

[1] In Luc. 10. tom. 2. Pygmæi gigantum humeris impositi plus quam ipsi
gigantes vident.   [2] Nec aranearum textus ideo melior, quia ex se fila gignuntur, nec noster ideo vilior, quia ex alienis libamus, ut apes. Lipsius adversus
dialogist.   [3] Uno absurdo dato, mille sequuntur.   [4] Non dubito multos
lectores hic fore stultos.   [5] Martial. 13. 2.

DEMOCRITUS TO THE READER. 13

am an inch, or so many feet, so many parasanges, after him
or him, I may be peradventure an ace before thee. Be it
therefore as it is, well or ill, I have assayed, put my self upon
the stage : I must abide the censure ; I may not escape it. It
is most true, *stylus virum arguit,* our style bewrayes us, and as
[1] hunters find their game by the trace, so is a mans genius
descried by his works: *multo melius ex sermone quam linea-
mentis, de moribus hominum judicamus;* 'twas old Cato's rule.
I have laid my self open (I know it) in this treatise, turned
mine inside outward : I shall be censured, I doubt not ; for,
to say truth with Erasmus, *nihil morosius hominum judiciis,*
there's nought so peevish as mens judgments: yet this is some
comfort—*ut palata, sic judicia,* our censures are as various as
our palats.

> [2] Tres mihi convivæ prope dissentire videntur,
> Poscentes vario multum diversa palato, &c.

Our writings are as so many dishes, our readers guests ; our
books like beauty; that which one admires, another rejects ;
so are we approved as mens fancies are inclined.

> Pro captu lectoris habent sua fata libelli.

That which is most pleasing to one is *amaracum sui,* most
harsh to another. *Quot homines, tot sententiæ,* so many men,
so many minds: that which thou condemnest, he commends.

> [3] Quod petis, id sane est invisum acidumque duobus.

He respects matter; thou art wholly for words; he loves a
loose and free stile ; thou art all for neat composition, strong
lines, hyperboles, allegories : he desires a fine frontispiece, en-
ticing pictures, such as Hieron. Natali [4] the Jesuit hath cut
to the Dominicals, to draw on the readers attention, which
thou rejectest; that which one admires, another explodes as
most absurd and ridiculous. If it be not point-blank to his
humour, his method, his conceit, [5] *si quid forsan omissum,
quod is animo conceperit, si quæ dictio, &c.* if ought be omitted,
or added, which he likes, or dislikes, thou art *mancipium
paucæ lectionis,* an ideot, an ass, *nullus es,* or *plagiarius,* a
trifler, a trivant, thou art an idle fellow ; or else 'tis a thing
of meer industry, a collection without wit or invention, a
very toy. [6] *Facilia sic putant omnes quæ jam facta, nec de
salebris cogitant, ubi via strata;* so men are valued, their labours vilified, by fellows of no worth themselves, as things of
nought: who could not have done as much ? *unusquisque
abundat sensu suo,* every man abounds in his own sense; and

---

[1] Ut venatores feram e vestigio impresso, virum scriptiunculâ. Lips.   [2] Hor.
[3] Hor.   [4] Antwerp. fol. 1607.   [5] Muretus.   [6] Lipsius.

14   DEMOCRITUS TO THE READER.

whilest each particular party is so affected, how should one please all?

[1] Quid dem? quid non dem? Renuis tu, quod jubet ille.

How shall I hope to express my self to each mans humor and [2] conceit, or to give satisfaction to all? Some understand too little, some too much, *qui similiter in legendos libros, atque in salutandos homines irruunt, non cogitantes quales, sed quibus vestibus induti sint,* as [3] Austin observes, not regarding what, but who write, [4] *orexin habet auctoris celebritas,* not valuing the mettal, but the stamp that is upon it; *cantharum aspiciunt, non quid in eo.* If he be not rich, in great place, polite and brave, a great doctor, or full fraught with grand titles, though never so well qualified, he is a dunce. But as [5] Baronius hath it of cardinal Caraffa's works, he is a meer hog that rejects any man for his poverty. Some are too partial, as friends to overween; others come with a prejudice to carp, vilifie, detract and scoff; *(qui de me forsan quidquid est, omni contemptu contemptius judicant)* some as bees for honey, some as spiders to gather poyson. What shall I do in this case? As a Dutch host, if you come to an inn in Germany, and dislike your fare, diet, lodging, &c. replyes in a surly tone, [6] *aliud tibi quæras diversorium,* if you like not this, get you to another inn: I resolve, if you like not my writing, go read something else. I do not much esteem thy censure: take thy course: 'tis not as thou wilt, nor as I will: but when we have both done, that of [7] Plinius Secundus to Trajan will prove true, *Every mans witty labour takes not, except the matter, subject, occasion, and some commending favourite happen to it.* If I be taxed, exploded by thee and some such, I shall haply be approved and commended by others, and so have been *(expertus loquor);* and may truly say with [8] Jovius in like case *(absit verbo jactantia) heroum quorundam, pontificum, et virorum nobilium familiaritatem et amicitiam, gratasque gratias, et multorum [9] bene laudatorum laudes sum inde promeritus:* as I have been honoured by some worthy men, so have I been vilified by others, and shall be. At the first publishing of this book, (which [10] Probus of Persius satyrs) *editum librum continuo mirari homines, atque avide deripere cœperunt,* I may in some-sort apply to this my work. The first, second, and third edition were suddenly gone, eagerly read, and,

[1] Hor.   [2] Fieri non potest, ut quod quisque cogitat, dicat unus. Muretus.
[3] Lib. 1. de ord. cap. 11.   [4] Erasmus.   [5] Annal. tom. 3. ad annum 360.
Est porcus ille qui sacerdotem ex amplitudine redituum sordide demetitur.
[6] Erasm. dial.   [7] Epist. l. 6. Cujusque ingenium non statim emergit, nisi materiæ fautor, occasio, commendatorque contingat.   [8] Præf. hist.   [9] Laudari a laudato laus est.   [10] Vit. Persii.

DEMOCRITUS TO THE READER.   15

as I have said, not so much approved by some, as scornfully
rejected by others. But it was Democritus his fortune, *Idem
admirationi et* [1]*irrisioni habitus.* 'Twas Seneca's fate: that
superintendant of wit, learning, judgement, [2] *ad stuporem
doctus,* the best of Greek and Latin writers, in Plutarch's
opinion; that *renowned corrector of vice,* as [3]Fabius terms
him, *and painful omniscious philosopher that writ so excellently and admirably well,* could not please all parties, or
escape censure. How is he vilified by [4] Caligula, Agellius,
Fabius, and Lipsius himself, his chief propugner ? *In eo pleraque perniciosa,* saith the same Fabius : many childish tracts
and sentences he hath, *sermo illaboratus,* too negligent often
and remiss, as Agellius observes, *oratio vulgaris et protrita,
dicaces et ineptæ sententiæ, eruditio plebeia,* an homely shallow writer as he is. *In partibus spinas et fastidia habet,* saith
[5] Lipsius; and, as in all his other works, so especially in his
Epistles, *aliæ in argutiis et ineptiis occupantur: intricatus
alicubi, et parum compositus, sine copiâ rerum hoc fecit :* he
jumbles up many things together inmethodically, after the
Stoicks fashion : *parum ordinavit, multa accumulavit, &c.* If
Seneca be thus lashed, and many famous men that I could
name, what shall I expect? How shall I that am *vix umbra
tanti philosophi,* hope to please? *No man so absolute,* [6] Erasmus holds, *to satisfie all, except antiquity, prescription, &c. set
a bar.* But, as I have proved in Seneca, this will not always
take place, how shall I evade? 'Tis the common doom of
all writers : I must (I say) abide it : I seek not applause;
[7] *Non ego ventosæ venor suffragia plebis;* again, *non sum adeo
informis :* I would not be vilified [8] ;

———————————— [9]laudatus abunde,
Non fastiditus si tibi, lector, ero.

I fear good mens censures; and to their favourable acceptance
I submit my labours,

——— [10] et linguas mancipiorum
Contemno———

As the barking of a dog, I securely contemn those malicious
and scurrile obloquies, flouts, calumnies of railers and detractors; I scorn the rest. What therefore I have said, *pro tenui-
tate meâ* I have said.

[1] Minuit præsentia famam.   [2] Lipsius, Judic. de Senecâ.   [3] Lib. 10.
Plurimum studii, multam rerum cognitionem, omnem studiorum materiam, &c.
multa in eo probanda, multa admiranda.   [4] Suet. Arena sine calce.
[5] Introduc. ad Sen.   [6] Judic. de Sen.   Vix aliquis tam absolutus, ut alteri
per omnia satisfaciat, nisi longa temporis præscriptio, semotâ judicandi libertate,
religione quâdam animos occupârit.   [7] Hor. Ep. 1. lib. 29.   [8] Æque
turpe frigide laudari ac insectantes vituperari. Phavorinus. A. Gel. lib. 19. c. 2.
[9] Ovid. Trist. 1. eleg. 6.   [10] Juven. Sat. 5.

DEMOCRITUS TO THE READER.

One or two things yet I was desirous to have amended, if I could, concerning the manner of handling this my subject, for which I must apologize, *deprecari*, and upon better advice give the friendly reader notice. It was not mine intent to prostitute my muse in English, or to divulge *secreta Minervæ*, but to have exposed this more contract in Latin, if I could have got it printed. Any scurrile pamphlet is welcome to our mercenary stationers in English: they print all,

—————————— cuduntque libellos,
In quorum foliis vix simia nuda cacaret:

but in Latin they will not deal: which is one of the reasons [1] Nicholas Car, in his Oration of the paucity of English writers, gives, that so many flourishing wits are smothered in oblivion, lye dead and buried, in this our nation. Another main fault is, that I have not revised the copy, and amended the style, which now flows remisly, as it was first conceived: but my leisure would not permit: *Feci nec quod potui, nec quod volui*, I confess it is neither as I would, or as it should be.

[2] Cum relego, scripsisse pudet, quia plurima cerno,
Me quoque quæ fuerant judice digna lini.

When I peruse this tract which I have writ,
I am abash'd, and much I hold unfit.

Et quod gravissimum, in the matter it self, many things I disallow at this present, which when I writ, [3]*Non eadem est ætas, non mens*. I would willingly retract much, &c. but 'tis too late. I can only crave pardon now for what is amiss.

I might indeed (had I wisely done) observed that precept of the poet,

——nonumque prematur in annum,

and have taken more care : or as Alexander the physician would have done by lapis lazuli, fifty times washed before it be used, I should have revised, corrected, and amended this tract; but I had not (as I said) that happy leisure, no amanuenses or assistants. Pancrates in [4]Lucian, wanting a servant as he went from Memphis to Coptus in Ægypt, took a door bar, and, after some superstitious words pronounced, (Eucrates the relator was then present) made it stand up like a serving man, fetch him water, turn the spit, serve in supper, and what work he would besides; and when he had done that service he desired, turn'd his man to a stick again. I have no

---

[1] Aut artis inscii, aut quæstui magis quam literis student. hab. Cantab. et Lond. excus. 1576.　　[2] Ovid. de Pont. eleg. 1. 6.　　[3] Hor.　　[4] Tom. 3. Philopseud. accepto pessulo, quum carmen quoddam dixisset, effecit ut ambularet, aquam hauriret, cœnam pararet, &c.

DEMOCRITUS TO THE READER.

such skill to make new men at my pleasure, or means to hire them, no whistle, to call, like the master of a ship, and bid them run, &c. I have no such authority, no such benefactors, as that noble [1] Ambrosius was to Origen, allowing him six or seven amanuenses to write out his dictates; I must, for that cause, do my business my self, and was therefore enforced, as a bear doth her whelps, to bring forth this confused lump : I had not time to lick it into form, as she doth her young ones, but even so to publish it, as it was first written, *quicquid in buccam venit :* in an extemporean style, (as [2] I do commonly all other exercises) *effudi quicquid dictavit genius meus;* out of a confused company of notes, and writ with as small deliberation as I do ordinarily speak, without all affectation of big words, fustian phrases, jingling terms, tropes, strong lines, (that like [3] Acestes arrows, caught fire as they flew) strains of wit, brave heats, elogies, hyperbolical exornations, elegancies, &c. which many so much affect. I am [4] *aquæ potor*, drink no wine at all, which so much improves our modern wits ; a loose, plain, rude, writer, *ficum voco ficum, et ligonem ligonem,* and as free, as loose; *idem calamo quod in mente :* [5] I call a spade a. spade ; *animis hæc scribo, non auribus,* I respect matter not words ; remembering that of Cardan, *verba propter res, non res propter verba ;* and seeking with Seneca, *quid scribam, non quemadmodum,* rather what, than how to write. For, as Philo thinks, [6] *he that is conversant about matter, neglects words ; and those that excell in this art of speaking, have no profound learning :*

> [7] Verba nitent phaleris; at nullas verba medullas
> Intus habent——

Besides, it was the observation of that wise Seneca, [8] *when you see a fellow careful about his words, and neat in his speech, know this for a certainty, that mans mind is busied about toyes, there's no solidity in him. Non est ornamentum virile concinnitas ;* as he said of a nightingale,

> ——vox es, præterea nihil, &c.

I am therefore in this point a professed disciple of [9] Apollonius, a scholar of Socrates : I neglect phrases, and labour wholly to inform my readers understanding, not to please his ear; 'tis

---

[1] Eusebius, eccles. hist. lib. 6.   [2] Stans pede in uno, as he made verses.
[3] Virg.   [4] Non eadem a summo expectes, minimoque poëtâ.   [5] Stylus hic nullus præter parrhesiam.   [6] Qui rebus sé exercet, verba negligit : et qui callet artem dicendi, nullam disciplinam habet recognitam.   [7] Palingenius.
[8] Cujuscunque orationem vides politam et solicitam, scito animum in pusillis occupatum, in scriptis nil solidum. Epist. lib. l. 21.   [9] Philostratus, lib. 8. vit. Apol. Negligebat oratoriam facultatem, et penitus aspernabatur ejus professores, quod linguam duntaxat, non autem mentem, redderent eruditiorem.

VOL. I.   C

18   DEMOCRITUS TO THE READER.

not my study or intent to compose neatly, which an orator requires, but to express myself readily and plainly as it happens: so that, as a river runs, sometimes precipitate and swift, then dull and slow; now direct, then *per ambages;* now deep, then shallow; now muddy, then clear; now broad, then narrow, doth my style flow—now serious, then light; now comical, then satyrical; now more elaborate, then remiss, as the present subject required, or as at that time I was affected. And if thou vouchsafe to read this treatise, it shall seem no otherwise to thee, than the way to an ordinary traveller, sometimes fair, sometimes foul; here champion, there inclosed; barren in one place, better soil in another. By woods, groves, hills, dales, plains, &c. I shall lead thee *per ardua montium, et lubrica vallium, et roscida cespitum, et* [1]*glebosa camporum,* through variety of objects, that which thou shalt like, and surely dislike.

For the matter it self or method, if it be faulty, consider, I pray you, that of Columella: *nihil perfectum, aut a singulari consummatum industriâ:* no man can observe all; much is defective no doubt, may be justly taxed, altered, and avoided in Galen, Aristotle, those great masters. *Boni venatoris* ([2]one holds) *plures feras capere, non omnes.* He is a good huntsman can catch some, not all: I have done my endeavour. Besides, I dwell not in this study: *non hic sulcos ducimus; non hoc pulvere desudamus:* I am but a smatterer, I confess, a stranger: [3]here and there I pull a flower. I do easily grant, if a rigid censurer should criticize on this which I have writ, he should not find three sole faults, as Scaliger in Terence, but three hundred, so many as he hath done in Cardans Subtleties, as many notable errors as [4]Gul. Laurembergius, a late professor of Rustocke, discovers in that anatomy of Laurentius, or Barocius the Venetian in Sacroboscus. And although this be a sixth edition, in which I should have been more accurate, corrected all those former escapes, yet it was *magni laboris opus,* so difficult and tedious, that (as carpenters do find out of experience, 'tis much better build a new sometimes, than repair an old house) I could as soon write as much more, as alter that which is written. If ought therefore be amiss, (as I grant there is,) I require a friendly admonition, no bitter invective:

[5]Sint Musis sociæ Charites; Furia omnis abesto.

Otherwise, as in ordinary controversies, *funem contentionis*

---

[1] Hic enim, quod Seneca de Ponto, bos herbam, ciconia larisam, canis leporem, virgo florem legat.   [2] Pet. Nannius, not. in Hor.   [3] Non hic colonus domicilium habeo; sed, topiarii in morem, hinc inde florem vellico, ut canis Nilum lambens.   [4] Supra bis mille notabiles errores Laurentii demonstravi, &c.
[5] Philo, de Con.

2

DEMOCRITUS TO THE READER. 19

nectamus: sed cui bono? We may contend, and likely misuse each other: but to what purpose? We are both scholars,
say,

—————————[1]Arcades ambo,
Et cantare pares, et respondere parati.

If we do wrangle, what shall we get by it? Trouble and wrong
our selves, make sport to others. If I be convict of an error,
I will yield, I will amend. *Si quid bonis moribus, si quid
veritati dissentaneum, in sacris vel humanis literis a me dictum
sit, id nec dictum esto.* In the mean time I require a favourable censure of all faults omitted, harsh compositions, pleo-
nasmes of words, tautological repetitions, (though Seneca bear
me out, *nunquam nimis dicitur, quod nunquam satis dicitur)*
perturbations of tenses, numbers, printers faults, &c. My
translations are sometimes rather paraphrases, than interpretations; *non ad verbum;* but, as an author, I use more liberty,
and that's only taken, which was to my purpose. Quotations are often inserted in the text, which make the style
more harsh, or in the margent, as it hapned. Greek authors,
Plato, Plutarch, Athenæus, &c. I have cited out of their interpreters, because the original was not so ready. I have
mingled *sacra profanis,* but I hope not prophaned, and, in
repetition of authors names, ranked them *per accidens,* not
according to chronology; sometimes neotericks before ancients, as my memory suggested. Some things are here altered, expunged in this sixth edition, others amended, much
added, because many good [2]authors in all kinds are come to
my hands since ; and 'tis no prejudice, no such *indecorum,* or
oversight.

[3] Nunquam ita *quidquam* bene subductâ ratione ad vitam fuit,
Quin res, ætas, usus, semper aliquid apportent novi,
Aliquid moneant; ut illa, quæ scire te credas, nescias,
Et, quæ tibi putâris prima, in exercendo ut repudies.

Ne'er was ought yet at first contriv'd so fit,
But use, age, or something, would alter it;
Advise thee better, and, upon peruse,
Make thee not say, and, what thou tak'st, refuse.

But I am now resolved never to put this treatise out again:
ne quid nimis, I will not hereafter add, alter, or retract; I
have done.

The last and greatest exception is, that I, being a divine,
have medled with physick:

——[4] Tantumne est ab re tuâ otii tibi,
Aliena ut cures, eaque nihil quæ ad te attinent?

[1] Virg.　　[2] Frambesarius, Sennertus, Ferandus, &c.　　[3] Ter. Adelph.
[4] Heaut. act. 1. scen. 1.

c 2

DEMOCRITUS TO THE READER.

(which Menedemus objected to Chremes) have I so much
leisure or little business of mine own, as to look after other
mens matters, which concern me not? What have I to do
with physick? *quod medicorum est, promittant medici.* The
[1]Lacedæmonians were once in counsel about state-matters : a
debauched fellow spake excellent well, and to the purpose : his
speech was generally approved : a grave senator steps up, and
by all means would have it repealed, though good, because
dehonestabatur pessimo auctore, it had no better an author;
let some good man relate the same, and then it should pass.
This counsel was embraced, *factum est,* and it was registered
forthwith; *et sic bona sententia mansit, malus auctor mutatus
est.* Thou sayest as much of me, stomachous as thou art, and
grantest peradventure this which I have written in physick,
not to be amiss, had another done it, a professed physician,
or so; but why should I meddle with this tract? Hear me
speak : there be many other subjects, I do easily grant, both
in humanity and divinity, fit to be treated of, of which, had I
written *ad ostentationem* only, to shew my self, I should have
rather chosen, and in which I have been more conversant, I
could have more willingly luxuriated, and better satisfied my
self and others ; but that at this time I was fatally driven
upon this rock of melancholy, and carried away by this by-
stream, which, as a rillet, is deducted from the main chanel
of my studies, in which I have pleased and busied my self at
idle hours, as a subject most necessary and commodious:—
not that I prefer it before divinity, which I do acknowledge
to be the queen of professions, and to which all the rest are
as handmaids, but that in divinity I saw no such great need:
for, had I written positively, there be so many books in that
kind, so many commentators, treatises, pamphlets, expositions,
sermons, that whole teems of oxen cannot draw them; and,
had I been as forward and ambitious as some others, I might
have haply printed a sermon at Pauls Cross, a sermon in St.
Maries Oxon, a sermon in Christ-Church, or a sermon before the right honourable, right reverend, a sermon before the
right worshipful, a sermon in Latine, in English, a sermon with
a name, a sermon without, a sermon, a sermon, &c. But I
have been ever as desirous to suppress my labours in this kind,
as others have been to press and publish theirs. To have
written in controversie, had been to cut off an Hydras head :
[2]*lis litem generat;* one begets another; so many duplications,
triplications, and swarms of questions, *in sacro bello hoc quod
styli mucrone agitur,* that, having once begun, I should never

---

[1] Gellius, lib. 18. c. 3.   [2] Et inde catena quædam fit, quæ hæredes etiam
ligat. Cardan. Heinsius.

DEMOCRITUS TO THE READER.   21

make an end. One had much better, as [1] Alexander the
Sixth, pope, long since observed, provoke a great prince than
a begging friar, a Jesuite, or a seminary priest: I will add, for
inexpugnabile genus hoc hominum: they are an irrefragable
society; they must and will have the last word, and that
with such eagerness, impudence, abominable lying, falsifying,
and bitterness in their questions they proceed, that, as [2] he
said *furore cæcus, an rapit vis acrior, an culpa? responsum
date.* Blind fury or errour, or rashness, or what it is that
eggs them, I know not, I am sure, many times; which [3] Austin
perceived long since: *tempestate contentionis, serenitas charitatis obnubilatur:* with this tempest of contention, the serenity of charity is over-clouded: and there be too many
spirits conjured up already in this kind in all sciences, and
more than we can tell how to lay, which do so furiously rage,
and keep such a racket, that, as [4] Fabius said, *it had been
much better for some of them to have been born dumb, and
altogether illiterate, than so far to dote to their own destruction.*

> At melius fuerat non scribere; namque tacere
> Tutum semper erit.

'Tis a general fault—so Severinus the Dane complains [5] in
physick—*unhappy men as we are, we spend our daies in unprofitable questions and disputations,* intricate subtilties, *de land
caprinâ,* about moonshine in the water, *leaving in the mean
time those chiefest treasures of nature untouched, wherein the
best medicines for all manner of diseases are to be found, and
do not only neglect them our selves, but hinder, condemn, forbid,
and scoff at others, that are willing to enquire after them.*
These motives at this present have induced me to make choice
of this medicinal subject.

If any physician in the mean time shall infer, *ne sutor ultra
crepidam,* and find himself grieved that I have intruded into
his profession, I will tell him in brief, I do not otherwise by
them, than they do by us, if it be for their advantage.
I know many of their sect which have taken orders in
hope of a benefice: 'tis a common transition: and why may

---

[1] Malle se bellum cum magno principe gerere, quam cum uno ex fratrum men-
dicantium ordine.   [2] Hor. epod. lib. od. 7.   [3] Epist. 86. ad Casulam
presb.   [4] Lib. 12. cap. 1. Mutos nasci, et omni scientiâ egere, satius fuisset,
quam sic in propriam perniciem insanire.   [5] Infelix mortalitas! Inutilibus
quæstionibus ac disceptationibus vitam traducimus; naturæ principes thesauros,
in quibus gravissimæ morborum medicinæ collocatæ sunt, interim intactos relinquimus; nec ipsi solum relinquimus, sed et alios prohibemus, impedimus, con-
demnamus, ludibriis que afficimus.

DEMOCRITUS TO THE READER.

not a melancholy divine, that can get nothing but by simony, profess physick? Drusianus, an Italian, (Crusianus
but corruptly, Trithemius calls him) [1] *because he was not
fortunate in his practice, forsook his profession, and writ afterwards in divinity.* Marcilius Ficinus was *semel et simul,* a
priest and a physician at once; and [2] T. Linacer, in his old
age, took orders. The Jesuites profess both at this time:
divers of them, *permissu superiorum,* chirurgions, panders,
bawds, and midwives, &c. Many poor countrey-vicars, for
want of other means, are driven to their shifts; to turn
mountebanks, quacksalvers, empiricks: and if our greedy
patrons hold us to such hard conditions, as commonly they
do, they will make most of us work at some trade, as Paul did
—at last turn taskers, maltsters, costermongers, grasiers, sell
ale, as some have done, or worse. Howsoever, in undertaking this task, I hope I shall commit no great errour, or *indecorum,* if all be considered aright. I can vindicate my self
with Georgius Braunus, and Hieronymus Hemingius, those
two learned divines, who, (to borrow a line or two of mine
[3] elder brother) drawn by a *natural love, the one of pictures
and maps, prospectives and chorographical delights, writ that
ample Theatre of Cities; the other to the study of genealogies,
penned* Theatrum Genealogicum: or else I can excuse my
studies with [4] Lessius the Jesuite in like case—'Tis a disease of
the soul, on which I am to treat, and as much appertaining to
a divine as to a physician; and who knows not what an agreement there is betwixt these two professions? A good divine
either is, or ought to be, a good physician, a spiritual physician
at least, as our Saviour calls himself, and was indeed, Mat. 4.
23. Luke 5. 18. Luke 7. 8. They differ but in object, the
one of the body, the other of the soul, and use divers medicines to cure; one amends *animam per corpus,* the other *corpus
per animam,* as [5] our regius professour of physick well informed
us in a learned lecture of his not long since. One helps the
vices and passions of the soul, anger, lust, desperation, pride,
presumption, &c. by applying that spiritual physick, as the
other uses proper remedies in bodily diseases. Now, this being
a common infirmity of body and soul, and such a one that hath
as much need of a spiritual as a corporal cure, I could not find
a fitter task to busie my self about—a more apposite theam,
so necessary, so commodious, and generally concerning all

---

[1] Quod in praxi minime fortunatus esset, medicinam reliquit, et, ordinibus ini-
tiatus, in theologiâ postmodum scripsit. Gesner, Bibliotheca.   [2] P. Jovius.
[3] M. W. Burton, Preface to his Description of Leicestershire, printed at London
by W. Jaggard for J. White, 1622.   [4] In Hygiasticon; neque enim hæc
tractatio aliena videri debet a theologo, &c. agitur de morbo animæ.   [5] D.
Clayton, in comitiis, anno 1621.

DEMOCRITUS TO THE READER.

sorts of men, that should so equally participate of both, and require a whole physician. A divine, in this compound mixt malady, can do little alone: a physician, in some kinds of melancholy, much less: both make an absolute cure:

[1] Alterius sic altera poscit opem:

and 'tis proper to them both, and, I hope, not unbeseeming me, who am by my profession a divine, and by mine inclination a physician. I had Jupiter in my sixth house; I say, with [2] Beroaldus, *non sum medicus, nec medicinæ prorsus expers ;* in the theorick of physick I have taken some pains, not with an intent to practise, but to satisfie my self; which was a cause likewise of the first undertaking of this subject.

If these reasons do not satisfie thee, good reader—as Alexander Munificus, that bountiful prelate, sometime bishop of Lincoln, when he had built six castles, *ad invidiam operis eluendam*, saith [3] Mr. Cambden, to take away the envy of his work, (which very words Nubrigensis hath of Roger the rich bishop of Salisbury, who, in king Stephens time, built Shirburn castle, and that of Devises) to divert the scandal or imputation which might be thence inferred, built so many religious houses—If this my discourse be over medicinal, or savour too much of humanity, I promise thee that I will hereafter make thee amends in some treatise of divinity. But this, I hope, shall suffice, when you have more fully considered of the matter of this my subject, *rem substratam*, melancholy madness, and of the reasons following, which were my chief motives— the generality of the disease, the necessity of the cure, and the commodity or common good that will arise to all men by the knowledge of it, as shall at large appear in the ensuing preface. And I doubt not but that in the end you will say with me, that to anatomise this humour aright through all the members of this our *microcosmus*, is as great a task as to reconcile those chronological errours in the Assyrian monarchy, find out the quadrature of a circle, the creeks and sounds of the north-east or north-west passages, and, all out, as good a discovery as that hungry [4] Spaniards of Terra Australis Incognita—as great trouble as to perfect the motion of Mars and Mercury, which so crucifies our astronomers, or to rectifie the Gregorian kalendar. I am so affected, for my part, and hope, as [5] Theophrastus did by his Characters, *that our posterity,*

---

[1] Hor.   [2] Lib. de pestil.   [3] In Newark in Nottinghamshire. Cum duo ædificâsset castella, ad tollendam structionis invidiam, et expiandam maculam, duo instituit cœnobia, et collegis religiosis implevit.   [4] Ferdinando de Quir. anno 1612. Amsterdami impress.   [5] Præfat. ad Characteres. Spero enim, O Polycles, liberos nostros meliores inde futuros, quod istiusmodi memoriæ mandata reliquerimus, ex præceptis et exemplis nostris ad vitam accommodatis, ut se inde corrigant.

DEMOCRITUS TO THE READER.

friend Polycles, shall be the better for this which we have written, by correcting and rectifying what is amiss in themselves by our examples, and applying our precepts and cautions to their own use. And, as that great captain, Zisca, would have a drum made of his skin when he was dead, because he thought the very noise of it would put his enemies to flight, I doubt not but that these following lines, when they shall be recited, or hereafter read, will drive away melancholy (though I be gone), as much as Zisca's drum could terrifie his foes. Yet one caution let me give by the way to my present or future reader, who is actually melancholy—that he read not the [1] symptomes or prognosticks in this following tract, lest, by applying that which he reads to himself, aggravating, appropriating things generally spoken, to his own person (as melancholy men for the most part do), he trouble or hurt himself, and get, in conclusion, more harm than good. I advise them therefore warily to peruse that tract. *Lapides loquitur* (so said [2] Agrippa, de occ. Phil.) *et caveant lectores ne cerebrum iis excutiat.* The rest, I doubt not, they may securely read, and to their benefit. But I am over-tedious : I proceed.

Of the necessity and generality of this which I have said, if any man doubt, I shall desire him to make a brief survey of the world, as [3] Cyprian adviseth Donate—*Supposing himself to be transported to the top of some high mountain, and thence to behold the tumults and chances of this wavering world, he cannot chuse but either laugh at, or pity it.* St. Hierom, out of a strong imagination, being in the wilderness, conceived with himself that he then saw them dancing in Rome: and if thou shalt either conceive, or climb to see, thou shalt soon perceive that all the world is mad, that it is melancholy, dotes; that it is (which Epichthonius Cosmopolites expressed not many years since in a map) made like a fools head (with that motto, *caput helleboro dignum*) a crased head, *cavea stultorum*, a fools paradise, or (as Apollonius) a common prison of gulls, cheaters, flatterers, &c. and needs to be reformed. Strabo, in the ninth book of his Geography, compares Greece to the picture of a man; which comparison of his Nic. Gerbelius, in his exposition of Sophianus map, approves—The breast lies open from those Acroceraunian hills in Epirus, to the Sunian promontory in Attica; Pagæ and Megara are the two shoulders; that Isthmos of Corinth the neck; and Peloponnesus the head. If this allusion hold, 'tis, sure, a mad

---

[1] Part I. sect. 3.   [2] Præf. Lectori.   [3] Ep. 2. l. 2. ad Donatum. Paullisper te crede subduci in ardui montis verticem celsiorem: speculare inde rerum jacentium facies; et, oculis in diversa porrectis, fluctuantis mundi turbines intuere: jam simul aut ridebis aut misereberis, &c.

DEMOCRITUS TO THE READER.

head—*Morea* may be *Moria;* and, to speak what I think, the inhabitants of modern Greece swerve as much from reason and true religion at this day, as that Morea doth from the picture of a man. Examine the rest in like sort; and you shall find that kingdoms and provinces are melancholy, cities and families, all creatures, vegetal, sensible, and rational—that all sorts, sects, ages, conditions, are out of tune: as in Cebes table, *omnes errorem bibunt :* before they come into the world, they are intoxicated by errours cup—from the highest to the lowest, have need of physick; and those particular actions in [1]Seneca, where father and son prove one another mad, may be general : Porcius Latro shall plead against us all. For indeed who is not a fool, melancholy, mad?—[2] *Qui nil molitur inepte ;* who is not brain-sick ? Folly, melancholy, madness, are but one disease: *delirium* is a common name to all. Alexander Gordonius, Jason Pratensis, Savanarola, Guianerius, Montaltus, confound them, as differing *secundum magis et minus;* so doth David, Psal. 37. 5. *I said unto the fools, deal not so madly :* and 'twas an old Stoical paradox, *omnes stultos insanire,*—[3]all fools are mad, though some madder than others. And who is not a fool ? who is free from melancholy ? who is not touched more or less in habit or disposition ? If in disposition, ill dispositions beget habits: if they persevere, saith [4]Plutarch, habits either are or turn to diseases. 'Tis the same which Tully maintains in the second of his Tusculanes, *omnium insipientum animi in morbo sunt, et perturbatorum :* fools are sick, and all that are troubled in mind : for what is sickness, but, as [5]Gregory Tholosanus defines it, *a dissolution or perturbation of the bodily league which health combines?* and who is not sick, or ill disposed? in whom doth not passion, anger, envy, discontent, fear, and sorrow, reign? who labours not of this disease? Give me but a little leave, and you shall see by what testimonies, confessions, arguments, I will evince it, that most men are mad, that they had as much need to go a pilgrimage to the Anticyræ (as in [6]Strabo's time they did), as in our dayes they run to Compostella, our Lady of Sichem or Lauretta, to seek for help—that it is like to be as prosperous a voyage as that of Guiana, and that there is much more need of hellebore than of tobacco.

That men are so misaffected, melancholy, mad, giddy-

---

[1] Controv. l. 2. cont. 7. et l. 6. cont.   [2] Horatius.   [3] Idem Hor. l. 2. sat. 3. Damasippus Stoicus probat omnes stultos insanire.   [4] Tom. 2. sympos. lib. 5, c. 6. Animi affectiones, si diutius inhæreant, pravos generant habitus. [5] Lib. 28. cap. 1. Synt. art. mir. Morbus nihil est aliud quam dissolutio quædam ac perturbatio fœderis in corpore existentis, sicut et sanitas est consentientis bene corporis consummatio quædam.   [6] Lib. 9. Geogr. Plures olim gentes navigabant illuc sanitatis caussà.

26   DEMOCRITUS TO THE READER.

headed, hear the testimony of Solomon, Eccles. 2. 12. *And
I turned to behold wisdom, madness, and folly, &c.* And
ver. 23. *All his dayes are sorrow, his travel grief, and his
heart taketh no rest in the night.* So that, take melancholy
in what sense you will, properly or improperly, in disposition
or habit, for pleasure or for pain, dotage, discontent, fear,
sorrow, madness, for part, or all, truly, or metaphorically, 'tis
all one. Laughter it self is madness, according to Solomon;
and, as St. Paul hath it, *worldly sorrow brings death. The
hearts of the sons of men are evil; and madness is in their
hearts while they live,* Eccles. 9. 3. *Wise men themselves are
no better,* Eccles. 1. 18. *In the multitude of wisdom is much
grief; and he that increaseth wisdom, increaseth sorrow,* cap.
2. 17. He hated life it self; nothing pleased him; he hated
his labour; all, as [1]he concludes, is *sorrow, grief, vanity,
vexation of spirit.* And, though he were the wisest man in the
world, *sanctuarium sapientiæ,* and had wisdom in abundance,
he will not vindicate himself, or justifie his own actions.
*Surely I am more foolish than any man, and have not the
understanding of a man in me,* Prov. 30. 2. Be they Solomons words, or the words of Agur the son of Jakeh, they are
canonical. David, a man after Gods own heart, confesseth as
much of himself, Psal. 37. 21, 22. *So foolish was I and
ignorant, I was even as a beast before thee*—and condemns all
for fools, Psal. 93. and 32. 9. and 49. 20. He compares them
to *beasts, horses, and mules, in which there is no understanding.* The Apostle Paul accuseth himself in like sort,
2 Cor. 11. 21. *I would you would suffer a little my foolishness; I speak foolishly. The whole head is sick,* saith
Esay; *and the heart is heavy,* cap. 1. 5. and makes lighter
of them *than of oxen and asses; the ass knows his owner, &c.*
read Deut. 32. 6. Jer. 4. Amos 3. 1. Ephes. 5. 6. *Be
not mad, be not deceived: foolish Galatians, who hath bewitched you?* How often are they branded with this epithet
of madness and folly! No word so frequent amongst the
fathers of the church and divines. You may see what an
opinion they had of the world, and how they valued mens
actions.

I know that we think far otherwise, and hold them, most
part, wise men that are in authority—princes, magistrates,
[2] rich men—they are wise men born: all politicians and statesmen must needs be so; for who dare speak against them?
And on the other, so corrupt is our judgement, we esteem wise
and honest men fools; which Democritus well signified in an

---

[1] Eccles. 1. 24.   [2] Jure hæreditario sapere jubentur. Euphormio. Satyr.

DEMOCRITUS TO THE READER. 27

epistle of his to Hippocrates; [1] the *Abderites account vertue madness;* and so do most men living. Shall I tell you the reason of it? [2] *Fortune* and *Vertue (Wisdom* and *Folly* their seconds) upon a time contended in the Olympicks; every man thought that *Fortune* and *Folly* would have the worst, and pittied their cases. But it fell out otherwise. *Fortune* was blind, and cared not where she stroke, nor whom, without laws, *andabatarum instar, &c. Folly,* rash and inconsiderate, esteemed as little what she said or did. *Vertue* and *Wisdom* gave place, [3] were hissed out, and exploded by the common people—*Folly* and *Fortune* admired; and so are all their followers ever since. Knaves and fools commonly fare and deserve best in worldlings eyes and opinions. Many good men have no better fate in their ages. Achish, 1 Sam. 21. 14. held David for a madman. [4] Elisha and the rest were no otherwise esteemed. David was derided of the common people, Psal. 9. 7. *I am become a monster to many.* And generally we are accounted fools for Christ, 1 Cor. 14. *We fools thought his life madness, and his end without honour,* Wisd. 5. 4. Christ and his Apostles were censured in like sort, John 10. Mark 3. Acts 26. And so were all Christians in [5]Plinys time: *fuerunt et alii similis dementiæ, &c.* and called not long after, [6] *vesaniæ sectatores, eversores hominum, polluti novatores, fanatici, canes, malefici, venefici, Gallilæi homunciones, &c.* 'Tis an ordinary thing with us to account honest, devout, orthodox, divine, religious, plain-dealing men, ideots, asses, that cannot or will not lye and dissemble, shift, flatter, *accommodare se ad eum locum ubi nati sunt,* make good bargains, supplant, thrive, *patronis inservire, solennes ascendendi modos apprehendere, leges, mores, consuetudines recte observare, candide laudare, fortiter defendere, sententias amplecti, dubitare de nullis, credere omnia, accipere omnia, nihil reprehendere, cæteraque quæ promotionem ferunt et securitatem, quæ sine ambage felicem reddunt hominem, et vere sapientem apud nos* —that cannot temporize as other men do, [7] hand and take bribes, &c.—but fear God, and make a conscience of their doings. But the Holy Ghost, that knows better how to judge —he calls them fools. *The fool hath said in his heart,* Psal. 53. 1. *And their wayes utter their folly,* Psal. 49. 14. [8] *For what can be more mad, than, for a little worldly pleasure, to*

---

[1] Apud quos virtus, insania et furor esse dicitur.   [2] Calcagninus, Apol. Omnes mirabantur, putantes illisum iri Stultitiam. Sed præter expectationem res evenit. Audax Stultitia in eam irruit, &c. illa cedit irrisa; et plures hinc habet sectatores Stultitia.   [3] Non est respondendum stulto secundum stultitiam.   [4] 2 Reg. 7.   [5] Lib. 10. ep. 97.   [6] Aug. ep. 178.   [7] Quis, nisi mentis inops, &c.   [8] Quid insanius quam pro momentaneâ felicitate æternis te mancipare suppliciis?

28   DEMOCRITUS TO THE READER.

procure unto themselves eternal punishment? as Gregory and
others inculcate unto us.

Yea even all those great philosophers the world hath ever
had in admiration, whose works we do so much esteem, that
gave precepts of wisdom to others, inventers of arts and sciences
—Socrates, the wisest man of his time by the oracle of Apollo,
whom his two scholars [1]Plato and [2]Xenophon so much extol
and magnifie with those honourable titles, *best and wisest of
all mortal men, the happiest, and most just;* and as [3]Alcibiades
incomparably commends him; " Achilles was a worthy man,
but Brasidas and others were as worthy as himself; Antenor
and Nestor were as good as Pericles: and so of the rest: but
none present, before, or after Socrates, *nemo veterum neque
eorum qui nunc sunt,* were ever such, will match, or come near
him"—those seven wise men of Greece, those Britain Druides,
Indian Brachmanni, Æthiopian Gymnosophists, Magi of the
Persians—Apollonius, of whom Philostratus, *non doctus, sed
natus sapiens,* wise from his cradle—Epicurus, so much admired by his scholar Lucretius;

> Qui genus humanum ingenio superavit, et omnes
> Perstrinxit, stellas exortus ut ætherius Sol——
> Whose wit excell'd the wits of men as far
> As the Sun rising doth obscure a star——

or that so much renowned Empedocles,

> [4]Ut vix humanâ videatur stirpe creatus——

all those, of whom we read such [5]hyperbolical eulogiums; as
of Aristotle, that he was wisdom itself in the abstract, [6]a miracle of nature, breathing libraries, (as Eunapius of Longinus)
lights of nature, gyants for wit, quintessence of wit, divine
spirits, eagles in the clouds, fallen from heaven, gods, spirits,
lamps of the world, dictators,

> (Nulla ferant talem secla futura virum)

monarchs, miracles, superintendents of wit and learning,
*Oceanus, phœnix, Atlas, monstrum, portentum hominis, orbis
universi musæum, ultimus humanæ naturæ conatus, naturæ
maritus,*

> ——— merito cui doctior orbis
> Submissis defert fascibus imperium,

---

[1] In fine Phædonis. Hic finis fuit amici nostri, o Eucrates, nostro quidem
judicio, omnium quos experti sumus optimi et apprime sapientissimi, et justis-
simi.   [2] Xenoph. l. 4. de dictis Socratis, ad finem. Talis fuit Socrates, quem
omnium optimum et felicissimum statuam.   [3] Lib. 25. Platonis Convivio.
[4] Lucretius.   [5] Anaxagoras olim Mens dictus ab antiquis.   [6] Regula
naturæ, naturæ miraculum, ipsa eruditio, dæmonium hominis, sol scientiarum,
mare, sophia, antistes literarum et sapientiæ, ut Scioppius olim de Scal. et Heinsius. Aquila in nubibus, imperator literatorum, columen literarum, abyssus eruditionis, ocellus Europæ. Scaliger.

DEMOCRITUS TO THE READER.

as Ælian writ of Protagoras and Gorgias—we may say of them all, *tantum a sapientibus abfuerunt, quantum a viris pueri*, they were children in respect, infants, not eagles but kites, novices, illiterate *eunuchi sapientiæ*. And, although they were the wisest, and most admired in their age, as he censured Alexander, I do them: there were 10,000 in his army as worthy captains (had they been in place of command), as valiant as himself; there were myriads of men wiser in those dayes, and yet all short of what they ought to be. [1] Lactantius, in his book of Wisdom, proves them to be dizards, fools, asses, mad-men, so full of absurd and ridiculous tenents and brain-sick positions, that, to his thinking, never any old woman or sick person doted worse. [2] Democritus took all from Leucippus, and left, saith he, *the inheritance of his folly to* Epicurus : [3] *insanienti dum sapientiæ, &c* The like he holds of Plato, Aristippus, and the rest, making no difference [4] *betwixt them and beasts, saving that they could speak*. [5] Theodoret, in his tract *De Cur. Græc. Affect.* manifestly evinces as much of Socrates, whom though that oracle of Apollo confirmed to be the wisest man then living, and saved him from the plague, whom 2000 years have admired, of whom some will as soon speak evil as of Christ, yet *re verâ*, he was an illiterate ideot, as [6] Aristophanes calls him—*irrisor et ambitiosus*, as his master Aristotle terms him, *scurra Atticus*, as Zeno, an [7] enemy to all arts and sciences, as Athenæus, to philosophers and travellers, an opinionative asse, a caviller, a kind of pedant; for his manners, (as Theod. Cyrensis describes him) a [8] Sodomite, an atheist, (so convict by Anytus) *iracundus et ebrius, dicax, &c.* a pot-companion, by Plato's own confession, a sturdy drinker; and that of all others he was most sottish, a very mad-man in his actions and opinions. Pythagoras was part philosopher, part magician, or part witch. If you desire to hear more of Apollonius, a great wise man, sometime parallel'd by Julian the apostate to Christ, I refer you to that learned tract of Eusebius against Hierocles—and, for them all, to Lucian's *Piscator, Icaromenippus, Necyomantia*. Their actions, opinions in general, were so prodigious, absurd, ridiculous, which they broached and maintained; their books and elaborate treatises were full of dotage; which Tully *(ad Atticum)* long since observed—*delirant plerumque scriptores in libris suis*—their lives being opposite to their words, they com-

---

[1] Lib. 3. de sap. c. 17. et 20. Omnes philosophi aut stulti aut insani: nulla anus, nullus æger, ineptius deliravit. [2] Democritus, a Leucippo doctus, hæreditatem stultitiæ reliquit Epicuro. [3] Hor. car. lib. 1. od. 34. [4] Nihil interest inter hos et bestias, nisi quod loquantur. De sa. 1. 26. c. 8. [5] Cap. de virt. [6] Neb. et Ranis. [7] Omnium disciplinarum ignarus. [8] Pulchrorum adolescentum caussâ frequenter gymnasium obibat, &c.

30 DEMOCRITUS TO THE READER.

mended poverty to others, and were most covetous themselves, extolled love and peace, and yet persecuted one another with virulent hate and malice. They could give precepts for verse and prose; but not a man of them (as [1] Seneca tells them home) could moderate his affections. Their musick did shew us *flebiles modos, &c.* how to rise and fall; but they could not so contain themselves, as in adversity not to make a lamentable tone. They will measure ground by geometry, set down limits, divide and subdivide, but cannot yet prescribe *quantum homini satis*, or keep within compass of reason and discretion. They can square circles, but understand not the state of their own souls—describe right lines, and crooked, &c. but know not what is right in this life—*quid in vitâ rectum sit, ignorant:* so that, as he said,

Nescio, an Anticyram ratio illis destinet omnem.

I think all the Anticyræ will not restore them to their wits. [2] If these men now, that held [3] Zenodotus heart, Crates liver, Epictetus lanthorn, were so sottish, and had no more brains than so many beetles, what shall we think of the commonalty? what of the rest?

Yea, but (will you infer) that is true of heathens, if they be conferred with Christians, 1 Cor. 3. 19. *The wisdom of this world is foolishness with God, earthly and devilish*, as James calls it, 3. 15. *They were vain in their imaginations; and their foolish heart was full of darkness.* Rom. 1. 21, 22. *When they professed themselves wise, became fools.* Their witty works are admired here on earth, whilst their souls are tormented in hell fire. In some sense, *Christiani Crassiani*, Christians are Crassians, and, if compared to that wisdom, no better than fools. *Quis est sapiens? Solus Deus*, [4] Pythagoras replies; *God is only wise.*—Rom. 16. Paul determines, *only good*, as Austin well contends; *and no man living can be justified in his sight. God looked down from heaven upon the children of men, to see if any did understand*, Psal. 53. 2, 3. but all are corrupt, erre. Rom. 3. 12. *None doth good, no not one.* Job aggravates this, 4. 18. *Behold, he found no steadfastness in his servants, and laid folly upon his angels*, 19. *How much more on them that dwell in houses of clay!* In this sense, we are all as fools; and the [5] Scripture alone is *arx Minervæ;* we and our writings are shallow and unperfect. But I do not so mean: even in our ordinary dealings, we are

[1] Seneca. Scis rotunda metiri, sed non tuum animum.   [2] Ab uberibus sapientiâ lactati, cæcutire non possunt.   [3] Cor Zenodoti, et jecur Cratetis. [4] Lib. de nat. boni.   [5] Hic profundissimæ sophiæ fodinæ.

DEMOCRITUS TO THE READER. 31

no better than fools. All our actions, as [1] Pliny told Trajan, *upbraid us of folly :* our whole course of life is but matter of laughter : we are not soberly wise ; and the world it self, which ought at least to be wise by reason of his antiquity, as [2] Hugo de Prato Florido will have it, *semper stultizat, is every day more foolish than other: the more it is whipped, the worse it is ; and as a child will still be crowned with roses and flowers.* We are apish in it, *asini bipedes;* and every place is full *inversorum Apuleiorum,* of metamorphosed and two-legged asses, *inversorum Silenorum,* childish, *pueri instar bimuli, tremulâ patris dormientis in ulnâ.* Jovianus Pontanus (Antonio Dial.) brings in some laughing at an old man, that by reason of his age was a little fond : but, as he admonisheth there, *ne mireris, mi hospes, de hoc sene,* marvel not at him only ; for *tota hæc civitas delirium,* all our town dotes in like sort ; [3] we are a company of fools. Ask not, with him in the poet, [4] *Larvæ hunc, intemperiæ insaniæque, agitant senem ?* What madness ghosts this old man ; but what madness ghosts us all ? For we are, *ad unum omnes,* all mad ; *semel insanivimus omnes,* not once, but always so, *et semel, et simul, et semper,* ever and altogether as bad as he ; and not *senex bis puer, delira anus ;* but say it of us all, *semper pueri ;* young and old, all dote, as Lactantius proves out of Seneca ; and no difference betwixt us and children, saving that *majora ludimus, et grandioribus pupis,* they play with babies cf clouts, and such toys, we sport with greater bables. We cannot accuse or condemn one another, being faulty ourselves, *deliramenta loqueris,* you talk idly, or, as [5] Micio upbraided Demea, *insanis? aufer;* for we are as mad our own selves ; and it is hard to say which is the worst. Nay, 'tis universally so,

[6] Vitam regit fortuna, non sapientia.

When [7] Socrates had taken great pains to find out a wise man, and, to that purpose, had consulted with philosophers, poets, artificers, he concludes all men were fools ; and, though it procured him both anger and much envy, yet in all companies he would openly profess it. When [8] Supputius in Pontanus had travelled all over Europe to conferr with a wise man, he returned at last without his errand, and could find none. [9] Cardan concurs with him : *Few there are (for ought*

---

[1] Panegyr. Trajano. Omnes actiones exprobrare stultitiam videntur. [2] Ser. 4. in domi Pal. Mundus, qui ob antiquitatem deberet esse sapiens, semper stultizat, et nullis flagellis alteratur; sed, ut puer, vult rosis et floribus coronari. [3] Insanum te omnes pueri, clamantque puellæ. Hor. [4] Plautus, Aulular. [5] Adelph. act. 5. scen. 8. [6] Tully, Tusc. 5. [7] Plato, Apologia Socratis. [8] Ant. Dial. [9] Lib. 3. de sap. Pauci, ut video, sanæ mentis sunt.

32   DEMOCRITUS TO THE READER.

I can perceive) well in their wits. So doth [1] Tully : *I see every thing to be done foolishly and unadvisedly.*

> Ille sinistrorsum, hic dextrorsum abit: unus utrique
> Error; sed variis illudit partibus omnes.

> One reels to this, another to that wall;
> 'Tis the same errour that deludes them all.

[2] They dote all, but not alike, (Μανια γ᾽ ου πασιν ὁμοια) not in the same kind. *One is covetous, a second lascivious, a third ambitious, a fourth envious, &c.* as Damasippus the Stoick hath well illustrated in the poet,

> [3] Desipiunt omnes æque ac tu.

'Tis an inbred maladie : in every one of us, there is *seminarium stultitiæ,* a seminary of folly, *which, if it be stirred up, or get a head, will run* in infinitum, *and infinitely varies, as we our selves are severally addicted,* (saith [4] Balthazar Castilio) and cannot so easily be rooted out ; it takes such fast hold, as Tully holds, *altæ radices stultitiæ;* [5] so we are bred, and so we continue. Some say there be two main defects of wit—errour and ignorance—to which all others are reduced. By ignorance we know not things necessary ; by errour we know them falsely. Ignorance is a privation, errour a positive act. From ignorance comes vice, from errour heresie, &c. But make how many kinds you will, divide and subdivide ; few men are free, or that do not impinge on some one kind or other. [6] *Sic plerumque agitat stultos inscitia,* as he that examines his own and other mens actions shall find.

[7] Charon, in Lucian, (as he wittily feigns) was conducted by Mercury to such a place, where he might see all the world at once. After he had sufficiently viewed and looked about, Mercury would needs know of him what he had observed. He told him, that he saw a vast multitude, and a promiscuous : their habitations like mole-hills ; the men as emmets : *he could discern cities like so many hives of bees, wherein every bee had a sting ; and they did nought else but sting one another ; some domineering like hornets, bigger than the rest, some like filching wasps, others as drones.* Over their heads were hovering a confused company of perturbations, hope, fear, anger, avarice, ignorance, &c. and a multitude of diseases hanging, which they still pulled on their pates. Some were

---

[1] Stulte et incaute omnia agi video.   [2] Insania non omnibus eadem. Erasm. chil. 3. cent. 10. Nemo mortalium qui non aliquâ in re desipit, licet alius alio morbo laboret, hic libidinis, ille avaritiæ, ambitionis, invidiæ.   [3] Hor. l. 2. sat. 3. [4] Lib. 1. de aulico. Est in unoquoque nostrûm seminarium aliquod stultitiæ, quod si quando excitetur, in infinitum facile excrescit.   [5] Primaque lux vitæ prima furoris erat.   [6] Tibullus. Stulti prætereunt dies; their wits are a woolgathering. So fools commonly dote.   [7] Dial. contemplantes, tom. 2.

DEMOCRITUS TO THE READER. 33

brawling, some fighting, riding, running, *solicite ambientes, callide litigantes,* for toyes, and trifles, and such momentany things—their towns and provinces meer factions, rich against poor, poor against rich, nobles against artificers, they against nobles, and so the rest. In conclusion, he condemned them all for mad-men, fools, ideots, asses,— *O stulti! quænam hæc est amentia ?* O fools! O mad-men! he exclaims, *insana studia, insani labores, &c.* Mad endeavours! mad actions! mad! mad! mad! [1] *O seclum insipiens et inficetum!* a giddy-headed age. Heraclitus the philosopher, out of a serious meditation of mens lives, fell a weeping, and with continual tears bewailed their misery, madness, and folly. Democritus, on the other side, burst out a laughing; their whole life seemed to him so ridiculous : and he was so far carried with this ironical passion, that the citizens of Abdera took him to be mad, and sent therefore embassadors to Hippocrates the physician, that he would exercise his skill upon him. But the story is set down at large by Hippocrates, in his Epistle to Damegetus, which, because it is not impertinent to this discourse, I will insert *verbatim* almost, as it is delivered by Hippocrates himself, with all the circumstances belonging unto it.

When Hippocrates was come to Abdera, the people of the city came flocking about him, some weeping, some entreating of him that he would do his best. After some little repast, he went to see Democritus, the people following him, whom he found (as before) in his garden in the suburbs, all alone, [2] *sitting upon a stone under a plane tree, without hose or shoes, with a book on his knees, cutting up several beasts, and busie at his study.* The multitude stood gazing round about, to see the congress. Hippocrates, after a little pause, saluted him by his name, whom he re-saluted, ashamed almost that he could not call him likewise by his, or that he had forgot it. Hippocrates demanded of him what he was doing. He told him that he was [3] *busie in cutting up several beasts, to find out the cause of madness and melancholy.* Hippocrates commended his work, admiring his happiness and leisure. And why, quoth Democritus, have not you that leisure? Because, replyed Hippocrates, domestical affairs hinder, necessary to be done, for our selves, neighbours, friends—expences, diseases, frailties and mortalities which happen—wife, children, servants, and such businesses, which deprive us of our time.

---

[1] Catullus.   [2] Sub ramosâ platano sedentem, solum, discalceatum, super lapidem, valde pallidum ac macilentum, promissâ barbâ, librum super genibus habentem.   [3] De furore, maniâ, melancholiâ scribo, ut sciam quo pacto in hominibus gignatur, fiat, crescat, cumuletur, minuatur. Hæc (inquit) animalia, quæ vides, propterea seco, non Dei opera perosus, sed fellis bilisque naturam disquirens.

VOL. I.   D

34   DEMOCRITUS TO THE READER.

At this speech Democritus profusely laughed (his friends, and
the people standing by, weeping in the mean time, and lament-
ing his madness). Hippocrates asked the reason why he
laughed. He told him, at the vanities and fopperies of the
time, to see men so empty of all vertuous actions, to hunt so
far after gold, having no end of ambition—to take such infinite
pains for a little glory, and to be favoured of men—to make
such deep mines into the earth for gold, and many times to
find nothing, with loss of their lives and fortunes—some to
love dogs, others horses, some to desire to be obeyed in many
provinces, [1] and yet themselves will know no obedience—[2] some
to love their wives dearly at first, and, after a while, to forsake
and hate them—begetting children, with much care and cost
for their education, yet, when they grow to mans estate, [3] to
despise, neglect, and leave them naked to the worlds mercy.
[4] Do not these behaviours express their intolerable folly?
When men live in peace, they covet war, detesting quietness,
[5] deposing kings, and advancing others in their stead, murdering some men, to beget children of their wives. How many
strange humours are in men! When they are poor and needy,
they seek riches; and, when they have them, they do not enjoy
them, but hide them under ground, or else wastefully spend
them. O wise Hippocrates! I laugh at such things being
done, but much more when no good comes of them, and when
they are done to so ill purpose. There is no truth or justice
found amongst them: for they daily plead one against another,
[6] the son against the father and the mother, brother against
brother, kindred and friends of the same quality; and all this
for riches, whereof, after death, they cannot be possessors.
And yet—notwithstanding they will defame and kill one another, commit all unlawful actions, contemning God and men,
friends and countrey—they make great account of many senseless things, esteeming them as a great part of their treasure,
statues, pictures, and such like moveables, dear bought, and so
cunningly wrought, [7] as nothing but speech wanteth in them;
[8] and yet they hate living persons speaking to them. Others
affect difficult things: if they dwell on firm land, they will remove to an island, and thence to land again, being no way constant to their desires. They commend courage and strength in
wars, and let themselves be conquered by lust and avarice.
They are, in brief, as disordered in their minds, as Thersites was

---

[1] Aust. l. 1. in Gen. Jumenti et servi tui obsequium rigide postulas; et tu nullum præstas aliis, nec ipsi Deo.   [2] Uxores ducunt, mox foras ejiciunt.
[3] Pueros amant, mox fastidiunt.   [4] Quid hoc ab insaniâ deest?   [5] Reges
eligunt, deponunt.   [6] Contra parentes, fratres, cives, perpetuo rixantur, et
inimicitias agunt.   [7] Credo equidem, vivos ducent de marmore vultus.
[8] Idola inanimata amant; animata odio habent; sic pontificii.

2

DEMOCRITUS TO THE READER. 35

in his body. And now methinks, O most worthy Hippocrates! you should not reprehend my laughing, perceiving so many fooleries in men; [1] for no man will mock his own folly, but that which he seeth in a second; and so they justly mock one another. The drunkard calls him a glutton, whom he knows to be sober. Many men love the sea, others husbandry : briefly, they cannot agree in their own trades and professions, much less in their lives and actions.

When Hippocrates heard these words so readily uttered, without premeditation, to declare the worlds vanity, full of ridiculous contrariety, he made answer, that necessity compelled men to many such actions, and divers wills ensuing from divine permission, that we might not be idle, being nothing is so odious to them as sloth and negligence. Besides, men cannot foresee future events, in this uncertainty of humane affairs ; they would not so marry, if they could foretel the causes of their dislike and separation ; or parents, if they knew the hour of their childrens death, so tenderly provide for them ; or an husbandman sow, if he thought there would be no increase ; or a merchant adventure to sea, if he foresaw shipwrack ; or be a magistrate, if presently to be deposed. Alas! worthy Democritus, every man hopes the best ; and to that end he doth it ; and therefore no such cause, or ridiculous occasion of laughter.

Democritus, hearing this poor excuse, laughed again aloud, perceiving he wholly mistook him, and did not well understand what he had said concerning perturbations, and tranquillity of the mind—insomuch, that if men would govern their actions by discretion and providence, they would not declare themselves fools, as now they do ; and he should have no cause of laughter : but (quoth he) they swell in this life, as if they were immortal, and demi-gods, for want of understanding. It were enough to make them wise, if they would but consider the mutability of this world, and how it wheels about, nothing being firm and sure. He that is now above, to morrow is beneath ; he that sate on this side to day, to morrow is hurled on the other ; and, not considering these matters, they fall into many inconveniencies and troubles, coveting things of no profit, and thirsting after them, tumbling headlong into many calamities—so that, if men would attempt no more than what they can bear, they should lead contented lives—and, learning to know themselves, would limit their ambition, [2] they would perceive then that nature hath enough, without seeking such

---

[1] Suam stultitiam perspicit nemo, sed alter alterum deridet.　　[2] Denique sit finis quærendi : cumque habeas plus, Pauperiem metuas minus, et finire laborem Incipias, parto quod avebas ; utere. Hor.

D 2

DEMOCRITUS TO THE READER.

superfluities and unprofitable things, which bring nothing with them but grief and molestation. As a fat body is more subject to diseases, so are rich men to absurdities and fooleries, to many casualties and cross inconveniencies. There are many that take no heed what happeneth to others by bad conversation, and therefore overthrow themselves in the same manner through their own fault, not foreseeing dangers manifest. These are things (O more than mad! quoth he) that give me matter of laughter, by suffering the pains of your impieties, as your avarice, envy, malice, enormous villanies, mutinies, unsatiable desires, conspiracies, and other incurable vices— besides your [1]dissimulation and hypocrisie, bearing deadly hatred one to the other, and yet shadowing it with a good face— flying out into all filthy lusts, and transgressions of all laws, both of nature and civility. Many things, which they have left off, after a while they fall to again—husbandry, navigation—and leave again, fickle and unconstant as they are. When they are young, they would be old, and old, young. [2]Princes commend a private life; private men itch after honour: a magistrate commends a quiet life; a quiet man would be in his office, and obeyed as he is: and what is the cause of all this, but that they know not themselves? Some delight to destroy, [3]one to build, another to spoil one countrey to enrich another and himself. [4]In all these things they are like children, in whom is no judgement or counsel, and resemble beasts, saving that beasts are better than they, as being contented with nature. [5]When shall you see a lion hide gold in the ground, or a bull contend for a better pasture? When a boar is thirsty, he drinks what will serve him, and no more; and, when his belly is full, he ceaseth to eat: but men are immoderate in both, as in lust— they covet carnal copulation at set times; men always, ruinating thereby the health of their bodies. And doth it not deserve laughter to see an amorous fool torment himself for a wench, weep, howl for a mis-shapen slut, a dowdy sometimes, that might have his choice of the finest beauties? Is there any remedy for this in physick? [6]I do anatomize and cut up these poor beasts, to see these distempers, vanities, and follies: yet such proof were better made on man's body, (if my

---

[1] Astutam vapido servat sub pectore vulpem.—Et, cum vulpe positus, pariter vulpinarier.—Cretizandum cum Crete. [2] Qui fit, Mæcenas, ut nemo, quam sibi sortem, Seu ratio dederit, seu sors objecerit, illâ Contentus vivat? &c. Hor. [3] Diruit, ædificat, mutat quadrata rotundis.—Trajanus pontem struxit super Danubium, quem successor ejus Adrianus statim demolitus. [4] Quâ quid in re ab infantibus differunt, quibus mens et sensus sine ratione inest? Quidquid sese his offert, volupe est. [5] Idem Plut. [6] Ut insaniæ causam disquiram, bruta macto et seco, cum hoc potius in hominibus investigandum esset.

DEMOCRITUS TO THE READER.

kind nature would endure it,) [1] who, from the hour of his birth, is most miserable, weak, and sickly : when he sucks, he is guided by others, when he is grown great, practiseth unhappiness, [2] and is sturdy, and, when old, a child again, and repenteth him of his life past. And here being interrupted by one that brought books, he fell to it again, that all were mad, careless, stupid. To prove my former speeches, look into courts or private houses. [3] Judges give judgement according to their own advantage, doing manifest wrong to poor innocents to please others. Notaries alter sentences, and, for money, lose their deeds. Some make false moneys : others counterfeit false weights. Some abuse their parents, yea corrupt their own sisters; others make long libels and pasquils, defaming men of good life, and extol such as are lewd and vicious. Some rob one, some another : [4] magistrates make laws against thieves, and are the veriest thieves themselves. Some kill themselves, others despair, not obtaining their desires. Some dance, sing, laugh, feast, and banquet, whilest others sigh, languish, mourn, and lament, having neither meat, drink, nor clothes. [5] Some prank up their bodies, and have their minds full of execrable vices. Some trot about, [6] to bear false witness, and say any thing for money ; and though judges know of it, yet for a bribe they wink at it, and suffer false contracts to prevail against equity. Women are all day a dressing to pleasure other men abroad, and go like sluts at home, not caring to please their own husbands whom they should. Seeing men are so fickle, so sottish, so intemperate, why should not I laugh at those to whom [7] folly seems wisdom, will not be cured, and perceive it not ?

It grew late : Hippocrates left him ; and no sooner was he come away, but all the citizens came about flocking, to know how he liked him. He told them in brief, that, notwithstanding those small neglects of his attire, body, diet, [8] the world had not a wiser, a more learned, a more honest man ; and they were much deceived to say that he was mad.

Thus Democritus esteemed of the world in his time ; and this was the cause of his laughter ; and good cause he had.

---

[1] Totus a nativitate morbus est.   [2] In vigore furibundus, quum decrescit insanabilis.   [3] Cyprian. ad Donatum Qui sedet, crimina judicaturus, &c. [4] Tu pessimus omnium latro es, as a thief told Alexander in Curtius.—Damnat foras judex, quod intus operatur. Cyprian.   [5] Vultûs magna cura; magna animi incuria. Am. Marcel.   [6] Horrenda res est! vix duo verba sine mendacio proferuntur: et, quamvis solenniter homines ad veritatem dicendam invitentur, pejerare tamen non dubitant; ut ex decem testibus vix unus verum dicat. Calv. in 8. Joh. Serm. 1.   [7] Sapientiam insaniam esse dicunt.   [8] Siquidem sapientiæ suæ admiratione me complevit; offendi sapientissimum virum qui salvos potest omnes homines reddere.

DEMOCRITUS TO THE READER.

[1] Olim jure quidem, nunc plus, Democrite, ride.
Quin rides? vita hæc nunc mage ridicula est.

Democritus did well to laugh of old:
Good cause he had, but now much more:
This life of ours is more ridiculous
Than that of his, or long before.

Never so much cause of laughter, as now; never so many fools and mad men. 'Tis not one [2] Democritus will serve turn to laugh in these days: we have now need of a *Democritus to laugh at Democritus,* one jester to flout at another, one fool to flear at another—a great Stentorian Democritus, as big as that Rhodian Colossus; for now, as [3] Salisburiensis said in his time, *totus mundus histrionem agit*—the whole world plays the fool: we have a new theatre, a new scene, a new comedy of errours, a new company of personate actors: *Volupiæ sacræ* (as Calcagninus wittily feigns in his Apologues) are celebrated all the world over, [4] where all the actors were mad men and fools, and every hour changed habits, or took that which came next. He that was a marriner to day, is an apothecary to morrow, a smith one while, a philosopher another, *in his Volupiæ ludis*—a king now with his crown, robes, scepter, attendants, by and by drove a loaded asse before him like a carter, &c. If Democritus were alive now, he should see strange alterations, a new company of counterfeit vizards, whiflers, Cumane asses, maskers, mummers, painted puppets, outsides, phantastick shadows, guls, monsters, giddy-heads, butter-flies: and so many of them are indeed ([5] if all be true that I have read); for, when Jupiter and Junos wedding was solemnised of old, the gods were all invited to the feast, and many noble men besides: amongst the rest came Chrysalus, a Persian prince, bravely attended, rich in golden attires, in gay robes, with a majestical presence, but otherwise an asse. The gods, seeing him come in such pomp and state, rose up to give him place, *ex habitu hominem metientes;* [6] but Jupiter, perceiving what he was—a light, phantastick, idle fellow—turned him and his proud followers into butter-flies: and so they continue still (for ought I know to the contrary) roving about in

---

[1] E Græc. epig.   [2] Plures Democriti nunc non sufficiunt. Opus Democrito, qui Democritum rideat. Eras. Moria.   [3] Polycrat. lib. 3. cap. 8. e Petron.   [4] Ubi omnes delirabant, omnes insani, &c. hodie nauta, cras philosophus; hodie faber, cras pharmacopola; hic modo regem agebat multo satellitio, tiarâ, et sceptro ornatus, nunc vili amictus centiculo, asinum clitellarium impellit.   [5] Calcagninus, Apol. Chrysalus e cæteris, auro dives, manicato peplo et tiarâ conspicuus, levis alioquin et nullius consilii, &c. Magno fastu ingredienti assurgunt Dii, &c.   [6] Sed hominis levitatem Jupiter perspiciens, at tu (inquit) esto bombilio, &c. protinusque vestis illa manicata in alas versa est; et mortales inde Chrysalides vocant hujusmodi homines.

DEMOCRITUS TO THE READER.

pied-coats, and are called Chrysalides by the wiser sort of men
—that is, golden outsides, drones, flies, and things of no
worth. Multitudes of such, &c.

—————ubique invenies
Stultos avaros, sycophantas prodigos.

Many additions, much increase of madness, folly, vanity, should
Democritus observe, were he now to travel, or could get leave
of Pluto to come see fashions, (as Charon did in Lucian) to
visit our cities of Moronia Pia, and Moronia Felix—sure I
think he would break the rim of his belly with laughing.

[1]Si foret in terris, rideret Democritus, seu, &c.

A satyrical Roman, in his time, thought all vice, folly, and
madness, were all at full sea,

[2]Omne in præcipiti vitium stetit.——

[3]Josephus the historian taxeth his countreymen Jews for
bragging of their vices, publishing their follies, and that they did
contend amongst themselves, who should be most notorious in
villanies: but we flow higher in madness, far beyond them,

[4]Mox daturi progeniem vitiosiorem;

and the latter end (you know, whose oracle it is) is like to be
worst. 'Tis not to be denied; the world alters every day.
*Ruunt urbes, regna transferuntur, &c. variantur habitus, leges
innovantur,* as [5]Petrarch observes—we change language, habits, laws, customs, manners, but not vices, not diseases, not
the symptoms of folly and madness: they are still the same.
And, as a river (we see) keeps the like name and place, but
not water, and yet ever runs,

([6]Labitur et labetur in omne volubilis ævum)

our times and persons alter, vices are the same, and ever will
be. Look how nightingales sang of old, cocks crowed, kine
lowed, sheep bleated, sparrows chirped, dogs barked; so they
do still: we keep our madness still, play the fools still, *nec
dum finitus Orestes* we are of the same humours and inclinations as our predecessors were; you shall find us all alike,
much at one, we and our sons,

Et nati natorum, et qui nascentur ab illis;

and so shall our posterity continue to the last. But, to speak
of times present—

---

[1] Juven.   [2] Idem.   [3] De bello Jud. l. 8. c. 11.   Iniquitates vestræ
neminem latent; inque dies singulos certamen habetis, quis pejor sit.   [4] Hor.
[5] Lib. 5. Epist. 8.   [6] Hor.

40   DEMOCRITUS TO THE READER.

If Democritus were alive now, and should but see the
superstition of our age, our [1] religious madness, as [2] Meteran
calls it, *religiosam insaniam*—so many professed Christians,
yet so few imitators of Christ, so much talk of religion, so
much science, so little conscience, so much knowledge, so
many preachers, so little practice—such variety of sects, such
have and hold of all sides,

———[3] obvia signis signa, &c.——

such absurd and ridiculous traditions and ceremonies—if he
should meet a [4] Capouchin, a Franciscan, a pharisaical Jesuit,
a man-serpent, a shave-crowned monk in his robes, a begging
frier, or see their three-crowned soveraign lord the pope, poor
Peter's successour, *servus servorum Dei*, to depose kings with
his foot, to tread on emperours necks, make them bare-foot
and bare-legg'd at his gates, hold his bridle and stirrup, &c.
(O that Peter and Paul were alive to see this!)—if he should
observe a [5] prince creep so devoutly to kiss his toe, and those
red-cap cardinals, poor parish priests of old, now princes companions—what would he say? *Cœlum ipsum petitur stultitiâ.*
Had he met some of our devout pilgrims going bare-foot to
Jerusalem, our lady of Lauretto, Rome, St. Iago, St. Thomas
shrine, to creep to those counterfeit and maggot-eaten reliques
—had he been present at a masse, and seen such kissing of
paxes, crucifixes, cringes, duckings, their several attires and
ceremonies, pictures of saints, [6] indulgencies, pardons, vigils,
fasting, feasts, crossing, knocking, kneeling at *Ave Maries,*
bells, with many such

———jucunda rudi spectacula plebi,

praying in gibberish, and mumbling of beads—had he heard
an old woman say her prayers in Latine, their sprinkling of
holy water, and going a procession,

(———[7] monachorum incedunt agmina mille;
Quid memorem vexilla, cruces, idolaque culta, &c.)

their breviaries, bulls, hallowed beads, exorcisms, pictures,
curious crosses, fables, and bables—had he read the Golden
Legend, the Turks Alcoran, or Jews Talmud, the Rabbins

---

[1] Superstitio est insanus error.   [2] Lib. 8. hist. Belg.   [3] Lucan.
[4] Father Angelo, the Duke of Joyeuse, going bare-foot over the Alps to Rome. &c.
[5] Si cui intueri vacet quæ patiuntur superstitiosi, invenies tam indecora honestis, tam indigna liberis, tam dissimilia sanis, ut nemo fuerit dubitaturus furere
eos, si cum paucioribus furerent. Senec.   [6] Quid dicam de eorum indul-
gentiis, oblationibus, votis, solutionibus, jejuniis, cœnobiis, vigiliis, somniis, horis,
organis, cantilenis, campanis, simulacris, missis, purgatoriis, mitris, breviariis,
bullis, lustralibus aquis, rasuris, unctionibus, candelis, calicibus, crucibus, map-
pis, cereis, thuribulis, incantationibus, exorcismis, sputis, legendis, &c. Baleus,
de actis Rom. Pont.   [7] Th. Nauger.

DEMOCRITUS TO THE READER.

Comments, what would he have thought? How dost thou think he might have been affected? Had he more particularly examined a Jesuits life amongst the rest, he should have seen an hypocrite profess poverty, [1] and yet possess more goods and lands than many princes, to have infinite treasures and revenues—teach others to fast, and play the gluttons themselves ; like watermen, that rowe one way and look another—[2] vow virginity, talk of holiness, and yet indeed a notorious bawd, and famous fornicator, *lascivum pecus*, a very goat—monks by profession [3], such as give over the world, and the vanities of it, and yet a *Machiavellian* rout [4] interested in all maner of state—holy men, peace-makers, and yet composed of envy, lust, ambition, hatred and malice, fire-brands, *adulta patriæ pestis*, traitours, assassinates—*hac itur ad astra ;* and this is to supererogate, and merit heaven for themselves and others ! Had he seen, on the adverse side, some of our nice and curious schismaticks, in another extream, abhor all ceremonies, and rather lose their lives and livings, than do or admit any thing papists have formerly used, though in things indifferent (they alone are the true church, *sal terræ, cum sint omnium insulsissimi)*—formalists, out of fear and base flattery, like so many weather-cocks, turn round—a rout of temporisers, ready to embrace and maintain all that is or shall be proposed, in hope of preferment—another Epicurean company, lying at lurch as so many vultures, watching for a prey of church goods, and ready to rise by the down-fall of any—as [5] Lucian said in like case, what dost thou think Democritus would have done, had he been spectatour of these things—or, had he but observed the common people follow like so many sheep one of their fellows drawn by the horns over a gap, some for zeal, some for fear, *quo se cumque rapit tempestas,* to credit all, examine nothing, and yet ready to dye before they will abjure any of those ceremonies, to which they have been accustomed —others out of hypocrisie frequent sermons, knock their breasts, turn up their eyes, pretend zeal, desire reformation, and yet professed usurers, gripers, monsters of men, harpies, devils, in their lives, to express nothing less?

What would he have said, to see, hear, and read so many bloody battels, so many thousands slain at once, such streams of blood able to turn mills, *unius ob noxam furiasque,* or to

---

[1] Dum simulant spernere, acquisiverunt sibi 30 annorum spatio bis centena millia librarum annua. Arnold. [2] Et quum interdin de virtute loquuti sunt, sero in latibulis clunes agitant labore nocturno. Agrippa. [3] 2 Tim. 3. 9. But they shall prevail no longer: their madness shall be evident to all men. [4] Benignitatis sinus solebat esse, nunc litium officina, curia Romana. Budæus. [5] Quid tibi videtur facturus Democritus, si horum spectator contigisset?

DEMOCRITUS TO THE READER.

make sport for princes, without any just cause, [1] *for vain titles* (saith Austin) *precedency, some wench, or such like toy, or out of desire of domineering, vain-glory, malice, revenge, folly, madness,* (goodly causes all, *ob quas universus orbis bellis et cædibus misceatur)* whilest statesmen themselves in the mean time are secure at home, pampered with all delights and pleasures, take their ease, and follow their lusts, not considering what intolerable misery poor souldiers endure, their often wounds, hunger, thirst, &c. ? The lamentable cares, torments, calamities, and oppressions, that accompany such proceedings, they feel not, take no notice of it. *So wars are begun, by the perswasion of a few debauched, hair-brain'd, poor, dissolute, hungry captains, parasitical fawners, unquiet hotspurs, restless innovators, green heads, to satisfie one mans private spleen, lust, ambition, avarice, &c. tales rapiunt scelerata in prælia causæ. Flos hominum,* proper men, well proportioned, carefully brought up, able both in body and mind, sound, led like so many [2] beasts to the slaughter in the flower of their years, pride, and full strength, without all remorse and pitty, sacrificed to Pluto, killed up as so many sheep, for devils food, 40000 at once. At once, said I?—that were tolerable : but these wars last alwayes ; and for many ages, nothing so familiar as this hacking and hewing, massacres, murders, desolations—

(————ignoto cœlum clangore remugit)

they care not what mischief they procure, so that they may enrich themselves for the present : they will so long blow the coals of contention, till all the world be consumed with fire. The [3] siege of Troy lasted ten years, eight months : there died 870000 Grecians, 670000 Trojans : at the taking of the city, and after, were slain 276000 men, women, and children, of all sorts. Cæsar killed a million, Mahomet the [4] Second Turk 300000 persons ; Sicinius Dentatus fought in an hundred battels ; eight times in single combat he overcame, had forty wounds before, was rewarded with 140 crowns, triumphed nine times for his good service. M. Sergius had 32 wounds ; Scæva the centurion, I know not how many ; every nation hath their Hectors, Scipios, Cæsars and Alexanders. Our [5] Edward the Fourth was in 26 battles afoot : and, as they do all, he glories in it ; 'tis related to his honour. At the siege of Hierusalem, 1100000 died with sword and famine. At the battel of Cannas, 70000 men were

---

[1] Ob inanes ditionum titulos, ob præreptum locum, ob interceptam mulierculam, vel quod e stultitiâ natum, vel e malitiâ, quod cupido dominandi, libido nocendi, &c.   [2] Bellum rem plane belluinam vocat Morus, Utop. lib. 2. [3] Munster. Cosmog. l. 5. c. 3. E Dict. Cretens.   [4] Jovius, vit. ejus.   [5] Comineus.

DEMOCRITUS TO THE READER.
43

slain, [1]as Polybius records, and as many at Battle Abbye with us ; and 'tis no news to fight from sun to sun, as they did, as Constantine and Licinius, &c. At the siege of Ostend, (the devils academy) a poor town in respect, a small fort, but a great grave, 120000 men lost their lives, besides whole towns, dorpes, and hospitals, full of maimed souldiers. There were engines, fire-works, and whatsoever the devil could invent to do mischief, with 2500000 iron bullets shot of 40 pounds weight, three or four millions of gold consumed. [2]*Who* (saith mine author) *can be sufficiently amazed at their flinty hearts, obstinacy, fury, blindness, who, without any likelyhood of good success, hazard poor souldiers, and lead them without pitty to the slaughter, which may justly be called the rage of furious beasts, that run without reason upon their own deaths?* [3]*quis malus genius, quæ Furia, quæ pestis,* &c. what plague, what Fury, brought so devillish, so bruitish a thing as war first into mens minds? Who made so soft and peaceable a creature, born to love, mercy, meekness, so to rave, rage like beasts, and run on to their own destruction? how may Nature expostulate with mankind, *Ego te divinum animal finxi, &c.* I made thee an harmless, quiet, a divine creature! how may God expostulate, and all good men! yet, *horum facta* (as [4]one condoles) *tantum admirantur, et heroum numero habent:* these are the brave spirits, the gallants of the world, these admired alone, triumph alone, have statues, crowns, pyramids, obelisks to their eternal fame, that immortal genius attends on them : *hac itur ad astra.* When Rhodes was besieged, [5]*fossæ urbis cadaveribus repletæ sunt,* the ditches were full of dead carcases; and (as when the said Solyman great Turk beleagred Vienna) they lay level with the top of the walls. This they make a sport of, and will do it to their friends and confederates, against oaths, vows, promises, by treachery or otherwise—

[6]dolus an virtus, quis in hoste requirat?

leagues and laws of arms ([7]*silent leges inter arma:* for their advantage, *omnia jura, divina, humana, proculcata plerumque sunt).* Gods and mens laws, are trampled under foot; the sword alone determines all; to satisfie their lust and spleen, they care not what they attempt, say, or do:

[8]Rara fides, probitasque, viris qui castra sequuntur.

---

[1] Lib. 3.   [2] Hist. of the Siege of Ostend, fol. 23.   [3] Erasmus de bello. Ut placidum illud animal benevolentiæ natum tam ferinâ vecordiâ in mutuam rueret perniciem.   [4] Rich. Dinoth. præfat. Belli civilis Gal. [5] Jovius.   [6] Dolus, asperitas, injustitia, propria bellorum negotia. Tertul. [7] Tully.   [8] Lucan.

DEMOCRITUS TO THE READER.

Nothing so common as to have [1]*father fight against the son, brother against brother, kinsman against kinsman, kingdom against kingdom, province against province, Christians against Christians, a quibus nec unquam cogitatione fuerunt læsi*, of whom they never had offence in thought, word, or deed. Infinite treasures consumed, towns burned, flourishing cities sacked and ruinated—*quodque animus meminisse horret*, goodly countries depopulated, and left desolate, old inhabitants expelled, trade and traffick decayed, maids defloured,

Virgines nondum thalamis jugatæ,
Et comis nondum positis ephebi;

chast matrons cry out with Andromache, [2]*Concubitum mox cogar pati ejus, qui interemit Hectorem*, they shall be compelled peradventure to lye with them that erst killed their husbands—to see rich, poor, sick, sound, lords, servants, *eodem omnes incommodo mactati*, consumed all or maimed, &c. *et quidquid gaudens scelere animus audet, et perversa mens*, saith Cyprian, and whatsoever torment, misery, mischief, hell it self, the devil, [3]fury and rage can invent to their own ruine and destruction: so abominable a thing [4]is war, as Gerbelius concludes—*adeo fœda et abominanda res est bellum, ex quo hominum cædes, vastationes, &c.*—the scourge of God, cause, effect, fruit and punishment of sin, and not *tonsura humani generis*, as Tertullian calls it, but *ruina*. Had Democritus been present at the late civil wars in France, those abominable wars,

(———bellaque matribus detestata)

[5]*where, in less than ten years, ten hundred thousand men were consumed*, saith Collignius, 20 thousand churches overthrown, nay the whole kingdom subverted (as [6]Richard Dinoth adds) so many myriades of the commons were butchered up, with sword, famine, war, *tanto odio utrinque, ut barbari ad abhorrendam lanienam obstupescerent*, with such feral hatred, the world was amazed at it—or at our late Pharsalian fields in the time of Henry the Sixth, betwixt the houses of Lancaster and York, an hundred thousand men slain, [7]one writes, [8]another, ten thousand families were rooted out, *that no man can but marvel, (saith Comineus,) at that barbarous immanity,*

---

[1] Pater in filium, affinis in affinem, amicus in amicum, &c. Regio cum regione, regnum regno colliditur. Populus populo, in mutuam perniciem, belluarum instar sanguinolente ruentium.   [2] Libanii declam.   [3] Ira enim et furor Bellonæ consultores, &c. dementes sacerdotes sunt.   [4] Bellum quasi bellua, et ad omnia scelera furor immissus.   [5] Gallorum decies centum millia ceciderunt, ecclesiarum 20 millia fundamentis excisa.   [6] Belli civilis Gal. l. 1. hoc ferali bello et cædibus omnia repleverunt, et regnum amplissimum a fundamentis pene everterunt; plebis tot myriades gladio, bello, fame miserabiliter perierunt.   [7] Pont. Huterus.   [8] Comineus. Ut nullus non execretur et admiretur crudelitatem, et barbaram insaniam, quæ inter homines eodem sub cœlo natos, ejusdem linguæ, sanguinis, religionis, exercebatur.

DEMOCRITUS TO THE READER.

*feral madness, committed betwixt men of the same nation,
language, and religion.* [1] *Quis furor, O cives?* Why do the
gentiles so furiously rage? saith the prophet David, Psal. 2. 1.
But we may ask, why do the Christians so furiously rage?

[2]Arma volunt quare, poscunt, rapiuntque juventus?

Unfit for gentiles, much less for us, so to tyrannize, as the
Spaniard in the West Indies, that killed up in 42 years (if we
may believe [3]Bartholomæus a Casa their own bishop) 12 millions of men, with stupend and exquisite torments; neither
should I lye, (said he) if I said 50 millions. I omit those
French massacres, Sicilian evensongs, [4]the duke of Alva's
tyrannies, our gun-powder machinations, and that fourth
Fury (as [5]one calls it), the Spanish inquisition, which quite
obscures those ten persecutions—

———[6]sævit toto Mars impius orbe.

Is not this [7]*mundus furiosus,* a mad world, as he terms it, *insanum bellum?* are not these mad men, as [8]Scaliger concludes,
*qui in prælio, acerbâ morte, insaniæ suæ memoriam pro per-
petuo teste relinquunt posteritati*—which leave so frequent
battels, as perpetual memorials of their madness to all succeeding ages? Would this, think you, have enforced our Democritus
to laughter, or rather made him turn his tune, alter his tone,
and weep with [9]Heraclitus, or rather howl, [10]roar, and tear his
hair, in commiseration—stand amazed ; or as the poets faign,
that Niobe was for grief quite stupified, and turned to a stone?
I have not yet said the worst. That which is more absurd and
[11]mad—in their tumults, seditions, civil and unjust wars, [12]*quod
stulte suscipitur, impie geritur, misere finitur*—such wars, I
mean ; for all are not to be condemned, as those phantastical
Anabaptists vainly conceive. Our Christian tacticks are, all
out, as necessary as the Roman *acies,* or Grecian *phalanx.*
To be a souldier is a most noble and honourable profession, (as
the world is) not to be spared. They are our best walls and bul-
warks; and I do therefore acknowledge that of [13]Tully to be
most true, *All our civil affairs, all our studies, all our pleading, industry, and commendation, lies under the protection of
warlike vertues; and, whensoever there is any suspicion of*

---

[1] Lucan.   [2] Virg.   [3] Bishop of Cusco, an eye witness.   [4] Read
Meteran, of his stupend cruelties.   [5] Heinsius, Austriaco.   [6] Virg. Georg.
[7] Jansenius Gallobelgicus, 1596. Mundus furiosus, inscriptio libri.   [8] Exercitat. 250. serm. 4.   [9] Fleat Heraclitus, an rideat Democritus?   [10] Curæ
leves loquuntur, ingentes stupent.   [11] Arma amens capio, nec sat rationis in
armis.   [12] Erasmus.   [13] Pro Murænâ. Omnes urbanæ res, omnia studia, omnis forensis laus et industria latet in tutelâ et præsidio bellicæ virtutis; et,
simul atque increpuit suspicio tumultûs, artes illico nostræ conticescunt.

DEMOCRITUS TO THE READER.

tumult, all our arts cease : wars are most behoveful; *et bella-tores agricolis civitati sunt utiliores,* as [1] Tyrius defends: and valour is much to be commended in a wise man: but they mistake most part; *auferre, trucidare, rapere, falsis nominibus virtutem vocant, &c.* ('Twas Galgacus observation in Tacitus) they term theft, murder, and rapine, vertue, by a wrong name: rapes, slaughters, massacres, &c. *jocus et ludus,* are pretty pastimes, as Ludovicus Vives notes. [2] *They commonly call the most hair-brain blood-suckers, strongest thieves, the most desperate villains, trecherous rogues, inhumane murderers, rash, cruel and dissolute caitiffs, couragious and generous spirits, heroical and worthy captains,* [3] *brave men at arms, valiant and renowned souldiers,—possessed with a brute perswasion of false honour,* as Pontus Huter in his Burgundian history complains: by means of which, it comes to pass that daily so many voluntaries offer themselves, leaving their sweet wives, children, friends,—for sixpence (if they can get it) a day, prostitute their lives and limbs, desire to enter upon breaches, lye sentinel, perdue, give the first onset, stand in the fore-front of the battel, marching bravely on, with a cheerful noise of drums and trumpets, such vigour and alacrity, so many banners streaming in the ayr, glittering armours, motions of plumes, woods of pikes, and swords, variety of colours, cost, and magnificence, as if they went in triumph, now victors, to the Capitol, and with such pomp, as when Darius army marched to meet Alexander at Issus. Void of all fear, they run into eminent dangers, canons mouth, &c. *ut vulneribus suis ferrum hostium hebetent,* saith [4] Barletius, to get a name of valour, honour and applause, which lasts not neither ; for it is but a mere flash, this fame, and, like a rose, *intra diem unum extinguitur,* 'tis gone in an instant. Of 15000 proletaries slain in a battel, scarce fifteen are recorded in history, or one alone, the general perhaps; and, after a while, his and their names are likewise blotted out ; the whole battel it self is forgotten. Those Grecian orators, *summâ vi ingenii et eloquentiæ,* set out the renowned overthrows at *Thermopylæ, Salamine, Marathon, Mycale, Mantinea, Chæronea, Platea :* the Romans record their battel at Cannas, and Pharsalian fields ; but they do but record; and we scarce hear of them. And yet this supposed honour, popular applause, desire of immortality by this means, pride and vain-glory, spurs them on many times

---

[1] Ser. 13. [2] Crudelissimos sævissimosque latrones, fortissimos propugnatores, fidelissimos duces, habent, brutâ persuasione donati. [3] Eobanus Hessus. Quibus omnis in armis Vita placet, non ulla juvat, nisi morte; nec ullam Esse putant vitam, quæ non assueverit armis. [4] Lib. 10. vit. Scanderbeg.

DEMOCRITUS TO THE READER. 47

rashly and unadvisedly to make away themselves and multitudes of others. Alexander was sorry, because there were no more worlds for him to conquer: he is admired by some for it: *animosa vox videtur, et regia:* 'twas spoken like a prince: but (as wise [1] Seneca censures him) 'twas *vox iniquissima et stultissima*: 'twas spoken like a bedlam fool; and that sentence which the same [2] Seneca appropriates to his father Philip and him, I apply to them all—*Non minores fuére pestes mortalium quam inundatio, quam conflagratio, quibus, &c.* they did as much mischief to mortal men, as fire and water, those merciless elements when they rage. [3] Which is yet more to be lamented, they perswade them this hellish course of life is holy: they promise heaven to such as venture their lives *bello sacro*, and that by these bloody wars, (as Persians, Greeks, and Romans of old, as modern Turks do now their commons, to encourage them to fight, *ut cadant infeliciter,*) *if they die in the field they go directly to heaven, and shall be canonized for saints,* (O diabolical invention!) put in the chronicles, *in perpetuam rei memoriam,* to their eternal memory; when as in truth, as [4] some hold, it were much better (since wars are the scourge of God for sin, by which he punisheth mortal mens pievishness and folly) such brutish stories were suppressed, because *ad morum institutionem nihil habent,* they conduce not at all to manners or good life. But they will have it thus nevertheless; and so they put a note of [5] *divinity upon the most cruel and pernicious plague of humane kind,* adorn such men with grand titles, degrees, statues, images—[6] honour, applaud and highly reward them for their good service—no greater glory than to dye in the field. So Africanus is extolled by Ennius: Mars, and [7] Hercules, and I know not how many besides, of old were deified, went this way to heaven, that were indeed bloody butchers, wicked destroyers, and troublers of the world, prodigious monsters, hell-hounds, feral plagues, devourers, common executioners of humane kind, (as Lactantius truly proves, and Cyprian to Donat) such as were desperate in wars and precipitately made

---

[1] Nulli beatiores habiti, quam qui in prœliis cecidissent. Brisonius, de rep. Persarum. l. 3. fol. 3. 44. Idem Lactantius de Romanis et Græcis. Idem Ammianus, lib. 23. de Parthis. Judicatur is solus beatus apud·eos, qui in prœlio fuderit animam. De Benef. lib. 2. c. 1.   [2] Nat. quæst. lib. 3.   [3] Boterus Amphitridrion. Busbequius, Turc. hist. Per cædes et sanguinem parare hominibus ascensum in cœlum putant. Lactant. de falsâ relig. l. 1. cap. 8.   [4] Quoniam bella acerbissima Dei flagella sunt, quibus hominum pertinaciam punit, ea perpetuâ oblivione sepelienda potius quam memoriæ mandanda plerique judicant. Rich. Dinoth. præf. hist. Gall.   [5] Cruentam humani generis pestem et perniciem divinitatis notâ insigniunt.   [6] Et (quod dolendum) applausum habent et occursum viri tales.   [7] Herćuli eadem porta ad cœlum patuit, qui magnam generis humani partem perdidit.

48   DEMOCRITUS TO THE READER.

away themselves, like those Celtes in Damascen, with ridiculous valour, *ut dedecorosum putarent muro ruenti se subducere*, a disgrace to run away from a rotten wall, now ready to fall on their heads. Such as will not rush on a swords point, or seek to shun a canons shot, are base cowards, and no valiant men. By which means, *Madet orbis mutuo sanguine*, the earth wallows in her own blood: [1] *Sævit amor ferri et sceleratæ insania belli ;* and for that which if it be done in private, a man shall be rigorously executed, [2] *and which is no less than murder it self, if the same fact be done in publick in wars, it is called manhood, and the party is honoured for it.*——— [3] *prosperum et felix scelus virtus vocatur*———We measure all, as Turks do, by the event ; and most part, as Cyprian notes, in all ages, countreys, places, *sævitiæ magnitudo impunitatem sceleris acquirit*—the foulness of the fact vindicates the offender. [4] One is crowned for that which another is tormented :

(Ille crucem sceleris pretium tulit, hic diadema)

made a knight, a lord, an earl, a great duke, (as [5] Agrippa notes) for which another should have hung in gibbets, as a terror to the rest—

———————[6] et tamen alter,
Si fecisset idem, caderet sub judice morum.

A poor sheep-stealer is hanged for stealing of victuals, compelled peradventure by necessity of that intolerable cold, hunger, and thirst, to save himself from starving : but a [7] great man in office may securely rob whole provinces, undo thousands, pill and pole, oppress *ad libitum*, fley, grind, tyrannize, enrich himself by spoils of the commons, be uncontrollable in his actions, and, after all, be recompensed with turgent titles, honoured for his good service ; and no man dare find fault or [8] mutter at it.

How would our Democritus have been affected, to see a wicked caitiff, or [9] *fool, a very ideot, a funge, a golden ass, a monster of men, to have many good men, wise men,*

---

[1] Virg. Æneïd. 7.   [2] Homicidium quum committunt singuli, crimen est, quum publice geritur, virtus vocatur. Cyprianus.   [3] Seneca.   [4] Juven.   [5] De vanit. scient. de princip. nobilitatis.   [6] Juven. Sat. 4.   [7] Pansa rapit, quod Natta reliquit.—Tu pessimus omnium latro es, as Demetrius the Pyrat told Alexander in Curtius.   [8] Non ausi mutire, &c. Æsop.   [9] Improbum et stultum si divitem, multos bonos viros in servitute habentem, (ob id duntaxat quod ei contingat aureorum numismatum cumulus) ut appendices et additamenta numismatum. Morus, Utopia.

DEMOCRITUS TO THE READER.

learned men to attend upon him with all submission, as an appendix to his riches, for that respect alone, because he hath more wealth and money, [1] *and to honour him with divine titles, and bumbast epithets,* to smother him with fumes and eulogies, whom they knew to be a dizard, a fool, a covetous wretch, a beast, &c. *because he is rich!*—to see *sub exuviis leonis onagrum,* a filthy loathsome carkass, a Gorgons head puffed up by parasites, assume thus unto himself glorious titles, in worth an infant, a Cuman ass, a painted sepulchre, an Egyptian temple!—to see a withered face, a diseased, deformed, cankered complexion, a rotten carkass, a viperous mind, and Epicurean soul, set out with orient pearls, jewels, diadems, perfumes, curious, elaborate works, as proud of his clothes as a child of his new coats—and a goodly person, of an angelick divine countenance, a saint, an humble mind, a meek spirit, clothed in rags, beg, and now ready to be starved! —to see a silly contemptible sloven in apparel, ragged in his coat, polite in speech, of a divine spirit, wise! another neat in clothes, spruce, full of courtesie, empty of grace, wit, talk non-sense!

To see so many lawyers, advocates, so many tribunals, so little justice: so many magistrates, so little care of common good; so many laws, yet never more disorders—*tribunal litium segetem,* the tribunal a labyrinth—so many thousand suits in one court sometimes, so violently followed!—to see *injustissimum sæpe juri præsidentem, impium religioni, imperitissimum eruditioni, otiosissimum labori, monstrosum humanitati!* To see a lamb [2] executed, a woolf pronounce sentence, *Latro* arraigned, and *Fur* sit on the bench, the judge severely punish others, and do worse himself, [3] *eundem furtum facere et punire,* [4] *rapinam plectere, quum sit ipse raptor!*—Laws altered, misconstrued, interpreted *pro* and *con,* as the [5] judge is made by friends, bribed, or otherwise affected as a nose of wax, good to day, none to morrow; or firm in his opinion, cast in his! Sentence prolonged, changed, *ad arbitrium judicis;* still the same case [6] *one thrust out of his inheritance, another falsly put in by favour, false forged deeds or wills. Incisæ leges negliguntur,* laws are made and not kept; or, if put in execution, [7] they be some silly ones that are

---

[1] Eorumque detestantur Utopienses insaniam, qui divinos honores iis impendunt, quos sordidos et avaros agnoscunt: non alio respectu honorantes, quam quod dites sint. Idem. lib. 2.　　[2] Cyp. 2. ad Donat. ep. ut reus innocens pereat, fit nocens. Judex damnat foris, quod intus operatur.　　[3] Sidonius Apo. [4] Salvianus, l. 3. de provid.　　[5] Ergo judicium nihil est nisi publica merces. Petronius. Quid faciant leges, ubi sola pecunia regnat? Idem.　　[6] Hic arcentur hæreditatibus liberi; hic donatur bonis alienis; falsum consulit; alter testamentum corrumpit, &c. Idem.　　[7] Vexat censura columbas.

VOL. 1.　　　　　　　　　　　　　E

50   DEMOCRITUS TO THE READER.

punished.   As, put case it be fornication, the father will dis-
inherit or abdicate his child, quite casheer him (out, villain!
be gone! come no more in my sight): a poor man is miserably
tormented with loss of his estate perhaps, goods, fortunes,
good name, for ever disgraced, forsaken, and must do penance
to the utmost:—a mortal sin! and yet, make the worst of it,
numquid aliud fecit, saith Tranio in the [1] poet, *nisi quod faciunt summis nati generibus;* he hath done no more than what
gentlemen usually do—

　　([2] Neque novum, neque mirum, neque secus quam alii solent)

for, in a great person, right worshipful sir, a right honourable
grandee, 'tis not a venial sin, no not a *peccadillo:* 'tis no offence at all, a common and ordinary thing: no man takes
notice of it; he justifies it in publick, and peradventure brags
of it;

　　[3] Nam quod turpe bonis, Titio, Seioque, decebat
　　Crispinum ————————

[4] many poor men, younger brothers, &c. by reason of bad
policy, and idle education (for they are, likely, brought up in
no calling), are compelled to beg or steal, and then hanged for
theft; than which, what can be more ignominious? *non minus
enim turpe principi multa supplicia, quam medico multa
funera:* 'tis the governours fault. *Libentius verberant quam
docent,* as school-masters do rather correct their pupils, than
teach them when they do amiss.   [5] *They had more need
provide there should be no more thieves and beggars, as they
ought with good policy, and take away the occasions, than
let them run on, as they do, to their own destruction*—root out
likewise those causes of wrangling, a multitude of lawyers, and
compose controversies, *lites lustrales et seculares,* by some
more compendious means; whereas now, for every toy and
trifle, they go to law, ([6] *Mugit litibus insanum forum, et sævit
invicem discordantium rabies)* they are ready to pull out
one anothers throats; and, for commodity [7] *to squeeze blood*
(saith Hierom) *out of their brothers heart,* defame, lye, disgrace, backbite, rail, bear false witness, swear. forswear, fight
and wrangle, spend their goods, lives, fortunes, friends, undo
one another, to enrich an *harpy* advocate, that preys upon
them both, and cryes, *eia, Socrates! eia, Xanthippe!* or some

---

　　[1] Plaut. Mostel.   [2] Idem.   [3] Juven. Sat. 4.   [4] Quod tot sint fures
et mendici, magistratuum culpâ fit, qui malos imitantur præceptores, qui disci-
pulos libentius verberant quam docent. Morus, Utop. lib. 1.   [5] Decernuntur
furi gravia et horrenda supplicia, quum potius providendum multo foret ne fures
sint, ne cuiquam tam dira furandi aut pereundi sit necessitas. Idem.   [6] Boterus, de augmen. urb. lib. 3. cap. 3.   [7] E fraterno corde sanguinem
eliciunt.

DEMOCRITUS TO THE READER.

corrupt judge, that like the [1]kite in Æsop, while the mouse and frog fought, carryed both away. Generally they prey one upon another, as so many ravenous birds, brute beasts, devouring fishes: no *medium; omnes* [2] *hic aut captantur aut captant; aut cadavera quæ lacerantur, aut corvi qui lacerant*—either deceive or be deceived—tear others, or be torn in pieces themselves; like so many buckets in a well, as one riseth, another falleth; one's empty, another's full; his ruine is a ladder to the third: such are our ordinary proceedings. What's the market? a place (according to [3]Anacharsis) wherein they cozen one another, a trap; nay, what's the world it self? [4] a vast *chaos*, a confusion of manners, as fickle as the air, *domicilium insanorum*, a turbulent troop full of impurities, a mart of walking spirits, goblins, the theatre of hypocrisie, a shop of knavery, flattery, a nursery of villany, the scene of babling, the school of giddiness, the academy of vice: a warfare *ubi (velis, nolis) pugnandum; aut vincas aut succumbas*, in which kill or be killed; wherein every man is for himself, his private ends, and stands upon his own guard. No charity, [5]love, friendship, fear of God, alliance, affinity, consanguinity, christianity, can contain them; but if they be any wayes offended, or that string of commodity be touched, they fall foul. Old friends become bitter enemies on a suddain, for toyes and small offences; and they that erst were willing to do all mutual offices of love and kindness, now revile, and persecute one another to death, with more than Vatinian hatred, and will not be reconciled. So long as they are behoveful, they love, or may bestead each other; but, when there is no more good to be expected, as they do by an old dog, hang him up or casheer him; which [6] Cato counts a great *indecorum*, to use men like old shoos or broken glasses, which are flung to the dunghil: he could not find in his heart to sell an old ox, much less, to turn away an old servant: but they in stead of recompence, revile him: and when they have made him an instrument of their villany, (as [7] Bajazet the second, emperour of the Turks, did by Acomethes Bassa) make him away, or, in stead of [8]reward, hate him to death, as Silius was served by Tiberius. In a word, every man for his own ends. Our *summum bonum* is

---

[1] Milvus rapit ac deglubit.   [2] Petronius, de Crotone civit.   [3] Quid forum? locus quo alius alium circumvenit.   [4] Vastum chaos, larvarum emporium, theatrum hypocrisios, &c.   [5] Nemo cœlum, nemo jusjurandum, nemo Jovem, pluris facit; sed omnes apertis oculis bona sua computant. Petron.   [6] Plutarch. vit. ejus. Indecorum animatis ut calceis uti aut vitris, quæ, ubi fracta, abjicimus; nam, ut de me ipso dicam, nec bovem senem vendiderim, nedum hominem natu grandem, laboris socium.   [7] Jovius. Cum innumera illius beneficia rependere non posset aliter, interfici jussit.   [8] Beneficia eousque lata sunt, dum videntur solvi posse: ubi multum antevenere, pro gratiâ odium redditur. Tac.

E 2

52 DEMOCRITUS TO THE READER.

commodity ; and the goddess we adore, *Dea moneta*, queen money, to whom we daily offer sacrifice; which steers our hearts, hands, [1] affections, all—that most powerful goddess, by whom we are reared, depressed, elevated, [2] esteemed the sole commándress of our actions—for which we pray, run, ride, go, come, labour, and contend as fishes do for a crum that falleth into the water. It's not worth, vertue, (that's *bonum theatrale*) wisdom, valour, learning, honesty, religion, or any sufficiency, for which we are respected, but [3] money, greatness, office, honour, authority. Honesty is accounted folly : knavery, policy; [4] men admired out of opinion, not as they are, but as they seem to be: such shifting, lying, cogging, plotting, counterplotting, temporizing, flattering, cozening, dissembling, [5] *that of necessity one must highly offend God, if he be conformable to the world*, (Cretizare cum Crete) *or else live in contempt, disgrace, and misery.* One takes upon him temperance, holiness; another, austerity; a third, an affected kind of simplicity ; when as indeed he, and he, and he, and the rest, are [6] hypocrites, ambodexters, out-sides, so many turning pictures, a [7] lion on the one side, a lamb on the other. How would Democritus have been affected to see these things ?

To see a man turn himself into all shapes like a camelion, or, as Proteus, *omnia transformans sese in miracula rerum*, to act twenty parts and persons at once, for his advantage—to temporize and vary like Mercury the planet, good with good, bad with bad : having a several face, garb, and character for every one he meets—of all religions, humours, inclinations— to fawn like a spaniel, *mentitis et mimicis obsequiis*, rage like a lion, bark like a cur, fight like a dragon, sting like a serpent, as meek as a lamb, and yet again grin like a tygre, weep like a crocodile, insult over some, and yet others domineer over him, here command, there crouch ; tyrannize in one place, be baffled in another: a wise man at home, a fool abroad to make others merry.

To see so much difference betwixt words and deeds, so many parasanges betwixt tongue and heart—men, like stageplayers, act variety of parts, [8] give good precepts to others to soar aloft, whilest they themselves grovel on the ground.

---

[1] Paucis carior est fides quam pecunia. Sallust. [2] Prima fere vota et cunctis, &c. [3] Et genus et formam regina pecunia donat. Quantum quisque suâ nummorum servat in arcâ, Tantum habet et fidei. [4] Non a peritiâ, sed ab ornatu et vulgi vocibus, habemur excellentes. Cardan. l. 2. de cons. [5] Perjurata suo postponit numina lucro Mercator.—Ut necessarium sit vel Deo displicere, vel ab hominibus contemni, vexari, negligi. [6] Qui Curios simulant, et Bacchanalia vivunt. [7] Tragelapho similes vel Centauris, sursum homines, deorsum equi. [8] Præceptis suis cœlum promittunt, ipsi interim pulveris terreni vilia mancipia.

DEMOCRITUS TO THE READER.   53

To see a man protest friendship, kiss his hand, [1] *quem mallet truncatum videre,* [2] smile with an intent to do mischief, or cozen him whom he salutes, [3] magnifie his friend unworthy with hyperbolical elogiums—his enemy albeit a good man, to vilifie, and disgrace him, yea, all his actions, with the utmost livor and malice can invent.

To see a [4] servant able to buy out his master, him that carries the mace more worth than the magistrate; which Plato *(lib.* 11. *de leg.)* absolutely forbids, Epictetus abhors. An horse that tills the [5] land fed with chaff, an idle jade have provender in abundance ; him that makes shoos go bare-foot himself, him that sells meat almost pined ; a toiling drudge starve, a drone flourish.

To see men buy smoke for wares, castles built with fools heads, men like apes follow the fashions, in tires, gestures, actions : if the king laugh, all laugh ;

> ———————[6] Rides ? majore cachinno
> Concutitur : flet, si lacrymas conspexit amici.

[7] Alexander stooped ; so did his courtiers : Alphonsus turned his head ; and so did his parasites. [8] Sabina Poppæa, Neros wife, wore amber-coloured hair ; so did all the Roman ladies in an instant ; her fashion was theirs.

To see men wholly led by affection, admired and censured out of opinion without judgement : an inconsiderate multitude, like so many dogs in a village, if one bark, all bark without a cause : as fortunes fan turns, if a man be in favour, or commended by some great one, all the world applauds him : [9] if in disgrace, in an instant all hate him, and as the sun when he is eclipsed, that erst took no notice, now gaze, and stare upon him.

To see a [10] man wear his brains in his belly, his guts in his head, an hundred oaks on his back, to devour an hundred oxen at a meal ; nay more, to devour houses and towns, or as those anthropophagi, [11] to eat one another.

To see a man roll himself up, like a snow-ball, from base beg - gary to right worshipful and right honourable titles, unjustly to

---

[1] Æneas Sylv.   [2] Arridere homines, ut sæviant: blandiri ut fallant. Cyp. ad Donatum.   [3] Love and hate are like the two ends of a perspective glass : the ne multiplies , the other makes less.   [4] Ministri locupletiores iis quibus ministratur ; servus majores opes habens quam patronus.   [5] Qui terram colunt equi paleis pascuntur ; qui otiantur caballi avenâ saginantur : discalceatus discurrit, qui calceos aliis facit.   [6] Juven.   [7] Bodin. lib. 4. de repub. c. 6. [8] Plinius, l. 37. c. 3. Capillos habuit succineos : exinde factum ut omnes puellæ Romanæ colorem illum affectarent.   [9] Odit damnatos. Juv.   [10] Agrippa ep. 28. l. 7. Quorum cerebrum est in ventre, ingenium in patinis.   [11] Psal. They eat up my people as bread.

DEMOCRITUS TO THE READER.

screw himself into honours and offices ; another to starve his *genius,* damn his soul, to gather wealth, which he shall not enjoy, which his prodigal [1] son melts and consumes in an instant.

To see the κακοζηλιαν of our times, a man bend all his forces, means, time, fortunes, to be a favourites favourites favourite, &c. a parasites parasites parasite, that may scorn the servile world, as having enough already.

To see an hirsute beggars brat, that lately fed on scraps, crept and whin'd, crying to all, and for an old jerkin ran of errands, now ruffle in silk and satten, bravely mounted, jovial and polite, now scorn his old friends and familiars, neglect his kindred, insult over his betters, domineer over all.

To see a scholar crouch and creep to an illiterate peasant for a meals meat; a scrivener better paid for an obligation, a faulkner receive greater wages, than a student: a lawyer get more in a day, than a philosopher in a year; better reward for an hour, than a scholar for a twelve moneths study; him that can [2] paint Thaïs, play on a fiddle, curl hair, &c. sooner get preferment than a philologer or a poet.

To see a fond mother, like Æsops ape, hug her child to death, a [3] wittal wink at his wives honesty, and too perspicuous in all other affairs; one stumble at a straw, and leap over a block; rob Peter, and pay Paul; scrape unjust summs with one hand, purchase great mannors by corruption, fraud, and cozenage, and liberally to distribute to the poor with the other, give a remnant to pious uses, &c.—penny wise, pound foolish ; blind men judge of colours, wise men silent, fools talk; [4] find fault with others, and do worse themselves; [5] denounce that in publick which he doth in secret; and (which Aurelius Victor gives out of Augustus) severely censure that in a third, of which he is most guilty himself.

To see a poor fellow, or an hired servant, venture his life for his new master, that will scarce give him his wages at years end ; a countrey colone toil and moil, till and drudge for a prodigal idle drone, that devours all the gain, or lasciviously consumes with phantastical expences ; a noble man in a bravado to encounter death, and, for a small flash of honour, to cast away himself; a worldling tremble at an executer, and yet not fear hell-fire; to wish and hope for immortality, desire to be

---

[1] Absumet hæres Cæcuba dignior servata centum clavibus, et mero distinguet pavimentum superbis pontificum potiore cœnis. Hor.   [2] Qui Thaïdem pingere, inflare tibiam, crispare crines.   [3] Doctus spectare lacunar.   [4] Tullius. Est enim proprium stultitiæ aliorum cernere vitia, oblivisci suorum. Idem Aristippus Charidemo apud Lucianum. Omnino stultitiæ cujusdam esse puto, &c.   [5] Execrari publice quod occulte agat. Salvianus, lib. de pro. Acres ulciscendis vitiis quibus ipsi vehementer indulgent.

DEMOCRITUS TO THE READER. 55

happy, and yet by all means avoid death, a necessary passage
to bring him to it.

To see a fool-hardy fellow like those old Danes, *qui decol-
lari malunt quam verberari*, dye rather than be punished, in
a sottish humour imbrace death with alacrity, [1] yet scorn to
lament his own sins and miseries, or his dearest friends de-
partures.

To see wise men degraded, fools preferred, one govern
towns and cities, and yet a silly woman over-rules him at
home; command a province, and yet his own [2] servants or
children prescribe laws to him, as Themistocles son did in
Greece; [3] *What I will* (said he) *my mother will, and what
my mother will, my father doth.* To see horses ride in a
coach, men draw it; dogs devour their masters; towers build
masons; children rule; old men go to school; women wear
the breeches; [4] sheep demolish towns, devour men, &c. and
in a word, the world turned upside downward. *O! viveret
Democritus!*

[5] To insist in every particular, were one of Hercules labours;
there 's so many ridiculous instances, as motes in the sun.
Quantum est in rebus inane! And who can speak of all?
Crimine ab uno disce omnes; take this for a taste.

But these are obvious to sense, trivial and well known, easie
to be discerned. How would Democritus have been moved,
had he seen [6] the secrets of their hearts! If every man had a
window in his breast, which Momus would have had in Vulcan's
man, or (that which Tully so much wisht) it were written
in every mans forehead, *Quid quisque de republicâ sentiret,*
what he thought; or that it could be effected in an instant,
which Mercury did by Charon in Lucian, by touching of his
eyes to make him discern *semel et simul rumores et susurros,*

Spes hominum cæcas, morbos, votumque, labores,
Et passim toto volitantes æthere curas—

Blind hopes and wishes, their thoughts and affairs,
Whispers and rumours, and those flying cares—

---

[1] Adamus, eccl. hist. cap. 212. Siquis damnatus fuerit, lætus esse gloria est;
nam lacrymas, et planctum, cæteraque compunctionum genera, quæ nos salubria
censemus, ita abominantur Dani, ut nec pro peccatis nec pro defunctis amicis ulli
flere liceat.   [2] Orbi dat leges foris, vix famulum regit sine strepitu domi.
[3] Quidquid ego volo, hoc vult mater mea, et quod mater vult, facit pater.   [4] Oves,
olim mite pecus, nunc tam indomitum et edax, ut homines devorent, &c. Morus,
Utop. lib. 1.   [5] Diversos variis tribuit natura furores.   [6] Democrit. ep.
præd. Hos dejerantes et potantes deprehendet, hos vomentes, illos litigantes, insidias molientes, suffragantes, venena miscentes, in amicorum accusationem sub-
scribentes, hos gloriâ, illos ambitione, cupiditate, mente captos, &c.

that he could *cubiculorum obductas fores recludere, et secreta cordium penetrare,* (which [1] Cyprian desired) open doors and locks, shoot bolts, as Lucians Gallus did with a feather of his tail; or Gyges invisible ring, or some rare perspective glass, or *otacousticon,* which would so multiply species, that a man might hear and see all at once (as [2] Martianus Capellas Jupiter did in a spear, which he held in his hand, which did present unto him all that was daily done upon the face of the earth) observe cuckolds horns, forgeries of alchymists, the philosopher's stone, new projectors, &c. and all those works of darkness, foolish vows, hopes, fears, and wishes, what a deal of laughter would it have afforded! He should have seen wind-mills in one mans head, an hornets nest in another. Or, had he been present with Icaromenippus in Lucian at Jupiters whispering place, [3] and heard one pray for rain, another for fair weather; one for his wives, another for his fathers death, &c. *to ask that at Gods hand, which they are abashed any man should hear;* how would he have been confounded! would he, think you, or any man else, say that these men were well in their wits?

Hæc sani esse hominis qui sanus juret Orestes?

Can all the hellebore in the Anticyræ cure these men? No, sure, [4] *an acre of hellebore will not do it.*

That which is more to be lamented, they are mad like Senecas blind woman, and will not acknowledge, or [5] seek for any cure of it; for *pauci vident morbum suum, omnes amant.* If our [6] leg or arm offend us, we covet by all means possible to redress it; [7] and, if we labour of a bodily disease, we send for a physician; but, for the diseases of the mind, we take no notice of them. Lust harrows us on the one side, envy, anger, ambition on the other. We are torn in pieces by our passions, as so many wild horses, one in disposition, another in habit; one is melancholy, another mad; [8] and which of us all seeks

---

[1] Ad Donat. ep. 2. lib. 1. O si posses in speculâ sublimi constitutus, &c. [2] Lib. 1. de nup. Philol. in quâ, quid singuli nationum populi quotidianis motibus agitarent, relucebat. [3] O Jupiter! contingat mihi aurum, hæreditas, &c. Multos da, Jupiter, annos! Dementia quanta est hominum! turpissima vota Diis insusurrant: si quis admoverit aurem, conticescunt; et quod scire homines nolunt, Deo narrant. Senec. ep. 10. lib. 1. [4] Plautus, Menæch. Non potest hæc res hellebori jugere obtinerier. [5] Eoque gravior morbus, quo ignotior periclitanti. [6] Quæ lædunt oculos, festinas demere; si quid Est animum, differs curandi tempus in annum. Hor. [7] Si caput, crus dolet, brachium, &c. medicum accersimus, recte et honeste, si par etiam industria in animi morbis poneretur. Joh. Peletius Jesuita, lib. 2. de hum. affec. morborumque curâ. [8] Et quotusquisque tamen est, qui contra tot pestes medicum requirat, vel ægrotare se agnoscat? ebullit ira, &c. Et nos tamen ægros esse negamus. Incolumes medicum recusant.

DEMOCRITUS TO THE READER.

for help, doth acknowledge his error, or knows he is sick ?
As that stupid fellow put out the candle, because the biting
fleas should not find him; he shrouds himself in an unknown
habit, borrowed titles, because no body should discern him.
Every man thinks with himself, *egomet videor mihi sanus.* I
am well, I am wise, and laughs at others. And 'tis a general
fault amongst them all, that [1] which our fore-fathers have approved, diet, apparel, opinions, humours, customs, manners,
we deride and reject in our time as absurd. [2] Old men account juniors all fools, when they are meer dizards; and (as,
to sailers,

——terræque urbesque recedunt——

they move; the land stands still) the world hath much more
wit; they dote themselves. Turks deride us, we them;
Italians Frenchmen, accounting them light headed fellows;
the French scoff again at Italians, and at their several customs: Greeks have condemned all the world but themselves
of barbarism; the world as much vilifies them now: we account Germans heavy, dull fellows, explode many of their
fashions; they as contemptibly think of us; Spaniards laugh
at all, and all again at them. So are we fools and ridiculous,
absurd in our actions, carriages, dyet, apparel, customs and
consultations; [3] we scoff and point one at another, when as, in
conclusion, all are fools [4] *and they the veriest asses that hide
their ears most.* A private man, if he be resolved with himself
or set on an opinion, accounts all ideots and asses that are not
affected as he is,

[5] ——(nil rectum, nisi quod placuit sibi, ducit)

that are not so minded, [6] *(quodque volunt homines, se bene velle
putant)* all fools that think not as he doth. He will not say
with Atticus, *suam quisque sponsam, mihi meam,* let every
man enjoy his own spouse; but his alone is fair, *suus amor,
&c.* and scorns all in respect of himself, [7] will imitate none, hear
none [8] but himself, as Pliny said, a law and example to himself. And that which Hippocrates, in his epistle to Dionysius,
reprehended of old, is verified in our times, *Quisque in alio
superfluum esse censet, ipse quod non habet, nec curat;* that
which he hath not himself or doth not esteem, he accounts
superfluity, an idle quality, a meer foppery in another; like
Æsops fox when he had lost his tail, would have all his

---

[1] Præsens ætas stultitiam priscis exprobrat. Bud. de affec. lib. 5. [2] Senes
pro stultis habent juvenes. Balth. Cast. [3] Clodius accusat mœchos.
[4] Omnium stultissimi qui auriculas studiose tegunt. Sat. Menip. [5] Hor.
Epist. 2. [6] Prosper. [7] Statim sapiunt, statim sciunt, neminem reve-
rentur, neminem imitantur, ipsi sibi exemplo. Plin. ep. lib. 8. [8] Nulli
alteri sapere concedit, ne desipere videatur. Agrip.

58   DEMOCRITUS TO THE READER.

fellow foxes cut off theirs. The Chineses say, that we Europeans have one eye, they themselves two, all the world else is blind (though [1] Scaliger accounts them brutes too, *merum pecus*): so thou and thy sectaries are only wise, others indifferent; the rest, beside themselves, meer ideots and asses. Thus not acknowledging our own errors and imperfections, we securely deride others, as if we alone were free, and spectators of the rest, accounting it an excellent thing, as indeed it is, *alienâ optimum frui insaniâ*, to make our selves merry with other mens obliquities, when as he himself is more faulty than the rest: *mutato nomine, de te fabula narratur:* he may take himself by the nose for a fool; and, which one calls *maximum stultitiæ specimen*, to be ridiculous to others, and not to perceive or take notice of it, as Marsyas when he contended with Apollo, *non intelligens se deridiculo haberi*, saith [2] Apuleius; 'tis his own cause; he is a convict mad-man, as [3] Austin well infers: *In the eyes of wise men and angels he seems like one, that to our thinking walks with his heels upward.* So thou laughest at me, and I at thee, both at a third; and he returns that of the poet upon us again, [4] *Hei mihi! insanire me aiunt, quum ipsi ultro insaniant.* We accuse others of madness, of folly, and are the veriest dizards our selves: for it is a great sign and property of a fool (which Eccles. 10. 3. points at), out of pride and self-conceit, to insult, vilifie, condemn, censure, and call other men fools *(Non videmus manticæ quod a tergo est)*; to tax that in others of which we are most faulty; teach that which we follow not our selves; for an inconstant man to write of constancy, a prophane liver prescribe rules of sanctity and piety, a dizard himself make a treatise of wisdom, or, with Sallust, to rail down-right, at spoilers of countreys, and yet in [5] office to be a most grievous poller himself. This argues weakness, and is an evident sign of such parties indiscretion. [6] *Peccat uter nostrûm cruce dignius? Who is the fool now?* Or else peradventure in some places we are [7] all mad for company; and so 'tis not seen: *societas erroris et dementiæ pariter absurditatem et admirationem tollit.* 'Tis with us, as it was of old (in [8] Tullies censure at least) with C. Fimbria in Rome, a bold, hair-brained, mad fellow, and so esteemed of all, such only excepted, that were as mad as himself: now in such a case there is no notice taken of it.

[1] Omnis orbis........a Persis ad Lusitaniam.   [2] 2 Florid.   [3] August. Qualis in oculis hominum qui inversis pedibus ambulat, talis in oculis sapientum et angelorum qui sibi placet, aut cui passiones dominantur.   [4] Plautus, Menæchmi.   [5] Governour of Africk by Cæsar's appointment.   [6] Nunc sanitatis patrocinium est insanientium turba. Sen.   [7] Pro Roscio Amerino; et, quod inter omnes constat, insanissimus, nisi inter eos, qui ipsi quoque insaniunt.   [8] Necesse est cum insanientibus furere, nisi solus relinqueris. Petronius.

DEMOCRITUS TO THE READER.

Nimirum insanus paucis videatur, eo quod
Maxima pars hominum morbo jactatur eodem.

When all are mad, where all are like opprest,
Who can discern one mad man from the rest?

But put the case they do perceive it and some one be manifestly convict of madness; [1] he now takes notice of his folly, be it in action, gesture, speech, a vain humour he hath in building, bragging, jangling, spending, gaming, courting, scribling, prating, for which he is ridiculous to others, [2] on which he dotes; he doth acknowledge as much: yet, with all the rhetorick thou hast, thou canst not so recal him, but, to the contrary, notwithstanding, he will persevere in his dotage. 'Tis *amabilis insania, et mentis gratissimus error*, so pleasing, so delicious, that he [3] cannot leave it. He knows his error, but will not seek to decline it. Tell him what the event will be, beggary, sorrow, sickness, disgrace, shame, loss, madness; yet [4] *an angry man will prefer vengeance, a lascivious his whore, a thief his booty, a glutton his belly, before his welfare.* Tell an epicure, a covetous man, an ambitious man, of his irregular course; wean him from it a little, *(Pol! me occidistis, amici!)* he cryes anon, you have undone him; and, as [5] a *dog to his vomit*, he returns to it again; no perswasion will take place, no counsel: say what thou canst,

——Clames, licet, et mare cœlo
Confundas,——surdo narras:

demonstrate as Ulysses did to [6] Elpenor and Gryllus and the rest of his companions *those swinish men*, he is irrefragable in his humour; he will be a hog still: bray him in a morter; he will be the same. If he be in an heresie, or some perverse opinion, setled as some of our ignorant papists are, convince his understanding, shew him the several follies and absurd fopperies of that sect, force him to say, *veris vincor*, make it as clear as the sun, [7] he will err still, peevish and obstinate as he is; and as he said, [8] *si in hoc erro, libenter erro, nec hunc errorem auferri mihi volo;* I will do as I have done, as my predecessors have done, [9] and as my friends now do: I will dote for company. Say now, are these men [10] mad or

---

[1] Quoniam non est genus unum stultitiæ, quâ me insanire putas? [2] Stultum me fateor, liceat concedere verum, Atque etiam insanum. Hor. [3] Odi; nec possum cupiens non esse quod odi. Ovid. Errore grato libenter omnes insanimus. [4] Amator scortum vitæ præponit, iracundus vindictam, fur prædam, parasitus gulam, ambitiosus honores, avarus opes, &c. odimus hæc et accersimus. Cardan. 1. 2. de conso. [5] Prov. 26. 11. [6] Plutarch. Gryllo. suilli homines, sic Clem. Alex. vo. [7] Non persuadebis, etiamsi persuaseris. [8] Tully. [9] Malo cum illis insanire, quam cum aliis bene sentire. [10] Qui inter hos enutriuntur, non magis sapere possunt, quam qui in culinâ bene olere. Petron.

60 DEMOCRITUS TO THE READER.

no? [1] *Heus, age, responde!* are they ridiculous? *cedo quemvis arbitrum;* are they *sanæ mentis,* sober, wise, and discreet? have they common sense?

[2]———— uter est insanior horum?

I am of Democritus opinion, for my part; I hold them worthy to be laughed at: a company of brain-sick dizards, as mad as [3] Orestes and Athamas, that they may *go ride the ass,* and all sail along to the Anticyræ, in the *ship of fools,* for company together. I need not much labour to prove this which I say, otherwise than thus, make any solemn protestation, or swear; I think you will believe me without an oath: say at a word, are they fools? I refer it to you, though you be likewise fools and madmen your selves, and I as mad to ask the question: for what said our comical Mercury?

[4] Justum ab injustis petere insipientia est.
I'le stand to your censure yet, what think you?

But, for as much as I undertook at first, that kingdoms, provinces, families, were melancholy as well as private men, I will examine them in particular, and that which I have hitherto dilated at random in more general terms, I will particularly insist in, prove with more special and evident arguments, testimonies, illustrations, and that in brief.

[5]————Nunc accipe, quare
Desipiant omnes æque ac tu.

My first argument is borrowed from Solomon, an arrow drawn out of his sententious quiver, Prov. 3. 7. *Be not wise in thine own eyes.* And 26. 12, [6] *Seest thou a man wise in his own conceit? more hope is of a fool than of him.* Isaiah pronounceth a woe against such men, (cap. 5. 21.) *that are wise in their own eyes, and prudent in their own sight.* For hence we may gather, that it is a great offence, and men are much deceived that think too well of themselves, an especial argument to convince them of folly. Many men (saith [7] Seneca) *had been without question wise, had they not had an opinion that they had attained to perfection of knowledge already, even before they had gone half way,* too forward, too ripe, *præproperi,* too quick and ready, [8] *cito prudentes, cito pii, cito mariti, cito patres, cito sacerdotes, cito omnis officii capaces et curiosi:* they had too good a conceit of themselves, and that marred all—of their worth, valour, skill, art, learn-

---

[1] Persius.   [2] Hor. 2. ser.   [3] Vesanum exagitant pueri, inuptæque puellæ.
[4] Plautus.   [5] Hor. l. 2. sat. 2.   [6] Superbam stultitiam Plinius vocat. 7. ep.
21. quod semel dixi, fixum ratumque sit.   [7] Multi sapientes proculdubio fuissent, si sese non putâssent ad sapientiæ summum pervenisse.   [8] Idem.

DEMOCRITUS TO THE READER. 61

ing, judgment, eloquence, their good parts : all their geese
are swans : and that manifestly proves them to be no better
than fools. In former times they had but seven wise men ;
now you can scarce find so many fools. Thales sent the
golden *tripos*, which the fisherman found, and the oracle
commanded to be [1] *given to the wisest*, to Bias, Bias to Solon, &c. If such a thing were now found, we should all
fight for it, as the three goddesses did for the golden apple
—we are so wise : we have women-politicians, children meta-
physicians : every silly fellow can square a circle, make perpetual motions, find the philosophers stone, interpret Apo-
calypsis, make new theoricks, a new systeme of the world,
new logick, new philosophy, &c. *Nostra utique regio*, saith
[2] Petronius, *our countrey is so full of deified spirits, divine
souls, that you may sooner find a God than a man amongst us ;*
we think so well of our selves, and that is an ample testimony
of much folly.

My second argument is grounded upon the like place of
Scripture, which, though before mentioned in effect, yet for
some reasons is to be repeated (and, by Platos good leave, I
may do it : [3] δις το καλον ρηθεν ουδεν βλαπτει) *Fools*, (saith David) *by reason of their transgressions, &c.* Psal. 107. 17. Hence
Musculus inferrs, all transgressors must needs be fools. So
we read Rom. 2. *Tribulation and anguish on the soul of
every man that doth evil ;* but all do evil. And Isai. 65. 14.
*My servants shall sing for joy, and [4] ye shall cry for sorrow
of heart, and vexation of mind.* 'Tis ratified by the common consent of all philosophers. *Dishonesty* (saith Cardan)
is nothing else but folly and madness. [5] *Probus quis nobiscum
vivit ?* Shew me an honest man. *Nemo malus, qui non
stultus :* 'tis Fabius aphorism to the same end. If none
honest, none wise, then all fools. And well may they be so
accounted : for who will account him otherwise, *qui iter
adornat in occidentem, quum properaret in orientem ?* that goes
backward all his life, westward, when he is bound to the east ?
or hold him a wise man (saith [6] Musculus) *that prefers momentary pleasures to eternity, that spends his masters goods in
his absence, forthwith to be condemned for it ? Nequidquam
sapit qui sibi non sapit.* Who will say that a sick man is
wise, that eats and drinks to overthrow the temperature
of his body ? Can you account him wise or discreet that

---

[1] Plutarchus, Solone. Detur sapientiori. [2] Tam præsentibus plena est numinibus, ut facilius possis Deum quam hominem invenire. [3] Pulchrum bis
dicere non nocet. [4] Malefactors. [5] Who can find a faithful man ?
Prov. 20. 6. [6] In Psal. 49. Qui præfert momentanea sempiternis, qui di-
lapidat heri absentis bona, mox in jus vocandus et damnandus.

DEMOCRITUS TO THE READER.

would willingly have his health, and yet will do nothing that should procure or continue it? [1] Theodoret, (out of Plotinus the Platonist) *holds it a ridiculous thing for a man to live after his own laws, to do that which is offensive to God, and yet to hope that he should save him; and, when he voluntarily neglects his own safety, and contemns the means, to think to be delivered by another.* Who will say these men are wise?

A third argument may be derived from the precedent. [2] All men are carried away with passion, discontent, lust, pleasures, &c. They generally hate those vertues they should love, and love such vices they should hate. Therefore more than melancholy, quite mad, bruit beasts, and void of all reason, (so Chrysostome contends) *or rather dead and buried alive, as* [3] Philo Judæus concludes it for a certainty, *of all such that are carried away with passions, or labour of any disease of the mind. Where is fear and sorrow, there* ([4] Lactantius stifly maintains) *wisdom cannot dwell.*

———qui cupiet, metuet quoque; porro
Qui metuens vivit, liber mihi non erit unquam.

Seneca and the rest of the Stoicks are of opinion, that, where is any the least perturbation, wisdom may not be found. *What more ridiculous,* (as [5] Lactantius urgeth) than to hear how Xerxes whipped the Hellespont, threatned the mountain Athos, and the like? To speak *ad rem,* who is free from passion? [6] *Mortalis nemo est, quem non attingat dolor morbusve,* (as [7] Tully determines out of an old poem) no mortal men can avoid sorrow and sickness; and sorrow is an unseparable companion of melancholy. [8] Chrysostome pleads farther yet, that they are more than mad, very beasts, stupified, and void of common sense: *for how* (saith he) *shall I know thee to be a man, when thou kickest like an ass, neighest like an horse after women, ravest in lust like a bull, ravenest like a bear, stingest like a scorpion, rakest like a wolf,*

---

[1] Perquam ridiculum est homines ex animi sententiâ vivere, et, quæ Diis ingrata sunt, exequi, et tamen a solis Diis velle salvos fieri, quum propriæ salutis curam abjecerint. Theod. c. 6. de provid. lib. de curat. Græc. affect. [2] Sapiens, sibi qui imperiosus, &c. Hor. 2. ser. 7. [3] Conclus. lib. de vic. offer. Certum est animi morbis laborantes pro mortuis censendos. [4] Lib. de sap. Ubi timor adest, sapientia adesse nequit. [5] Quid insanius Xerxe Hellespontum verberante? &c. [6] Eccles. 21. 12. Where is bitterness, there is no understanding. Prov. 12. 16. An angry man is a fool. [7] 3 Tusc. Injuria in sapientem non cadit. [8] Hom. 6. in 2 Epist. ad Cor. Hominem te agnoscere nequeo, cum tamquam asinus recalcitres, lascivias ut taurus, hinnias ut equus post mulieres, ut ursus ventri indulgeas, quum rapias ut lupus, &c. At (inquis) formam hominis habeo. Id magis terret, quum feram humanâ specie videre me putem.

DEMOCRITUS TO THE READER.

as subtile as a fox, as impudent as a dog? Shall I say thou art a man, that hast all the symptomes of a beast? How shall I know thee to be a man? By thy shape? That affrights me more when I see a beast in likeness of a man.

[1] Seneca calls that of Epicurus, *magnificam vocem*, an heroical speech, *a fool still begins to live*, and accounts it a filthy lightness in men, every day to lay new foundations of their life: but who doth otherwise? One travels; another builds; one for this, another for that business; and old folks are as far out as the rest: *O dementem senectutem!* Tully exclaims. Therefore young, old, middle age, all are stupid, and dote.

[2] Æneas Sylvius, amongst many others, sets down three special wayes to find a fool by. He is a fool that seeks that he can not find: he is a fool that seeks that, which, being found, will do him more harm than good: he is a fool, that, having variety of ways to bring him to his journeys end, takes that which is worst. If so, me thinks most men are fools. Examine their courses, and you shall soon perceive what dizards and mad men the major part are.

Beroaldus will have drunkards, afternoon-men, and such as more than ordinarily delight in drink, to be mad. The first pot quencheth thirst (so Panyasis the poet determines in Athenæus): *secunda Gratiis, Horis, et Dionysio*—the second makes merry: the third for pleasure: *quarta ad insaniam*, the fourth makes them mad. If this position be true, what a catalogue of mad men shall we have! what shall they be that drink four times four? *Nonne supra omnem furorem, supra omnem insaniam, reddunt insanissimos?* I am of his opinion, they are more than mad, much worse than mad.

The [3] Abderites condemned Democritus for a mad man, because he was sometimes sad, and sometimes again profusely merry. *Hac patriâ* (saith Hippocrates) *ob risum furere et insanire dicunt:* his countrey men hold him mad, because he laughs; [4] and therefore *he desires him to advise all his friends at Rhodes, that they do not laugh too much, or be over sad.* Had those Abderites been conversant with us, and but seen what [5] fleering and grinning there is in this age, they would certainly have concluded, we had been all out of our wits.

---

[1] Epist. 1, 2. 13. Stultus semper incipit vivere. Fœda hominum levitas! nova quotidie fundamenta vitæ ponere, novas spes, &c. [2] De curial. miser. Stultus qui quærit quod nequit invenire, stultus qui quærit quod nocet inventum, stultus qui cum plures habet calles, deteriorem deligit. Mihi videntur omnes deliri, amentes, &c. [3] Ep. Damageto. [4] Amicis nostris Rhodi dicito, ne nimium rideant, aut nimium tristes sint. [5] Per multum risum poteris cognoscere stultum. Offic. 3. c. 9.

2

DEMOCRITUS TO THE READER.

Aristotle, in his Ethicks, holds, *felix idemque sapiens*, to be wise and happy, are reciprocal terms. *Bonus idemque sapiens honestus.* 'Tis [1] Tullies paradox: *wise men are free, but fools are slaves :* liberty is a power to live according to his own laws, as we will ourselves. Who hath this liberty? Who is free?

———————[2]sapiens sibique imperiosus,
Quem neque pauperies, neque mors, neque vincula terrent;
Responsare cupidinibus, contemnere honores
Fortis, et in seipso totus teres atque rotundus.

He is wise that can command his own will,
Valiant and constant to himself still,
Whom poverty, nor death, nor bands can fright,
Checks his desires, scorns honours, just and right.

But where shall such a man be found? if no where, then *e diametro*, we all are slaves, senseless, or worse. *Nemo malus felix.* But no man is happy in this life, none good; therefore no man wise.

[3] Rari quippe boni——

For one vertue, you shall find ten vices in the same party— *pauci Promethei, multi Epimethei.* We may peradventure usurp the name, or attribute it to others for favour, as Carolus Sapiens, Philippus Bonus, Ludovicus Pius, &c. and describe the properties of a wise man, as Tully doth an orator, Xenophon Cyrus, Castilio a courtier, Galen temperament; an aristocracy is described by politicians. But where shall such a man be found?

Vir bonus et sapiens, qualem vix repperit unum
Millibus e multis hominum consultus Apollo.

A wise, a good man in a million,
Apollo consulted could scarce find one.

A man is a miracle of himself; but Trismegistus adds, *maximum miraculum homo sapiens;* a wise man is a wonder: *multi thyrsigeri, pauci Bacchi.*

Alexander, when he was presented with that rich and costly casket of king Darius, and every man advised him what to put in it, he reserved it to keep Homers works, as the most precious jewel of humane wit: and yet [4] Scaliger upbraids Homers Muse, *nutricem insanæ sapientiæ*, a nursery of madness, [5] impudent as a court lady, that blushes at nothing. Jacobus Micyllus, Gilbertus Cognatus, Erasmus, and almost

---

[1] Sapientes liberi, stulti servi.   Libertas est potestas, &c.   [2] Hor. 2. ser. 7.
[3] Juven.   [4] Hypercrite.   [5] Ut mulier aulica nullius pudens.

DEMOCRITUS TO THE READER. 65

all posterity, admire Lucians luxuriant wit: yet Scaliger rejects him in his censure, and calls him the Cerberus of the Muses. Socrates, whom all the world so much magnified, is, by Lactantius and Theodoret, condemned for a fool. Plutarch extols Senecas wit beyond all the Greeks—*nulli secundus:* yet [1]Seneca saith of himself, *when I would solace my self with a fool, I reflect upon my self; and there I have him.* Cardan, in his sixteenth book of Subtilties, reckons up twelve supereminent, acute philosophers, for worth, subtlety, and wisdom—Archimedes, Galen, Vitruvius, Archytas Tarentinus, Euclide, Geber, that first inventer of algebra, Alkindus the mathematician, both Arabians, with others. But his *triumviri terrarum*, far beyond the rest, are Ptolemæus, Plotinus, Hippocrates. Scaliger (*exercitat.* 224) scoffs at this censure of his, calls some of them carpenters, and mechanicians: he makes Galen *fimbriam Hippocratis,* a skirt of Hippocrates: and the said [2]Cardan himself elsewhere condemns both Galen and Hippocrates for tediousness, obscurity, confusion. Paracelsus will have them both meer ideots, infants in physick and philosophy. Scaliger and Cardan admire Suisset the calculator, *qui pene modum excessit humani ingenii;* and yet [3]Lud. Vives calls them *nugas Suisseticas:* and Cardan opposite to himself in another place, contemns those antients in respect of times present, [4]*majoresque nostros, ad præsentes collatos, juste pueros appellari.* In conclusion, the said [5]Cardan and Saint Bernard will admit none into this catalogue of wise men, [6] but only prophets and apostles:—how they esteem themselves, you have heard before. We are worldly-wise, admire our selves, and seek for applause: but hear Saint [7]Bernard, *quanto magis foras es sapiens, tanto magis intus stultus efficeris, &c. in omnibus es prudens, circa teipsum insipiens:* the more wise thou art to others, the more fool to thy self. I may not deny but that there is some folly approved, a divine fury, a holy madness, even a spiritual drunkenness in the saints of God themselves: *Sanctam insaniam* Bernard calls it, (though not, as blaspheming [8]Vorstius would inferr it as a passion incident to God himself, but) familiar to good men, as that of Paul, 2 Cor. *he was a fool, &c.* and Rom. 9. he wisheth himself *to be anathematized for them.* Such is that drunkenness which Ficinus speaks of, when the

---

[1] Epist. 33. Quando fatuo delectari volo, non est longe quærendus; me video. [2] Primo contradicentium. [3] Lib. de caussis corrupt. artium. [4] Actione ad subtil. in Scal. fol. 12. 26. [5] Lib. 1. de sap. [6] Vide, miser homo, quia totum est vanitas, totum stultitia, totum dementia, quidquid facis in hoc mundo, præter hoc solum quod propter Deum facis. Ser. de miser hom. [7] In 2 Platonis dial. 1. de justo. [8] Dum iram et odium in Deo reverâ ponit.

VOL. I. F

66   DEMOCRITUS TO THE READER.

soul is elevated and ravished with a divine taste of that heavenly
nectar, which the poets deciphered by the sacrifice of Dionysius,
and in this sense, with the poet, [1]*insanire lubet :* as Austin exhorts us, *ad ebrietatem se quisque paret ;* let's all be mad and
[2]drunk. But we commonly mistake and go beyond our com-
mission : we reel to the opposite part; [3]we are not capable of
it; [4]and, as he said of the Greeks, *Vos Græci semper pueri,
vos Britanni, Galli, Germani, Itali, &c.* you are a company
of fools.

Proceed now *a partibus ad totum,* or from the whole to
parts, and you shall find no other issue. The parts shall be
sufficiently dilated in this following preface. The whole must
needs follow by a *sorites* or induction. Every multitude is
mad, [5]*bellua multorum capitum,* precipitate and rash, without judgement, *stultum animal,* a roaring rout. [6]Roger Bacon
proves it out of Aristotle—*vulgus dividi in oppositum contra
sapientes : quod vulgo videtur verum, falsum est ;* that which
the commonalty accounts true, is most part false ; they are
still opposite to wise men : but all the world is of this humour
(vulgus) ; and thou thyself art *de vulgo,* one of the commonalty ; and he, and he ; and so are all the rest; and therefore
(as Phocion concludes) to be approved in nought you say or
do, meer ideots and asses. Begin then where you will, go
backward or forward, choose out of the whole pack, wink and
choose : you shall find them all alike—*never a barrel better
herring.*

Copernicus, Atlas his successor, is of opinion, the earth is
a planet, moves and shines to others, as the moon doth to us.
Digges, Gilbert, Keplerus, Origanus, and others, defend this
hypothesis of his in sober sadness, and that the moon is inhabited. If it be so that the earth is a moon, then are we
also giddy, vertiginous, and lunatick, within this sublunary
maze.

I could produce such arguments till dark night. If you
should hear the rest,

Ante diem clauso componet Vesper Olympo :

but, according to my promise, I will descend to particulars.
This melancholy extends it self not to men only, but even to
vegetals and sensibles. I speak not of those creatures which
are saturnine, melancholy by nature, (as lead, and such like
minerals, or those plants, rue, cypress, &c. and hellebore

---

[1] Virg. 1. Ecl. 3.   [2] Ps. inebriabuntur ab ubertate domûs.   [3] In Psal.
104. Aust.   [4] In Platonis Tim. sacerdos Ægyptius.   [5] Hor. Vulgus insanum.   [6] Patet ea divisio probabilis, &c. ex Arist. Top. lib. 1. c. 8. Rog. Bac.
Epist. de secret. art. et nat. c. 8. Non est judicium in vulgo.

DEMOCRITUS TO THE READER.   67

it self, of which [1]Agrippa treats, fishes, birds, and beasts,
hares, conies, dormice, &c. owls, bats, night-birds,) but that
artificial, which is perceived in them all. Remove a plant; it
will pine away; which is especially perceived in date trees,
as you may read at large in Constantines husbandry—that
antipathy betwixt the vine and the cabbage, vine and oyle.
Put a bird in a cage ; he will dye for sullenness ; or a beast in
a pen, or take his young ones or companions from him; and
see what effect it will cause. But who perceives not these
common passions of sensible creatures, fear, sorrow, &c. Of
all other, dogs are most subject to this malady, in so much,
some hold they dream as men do, and through violence of
melancholy, run mad. I could relate many stories of dogs,
that have dyed for grief, and pined away for loss of their
masters: but they are common in every [2]author.

Kingdoms, provinces, and politick bodies, are likewise sensible and subject to this disease, as [3]Boterus, in his Politicks,
hath proved at large. *As, in humane bodies*, (saith he) *there
be divers alterations proceeding from humours, so there be
many diseases in a common-wealth, which do as diversely
happen from several distempers*, as you may easily perceive
by their particular symptoms. For where you shall see the
people civil, obedient to God and princes, judicious, peaceable and quiet, rich, fortunate, [4]and flourish, to live in peace,
in unity, and concord, a countrey well tilled, many fair built
and populous cities, *ubi incolæ nitent*, as old [5]Cato said, the
people are neat, polite, and terse, *ubi bene, beateque vivunt*,
(which our politicians make the chief end of a common-wealth;
and which [6]Aristotle, Polit. lib. 3. cap. 4. calls *commune
bonum*, Polybius, lib. 6. *optabilem et selectum statum*,) that
countrey is free from melancholy ; as it was in Italy in the
time of Augustus, now in China, now in many other flourishing
kingdoms of Europe. But whereas you shall see many discontents, common grievances, complaints, poverty, barbarism,
beggary, plagues, wars, rebellions, seditions, mutinies, contentions, idleness, riot, epicurism, the land lye untilled, waste,
full of bogs, fens, desarts, &c. cities decayed, base and poor
towns, villages depopulated, the people squalid, ugly, uncivil ;
that kingdom, that countrey, must needs be discontent, melancholy, hath a sick body, and had need to be reformed.

---

[1] De occult. philosoph. l. 1. c. 25. et 19. ejusd. l. Lib. 10. cap. 4.   [2] See Lipsius, epist.   [3] De politiâ illustrium, lib. 1. cap. 4. Ut in humanis corporibus
variæ accidunt mutationes corporis animique, sic in republicâ, &c.   [4] Ubi reges
philosophantur.   Plato.   [5] Lib. de re rust.   [6] Vel publicam utilitatem.
Salus publica suprema lex esto. Beata civitas, non ubi pauci beati, sed tota
civitas beata. Plato, quarto de repub.

F 2

68 DEMOCRITUS TO THE READER.

Now that cannot well be effected, till the causes of these maladies be first removed, which commonly proceed from their own default, or some accidental inconvenience ; as to be site in a bad clime, too far north, steril, in a barren place, as the desart of Libya, desarts of Arabia, places void of waters, as those of Lop and Belgian in Asia, or in a bad air, as at Alexandretta, Bantam, Pisa, Durazzo, S. John de Ullua, &c. or in danger of the seas continual inundations, as in many places of the Low-Countreys and elsewhere, or near some bad neighbours, as Hungarians to Turks, Podolians to Tartars, or almost any bordering countreys, they live in fear still, and, by reason of hostile incursions, are oftentimes left desolate. So are cities by reason [1] of wars, fires, plagues, inundations, [2] wild beasts, decay of trades, barred havens, the seas violence, as Antwerp may witness of late, Syracuse of old, Brundusium in Italy, Rhye and Dover with us, and many that at this day suspect the seas fury and rage, and labour against it, as the Venetians to their inestimable charge. But the most frequent maladies are such as proceed from themselves, as, first, when religion and Gods service is neglected, innovated, or altered— where they do not fear God, obey their prince—where atheism, epicurism, sacrilege, simony, &c. and all such impieties are freely committed—that countrey cannot prosper. When Abraham came to Gerar, and saw a bad land, he said, sure the fear of God was not in that place. [3] Cyprian Echovius, a Spanish chorographer, above all other cities of Spain, commends Borcino, *in which there was no beggar, no man poor,* &c. *but all rich and in good estate :* and he gives the reason, because *they were more religious than their neighbours.* Why was Israel so often spoiled by their enemies, led into captivity, &c. but for their idolatry, neglect of Gods word, for sacrilege, even for one Achans fault? And what shall we expect, that have such multitudes of Achans, church-robbers, simoniacal patrons, &c.? how can they hope to flourish, that neglect divine duties, that live, most part, like epicures?

Other common grievances are generally noxious to a body politick ; alteration of laws and customs, breaking privileges, general oppressions, seditions, &c. observed by [4] Aristotle, Bodin, Boterus, Junius, Arniscus, &c. I will only point at some of the chiefest. [5] *Impotentia gubernandi, ataxia,* con-

---

[1] Mantua, væ! miseræ nimium vicina Cremonæ.   [2] Interdum a feris, ut olim Mauritania, &c.   [3] Deliciis Hispaniæ an. 1604. Nemo malus, nemo pauper ; optimus quisque atque ditissimus. Pie, sancteque vivebant ; summâque cum veneratione et timore, divino cultui, sacrisque rebus, incumbebant.   [4] Polit. l. 5. c. 3.   [5] Boterus, polit. lib. 1. c. 1. Cum nempe princeps rerum gerendarum imperitus, segnis, oscitans, suique muneris immemor, aut fatuus est.

DEMOCRITUS TO THE READER. 69

fusion, ill government, which proceeds from unskilful, slothful, griping, covetous, unjust, rash, or tyrannizing magistrates, when they are fools, ideots, children, proud, wilful, partial, undiscreet, oppressors, giddy heads, tyrants, not able or unfit to manage such offices. [1] Many noble cities and flourishing kingdoms by that means are desolate; the whole body groans under such heads; and all the members must needs be misaffected, as at this day those goodly provinces in Asia Minor, &c. groan under the burthen of a Turkish government; and those vast kingdoms of Muscovia, Russia, [2] under a tyrannizing duke. Who ever heard of more civil and rich populous countreys than those of Greece, Asia Minor, *abounding with all* [3] *wealth, multitude of inhabitants, force, power, splendor, and magnificence?* and that miracle of countreys, [4] the Holy Land, that, in so small a compass of ground, could maintain so many towns, cities, produce so many fighting men? Egypt another Paradise, now barbarous and desart, and almost waste, by the despotical government of an imperious Turk, *intolerabili servitutis jugo premitur* ([5] one saith) : not only fire and water, goods or lands, *sed ipse spiritus ab insolentissimi victoris pendet nutu :* such is their slavery, their lives and souls depend upon his insolent will and command—a tyrant that spoyls all wheresoever he comes ; insomuch that an [6] historian complains, *if an old inhabitant should now see them, he would not know them ; if a traveller, or stranger, it would grieve his heart to behold them*—whereas ([7] Aristotle notes) *novæ exactiones, nova onera imposita,* new burdens and exactions daily come upon them, (like those of which Zosimus, lib. 2.) so grievous *ut viri uxores, patres filias prostituerent, ut exactoribus e quæstu, &c.* they must needs be discontent: *hinc civitatum gemitus et ploratus,* as [8] Tully holds ; hence come those complaints and tears of cities *poor, miserable, rebellious, and desperate subjects,* as [9] Hippolytus adds : and, [10] as a judicious countrey-man of ours observed not long since in a survey of that great Duchy of Tuscany, the people lived much grieved and discontent, as appeared by their manifold and manifest complainings in that kind ; *that the state was like a sick body which had lately taken physick, whose humours are not yet well settled, and weakened so much by purging, that nothing was left but melancholy.*

[1] Non viget respublica cujus caput infirmatur. Salisburiensis, c. 22.   [2] See D. Fletchers relation, and Alexander Gagninus history.   [3] Abundans omni divitiarum affluentiâ, incolarum multitudine, splendore, ac potentiâ.   [4] Not above 200 miles in length, 60 in breadth, according to Adricomius.   [5] Romulus Amaseus.   [6] Sabellicus. Si quis incola vetus, non agnosceret ; si quis peregrinus, ingemisceret.   [7] Polit. l. 5. c. 6. Crudelitas principum, impunitas scelerum, violatio legum, peculatus pecuniæ publicæ, &c.   [8] Epist. [9] De increm. urb. cap. 20. Subditi miseri, rebelles, desperati, &c.   [10] R. Dalington, 1596, conclusio libri.

70   DEMOCRITUS TO THE READER.

Whereas the princes and potentates are immoderate in lust, hypocrites, epicures, of no religion, but in shew—*Quid hypocrisi fragilius?* what so brittle and unsure? what sooner subverts their estates, than wandering and raging lusts on their subjects wives, daughters? to say no worse. They that should *facem præferre*, lead the way to all vertuous actions, are the ringleaders oftentimes of all mischief and dissolute courses; and by that means their countreys are plagued, [1] *and they themselves often ruined, banished or murdered by conspiracy of their subjects*, as Sardanapalus was, Dionysius junior, Heliogabalus, Periander, Pisistratus, Tarquinius, Timocrates, Childericus, Appius Claudius, Andronicus, Galeacius Sforsia, Alexander Medices, &c.

Whereas the princes or great men are malicious, envious, factious, ambitious, emulators, they tear a common-wealth asunder, as so many *Guelfes* and *Gibellines*, disturb the quietness of it, [2] and, with mutual murders, let it bleed to death. Our histories are too full of such barbarous inhumanities, and the miseries that issue from them.

Whereas they be like so many horse-leeches, hungry, griping, corrupt, [3] covetous, *avaritiæ mancipia*, ravenous as wolves, (for, as Tully writes, *qui præest, prodest ; et qui pecudibus præest, debet eorum utilitati inservire*) or such as prefer their private before the public good (for, as [4] he said long since, *res privatæ publicis semper officere*)—or whereas they be illiterate, ignorant, empiricks in policy, *ubi deest facultas,* [5] *virtus,* (Aristot. *pol. 5. cap.* 8.) *et scientia*, wise only by inheritance, and in authority by birth-right, or for their wealth and titles— there must needs be a fault, [6] a great defect, because, as an [7] old philosopher affirms, such men are not alwayes fit—*of an infinite number, few alone are senators; and of those few, fewer good ; and of that small number of honest, good, and noble men, few that are learned, wise, discreet, and sufficient, able to discharge such places*—it must needs turn to the confusion of a state.

For, as the [8] princes are, so are the people; *qualis rex,*

---

[1] Boterus, l. 9. c. 4. Polit. Quo fit ut aut rebus desperatis exulent, aut conjuratione subditorum crudelissime tandem trucidentur.   [2] Mutuis odiis et cædibus exhausti, &c.   [3] Lucra ex malis, sceleratisque caussis.   [4] Sallust.
[5] For most part, we mistake the name of politicians, accounting such as read Machiavel and Tacitus, great statesmen, that can dispute of political precepts, supplant and overthrow their adversaries, enrich themselves, get honour, dissemble. But what is this to the *bene esse*, or preservation of a common-wealth?
[6] Imperium suâpte sponte corruit.   [7] Apul. Prim. Flor. Ex innumerabilibus, pauci senatores genere nobiles ; e consularibus pauci boni ; e bonis adhuc pauci eruditi.   [8] Non solum vitia concipiunt ipsi principes, sed etiam infundunt in civitatem ; plusque exemplo, quam peccato, nocent. Cic. l. de legibus.

DEMOCRITUS TO THE READER.

talis grex: and, which [1]Antigonus right well said of old, *qui Macedoniæ regem erudit, omnes etiam subditos erudit,* he that teacheth the king of Macedon, teacheth all his subjects, is a true saying still.

> For princes are the glass, the school, the book,
> Where subjects eyes do learn, do read, do look.

> ———————Velocius et citius nos
> Corrumpunt vitiorum exempla domestica, magnis
> Cum subeant animos auctoribus————

their examples are soonest followed, vices entertained : if they be prophane, irreligious, lascivious, riotous, epicures, factious, covetous, ambitious, illiterate, so will the commons most part be, idle, unthrifts, prone to lust, drunkards, and therefore poor and needy (ἡ πενια στασιν εμποιει, και κακουργιαν, for poverty begets sedition and villany) upon all occasions ready to mutiny and rebel, discontent, still complaining, murmuring, grudging, apt to all outrages, thefts, treasons, murders, innovations, in debt, shifters, cozeners, outlaws, *profligatæ famæ ac vitæ.* It was an old [2]politicians aphorism, *they that are poor and bad, envy rich, hate good men, abhor the present government, wish for a new, and would have all turned topsie turvy.* When Cataline rebelled in Rome, he got a company of such debauched rogues together : they were his familiars and coadjutors, and such have been your rebels, most part, in all ages— Jack Cade, Tom Straw, Kette, and his companions.

Where they be generally riotous and contentious, where there be many discords, many laws, many law-suits, many lawyers, and many physicians, it is a manifest sign of a distempered, melancholy state, as [3]Plato long since maintained : for, where such kind of men swarm, they will make more work for themselves, and that body politick diseased, which was otherwise sound—a general mischief in these our times, an unsensible plague, and never so many of them ; *which are now multiplyed* (saith Mat. Geraldus, [4] *a lawyer himself,) as so many locusts, not the parents, but the plagues of the countrey, and, for the most part, a supercilious, bad, covetous, litigious generation of men—*[5]*crumenimulga natio, &c.* a purse-milking nation, a clamorous company, gowned vultures, [6]*qui*

---

[1] Epist. ad Zen. Juven. Sat. 4. Paupertas seditionem gignit et maleficium. Arist. pol. 2. c. 7.   [2] Sallust. Semper in civitate, quibus opes nullæ sunt, bonis invident ; vetera odere ; nova exoptant ; odio suarum rerum mutari omnia petunt. [3] De legibus. Profligatæ in repub. disciplinæ est indicium jurisperitorum numerus, et medicorum copia.   [4] In præf. stud. juris. Multiplicantur nunc in terris, ut locustæ, non patriæ parentes, sed pestes, pessimi homines, majore ex parte supercontentiosi, &c.—licitum latrocinium exercent.   [5] Dousa, epid. Loqua turba, vultures togati.   [6] Barc. Argen.

DEMOCRITUS TO THE READER.

ex injuriâ vivunt et sanguine civium, thieves and seminaries of discord, worse than any polers by the high way side, *auri accipitres, auri exterebronides, pecuniarum hamiotæ, quadruplatores, curiæ harpagones, fori tintinnabula, monstra hominum, mangones, &c.* that take upon them to make peace, but are indeed the very disturbers of our peace, a company of irreligious harpyes, scraping, griping catch-poles, (I mean our common hungry petty-foggers, *rabulas forenses*—love and honour, in the mean time, all good laws, and worthy lawyers, that are so many [1] oracles and pilots of a well governed common-wealth) without art, without judgment, that do more harm, as [2] Livy saith, *quam bella externa, fames, morbive,* than sickness, wars, hunger, diseases; *and cause a most incredible destruction of a common-wealth,* saith [3] Sesellius, a famous civilian sometimes in Paris. As ivy doth by an oke, imbrace it so long, until it hath got the heart out of it, so do they by such places they inhabit: no counsel at all, no justice, no speech to be had, *nisi eum præmulseris:* he must be fed still, or else he is as mute as a fish; better open an oyster without a knife. *Experto crede,* (saith [4] Salisburiensis): *in manus eorum millies incidi; et Charon immitis, qui nulli pepercit unquam, his longe clementior est—I speak out of experience; I have been a thousand times amongst them; and Charon himself is more gentle than they;* [5] *he is contented with his single pay; but they multiply still: they are never satisfied:* besides they have *damnificas linguas,* (as he terms it) *nisi funibus argenteis vincias:* they must be feed to say nothing, and [6] get more to hold their peace, than we can to say our best. They will speak their clients fair, and invite them to their tables: but (as he follows it) [7] *of all injustice, there is none so pernicious as that of theirs, which, when they deceive most, will seem to be honest men.* They take upon them to be peace-makers, *et fovere caussas humilium,* to help them to their right: *patrocinantur afflictis;* [8] but all is for their own good, *ut loculos pleniorum exhauriant:* they plead for poor men gratis; but they are but as a stale to catch others. If there be no jar, [9] they can make a jar, out of the law it self find still some quirk or other, to set them at odds, and continue causes so long, *(lustra aliquot)* I know not how many

---

[1] Jurisconsulti domus oraculum civitatis. Tully. [2] Lib. 3. [3] Lib. 1. de rep. Gallorum. Incredibilem reipub. perniciem afferunt. [4] Polycrat. lib. [5] Is stipe contentus; at hi asses integros sibi multiplicari jubent. [6] Plus accipiunt tacere, quam nos loqui. [7] Totius injustitiæ nulla capitalior, quam eorum, qui, cum maxime decipiunt, id agunt ut boni viri esse videantur. [8] Nam, quocunque modo caussa procedat, hoc semper agitur, ut loculi impleantur, etsi avaritia nequit satiari. [9] Camden, in Norfolk. Qui, si nihil sit litium, e juris apicibus lites tamen serere callent.

DEMOCRITUS TO THE READER. 73

years, before the cause is heard : and when 'tis judged and determined, by reason of some tricks and errours, it is as fresh to
begin, after twice seven years sometimes, as it was at first ; and
so they prolong time, delay suits till they have enriched themselves, and beggared their clients. And, as [1] Cato inveighed
against Isocrates scholars, we may justly tax our wrangling
lawyers,—they do *consenescere in litibus,* are so litigious and
busie here on earth, that I think they will plead their clients
causes hereafter, some of them in hell. [2] Simlerus complains,
amongst the Suissers, of the advocates in his time, that, when
they should make an end, they begin controversies, and *protract their causes many years, perswading them their title is
good, till their patrimonies be consumed, and that they have
spent more in seeking, than the thing is worth, or they shall
get by the recovery.* So that he that goes to law (as the proverb is) [3] holds a wolf by the ears ; or, as a sheep in a storm
runs for shelter to a brier, if he prosecute his cause, he is consumed : if he surcease his suit, he loseth all : what difference ?
They had wont heretofore, saith [4] Austin, to end matters, *per
communes arbitros;* and so in Switzerland, (we are informed
by [5] Simlerus) *they had some common arbitrators or dayes-
men in every town, that made a friendly composition betwixt
man and man : and he much wonders at their honest simplicity,
that could keep peace so well, and end such great causes by
that means.* At [6] Fez in Africk, they have neither lawyers
nor advocates ; but, if there be any controversies amongst
them, both parties, plaintiff and defendant, come to their Alfa-
kins or chief judge ; *and at once, without any farther appeals
or pitiful delays, the cause is heard and ended.* Our fore-
fathers, (as [7] a worthy chorographer of ours observes) had wont,
pauculis cruculis aureis, with a few golden crosses, and lines in
verse, to make all conveyances, assurances. And such was the
candour and integrity of succeeding ages, that a deed, (as I have
oft seen) to convey a whole manor, was *implicite* contained in
some twenty lines, or thereabouts ; like that scede or *scytala
Laconica,* so much renowned of old in all contracts, which
[8] Tully so earnestly commends to Atticus, Plutarch in his

---

[1] Plutarch. vit. Cat. Caussas apud inferos, quas in suam fidem receperunt, pa-
trocinio suo tuebuntur. [2] Lib. 2. de Helvet. repub. Non explicandis, sed mo-
liendis controversiis operam dant, ita ut lites in multos annos extrahantur,
summâ cum molestiâ utriusque partis, et dum interea patrimonia exhauriuntur.
[3] Lupum auribus tenent. [4] Hor. [5] Lib. de Helvet. repub. Judices
quocunque pago constituunt, qui amicâ aliquâ transactione, si fieri possit, lites
tollant. Ego majorum nostrorum simplicitatem admiror, qui sic caussas gra-
vissimas composuerint, &c. [6] Clenard. l. 1. ep. Si quæ controversiæ,
utraque pars judicem adit : is semel et simul rem transigit, audit : nec, quid sit
appellatio, lacrymosæque moræ, noscunt. [7] Camden. [8] Lib. 10.
epist. ad Atticum, epist. 11.

74   DEMOCRITUS TO THE READER.

Lysander, Aristotle, *polit.* Thucydides, *lib.* 1, [1] Diodorus,
and Suidas, approve and magnifie, for that Laconick brevity in
this kind; and well they might; for, according to [2] Tertullian,
certa sunt paucis, there is much more certainty in fewer words.
And so was it of old throughout: but now many skins of
parchment will scarce serve turn: he that buys and sells a
house, must have a house full of writings; there be so many
circumstances, so many words, such tautological repetitions of
all particulars (to avoid cavillation they say): but we find, by
our woful experience, that, to subtle wits, it is a cause of much
more contention and variance; and scarce any conveyance so
accurately penned by one, which another will not find a crack
in, or cavil at: if any one word be misplaced, any little errour,
all is disannulled.   That which is law to day, is none to morrow: that which is sound in one mans opinion, is most faulty
to another; that, in conclusion, here is nothing amongst us but
contention and confusion.   We bandy one against another;
and that, which long since [3] Plutarch complained of them in
Asia, may be verified in our times—*These men, here assembled,
come not to sacrifice to their gods, to offer Jupiter their first
fruits, or merriments to Bacchus; but an yearly disease, exas-
perating Asia, hath brought them hither, to make an end of
their controversies and law suits.* 'Tis *multitudo perdentium
et pereuntium,* a destructive rout, that seek one anothers ruine.
Such, most part, are our ordinary suitors, termers, clients: new
stirs every day, mistakes, errours, cavils, and at this present,
(as I have heard) in some one court, I know not how many
thousand causes: no person free, no title almost good, with
such bitterness in following, so many slights, procrastinations,
delayes, forgery, such cost (for infinite sums are inconsiderately
spent), violence and malice, I know not by whose fault, lawyers, clients, laws, both or all: but, as Paul reprehended the
[4] Corinthians long since, I may more appositely infer now:
*There is a fault amongst you; and I speak it to your shame.
Is there not a* [5] *wise man amongst you, to judge between his
brethren? but that a brother goes to law with a brother?* And
* Christs counsel concerning law-suits was never so fit to be
inculcated, as in this age: [6] *Agree with thine adversary
quickly, &c.* Matth. 5. 25.

---

[1] Biblioth. l. 3.   [2] Lib. de anim.   [3] Lib. major. morb. corp. an animi. Hi
non conveniunt, ut diis more majorum sacra faciant, non ut Jovi primitias offe-
rant, aut Baccho comissationes; sed anniversarius morbus, exasperans Asiam,
huc eos coëgit, ut contentiones hîc peragant.   [4] 1 Cor. 6. 5, 6.   [5] Stulti,
quando demum sapietis? Psal. 49. 8.   [6] Of which text read two learned
Sermons, * so intituled, and preached by our Regius Professour, D. Prideaux:
printed at London by Fœlix Kingston, 1621.

DEMOCRITUS TO THE READER.

I could repeat many such particular grievances, which must disturb a body politick:—to shut up all in brief, where good government is, prudent and wise princes, there all things thrive and prosper : peace and happiness is in that land: where it is otherwise, all things are ugly to behold, incult, barbarous, uncivil; a paradise is turned to a wilderness. This island amongst the rest, our next neighbours the French and Germans, may be a sufficient witness, that in a short time, by that prudent policy of the Romans, was brought from barbarism: see but what Cæsar reports of us, and Tacitus of those old Germans: they were once as uncivil as they in Virginia ; yet, by planting of colonies and good laws, they became, from barbarous outlaws, [1] to be full of rich and populous cities, as now they are, and most flourishing kingdoms. Even so might Virginia, and those wild Irish, have been civilized long since, if that order had been heretofore taken, which now begins, of planting colonies, &c. I have read a [2] discourse, printed anno 1612, *discovering the true causes, why Ireland was never intirely subdued, or brought under obedience to the crown of England, until the beginning of his Majesties happy reign.* Yet, if his reasons were thoroughly scanned by a judicious politician, I am afraid he would not altogether be approved, but that it would turn to the dishonour of our nation, to suffer it to lye so long waste. Yea, and if some travellers should see (to come neerer home) those rich united Provinces of Holland, Zealand, &c. over against us, those neat cities and populous towns, full of most industrious artificers, [3] so much land recovered from the sea, and so painfully preserved by those artificial inventions, so wonderfully approved, as that of Bemster in Holland, *ut nihil huic par aut simile invenias in toto orbe,* saith Bertius the geographer—all the world cannot match it: [4] so many navigable channels from place to place, made by mens hands, &c. and, on the other side, so many thousand acres of our fens lie drowned, our cities thin, and those vile, poor, and ugly to behold in respect of theirs; our trades decayed, our still running rivers stopped, and that beneficial use of transportation wholly neglected; so many havens void of ships and towns, so many parks and forests for pleasure, barren heaths, so many villages depopulated, &c. I think sure he would find some fault.

I may not deny but that this nation of ours doth *bene audire apud exteros*—is a most noble, a most flourishing kingdom, by

---

[1] Sæpius bona materia cessat sine artifice. Sabellicus, de Germaniâ. Si quis videret Germaniam urbibus hodie excultam, non diceret, ut olim, tristem cultu, asperam cœlo, terram informem. [2] By his Majesties Attorney General there. [3] As Zeipland, Bemster in Holland, &c. [4] From Gaunt to Sluce, from Bruges to the sea, &c.

DEMOCRITUS TO THE READER.

common consent of all [1] geographers, historians, politicians:
'tis *unica velut arx,* and which Quintius in Livy said of the
inhabitants of Peloponnesus, may be well applyed to us, we are
testudines testâ suâ inclusæ—like so many tortoises in our
shells, safely defended by an angry sea, as a wall, on all sides:
our island hath many such honourable elogiums ; and, as a
learned countrey-man of ours right well hath it, [2] *Ever since
the Normans first coming into England, this countrey, both
for military matters and all other of civility, hath been parallel'd with the most flourishing kingdoms of Europe, and
our Christian world*—a blessed, a rich countrey, and one of
the fortunate isles; and, for some things, [3] preferred before
other countreys, for expert seamen, our laborious discoveries,
art of navigation, true merchants—they carry the bell away
from all other nations, even the Portugals and Hollanders
themselves—[4] *without all fear,* (saith Boterus) *furrowing the
ocean winter and summer; and two of their captains, with no
less valour than fortune, have sailed round about the world.*
[5] We have besides many particular blessings, which our neighbours want—the gospel truly preached, church discipline
established, long peace and quietness—free from exactions,
foraign fears, invasions, domestical seditions—well manured,
[6] fortified by art, and nature, and now most happy in that
fortunate union of England and Scotland, which our fore-
fathers have laboured to effect, and desired to see: but, in
which we excell all others, a wise, learned, religious king,
another Numa, a second Augustus, a true Josiah, most worthy
senators, a learned clergy, an obedient commonalty, &c. Yet,
amongst many roses, some thistles grow, some bad weeds and
enormities, which much disturb the peace of this body politick,
eclipse the honour and glory of it, fit to be rooted out, and
with all speed to be reformed.

The first is idleness, by reason of which we have many
swarms of rogues and beggers, theeves, drunkards, and discontented persons, (whom Lycurgus, in Plutarch, calls *morbos
reipub.* the boils of the common-wealth) many poor people in
all our towns, *civitates ignobiles,* as [7] Polydore calls them,
base built cities, inglorious, poor, small, rare in sight, ruinous,
and thin of inhabitants. Our land is fertile (we may not deny),
full of all good things ; and why doth it not then abound with
cities, as well as Italy, France, Germany, the Low-Countreys ?

[1] Ortelius, Boterus, Mercator, Meteranus, &c.   [2] Jam inde non belli gloriâ,
quam humanitatis cultu, inter florentissimas orbis Christiani gentes imprimis
floruit. Camden. Brit. de Normannis.   [3] Geog. Kecker.   [4] Tam hyeme
quam æstate intrepide sulcant oceanum ; et duo illorum duces, non minore au-
daciâ quam fortunâ, totius orbem terræ circumnavigârunt. Amphitheatro Boterus.   [5] A fertile soil, good air, &c. tin, lead, wool, saffron, &c.   [6] Tota
Britannia unica velut arx. Boter.   [7] Lib. 1. hist.

DEMOCRITUS TO THE READER.

because their policy hath been otherwise ; and we are not so thrifty, circumspect, industrious. Idleness is the *malus genius* of our nation : for, (as [1] Boterus justly argues) fertility of a countrey is not enough, except art and industry be joyned unto it. According to Aristotle, riches are neither natural or artificial : natural are good land, fair mines, &c. artificial are manufactures, coines, &c. Many kingdoms are fertile, but thin of inhabitants, as that duchy of Piedmont in Italy, which Leander Albertus so much magnifies for corn, wine, fruits, &c. yet nothing near so populous as those which are more barren. [2] *England*, saith he, *(London only excepted) hath never a populous city, and yet a fruitful countrey.* I find 46 cities and walled towns in Alsatia, a small province in Germany, 50 castles, an infinite number of villages, no ground idle—no, not rocky places, or tops of hills, are untilled, as [3] Munster informeth us. In [4] Greichgea, a small territory on the Necker, 24 Italian miles over, I read of 20 walled towns, innumerable villages, each one containing 150 houses most part, besides castles and noblemens palaces. I observe, in [5] Turinge in Dutchland, (twelve miles over by their scale) 12 counties, and in them 144 cities, 2000 villages, 144 towns, 250 castles —in [6] Bavaria, 34 cities, 46 towns, &c. [7] *Portugallia interamnis*, a small plot of ground, hath 1460 parishes, 130 monasteries, 200 bridges. Malta, a barren island, yields 20000 inhabitants. But of all the rest, I admire Luet Guicciardines relations of the Low-Countries. Holland hath 26 cities, 400 great villages —Zeland, 10 cities, 102 parishes—Brabant, 26 cities, 102 parishes—Flanders, 28 cities, 90 towns, 1154 villages, besides abbies, castles, &c. The Low-Countries generally have three cities at least for one of ours, and those far more populous and rich : and what is the cause, but their industry and excellency in all manner of trades, their commerce, which is maintained by a multitude of tradesmen, so many excellent channels made by art, and opportune havens, to which they build their cities? all which we have in like measure, or at least may have. But their chiefest loadstone, which draws all manner of commerce and merchandise, which maintains their present estate, is not fertility of soyl, but industry that enricheth them ; the gold mines of Peru or Nova Hispania may not compare with them. They have neither gold nor silver of their own, wine nor oyl, or scarce any corn growing in those United Provinces, little or

---

[1] Increment. urb. lib. 1. cap. 9.   [2] Angliæ, excepto Londino, nulla est civitas memorabilis, licet ea natio rerum omnium copiâ abundet.   [3] Cosmog. lib. 3. cap. 119. Villarum non est numerus ; nullus locus otiosus, aut incultus. [4] Chytreus, orat. edit. Francof. 1583.   [5] Maginus Geog.   [6] Ortelius e Vasco et Pet. de Medina.   [7] A hundred families in each.

78   DEMOCRITUS TO THE READER.

no wood, tin, lead, iron, silk, wooll, any stuff almost, or mettle ;
and yet Hungary, Transilvania, that brag of their mines, fertile
England, cannot compare with them. I dare boldly say, that
neither France, Tarentum, Apulia, Lombardy, or any part
of Italy, Valence in Spain, or that pleasant Andalusia, with
their excellent fruits, wine, and oyl, two harvests—no, not any
part of Europe, is so flourishing, so rich, so populous, so full
of good ships, of well built cities, so abounding with all things
necessary for the use of man. 'Tis our Indies, an epitome of
China, and all by reason of their industry, good policy, and
commerce. Industry is a loadstone to draw all good things ;
that alone makes countreys flourish, cities populous, [1] and will
enforce, by reason of much manure which necessarily follows,
a barren soyl to be fertile and good, as sheep (saith [2] Dion)
mend a bad pasture.

Tell me, politicians, why is that fruitful Palestina, noble
Greece, Ægypt, Asia Minor, so much decayed, and (meer
carcasses now) faln from that they were? The ground is the
same; but the government is altered; the people are grown
slothful, idle; their good husbandry, policy, and industry, is
decayed. *Non fatigata aut effeta humus ;* (as [3] Columella well
informs Sylvinus) *sed nostrâ fit inertiâ,* &c. May a man believe that which Aristotle in his Politicks, Pausanias, Stephanus, Sophianus, Gerbelius, relate of old Greece? I find heretofore 70 cities in Epirus (overthrown by Paulus Æmilius), a
goodly province in times past, [4] now left desolate of good
towns, and almost inhabitants—62 cities in Macedonia, in
Strabo's time. I find 30 in Laconia, but now scarce so many
villages, saith Gerbelius. If any man, from Mount Täygetus,
should view the countrey round about, and see *tot delicias,
tot urbes per Peloponnesum dispersas,* so many delicate and
brave built cities, with such cost and exquisite cunning, so
neatly set out in Peloponnesus, [5] he should perceive them now
ruinous and overthrown, burnt, waste, desolate, and laid level
with the ground. *Incredibile dictu, &c.* And as he laments,
*Quis, talia fando, Temperet a lacrymis? Quis tam durus aut
ferreus,* (so he prosecutes it) who is he that can sufficiently
condole and commiserate these ruines? Where are those 4000
cities of Ægypt, those 100 cities in Crete? Are they now come
to two? What saith Pliny, and Ælian, of old Italy? There were,
in former ages, 1166 cities: Blondus and Machiavel both grant

---

[1] Populi multitudo diligenti culturâ fecundat solum. Boter. l. 8. c. 3.   [2] Orat.
35. Terra ubi oves stabulantur, optima agricolis ob stercus.   [3] De re rust. l. 2.
cap. 1.   [4] Hodie urbibus desolatur, et magnâ ex parte incolis destituitur.
Gerbelius, desc. Græciæ, lib. 6.   [5] Videbit eas fere omnes aut eversas, aut
solo æquatas, aut in rudera fœdissime dejectas. Gerbelius.

2

DEMOCRITUS TO THE READER. 79

them now nothing near so populous and full of good towns, as
in the time of Augustus (for now Leander Albertus can find
but 300 at most), and, if we may give credit to [1] Livy, not then
so strong and puissant as of old: *They mustered* 70 *legions
in former times, which now the known world will scarce yield.*
Alexander built 70 cities in a short space for his part; our
sultans and Turks demolish twice as many, and leave all
desolate. Many will not believe but that our island of Great
Britain is now more populous than ever it was: yet let them
read Bede, Leland, and others; they shall find it most
flourished in the Saxon Heptarchy, and in the Conquerors
time was far better inhabited, than at this present. See that
Doomsday-Book: and shew me those thousands of parishes,
which are now decayed, cities ruined, villages depopulated,
&c. The lesser the territory is, commonly the richer it is—
parvus, sed bene cultus, ager—as those Athenian, Lacedæmonian, Arcadian, Elean, Sicyonian, Messenian, &c. common-
wealths of Greece make ample proof—as those imperial cities
and free states of Germany may witness—those cantons of
Switzers, Rhæti, Grisons, Walloons, territories of Tuscany,
Lucca and Sienna of old, Piedmont, Mantua, Venice in Italy,
Raguse, &c.

That prince, therefore, (as [2] Boterus adviseth) that will have
a rich countrey, and fair cities, let him get good trades, privileges, painful inhabitants, artificers, and suffer no rude matter
unwrought, as tin, iron, wool, lead, &c. to be transported out
of his countrey—[3] a thing in part seriously attempted amongst
us, but not effected. And, because industry of men, and
multitude of trade, so much avails to the ornament and en-
riching of a kingdom, those ancient [4] Massilians would admit
no man into their city that had not some trade. Selym the
First, Turkish emperour, procured a thousand good artificers
to be brought from Tauris to Constantinople. The Polanders
indented with Henry duke of Anjou, their new chosen king,
to bring with him an hundred families of artificers into Poland.
James the First in Scotland (as [5] Buchanan writes) sent for the
best artificers he could get in Europe, and gave them great
rewards to teach his subjects their several trades. Edward
the Third, our most renowned king, to his eternal memory,
brought cloathing first into this island, transporting some
families of artificers from Gaunt hither. How many goodly
cities could I reckon up, that thrive wholly by trade, where

[1] Lib. 7. Septuaginta olim legiones scriptæ dicuntur; quas vires hodie, &c.
[2] Polit. l. 3. c. 8.   [3] For dying of cloaths, and dressing, &c.   [4] Valer.
lib. 2. c. 1.   [5] Hist. Scot. lib. 10. Magnis propositis præmiis, ut Scoti ab
iis edocerentur.

80   DEMOCRITUS TO THE READER.

thousands of inhabitants live singular well by their fingers ends,
as Florence in Italy by making cloth of gold ; great Milan by
silk, and all curious works; Arras in Artois by those fair
hangings; many cities in Spain, many in France, Germany,
have none other maintenance, especially those within the land.
[1] Mecha, in Arabia Petræa, stands in a most unfruitful countrey, that wants water, amongst the rocks (as Vertomannus
describes it) ; and yet it is a most elegant and pleasant city,
by reason of the traffick of the east and west.   Ormus, in
Persia, is a most famous mart-town, hath nought else but
the opportunity of the haven to make it flourish.   Corinth,
a noble city, (*lumen Græciæ*, Tully calls it) the eye of
Greece, by reason of Cenchreas and Lecheus, those excellent ports, drew all the traffick of the Ionian and Ægean seas
to it; and yet the countrey about it was *curva et superciliosa*,
(as [2] Strabo terms it) rugged and harsh.   We may say the
same of Athens, Actium, Thebes, Sparta, and most of
those towns in Greece.   Noremberg in Germany is sited in a
most barren soil, yet a noble imperial city, by the sole industry of artificers, and cunning trades : they draw the riches
of most countreys to them ; so expert in manufactures, that, as
Sallust long since gave out of the like, *sedem animæ in extremis digitis habent ;* their soul, or *intellectus agens*, was
placed in their fingers ends; and so we may say of Basil, Spire,
Cambray, Francfurt, &c.   It is almost incredible to speak
what some write of Mexico, and the cities adjoyning to it:
no place in the world, at their first discovery, more populous.
[3] Mat. Riccius the Jesuite, and some others, relate of the industry of the Chinaes most populous countreys, not a beggar,
or an idle person to be seen, and how by that means they
prosper and flourish.   We have the same means—able bodies,
pliant wits, matter of all sorts, wooll, flax, iron, tin, lead,
wood, &c. many excellent subjects to work upon: only industry is wanting.   We send our best commodities beyond the
seas, which they can make good use of to their necessities, set
themselves a work about, and severally improve, sending the
same to us back at dear rates, or else make toyes and bables
of the tails of them, which they sell to us again, at as great a
reckoning as they bought the whole.   In most of our cities,
some few excepted, like [4] Spanish loyterers, we live wholly
by tipling : inns and ale-houses, malting, are their best

---

[1] Munst. cosm. l. 5. c. 74 : Agro omnium rerum infecundissimo, aquâ indigente
inter saxeta, urbs tamen elegantissima, ob orientis negotiationes et occidentis.
[2] Lib. 8. Geogr. ob asperum situm.   [3] Lib. Edit. a Nic. Tregant. Belg.
A. 1616 expedit. in Sinas.   [4] Ubi nobiles probri loco habent artem aliquam
profiteri.   Clenard. ep. l. 1.

DEMOCRITUS TO THE READER. 81

ploughs; their greatest traffick, to sell ale. [1]Meteran and some others object to us, that we are no whit so industrious as the Hollanders: *Manual trades,* (saith he) *which are more curious or troublesome, are wholly exercised by strangers: they dwell in a sea full of fish; but they are so idle, they will not catch so much as shall serve their own turns, but buy it of their neighbours.* Tush! [2]*Mare liberum:* they fish under our noses, and sell it to us, when they have done, at their own prices.

———Pudet hæc opprobria nobis
Et dici potuisse et non potuisse refelli.

I am ashamed to hear this objected by strangers; and know not how to answer it.

Amongst our towns there is only [3] London that bears the face of a city—[4] *epitome Britanniæ,* a famous *emporium,* second to none beyond seas, a noble mart: but *sola crescit, decrescentibus aliis;* and yet, in my slender judgment, defective in many things. The rest ([5]some few excepted) are in mean estate, ruinous most part, poor and full of beggars, by reason of their decayed trades, neglected or bad policy, idleness of their inhabitants, and riot, which had rather beg or loyter, and be ready to starve, than work.

I cannot deny, but that something may be said in defence of our cities, [6]that they are not so fair built, (for the sole magnificence of this kingdom, concerning buildings, hath been of old in those Norman castles and religious houses) so rich, thick sited, populous, as in some other countreys. Besides the reasons Cardan gives, (*Subtil. Lib.* 11.) we want wine and oyl, their two harvests; we dwell in a colder air, and, for that cause, must a little more liberally [7] feed of flesh, as all Northern countreys do. Our provision will not therefore extend to the maintenance of so many : yet, notwithstanding, we have matter of all sorts, an open sea for traffick, as well as the rest, goodly havens. And how can we excuse our negligence,

---

[1] Lib. 13. Belg. Hist. Non tam laboriosi, ut Belgæ, sed, ut Hispani, otiatores, vitam ut plurimum otiosam agentes: artes manuariæ, quæ plurimum habent in se laboris et difficultatis, majoremque requirunt industriam, a peregrinis et exteris exercentur: habitant in piscosissimo mari ; interea tantum non piscantur quantum insulæ suffecerit, sed a vicinis emere coguntur. [2] Grotii Liber. [3] Urbs animis numeroque potens, et robore gentis. Scaliger. [4] Camden. [5] York, Bristow, Norwich, Worcester, &c. [6] M. Gainsfords argument, "Because gentlemen dwell with us in the countrey villages, our cities are less," is nothing to the purpose. Put 300 or 400 villages in a shire, and every village yield a gentleman: what is 400 families to encrease one of our cities or to contend with theirs, which stand thicker? and whereas ours usually consist of 7000, theirs consist of 40000 inhabitants. [7] Maxima pars victûs in carne consistit. Polyd. Lib. 1. Hist.

VOL. I.   G

DEMOCRITUS TO THE READER.

our riot, drunkenness, &c. and such enormities that follow it? We have excellent laws enacted, (you will say) severe statutes, houses of correction, &c.—to small purpose, it seems; it is not houses will serve, but cities of correction : [1] our trades generally ought to be reformed, wants supplyed. In other countreys, they have the same grievances, I confess, (but that doth not excuse us) [2] wants, defects, enormities, idle drones, tumults, discords, contention, law-suits, many laws made against them to repress those innumerable brawls and law-suits, excess in apparel, diet, decay of tillage, depopulations, [3] especially against rogues, beggars, Ægyptian vagabonds (so termed at least) which have [4] swarmed all over Germany, France, Italy, Poland, (as you may read in [5] Munster, Cranzius, and Aventinus) as those Tartars and Arabians at this day do in the eastern countreys—yet, (such hath been the iniquity of all ages) as it seems, to small purpose. *Nemo in nostrâ civitate mendicus esto,* saith Plato : he will have them purged from a [6] common-wealth, [7] *as a bad humour from the body,* that are like so many ulcers and boils, and must be cured before the melancholy body can be eased.

What Carolus Magnus, the Chinese, the Spaniards, the duke of Saxony, and many other states, have decreed in this case, read *Arnisæus, cap.* 19. *Boterus, libro* 8, *cap.* 2. *Osorius de rebus gestis Eman. lib.* 11. When a countrey is overstored with people, as a pasture is oft over-laid with cattle, they had wont in former times to disburden themselves, by sending out colonies, or by wars, as those old Romans; or by employing them at home about some publick buildings, as bridges, rode-wayes, (for which those Romans were famous in this island) as Augustus Cæsar did in Rome, the Spaniards in their Indian mines, as at Potosa in Peru, where some thirty thousand men are still at work, six thousand furnaces ever boyling, &c. [8] aqueducts, bridges, havens, those stupend works of Trajan, Claudius at [9] Ostium, Dioclesiani Thermæ, Fucinus Lacus, that Piræeum in Athens, made by Themistocles, amphitheatrums of curious marble, as at Verona, Cevitas Philippi, and Heraclea in Thrace, those Appian and Flaminian wayes, prodigious works all may witness; and

---

[1] Refrænate monopolii licentiam ; pauciores alantur otio ; redintegretur agricolatio ; lanificium instauretur ; ut sit honestum negotium, quo se exerceat otiosa illa turba. Nisi his malis medentur, frustra exercent justitiam. Mor. Utop. Lib. I. [2] Mancipiis locuples, eget æris Cappadocum rex. Hor. [3] Regis dignitatis non est exercere imperium in mendicos, sed in opulentos. Non est regni decus, sed carceris esse custos. Idem. [4] Colluvies hominum mirabilis, excocti sole, immundi veste, fœdi visu, furtis imprimis acres, &c. [5] Cosmog. lib. 3. c. 5. [6] Seneca. Haud minus turpia principi multa supplicia, quam medico multa funera. [7] Ut pituitam et bilem a corpore, (11 de leg.) omnes vult exterminari. [8] See Lipsius, Admiranda. [9] De quo Suet. in Claudio ; et Plinius, c. 36.

DEMOCRITUS TO THE READER. 83

(rather than they should be [1] idle) as those [2] Ægyptian Pharaohs, Mœris, and Sesostris, did, to task their subjects to
build unnecessary pyramids, obelisks, labyrinths, chanels,
lakes, gigantian works all, to divert them from rebellion, riot,
drunkenness; [3] *quo scilicet alantur, et ne vagando laborare
desuescant.*

Another eye-sore is that want of conduct and navigable
rivers,—a great blemish, (as [4] Boterus, [5] Hippolytus a Collibus, and other politicians hold) if it be neglected in a common-wealth. Admirable cost and charge is bestowed in the
Low-Countreys on this behalf, in the Duchy of Milan, territory of Padua, in [6] France, Italy, China, and so likewise
about corrivations of waters, to moisten and refresh barren
grounds, to drean fens, bogs, and moors. Massinissa made
many inward parts of Barbary and Numidia in Africk (before his time incult and horrid) fruitful and bartable by this
means. Great industry is generally used all over the eastern
countreys in this kind, especially in Ægypt, about Babylon
and Damascus, (as Vertomannus and [7] Gotardus Arthus relate) about Barcelona, Segovia, Murcia, and many other
places of Spain, Milan in Italy: by reason of which, their
soil is much improved, and infinite commodities arise to the
inhabitants.

The Turks of late attempted to cut that Isthmos betwixt
Africk and Asia, which [8] Sesostris and Darius, and some Pharaohs of Ægypt had formerly undertaken, but with ill success
(as [9] Diodorus Siculus records, and Pliny); for that the Red-
sea, being three [10] cubits higher than Ægypt, would have
drowned all the countrey, *cœpto destiterant,* they left off.
Yet (as the same [11] Diodorus writes) Ptolemy renewed the
work many years after, and absolved it in a more opportune
place.

That Isthmos of Corinth was likewise undertaken to be made
navigable by Demetrius, by Julius Cæsar, Nero, Domitian,
Herodes Atticus, to make a speedy [12] passage, and less dangerous, from the Ionian and Ægæan seas: but, because it could
not be so well effected, the Peloponnesians built a wall, like our
Picts wall, about Schœnus where Neptunes temple stood, and

---

[1] Ut egestati simul et ignaviæ occurratur, opificia condiscantur, tenues suble-
ventur. Bodin. l. 6. c. 2. num. 6, 7.   [2] Amasis, Ægypti rex, legem promulga-
vit, ut omnes subditi quotannis rationem redderent unde viverent.   [3] Buscoldus,
discursu polit. cap. 2.   [4] Lib. 1. de increm. urb. cap. 6.   [5] Cap. 5. de increm.
urb. Quas flumen, lacus, aut mare, alluit.   [6] Incredibilem commoditatem,
vecturâ mercium, tres fluvii navigabiles, &c. Boterus, de Galliâ.   [7] Herodotus.
[8] Ind. Orient. cap. 2. Rotam in medio flumine constituunt, cui ex pellibus animalium consutos utres appendunt: hi, dum rota movetur, aquam per canales, &c.
[9] Centum pedes lata fossa, 30 alta.   [10] Contrary to that of Archimedes, who
holds the superficies of all waters even.   [11] Lib. 1. cap. 3.   [12] Dion.
Pausanias, et Nic. Gerbelius, Munster. Cosm. lib. 4. cap. 36. Ut brevior foret navigatio, et minus periculosa.

G 2

DEMOCRITUS TO THE READER.

in the shortest cut over the Isthmos, (of which Dicdorus, lib. 11. Herodotus, lib. 8. Uran.—our later writers call it Hexamilium) which Amurath the Turk demolished, the Venetians, anno 1453, repaired in fifteen dayes with thirty thousand men. Some, saith Acosta, would have a passage cut from Panama to Nombre de Dios in America: but Thuanus and Serres, the French historians, speak of a famous aqueduct in France, intended in Henry the Fourths time, from the Loyr to the Seine, and from Rhodanus to Loyr, the like to which was formerly assayed by Domitian the emperour, [1] from Arar to Mosella, (which Cornelius Tacitus speaks of in the thirteenth of his Annals), after by Charles the great, and others. Much cost hath in former times been bestowed in either new making or mending chanels of rivers, and their passages, (as Aurelianus did by Tiber to make it navigable to Rome, to convey corn from Ægypt to the city: *vadum alvei tumentis effodit,* saith Vopiscus, *et Tiberis ripas extruxit;* he cut fords, made banks, &c.) decayed havens, which Claudius the emperour, with infinite pains and charges, attempted at Ostia, (as I have said) the Venetians at this day, to preserve their city. Many excellent means, to enrich their territories, have been fostered, invented in most provinces of Europe, as planting some Indian plants amongst us; silk-worms; [2] the very mulberry leaves in the plains of Granado yield thirty thousand crowns *per annum* to the king of Spains coffers, besides those many trades and artificers that are busied about them in the kingdom of Granado, Murcia, and all over Spain. In France, a great benefit is raised by salt, &c. Whether these things might not be as happily attempted with us, and with like success, it may be controverted — silk-worms (I mean), vines, fir-trees, &c. Cardan exhorts Edward the Sixth to plant olives, and is fully perswaded they would prosper in this island. With us, navigable rivers are most part neglected. Our streams are not great, I confess, by reason of the narrowness of the island: yet they run smoothly and even, not headlong, swift, or amongst rocks and shelves, as foaming Rhodanus and Loyr in France, Tigris in Mesopotamia, violent Durius in Spain, with cataracts and whirl-pools, as the Rhine, and Danubius, about Schafhausen, Lausenburgh, Linz, and Cremmes, to endanger navigators; or broad shallow, as Neckar in the Palatinate, Tibris in Italy; but calm and fair as Arar in France, Hebrus in Macedonia, Eurotas in Laconia: they gently glide along, and might as well be repaired, many of them, (I mean Wie, Trent, Ouse, Thamisis at Oxford, the

---

[1] Charles the great went about to make a channel from Rhine to Danubius. Bil. Pirkimerus, descript. Ger. the ruins are yet seen about Wessemberg, from Rednich to Altemul. Ut navigabilia inter se Occidentis et Septentrionis litora fierent.   [2] Maginus, Geogr. Simlerus, de rep. Helvet. lib. 1. descript.

DEMOCRITUS TO THE READER. 85

defect of which we feel in the mean time) as the river of Lee
from Ware to London. B. Atwater of old, or (as some will)
Henry the first, [1] made a chanel from Trent to Lincoln,
navigable; which now, saith Mr. Cambden, is decayed: and
much mention is made of anchors, and such like monuments,
found about old [2] Verulamium: good ships have formerly come
to Exeter, and many such places, whose chanels, havens, ports,
are now barred and rejected. We contemn this benefit of
carriage by waters, and are therefore compelled, in the inner
parts of this island, because portage is so dear, to eat up our
commodities our selves, and live like so many boars in a sty,
for want of vent and utterance.

We have many excellent havens, royal havens, Falmouth,
Portsmouth, Milford, &c.—equivalent, if not to be preferred,
to that Indian Havana, old Brundusium in Italy, Aulis in
Greece, Ambracia in Acarnania, Suda in Crete,—which have
few ships in them, little or no traffick or trade, which have
scarce a village on them, able to bear great cities: *sed viderint politici.* I could here justly tax many other neglects,
abuses, errors, defects among us, and in other countreys—depopulations, riot, drunkenness, &c. and many such, *quæ nunc
in aurem susurrare non libet.* But I must take heed, *nequid
gravius dicam,* that I do not overshoot my self—*Sus Mi-
nervam*—I am forth of my element, as you peradventure suppose; and sometimes *veritas odium parit,* as he said; *verjuice
and oatmeal is good for a parret:* for, as Lucian said of an
historian, I say of a politician, he that will freely speak and
write, must be for ever no subject, under no prince or law, but
lay out the matter truly as it is, not caring what any can, will,
like or dislike.

We have good laws, (I deny not) to rectify such enormities; and so in all other countreys; but, it seems, not alwayes to good purpose. We had need of some general visitor
in our age that should reform what is amiss—a just army
of Rosie-cross men; for they will amend all matters, (they
say) religion, policy, manners, with arts, sciences, &c.—
another Attila, Tamberlane, Hercules, to strive with Ache-
loüs, *Augeæ stabulum purgare,* to subdue tyrants, as [3] he did
Diomedes and Busiris; to expel thieves, as he did Cacus and
Lacinius; to vindicate poor captives, as he did Hesione;
to pass the torrid zone, the desarts of Libya, and purge the
world of monsters and Centaures—or another Theban Crates
to reform our manners, to compose quarrels and controversies, as in his time he did, and was therefore adored for a god

---

[1] Camden, in Lincolnshire. Fossedike.   [2] Near S. Albons.   [3] Lilius
Girald. Nat. Comes.

86   DEMOCRITUS TO THE READER.

in Athens. *As Hercules [1] purged the world of monsters, and
subdued them, so did he fight against envy, lust, anger, avarice,
&c. and all those feral vices and monsters of the mind.* It
were to be wished we had some such visitor, or (if wishing
would serve) one had such a ring or rings, as Timolaüs desired in [2] Lucian, by vertue of which he should be as strong as
ten thousand men, or an army of gyants, go invisible, open
gates and castle doors, have what treasure he would, transport
himself in an instant to what place he desired, alter affections,
cure all manner of diseases, that he might range over the
world, and reform all distressed states and persons, as he
would himself. He might reduce those wandering Tartars in
order, that infest China on the one side, Muscovy, Poland,
on the other; and tame the vagabond Arabians that rob and
spoil those eastern countreys, that they should never use more
caravans, or janizaries to conduct them. He might root out
barbarism out of America, and fully discover *Terra Australis
Incognita;* find out the north-east and north-west passages;
drean those mighty Mæotian fens; cut down those vast Her-
cynian woods, irrigate those barren Arabian desarts, &c.
cure us of our epidemical diseases, *scorbutum, plica, morbus
Neapolitanus, &c.* end all our idle controversies; cut off our
tumultuous desires, inordinate lusts; root out atheism, im-
piety, heresie, schism and superstition, which now so crucifie the world; catechise gross ignorance, purge Italy of
luxury and riot, Spain of superstition and jealousie, Germany
of drunkenness, all our northern countreys of gluttony and intemperance; castigate our hard-hearted parents, masters, tutors; lash disobedient children, negligent servants; correct
these spendthrifts and prodigal sons; enforce idle persons to
work; drive drunkards off the ale-house; repress thieves, visit
corrupt and tyrannizing magistrates, &c. But, as L. Licinius
taxed Timolaüs, you may us. These are vain, absurd, and
ridiculous wishes; not to be hoped: all must be as it is.
[3] Boccalinus may cite common-wealths to come before Apollo,
and seek to reform the world it self by commissioners; but
there is no remedy; it may not be redressed: *desinent homines tum demum stultescere, quando esse desinent:* so long
as they can wag their beards, they will play the knaves and
fools.

Because, therefore, it is a thing so difficult, impossible, and
far beyond Hercules labours to be performed, let them be rude,

---

[1] Apuleius, lib. 4. Flor. Lar familiaris inter homines ætatis suæ cultus est, litium
omnium et jurgiorum inter propinquos arbiter et disceptator. Adversus iracundiam, invidiam, avaritiam, libidinem, cæteraque animi humani vitia et monstra
philosophus iste Hercules fuit. Pestes eas mentibus exegit omnes, &c.   [2] Votis
Navig.   [3] Ragguaglio, part 2. cap. 2. et part 3. c. 17.

DEMOCRITUS TO THE READER. 87

stupid, ignorant, incult: *lapis super lapidem sedeat;* and as
the [1] apologist will, *resp. tussi et graveolentiâ laboret, mundus vitio:* let them be barbarous as they are: let them [2] tyrannize, epicurize, oppress, luxuriate, consume themselves
with factions, superstitions, law-suits, wars and contentions,
live in riot, poverty, want, misery; rebel, wallow as so many
swine in their own dung, with Ulysses companions: *stultos
jubeo esse libenter.* I will yet, to satisfie and please my self,
make an Utopia of mine own, a new Atlantis, a poetical
common-wealth of mine own, in which I will freely domineer,
build cities, make laws, statutes, as I list my self. And why
may I not?

——————[3] pictoribus atque poëtis, &c.

You know what liberty poets ever had; and, besides, my predecessor Democritus was a politician, a recorder of Abdera, a
law-maker, as some say; and why may not I presume so much
as he did? Howsoever I will adventure. For the site, if you
will needs urge me to it, I am not fully resolved: it may be
in *Terra Australis Incognita;* there is room enough (for, of
my knowledge, neither that hungry Spaniard, [4] nor Mercurius
Britannicus, have yet discovered half of it) or else one of
those floating islands in *Mare del Zur,* which, like the Cyanean isles in the Euxine sea, alter their place, and are
accessible only at set times, and to some few persons; or one of
the Fortunate isles; for who knows yet where, or which they
are? There is room enough in the inner parts of America, and
northern coasts of Asia. But I will choose a site, whose
latitude shall be 45 degrees (I respect not minutes), in the
midst of the temperate zone, or perhaps under the æquator,
that [5] paradise of the world, *ubi semper virens laurus, &c.*
where is a perpetual spring. The longitude, for some reasons,
I will conceal. Yet *be it known to all men by these presents,*
that if any honest gentleman will send in so much money, as
Cardan allows an astrologer for casting a nativity, he shall be
a sharer; I will acquaint him with my project; or, if any
worthy man will stand for any temporal or spiritual office or
dignity, (for, as he said of his archbishoprick of Utopia, 'tis
sanctus ambitus, and not amiss to be sought after) it shall be
freely given, without all intercessions, bribes, letters, &c. his
own worth shall be the best spokesman; and (because we
shall admit of no deputies or advowsons) if he be sufficiently
qualified, and as able as willing to execute the place himself,
he shall have present possession. It shall be divided into

[1] Velent. Andreæ Apolog. manip. 604.   [2] Qui sordidus est, sordescat adhuc.
[3] Hor.   [4] Ferdinando Quir. 1612.   [5] Vide Acosta et Laet.

88   DEMOCRITUS TO THE READER.

twelve or thirteen provinces; and those, by hills, rivers, rode-
wayes, or some more eminent limits, exactly bounded. Each
province shall have a metropolis, which shall be so placed
as a center almost in a circumference, and the rest at equal
distances, some twelve Italian miles asunder, or thereabout;
and in them shall be sold all things necessary for the use
of man, *statis horis et diebus:* no market-towns, markets or
fairs; for they do but beggar cities (no village shall stand
above six, seven, or eight miles from a city) except those em-
poriums which are by the sea side, general staples, marts, as
Antwerp, Venice, Bergen of old, London, &c. Cities, most
part, shall be situate upon navigable rivers or lakes, creeks,
havens—and, for their form, regular, round, square, or long
square, [1]with fair, broad, and straight [2]streets, houses uniform,
built of brick and stone, like Bruges, Bruxels, Rhegium
Lepidi, Berna in Switzerland, Milan, Mantua, Crema, Cambalu in Tartary described by M. Polus, or that Venetian Palma.
I will admit very few or no suburbs, and those of baser
building, walls only to keep out man and horse, except it be
in some frontier towns, or by the sea side, and those to be
fortified [3]after the latest manner of fortification, and site upon
convenient havens, or opportune places. In every so built
city, I will have convenient churches, and separate places to
bury the dead in, not in church-yards—a citadella (in some,
not all) to command it, prisons for offenders, opportune
market-places of all sorts, for corn, meat, cattle, fuel, fish,
&c. commodious courts of justice, public halls for all societies, burses, meeting places, armories, [4]in which shall be
kept engines for quenching fire,—artillery gardens, publick
walks, theaters, and spacious fields allotted for all gymnicks,
sports, and honest recreations,—hospitals of all kinds for
children, orphans, old folks, sick men, mad men, souldiers,
—pest-houses, &c. (not built *precario*, or by gowty benefactors, who, when by fraud and rapine they have extorted all
their lives, oppressed whole provinces, societies, &c. give
something to pious uses, build a satisfactory alms-house,
school, or bridge, &c. at their last end, or before perhaps;
which is no otherwise than to steal a goose, and stick down
a feather, rob a thousand to relieve ten) and those hospitals
so built and maintained, not by collections, benevolences,
donaries, for a set number, (as in ours) just so many and no
more at such a rate, but for all those who stand in need, be
they more or less, and that *ex publico ærario*, and so still
maintained: *non nobis solum nati sumus, &c.* I will have

---

[1] Vide Patritium, lib. 8. tit. 10. de Instit. Reip.   [2] Sic olim Hippodamus
Milesius. Arist. polit. c. 11. et Vitruvius, l. 1. c. ult.   [3] With walls of earth, &c.
[4] De his. Plin. epist. 42. lib. 10. et Tacit. Annal. 13. lib.

DEMOCRITUS TO THE READER.   89

conduits of sweet and good water, aptly disposed in each
town, common [1] granaries, as at Dresden in Misnia, Stetein
in Pomerland, Noremberg, &c. colleges of mathematicians,
musicians, and actors, as of old at Lebedum in Ionia, [2] alchymists, physicians, artists and philosophers : that all arts and
sciences may sooner be perfected and better learned; and
publick historiographers, (as amongst those antient [3] Persians,
qui in commentarios referebant quæ memoratu digna gere-
bantur) informed and appointed by the state to register all
famous acts, and not by each insufficient scribler, partial or
parasitical pedant, as in our times. I will provide publick
schools, of all kinds, singing, dancing, fencing, &c. especially
of [4] grammar and languages, not to be taught by those tedious
precepts ordinarily used, but by use, example, conversation, as
travellers learn abroad, and nurses teach their children. As I
will have all such places, so will I ordain [5] publick governours,
fit officers to each place, treasurers, ædiles, quæstors, overseers of pupils, widows goods, and all publick houses, &c. and
those, once a year, to make strict accounts of all receipts,
expences, to avoid confusion; *et sic fiet ut non absumant,*
(as Pliny to Trajan) *quod pudeat dicere.* They shall be
subordinate to those higher officers, and governours of each
city, which shall not be poor tradesmen, and mean artificers,
but noblemen and gentlemen, which shall be tyed to residence
in those towns they dwell next, at such set times and seasons;
for I see no reason (which [6] Hippolytus complains of) *that it*
should be more dishonourable for noblemen to govern the city,
than the countrey, or unseemingly to dwell there now, than of
old. [7] I will have no bogs, fens, marishes, vast woods, desarts,
heaths, commons, but all inclosed (yet not depopulated, and
therefore take heed you mistake me not); for that which is
common, and every mans, is no mans : the richest countreys
are still inclosed, as Essex, Kent, with us, &c. Spain, Italy;
and where inclosures are least in quantity, they are best [8] hus-

---

[1] Vide Brisonium, de regno Pers. lib. 3. de his, et Vegetium, lib. 2. cap. 3. de
Annonâ.   [2] Not to make gold, but for matters of physick.   [3] Brisonius.
Josephus, lib. 21. antiq. Jud. cap. 6. Herod. lib. 3.   [4] So Lud. Vives thinks
best, Comminius, and others.   [5] Plato 3. de leg. Ædiles creari vult, qui fora,
fontes, vias, portus, plateas, et id genus alia procurent.—Vide Isaacum Ponta-
num, de civ. Amstel. hæc omnia, &c. Gotardum et alios.   [6] De increm. urb.
cap. 13. Ingenue fateor me non intelligere cur ignobilius sit urbes bene munitas
colere nunc quam olim, aut casæ rusticæ præesse quam urbi. Idem Ubertus
Foliot, de Neapoli.   [7] Ne tantillum quidem soli incultum relinquitur ; ut
verum sit ne pollicem quidem agri in his regionibus sterilem aut infecundum repe-
riri. Marcus Hemingius, Augustanus, de regno Chinæ, l.1. c. 3.   [8] M. Carew,
in his survey of Cornwall, saith, that, before that countrey was inclosed, the
husbandmen drank water, did eat little or no bread, fol. 66. lib. 1. their apparel
was coarse; they went bare-legged ; their dwelling was correspondent ; but since
inclosure, they live decently, and have money to spend : (fol. 23.) when their

90   DEMOCRITUS TO THE READER.

banded, as about Florence in Italy, Damascus in Syria, &c.
which are liker gardens than fields. I will not have a barren
acre in all my territories, no not so much as the tops of mountains : where nature fails, it shall be supplyed by art: [1]lakes
and rivers shall not be left desolate. All common high-wayes,
bridges, banks, corrivations of waters, aqueducts, chanels,
publick works, buildings, &c. out of a [2] common stock, curiously maintained and kept in repair; no depopulations, in-
grossings, alterations of wood, arable, but by the consent of
some supervisors, that shall be appointed for that purpose, to
see what reformation ought to be had in all places, what is
amiss, how to help it;

> Et quid quæque ferat regio, et quid quæque recuset;

what ground is aptest for wood, what for corn, what for cattle,
garden, orchyards, fishponds, &c. with a charitable division in
every village, (not one domineering house greedily to swallow
up all, which is too common with us) what for lords, [3]what for
tenants: and, because they shall be better encouraged to improve such lands they hold, manure, plant trees, drean, fence,
&c. they shall have long leases, a known rent, and known fine,
to free them from those intolerable exactions of tyrannizing
landlords. These supervisors shall likewise appoint what
quantity of land in each manor is fit for the lords demesns,
what for holding of tenants, how it ought to be husbanded,

> ([4] Ut Magnetes equis, Minyæ, gens cognita remis,)

how to be manured, tilled, rectified, [5] and what proportion is
fit for all callings, because private possessors are many times
idiots, ill husbands, oppressors, covetous, and know not how
to improve their own, or else wholly respect their own, and
not publick good.

Utopian parity is a kind of government, to be wished for,
[6]rather than effected, *Respub. Christianopolitana,* Campanellas
City of the Sun, and that new Atlantis, witty fictions, but meer
chimeras: and Platos community in many things is impious,

---

fields were common, their wooll was coarse Cornish hair : but, since inclosure,
it is almost as good as Cotswol, and their soil much mended. Tusser, c. 52.
of his Husbandry, is of his opinion, one acre inclosed is worth three common.
The countrey inclosed I praise : The other delighteth not me ; For nothing of
wealth it doth raise, &c.   [1] Incredibilis navigiorum copia : nihilo pauciores
in aquis quam in continenti commorantur. M. Riccius, expedit. in Sinas, l. 1.
c. 3.   [2] To this purpose, Arist. polit. 2. c. 6. allows a third part of·their
revenews, Hippodamus half.   [3] Ita lex agraria olim Romæ.   [4] Lu-
canus, l. 6.   [5] Hic segetes, illic veniunt felicius uvæ ; Arborei fetus alibi,
atque injussa virescunt Gramina. Virg. I. Georg.   [6] Joh. Valent. Andreas,
Lord Verulam.

DEMOCRITUS TO THE READER.

absurd and ridiculous ; it takes away all splendor and magnificence. I will have several orders, degrees of nobility, and those [1] hereditary, not rejecting younger brothers in the mean time; for they shall be sufficiently provided for by pensions, or so qualified, brought up in some honest calling, they shall be able to live of themselves. I will have such a proportion of ground belonging to every barony : he that buyes the land, shall buy the barony : he that by riot consumes his patrimony, and antient demesns, shall forfeit his honours. As some dignities shall be hereditary, so some again by election or gift (besides free offices, pensions, annuities) like our bishopricks, prebends, the Bassas palaces in Turky, the [2] procurators houses, and offices in Venice, which (like the golden apple) shall be given to the worthiest and best deserving both in war and peace, as a reward of their worth and good service, as so many goals for all to aim at, (honos alit artes) and encouragements to others. For I hate those severe, unnatural, harsh, German, French, and Venetian decrees, which exclude plebeians from honours: be they never so wise, rich, vertuous, valiant, and well qualified, they must not be patritians, but keep their own rank : this is naturæ bellum inferre, odious to God and men: I abhor it. My form of government shall be monarchical ;

(————[3] nunquam libertas gratior exstat,
Quam sub rege pio, &c.)

few laws, but those severely kept, plainly put down, and in the mother tongue, that every man may understand. Every city shall have a peculiar trade or privilege, by which it shall be chiefly maintained: [4] and parents shall teach their children, (one of three at least) bring up and instruct them in the mysteries of their own trade. In each town, these several tradesmen shall be so aptly disposed, as they shall free the rest from danger or offence. Fire-trades, as smiths, forge-men, brewers, bakers, metal-men, &c. shall dwell apart by themselves ; dyers, tanners, fel-mongers, and such as use water, in convenient places by themselves : noisome or fulsome for bad smells, as butchers slaughter-houses, chandlers, curriers, in remote places, and some back lanes. Fraternities and companies I approve of, as merchants burses, colleges of druggers, physicians, musicians, &c. but all trades to be rated in the sale of wares, as our clerks of the market do bakers and brewers;

[1] So is it in the kingdom of Naples, and France.   [2] See Contarenus and Osorius de rebus gestis Emanuelis.   [3] Claudian, l. 7.   [4] Herodotus, Erato l. 6. Cum Ægyptiis Lacedæmonii in hoc congruunt, quod eorum præcones, tibicines, coqui, et reliqui artifices, in paterno artificio succedunt, et coquus a coquo gignitur, et paterno opere perseverat. Idem Marcus Polus, de Quinzay. Idem Osorius, de Emanuele rege Lusitano. Riccius, de Sinis.

DEMOCRITUS TO THE READER.

corn it self, what scarcity soever shall come, not to exceed such a price. Of such wares as are transported or brought in, [1] if they be necessary, commodious, and such as nearly concern mans life, as corn, wood, cole, &c. and such provision we cannot want, I will have little or no custom paid, no taxes; but for such things as are for pleasure, delight, or ornament, as wine, spice, tobacco, silk, velvet, cloth of gold, lace, jewels, &c. a greater impost. I will have certain ships sent out for new discoveries every year, [2] and some discreet men appointed to travel into all neighbour kingdoms by land, which shall observe what artificial inventions and good laws are in other countreys, customs, alterations, or ought else, concerning war or peace, which may tend to the common good;—ecclesiastical discipline, *penes episcopos*, subordinate as the other: no impropriations, no lay patrons of church-livings, or one private man, but common societies, corporations, &c. and those rectors of benefices to be chosen out of the universities, examined and approved as the *literati* in China. No parish to contain above a thousand auditors. If it were possible, I would have such priests as should imitate Christ, charitable lawyers should love their neighbours as themselves, temperate and modest physicians, politicians contemn the world, philosophers should know themselves, noblemen live honestly, tradesmen leave lying and cozening, magistrates corruption, &c. But this is impossible; I must get such as I may. I will therefore have [3] of lawyers, judges, advocates, physicians, chyrurgions, &c. a set number; [4] and every man, if it be possible, to plead his own cause, to tell that tale to the judge, which he doth to his advocate, as at Fez in Africk, Bantam, Aleppo, Raguse, *suam quisque caussam dicere tenetur;*—those advocates, chyrurgions and [5] physicians, which are allowed to be maintained out of the [6] common treasure; no fees to be given or taken, upon pain of losing their places; or, if they do, very small fees, and when [7] the cause is fully ended. [8] He that sues any man shall put in a pledge, which if it be proved he hath wrongfully sued his

---

[1] Hippol. a Collibus, de increm. urb. c. 20. Plat. id. 7. de legibus. Quæ ad vitam necessaria, et quibus carere non possumus, nullum dependi vectigal, &c. [2] Plato, 12. de legibus, 40 annos natos vult, ut, si quid memorabile viderint apud exteros, hoc ipsum in rempub. recipiatur. [3] Simlerus, in Helvetiâ. [4] Utopienses caussidicos excludunt, qui caussas callide et vafre tractent et disputent. Iniquissimum censent hominem ullis obligari legibus, quæ aut numerosiores sunt quam ut perlegi queant, aut obscuriores quam ut a quovis possint intelligi. Volunt ut suam quisque caussam agat, eamque referat judici quam narraturus fuerat patrono: sic minus erit ambagum, et veritas facilius elicietur. Mor. Utop. l. 2. [5] Medici ex publico victum sumunt. Boter. l. l. c. 5. de Ægyptiis. [6] De his, lege Patrit. l. 3. tit. 8. de reip. Instit. [7] Nihil a clientibus patroni accipiant, priusquam lis finita est. Barcl. Argen. lib. 3. [8] It is so in most free cities in Germany.

DEMOCRITUS TO THE READER. 93

adversary, rashly or malitiously, he shall forfeit and lose. Or
else, before any suit begin, the plaintiff shall have his complaint approved by a set delegacy to that purpose : if it be of
moment, he shall be suffered, as before, to proceed; if otherwise, they shall determine it. All causes shall be pleaded *suppresso nomine*, the parties names concealed, if some circumstances do not otherwise require. Judges and other officers
shall be aptly disposed in each province, villages, cities, as
common arbitrators to hear causes, and end all controversies;
and those not single, but three at least on the bench at once, to
determine or give sentence; and those again to sit by turns or
lots, and not to continue still in the same office. No controversie
to depend above a year, but without all delayes and further
appeals, to be speedily dispatched, and finally concluded in that
time allotted. These and all other inferiour magistrates, to be
chosen [1] as the *literati* in China, or by those exact suffrages of
the [2] Venetians; and such again not be eligible, or capable of
magistracies, honours, offices, except they be sufficiently [3] qualified for learning, manners, and that by the strict approbation
of deputed examinators : [4] first, scholars to take place, then,
souldiers; for I am of Vegetius his opinion, a scholar deserves
better than a souldier, because *unius ætatis sunt quæ fortiter
fiunt, quæ vero pro utilitate reipub. scribuntur, æterna :* a
souldiers work lasts for an age, a scholars for ever. If they
[5] misbehave themselves, they shall be deposed, and accordingly punished; and, whether their offices be annual [6] or
otherwise, once a year they shall be called in question, and
give an account : for men are partial and passionate, merciless,
covetous, corrupt, subject to love, hate, fear, favour, &c. *omne
sub regno graviore regnum.* Like Solons Areopagites, or
those Roman censors, some shall visit others, and [7] be visited
invicem themselves ; [8] they shall oversee that no proling officer,
under colour of authority, shall insult over his inferiors, as so
many wild beasts, oppress, domineer, fley, grinde, or trample
on, be partial or corrupt, but that there be *æquabile jus,* justice equally done, live as friends and brethren together; and

---

[1] Matt. Riccius, exped. in Sinas, l. 1. c. 5, de examinatione electionum copiose
agit, &c. [2] Contar. de repub. Venet. l. 1. [3] Osor. l. 11. de reb. gest.
Eman. Qui in literis maximos progressus fecerint, maximis honoribus afficiuntur ;
secundus honoris gradus militibus assignatur ; postremi ordinis mechanicis. Doctorum hominum judiciis in altiorem locum quisque præfertur : et qui a plurimis
approbatur, ampliores in rep. dignitates consequitur. Qui in hoc examine primas
habet, insigni per totam vitam dignitate insignitur, marchioni similis, aut duci,
apud nos. [4] Cedant arma togæ. [5] As in Berna, Lucerne, Friburge
in Switzerland, a vitious liver is incapable of any office ; if a senator, instantly
deposed. Simlerus. [6] Not above three years, Aristot. polit. 5. c. 8.
[7] Nam quis custodiet ipsos custodes ? [8] Cytreus, in Greisgeia. Qui non
ex sublimi despiciant inferiores, nec ut bestias conculcent sibi subditos, auctori-
tatis nomini confisi, &c.

94 DEMOCRITUS TO THE READER.

(which [1] Sesellius would have and so much desires in his kingdom of France) *a diapason and sweet harmony of kings, princes, nobles, and plebeians, so mutually tyed and involved in love, as well as laws and authority, as that they never disagree, insult, or encroach one upon another.* If any man deserve well in his office, he shall be rewarded;

————quis enim virtutem amplectitur ipsam,
Præmia si tollas ?————

He that invents any thing for publick good in any art or science, writes a treatise, [2] or performs any noble exploit at home or abroad, [3] shall be accordingly enriched, [4] honoured, and preferred. I say, with Hannibal in Ennius, *Hostem qui feriet, mihi erit Carthaginiensis:* let him be of what condition he will in all offices, actions, he that deserves best shall have best.

Tilianus, in Philonius, (out of a charitable mind no doubt) wisht all his books were gold and silver, jewels and precious stones, [5] to redeem captives, set free prisoners, and relieve all poor distressed souls that wanted means: religiously done, I deny not; but to what purpose? Suppose this were so well done, within a little after, though a man had Crœsus wealth to bestow, there would be as many more. Wherefore I will suffer no [6] beggars, rogues, vagabonds, or idle persons at all, that cannot give an account of their lives, how they [7] maintain themselves. If they be impotent, lame, blind, and single, they shall be sufficiently maintained in several hospitals, built for that purpose; if married and infirm, past work, or, by inevitable loss or some such like misfortune, cast behind,—by distribution of [8] corn, house-rent free, annual pensions or money, they shall be relieved, and highly rewarded for their good service they have formerly done: if able, they shall be enforced

---

[1] Sesellius de rep. Gallorum, lib. 1. et 2.   [2] Si quis egregium aut bello aut pace perfecerit. Sesel. l. l.   [3] Ad regendam rempub. soli literati admittuntur; nec ad eam rem gratiâ magistratuum aut regis indigent; omnia ab exploratâ cujusque scientiâ et virtute pendent. Riccius, l. l. c. 5.   [4] In defuncti locum eum jussit subrogari, qui inter majores virtute reliquis præiret; non fuit apud mortales ullum excellentius certamen, aut cujus victoria magis esset expetenda; non enim inter celeres, celerrimo, non inter robustos, robustissimo, &c.   [5] Nullum videres vel in hac vel in vicinis regionibus pauperem, nullum obæratum, &c.   [6] Nullus mendicus apud Sinas; nemini sano, quamvis oculis orbatus sit, mendicare permittitur: omnes pro viribus laborare coguntur; cæci molis trusatilibus versandis addicuntur: soli hospitiis gaudent, qui ad labores sunt inepti. Osor. l. 11. de reb. gest. Eman. Heming. de reg. Chin. l. l. c. 3. Gotard. Arth. Orient. Ind. descr.   [7] Alex. ab Alex. 3. c. 12.   [8] Sic olim Romæ. Isaac. Pontan. de his optime. Amstol. l. 2. c. 9.

2

DEMOCRITUS TO THE READER. 95

to work. [1] *For I see no reason* (as [2] he said) *why an epicure or idle drone, a rich glutton, a usurer, should live at ease, and do nothing, live in honour, in all manner of pleasures, and oppress others, when as, in the mean time, a poor labourer, a smith, a carpenter, an husbandman—that hath spent his time in continual labour, as an asse to carry burdens, to do the common-wealth good, and without whom we cannot live—shall be left in his old age to begg or starve, and lead a miserable life, worse than a jument.* As [3] all conditions shall be tied to their task, so none shall be over-tired, but have their set times of recreations and holidayes, *indulgere genio*, feasts and merry meetings, even to the meanest artificer, or basest servant, once a week to sing or dance, (though not all at once) or do whatsoever he shall please, (like [4] that *Saccarum festum* amongst the Persians, those Saturnals in Rome) as well as his master. [5] If any be drunk, he shall drink no more wine or strong drink in a twelve moneth after. A bankrupt shall be [6] *catademiatus in amphitheatro*, publickly shamed; and he that cannot pay his debts, if by riot or negligence he hath been impoverished, shall be for a twelve moneth imprisoned: if in that space his creditours be not satisfied, [7] he shall be hanged. He [8] that commits sacrilege, shall lose his hands; he that bears false witness, or is of perjury convict, shall have his tongue cut out, except he redeem it with his head. Murder, [9] adultery, shall be punished by death, [10] but not theft, except it be some more grievous offence, or notorious offenders: otherwise they shall be condemned to the gallies, mines, be his slaves whom they offended during their lives. I hate all hereditary slaves, and that *duram Persarum legem*, as [11] Brisonius calls it; or as

---

[1] Idem Aristot. pol. 5. c. 8. Vitiosum, quum soli pauperum liberi educantur ad labores, nobilium et divitum in voluptatibus et deliciis. [2] Quæ hæc injustitia, ut nobilis quispiam, aut fœnerator, qui nihil agat, lautam et splendidam vitam agat, otio et deliciis, quum interim auriga, faber, agricola, quo respub. carere non potest, vitam adeo miseram ducat, ut pejor quam jumentorum sit ejus conditio? Iniqua resp. quæ dat parasitis, adulatoribus, inanium voluptatum artificibus, generosis et otiosis, tanta munera prodigit, at contra agricolis, carbonariis, aurigis, fabris, &c. nihil prospicit, sed eorum abusa labore florentis ætatis, fame penset et ærumnis. Mor. Utop. l. 2. [3] In Segovià nemo otiosus, nemo mendicus, nisi per ætatem aut morbum opus facere non potest : nulli deest unde victum quærat, aut quo se exerceat. Cypr. Echovius Delit. Hispan. Nullus Genevæ otiosus, ne Septennis puer. Paulus Heuzner, Itiner. [4] Athenæus, l. 22, [5] Simlerus, de repub. Helvet. [6] Spartian. olim Romæ sic. [7] He that provides not for his family is worse than a thief. Paul. [8] Alfredi lex. Utraque manus et lingua præcidatur, nisi eam capite redemerit. [9] Si quis nuptam stuprârit, virga virilis ei præcidatur ; si mulier, nasus et auricula præcidatur. Alfredi lex. En leges ipsi Veneri Martique timendas ! [10] Pauperes non peccant, quum extremâ necessitate coacti rem alienam capiunt. Maldonat. summula quæst. 8. art. 3. Ego cum illis sentio qui licere putant a divite clam accipere, qui tenetur pauperi subvenire. Emmanuel Sa. Aphor. confess. [11] Lib. 2. de reg. Persarum.

96   DEMOCRITUS TO THE READER.

[1] Ammianus, *impendio formidatas et abominandas leges, per quas, ob noxam unius, omnis propinquitas perit :* hard law, that wife and children, friends and allies, should suffer for the fathers offence!

No man shall marry until he [2] be 25, no woman till she be 20, [3] *nisi aliter dispensatum fuerit.* If one [4] die, the other party shall not marry till six months after; and because many families are compelled to live niggardly, exhaust and undone by great dowers, [5] none shall be given at all, or very little, and that by supervisors, rated : they that are foul shall have a greater portion; if fair, none at all, or very little; [6] however, not to exceed such a rate as those supervisors shall think fit. And when once they come to those years, poverty shall hinder no man from marriage, or any other respect; [7] but all shall be rather inforced than hindered, [8] except they be [9] dismembred, or grievously deformed, infirm, or visited with some enormous hereditary disease, in body or mind; in such cases, upon a great pain or mulct, [10] man or woman shall not marry; other order shall be taken for them to their content. If people overbound, they shall be eased by [11] colonies.

[12] No man shall wear weapons in any city. The same attire shall be kept, and that proper to several callings, by which they shall be distinguished. [13] *Luxus funerum* shall be taken away, that intempestive expence moderated, and many others. Brokers, takers of pawns, biting usurers, I will not admit; yet, because *hic cum hominibus non cum diis agitur,* [14] we converse here with men, not with gods, and for the hardness of mens hearts, I will tolerate some kind of usury. If we were honest, I confess, *(si probi essemus)* we should have no use of it; but, being as it is, we must necessarily admit it. Howsoever most divines contradict it,

(Dicimus inficias ; sed vox ea sola reperta est)

---

[1] Lib. 24.   [2] Aliter Aristoteles—a man at 25, a woman at 20. polit.   [3] Lex olim Lycurgi, hodie Chinensium ; vide Plutarchum, Riccium, Hemmingium, Arniseum, Nevisanum, et alios de hac quæstione.   [4] Alfredus.   [5] Apud Lacones olim virgines sine dote nubebant.   Boter. l. 3. c. 3.   [6] Lege cautum non ita pridem apud Venetos, ne quis patritius dotem excederet 1500 coron. [7] Bux. Synag. Jud. Sic Judæi. Leo Afer, Africæ descript. ne sint aliter incontinentes, ob reipub. bonum, ut August. Cæsar. orat. ad cœlibes Romanos olim edocuit.   [8] Morbo laborans, qui in prolem facile diffunditur, ne genus humanum fœdâ contagione lædatur, juventute castratur : mulieres tales procul a consortio virorum ab. legantur, &c. Hector Boëthius, hist. lib. 1. de vet. Scotorum moribus.   [9] Speciossimi juvenes liberis dabunt operam.   Plato, 5. de legibus.   [10] The Saxons exclude dumb, blind, leprous, and such like persons, from all inheritance, as we do fools.   [11] Ut olim Romani, Hispani hodie, &c. [12] Riccius, lib. 11. cap. 5. de Sinarum expedit. Sic Hispani cogunt Mauros arma deponere.   So it is in most Italian cities.   [13] Idem Plato, 12. de legibus. It hath ever been immoderate. Vide Guil. Stuckium, antiq. convival. lib. 1. cap. 26.   [14] Plato, 9. de legibus.

DEMOCRITUS TO THE READER. 97

it must be winked at by politicians. And yet some great doctors approve of it, Calvin, Bucer, Zanchius, P. Martyr, because, by so many grand lawyers, decrees of emperours, princes, statutes, customs of common-wealths, churches approbations, it is permitted, &c. I will therefore allow it: but to no private persons, not to every man that will; to orphans only, maids, widows, or such as by reason of their age, sex, education, ignorance of trading, know not otherwise how to employ it; and those, so approved, not to let it out apart, but to bring their money to [1] a common bank which shall be allowed in every city, as in Genoua, Geneva, Noremberg, Venice, at [2] 5, 6, 7, not above 8 *per centum*, as the supervisors, or *ærarii præfecti*, shall think fit. [3] And, as it shall not be lawful for each man to be an usurer that will, so shall it not be lawful for all to take up money at use—not to prodigals and spendthrifts, but to merchants, young tradesmen, and such as stand in need, or know honestly how to imploy it, whose necessity, cause, and condition, the said supervisors shall approve of.

I will have no private monopolies, to enrich one man, and beggar a multitude—[4] multiplicity of offices, of supplying by deputies: weights and measures the same throughout, and those rectified by the *primum mobile*, and suns motion; three-score miles to a degree, according to observation: 1000 geometrical paces to a mile, five foot to a pace, twelve inches to a foot, &c. and, from measures known, it is an easie matter to rectifie weights, &c. to cast up all, and resolve bodies by algebra, stereometry.

I hate wars, if they be not *ad populi salutem*, upon urgent occasion.

Odimus accipitrem, quia semper vivit in armis.

[5] Offensive wars, except the cause be very just, I will not allow of: for I do highly magnifie that saying of Hannibal to Scipio, in [6] Livy—*It had been a blessed thing for you and us, if God had given that mind to our predecessours, that you had*

---

[1] As those Lombards beyond seas, (though with some reformation) mons pietatis, or bank of charity, (as Malines terms it, cap. 33. Lex mercat. part 2.) that lend money upon easie pawns, or take money upon adventure for mens lives. [2] That proportion will make merchandise increase, land dearer, and better improved, as he hath judicially proved in his tract of usury, exhibited to the Parliament anno 1621. [3] Hoc fere Zanchius, com. in 4. cap. ad Ephes. æquissimam vocat usuram et charitati Christianæ consentaneam, modo non exigant, &c. nec omnes dent ad fœnus, sed ii qui in pecuniis bona habent, et ob ætatem, sexum, artis alicujus ignorantiam, non possunt uti. Nec omnibus, sed mercatoribus, et iis qui honeste impendent, &c. [4] Idem apud Persas olim. Lege Brisonium. [5] Idem Plato, de legibus. [6] Lib. 30. Optimum quidem fuerat eam patribus nostris mentem a Diis datam esse, ut vos Italiæ, nos Africæ imperio contenti essemus. Neque enim Sicilia aut Sardinia satis digna pretia sunt pro tot classibus, &c.

VOL. I. H

98   DEMOCRITUS TO THE READER.

*been content with Italy, we with Africk. For neither Sicily
nor Sardinia are worth such cost and pains, so many fleets
and armies, or so many famous captains lives.* Omnia prius
tentanda: fair means shall first be tried. [1] *Peragit tranquilla
potestas, Quod violenta nequit.* I will have them proceed
with all moderation ; but (hear you !) Fabius my general, not
Minutius ; *nam* [2] *qui consilio nititur, plus hostibus nocet,
quam qui, sine animi ratione, viribus:* and, in such wars, to
abstain as much as is possible from [3] depopulations, burning
of towns, massacring of infants, &c. For defensive wars, I
will have forces still ready at a small warning, by land and sea,
a prepared navy, souldiers *in procinctu, et, quam* [4] *Bonfinius
apud Hungaros suos vult, virgam ferream,* and money,
which is *nervus belli,* still in a readiness and a sufficient
revenue, a third part (as in old [5] Rome and Egypt) reserved
for the common-wealth; to avoid those heavy taxes and impositions, as well to defray this charge of wars, as also all
other publick defalcations, expences, fees, pensions, repara-
tions, chaste sports, feasts, donaries, rewards, and entertainments. All things in this nature especially I will have ma-
turely done, and with great [6] deliberation : *ne quid* [7] *temere, ne
quid remisse, ac timide fiat. Sed quo feror hospes?* To prosecute the rest would require a volume. *Manum de tabellâ !*
I have been over-tedious in this subject : I could have here
willingly ranged ; but these straits wherein I am included will
not permit.

From common-wealths and cities, I will descend to families,
which have as many corrosives and molestations, as frequent
discontents, as the rest. Great affinity there is betwixt a
political and œconomical body ; they differ only in magnitude
and proportion of business (so Scaliger [8] writes): as they
have both, likely, the same period, as [9] Bodin and [10] Peucer
hold, out of Plato, six or seven hundred years, so, many times,
they have the same means of their vexation and overthrows ;
as, namely, riot, a common ruine of both, riot in building,
riot in profuse spending, riot in apparel, &c. be it in what kind
soever, it produceth the same effects. A [11] chorographer of ours,
speaking *obiter* of ancient families, why they are so frequent
in the north, continue so long, are so soon extinguished in the
south, and so few, gives no other reason but this, *luxus omnia*

---

[1] Claudian.   [2] Thucydides.   [3] A depopulatione agrorum, incendiis,
et ejusmodi factis immanibus. Plato.   [4] Hungar. dec. 1. lib. 9.   [5] Sesellius, lib. 2. de repub. Gal. valde enim est indecorum, ubi quid præter opinionem
accidit, dicere, Non putâram, præsertim si res præcaveri potuerit. Livius, lib. 1.
Dion. l. 2. Diodorus Siculus, lib. 2.   [6] Peragit tranquilla potestas, Quod
violenta nequit. Claudian.   [7] Bellum nec timendum nec provocandum.
Plin. Panegyr. Trajan.   [8] Lib. 3. poët. cap. 19.   [9] Lib. 4 de repub.
cap. 2.   [10] Peucer. lib. 1. de divinat.   [11] Camden, in Cheshire.

DEMOCRITUS TO THE READER. 99

dissipavit, riot hath consumed all. Fine cloaths and curious
buildings came into this island, as he notes in his annals, not
so many years since, *non sine dispendio hospitalitatis*, to the
decay of hospitality. Howbeit, many times that word is mistaken; and, under the name of bounty and hospitality, is
shrowded riot and prodigality; and, that which is commendable
in it self well used, hath been mistaken heretofore, is become,
by its abuse, the bane and utter ruine of many a noble family :
for some men live like the rich glutton, consuming themselves
and their substance by continual feasting and invitations,—
with [1] Axylos in Homer, keep open house for all comers, giving entertainment to such as visit them, [2] keeping a table beyond
their means, and a company of idle servants (though not so
frequent as of old)—are blown up on a sudden, and (as Actæon
was by his hounds) devoured by their kinsmen, friends, and
multitude of followers. [3] It is a wonder that Paulus Jovius
relates of our northern countreys, what an infinite deal of
meat we consume on our tables: that I may truly say, 'tis not
bounty, not hospitality, as it is often abused, but riot in excess,
gluttony and prodigality; a meer vice: it brings in debt, want,
and beggary, hereditary diseases, consumes their fortunes, and
overthrows the good temperature of their bodies. To this I
might here well add their inordinate expence in building those
phantastical houses, turrets, walks, parks, &c. gaming, excess
of pleasure, and that prodigious riot in apparel, by which
means they are compelled to break up house, and creep into
holes. Sesellius, in his Common wealth of [4] France, gives three
reasons why the French nobility were so frequently bankrupts ;
*First, because they had so many law-suits and contentions,
one upon another, which were tedious and costly : by which
means it came to pass, that commonly lawyers bought them
out of their possessions. A second cause was their riot ; they
lived beyond their means, and were therefore swallowed up
by merchants.* (La-Nove, a French writer, yields five reasons
of his countrey-mens poverty, to the same effect almost, and
thinks verily, if the gentry of France were divided into ten parts,
eight of them would be found much impaired by sales, mort-
gages, and debts, or wholly sunk in their estates.) *The last
was immoderate excess in apparel, which consumed their reve-*

---

[1] Iliad. lib. 6.   [2] Vide Puteani Comum ; Goclenium de portentosis cœnis
nostrorum temporum.   [3] Mirabile dictu est, quantum opsoniorum una
domus singulis diebus absumat ; sternuntur mensæ in omnes pene horas, calenti-
bus semper eduliis. Descript. Britan.   [4] Lib. 1. de rep. Gallorum. Quod
tot lites et caussæ forenses aliæ serantur ex aliis, in immensum producantur, et
magnos sumptus requirant ; unde fit ut juris administri plerumque nobilium pos-
sessiones adquirant........ Tum quod sumptuose vivant, et splendidissime vesti-
antur, et a mercatoribus absorbeantur, &c.

H 2

100   DEMOCRITUS TO THE READER.

nues. How this concerns and agrees with our present state,
look you. But of this elsewhere. As it is in a mans body—
if either head, heart, stomach, liver, spleen, or any one part be
misaffected, all the rest suffer with it—so is it with this œconomical body : if the head be naught, a spendthrift, a drunkard, a whoremaster, a gamester, how shall the family live at
ease ? [1] *Ipsa, si cupiat, Salus servare prorsus non potest hanc
familiam;* (as Demea said in the comedy) Safety herself cannot save it. A good, honest, painful man many times hath a
shrew to his wife—a sickly, dishonest, slothful, foolish, careless
woman to his mate—a proud, peevish flurt, a liquorish, prodigal
quean ; and by that means all goes to ruine : or, if they differ in
nature—he is thrifty, she spends all ; he wise, she sottish and
soft—what agreement can there be ? what friendship ? Like
that of the thrush and swallow in Æsop; instead of mutual
love, kind compellations, whore and thief is heard ; they fling
stools at one anothers heads. [2] *Quæ intemperies vexat hanc
familiam?* All enforced marriages commonly produce such
effects; or, if on their behalfs it be well, as to live and agree
lovingly together, they may have disobedient and unruly children, that take ill courses to disquiet them : [3] *their son is a
thief, a spendthrift, their daughter a whore;* a [4] stepmother,
or a daughter in law, distempers all; [5] or else for want of means,
many torturers arise—debts, dues, fees, dowries, joyntures, legacies to be paid, annuities issuing out; by means of which, they
have not wherewithall to maintain themselves in that pomp as
their predecessors have done, bring up or bestow their children
to their callings, to their birth and quality, [6] and will not descend to their present fortunes. Oftentimes too, to aggravate
the rest, concurr many other inconveniences—unthankful
friends, decayed friends, bad neighbours, negligent servants,
[7] *servi furaces, versipelles, callidi, occlusa sibi mille clavibus
reserant, furtimque raptant, consumunt, liguriunt)* casualties,
taxes, mulcts, chargeable offices, vain expences, entertainments,
loss of stock, enmities, emulations, frequent invitations, losses,
suretiship, sickness, death of friends, and (that which is the
gulf of all) improvidence, ill husbandry, disorder and confusion ; by which means they are drenched on a sudden in their
estates, and at unawares precipitated insensibly into an inex-
tricable labyrinth of debts, cares, woes, want, grief, discontent,
and melancholy it self.

---

[1] Ter.   [2] Amphit. Plaut.   [3] Paling. Filius aut fur.   [4] Catus cum
mure, duo galli simul in æde, et glotes binæ, nunquam vivunt sine lite.   [5] Res
angusta domi.   [6] When pride and beggary meet in a family, they roar and
howl, and cause as many flashes of discontents, as fire and water, when they concur, make thunder-claps in the skies.   [7] Plautus, Aulular.

DEMOCRITUS TO THE READER. 101

I have done with families, and will now briefly run over some few sorts and conditions of men. The most secure, happy, jovial, and merry in the worlds esteem, are princes and great men, free from melancholy; but, for their cares, miseries, suspicions, jealousies, discontents, folly, and madness, I refer you to Xenophons Tyrannus, where king Hieron discourseth at large with Simonides the poet, of this subject. Of all others, they are most troubled with perpetual fears, anxieties, insomuch, that (as he said in [1] Valerius) if thou knewest with what cares and miseries this robe were stuffed, thou wouldst not stoop to take it up. Or, put case they be secure and free from fears and discontents, yet they are void [2] of reason too oft, and precipitate in their actions. Read all our histories, *quas de stultis prodidere stulti*—Iliades, Æneides, Annales—and what is the subject?

> Stultorum regum et populorum continet æstus.

How mad they are, how furious, and upon small occasions, rash and inconsiderate in their proceedings, how they dote, every page almost will witness :

> ————delirant reges, plectuntur Achivi.

Next in place, next in miseries and discontents, in all manner of hairbrain'd actions, are great men: *procul a Jove, procul a fulmine :* the nearer, the worse. If they live in court, they are up and down, ebb and flow with their princes favours, *(Ingenium vultu statque caditque suo)* now aloft, to morrow down, (as [3] Polybius describes them) *like so many casting counters, now of gold, to morrow of silver, that vary in worth as the computant will; now they stand for unites, to morrow for thousands; now before all, and anon behind.* Beside, they torment one another with mutual factions, emulations: one is ambitious, another enamoured ; a third, in debt; a prodigal, over-runs his fortunes ; a fourth, solicitous with cares, gets nothing, &c. But, for these mens discontents, anxieties, I refer you to Lucians tract, *de mercede conductis,* [4] Æneas Sylvius, *(libidinis et stultitiæ servos,* he calls them) Agrippa, and many others. Of philosophers and scholars, *priscæ sapientiæ dictatores,* I have already spoken in general terms. Those superintendents of wit and learning, men above men, those refined men, minions of the Muses,

---

[1] Lib. 7. cap. 6.   [2] Pellitur in bellis sapientia ; vi geritur res. Vetus proverbium, Aut regem aut fatuum nasci oportere.   [3] Lib. 1. hist. Rom. similes abaculorum calculis, secundum computantis arbitrium, modo ærei sunt, modo aurei ; ad nutum regis, nunc beati sunt, nunc miseri.   [4] Ærumnosique Solones, in Sa. 3. De miser. curialium.

102   DEMOCRITUS TO THE READER.

———[1] mentemque habere queis bonam,
    Et esse [2] corculis, datum est,———

[3] these acute and subtil sophisters, so much honoured, have as
much need of hellebor as others.

————[4] O medici, mediam pertundite venam.

Read Lucians Piscator, and tell how he esteemed them;
Agrippas tract of the Vanity of Sciences; nay read their own
works, their absurd tenents, prodigious paradoxes, *et risum teneatis, amici?* You shall find that of Aristotle true, *nullum
magnum ingenium sine mixturâ dementiæ;* they have a worm,
as well as others : you shall find a phantastical strain, a fustian,
a bombast, a vainglorious humour, an affected stile, &c. like a
prominent thred in an uneven woven cloth, run parallel throughout their works ; and they that teach wisdom, patience, meekness, are the veryest dizards, hairbrains, and most discontent.
[5] *In the multitude of wisdom is grief; and he that encreaseth
wisdom, encreaseth sorrow.* I need not quote mine author.
They that laugh and contemn others, condemn the world of
folly, deserve to be mocked, are as giddy-headed, and lie as
open, as any other. [6] Democritus, that common flouter of folly,
was ridiculous himself: barking Menippus, scoffing Lucian,
satyrical Lucilius, Petronius, Varro, Persius, &c. may be censured with the rest; *Loripedem rectus derideat, Æthiopem
albus.* Bale, Erasmus, Hospinian, Vives, Kimnisius, explode,
as a vast ocean of Obs, and Sols, school divinity; [7] a labyrinth
of intricable questions, unprofitable contentions : *incredibilem
delirationem,* one calls it. If school divinity be so censured,
subtilis [8] *Scotus lima veritatis, Occam irrefragabilis, cujus
ingenium vetera omnia ingenia subvertit, &c.* Baconthrope,
Doctor Resolutus, and *Corculum Theologiæ,* Thomas himself,
Doctor [9] *Seraphicus, cui dictavit Angelus, &c.* what shall become of humanity ? *Ars stulta,* what can she plead ? what can
her followers say for themselves ; Much learning [10] *cere-dimi-
nuit-brum,* hath crackt their skonce, and taken such root, that
tribus Anticyris caput insanabile, hellebore it self can do no
good, nor that renowned [11] lanthorn of Epictetus, by which if
any man studied he should be as wise as he was. But all will
not serve. Rhetoricians, *in ostentationem loquacitatis, multa
agitant*—out of their volubility of tongue, will talk much to

---

[1] F. Dousæ Epid. lib. 1. c. 13.   [2] Hoc cognomento cohonestati Romæ,
qui cæteros mortales sapientiâ præstarent. Testis Plin. lib. 7. cap. 34.   [3] Insanire parant certâ ratione modoque : mad by the book, they.   [4] Juvenal.
[5] Solomon.   [6] Communis irrisor stultitiæ.   [7] Wit, whither wilt?
[8] Scaliger, exercitat. 324.   [9] Vit. ejus.   [10] Ennius.   [11] Lucian.
Ter mille drachmis olim empta ; studens inde sapientiam adipiscetur.

DEMOCRITUS TO THE READER. 103

no purpose. Orators can perswade other men what they will, *quo volunt, unde volunt*, move, pacifie, &c. but cannot settle their own brains. What saith Tully? *Malo indisertam prudentiam, quam loquacem stultitiam ;* and (as [1] Seneca seconds him) a wise mans oration should not be polite or solicitous. [2] Fabius esteems no better of most of them, either in speech, action, gesture, than as men beside themselves, *insanos declamatores;* so doth Gregory; *non mihi sapit qui sermone, sed qui factis, sapit.* Make the best of him, a good oratour is a turn-coat, an evil-man; *bonus orator pessimus vir ;* his tongue is set to sale; he is a meer voice (as [3] he said of a nightingal); *dat sine mente sonum;* an hyperbolical liar, a flatterer, a parasite, and (as [4] Ammianus Marcellinus will) a corrupting cosener, one that doth more mischief by his fair speeches, than he that bribes by money; for a man may with more facility avoid him that circumvents by money, than him that deceives with glosing terms; which made [5] Socrates so much abhor and explode them. [6] Fracastorius, a famous poet, freely grants all poets to be mad ; so doth [7] Scaliger ; and who doth not? (*Aut insanit homo, aut versus facit. Hor. Sat. 7. l. 2. Insanire lubet, i. e. versus componere, Virg. Ecl. 3.* So Servius interprets) all poets are mad, a company of bitter satyrists, detractors, or else parasitical applauders; and what is poetry it self, but (as Austin holds) *vinum erroris ab ebriis doctoribus propinatum ?* You may give that censure of them in general, which Sir Thomas Moore once did of Germanus Brixius poems in particular.

―――――――――――――vehuntur
In rate stultitiæ : sylvam habitant Furiæ.

Budæus, in an epistle of his to Lupsetus, will have civil law to be the tower of wisdom ; another honours physick, the quintessence of nature ; a third tumbles them both down, and sets up a flag of his own peculiar science. Your supercilious criticks, grammatical triflers, note-makers, curious antiquaries, find out all the ruines of wit, *ineptiarum delicias,* amongst the rubbish of old writers: [8] *pro stultis habent, nisi aliquid sufficiant invenire, quod in aliorum scriptis vertant vitio :* all fools with them that cannot find fault : they correct others, and are hot in a cold cause, puzzle themselves to find out how many streets in Rome, houses, gates, towers, Homers countrey, Æneas mother, Niobes daughters, *an Sappho publica fuerit ?*

[1] Epist. 21. 1. lib. Non oportet orationem sapientis esse politam aut solicitam. [2] Lib. 3. cap. 13. Multo anhelitu, jactatione, furentes, pectus, frontem cædentes, &c. [3] Lipsius, Voces sunt, præterea nihil. [4] Lib 30. Plus mali facere videtur qui oratione quam qui pretio quemvis corrumpit; nam, &c. [5] In Gorg. Platonis. [6] In Naugerio. [7] Si furor sit Lyæus, &c. quoties furit, furit, furit, amans, bibens, et poëta, &c. [8] Morus, Utop. lib. 11.

DEMOCRITUS TO THE READER.

ovum [1] *prius extiterit, an gallina? &c. et alia, quæ dediscenda essent, si scires,* as [2] Seneca holds—what clothes the senators did wear in Rome, what shews, how they sate, where they went to the close stool, how many dishes in a mess, what sauce; which, for the present, for an historian to relate, ([3] according to Lodovic. Vives) is very ridiculous, is to them most precious elaborate stuff, they admired for it, and as proud, as triumphant in the mean time for this discovery, as if they had won a city, or conquered a province; as rich as if they had found a mine of gold ore. *Quosvis auctores absurdis commentis suis percacant et stercorant,* one saith: they bewray and daub a company of books and good authors, with their absurd comments, *(correctorum sterquilinia* [4] Scaliger calls them) and shew their wit in censuring others,—a company of foolish note-makers, humble-bees, dors or beetles: *inter stercora ut plurimum versantur,* they rake over all those rubbish and dunghills, and prefer a manuscript many times before the Gospel itself, [5] *thesaurum criticum,* before any treasure, and with their *deleaturs, alii legunt sic, meus codex sic habet,* with their *postremæ editiones,* annotations, castigations, &c. make books dear, themselves ridiculous, and do no body good: yet, if any man dare oppose or contradict, they are mad, up in arms on a sudden; how many sheets are written in defence, how bitter invectives, what apologies? [6] *Epiphyllides hæ sunt et meræ nugæ.* But I dare say no more of, for, with, or against them, because I am liable to their lash, as well as others. Of these and the rest of our artists and philosophers, I will generally conclude, they are a kind of mad men, (as [7] Seneca esteems of them) to make doubts and scruples, how to read them truly, to mend old authors, but will not mend their own lives, or teach us *ingenia sanare, memoriam officiorum ingerere, ac fidem in rebus humanis retinere,* to keep our wits in order, or rectify our manners. *Numquid tibi non demens videtur, si istis operam impenderit?* is not he mad that draws lines with Archimedes, whilest his house is ransacked, and his city besieged, when the whole world is in combustion,—or we, whilest our souls are in danger, *(mors sequitur, vita fugit)* to spend our time in toyes, idle questions, and things of no worth?

That [8] lovers are mad, I think no man will deny. *Amare simul et sapere ipsi Jovi non datur;* Jupiter himself cannot intend both at once.

---

[1] Macrob. Satur. 7. 16. [2] Epist. 16. [3] Lib. de caussis corrup. artium.
[4] Lib. 2. in Ausonium, cap. 19. et 32. [5] Edit. 7. volum. Iano Grutero.
[6] Aristophanis Ranis. [7] Lib. de beneficiis. [8] Delirus et amens dicatur merito. Hor. Sene ca.

DEMOCRITUS TO THE READER.   105

[1] Non bene conveniunt, nec in unâ sede morantur,
     Majestas et amor.

Tully, when he was invited to a second marriage, replied,
he could not *simul amare et sapere,* be wise and love both
together.   [2] *Est Orcus ille; vis est immedicabilis; est rabies
insana:* love is madness, a hell, an incurable disease; *impo-
tentem et insanam libidinem* [3] Seneca calls it, an impotent and
raging lust.   I shall dilate this subject apart: in the mean
time let lovers sigh out the rest.

[4] Nevisanus the lawyer holds it for an axiome, *most women
are fools,* ([5] *consilium feminis invalidum*) Seneca, men, be they
young or old; who doubts it ? youth is mad, as Elius in Tully,
Stulti adolescentuli, old age little better, *deliri senes, &c.* Theophrastus, in the 107 year of his age, [6] said he then began to be
wise, *tum sapere cœpit,* and therefore lamented his departure.
If wisdom come so late, where shall we find a wise man ? our
old ones dote at threescore and ten.   I would cite more proofs
and a better author; but, for the present, let one fool point at
another.   [7] Nevisanus hath as hard an opinion of [8] rich men—
*wealth and wisdom cannot dwell together; stultitiam patiuntur
opes;* [9] and they do commonly [10] *infatuare cor hominis,* besot
men; and, as we see it, *fools have fortune:* [11] *sapientia non invenitur in terrâ suaviter viventium.*   For, beside a natural
contempt of learning, which accompanies such kind of men,
innate idleness, (for they will take no pains) and which [12] Aristotle observes, *ubi mens plurima, ibi minima fortuna; ubi
plurima fortuna, ibi mens perexigua;* great wealth and little
wit go commonly together : they have as much brains, some of
them, in their heads as in their heels; besides this inbred neglect
of liberal sciences, and all arts, which should *excolere mentem,*
polish the mind, they have most part some gullish humour or
other, by which they are led; one is an Epicure, an atheist, a
second a gamester, a third a whoremaster, (fit subjects all for
a satyrist to work upon)

———[13] Hic nuptarum insanit amoribus, hic puerorum ;—

[14] one is mad of hawking, hunting, cocking; another of ca-
rousing, horse-riding, spending; a fourth, of building, fighting, &c.

---

[1] Ovid. Met.   [2] Plutarch. Amatorio est amor insanus.   [3] Epist. 39.
[4] Sylvæ nuptialis. l. 1. num. 11. Omnes mulieres, ut plurimum, stultæ.   [5] Aristotle.   [6] Dolere se dixit, quod tum vitâ egrederetur.   [7] Lib. 1. num. 11.
Sapientia et divitiæ vix simul possideri possunt.   [8] They get their wisdom by
eating pie-crust, some.   [9] Χρηματα τοις θνητοις γινεται αφροσυνη. Opes quidem mortalibus sunt amentia. Theognis.   [10] Fortuna, nimium quem fovet,
stultum facit.   [11] Joh. 28.   [12] Mag. moral. lib. 2. et lib. 1. sat. 4.   [13] Hor.
ser. 1. sat. 4.   [14] Insana gula, insanæ obstructiones, insanum venandi
studium—Discordia demens. Virg. Æn.

Insanit veteres statuas Damasippus emendo ;

Damasippus hath an humour of his own, to be talkt of; [1] Heliodorus the Carthaginian, another. In a word, as Scaliger concludes of them all, they are *statuæ erectæ stultitiæ*, the very statues or pillars of folly. Chuse, out of all stories, him that hath been most admired ; you shall still find *multa ad laudem, multa ad vituperationem magnifica*, as [2] Berosus of Semiramis : *omnes mortales militiâ, triumphis, divitiis, &c. tum et luxu, cæde, cæterisque vitiis, antecessit :* as she had some good, so had she many bad parts.

Alexander, a worthy man, but furious in his anger, overtaken in drink: Cæsar and Scipio valiant and wise, but vainglorious, ambitious: Vespasian a worthy prince, but covetous: [3] Hannibal, as he had mighty vertues, so had he many vices ; *unam virtutem mille vitia comitantur*, as Machiavel of Cosmus Medices, he had two distinct persons in him. I will determine of them all, they are like these double or turning pictures ; stand before which, you see a fair maid on the one side, an ape on the other, an owle : look upon them at the first sight, all is well ; but farther examine, you shall find them wise on the one side, and fools on the other ; in some few things praise-worthy, in the rest incomparably faulty. I will say nothing of their diseases, emulations, discontents, wants, and such miseries ; let Poverty plead the rest in Aristophanes Plutus.

Covetous men, amongst others, are most mad ; [4] they have all the symptomes of melancholy—fear, sadness, suspicion, &c. as shall be proved in his proper place :

Danda est hellebori multo pars maxima avaris.

And yet, methinks, prodigals are much madder than they, be of what condition they will, that bear a publick, or private purse ; as a [5] Dutch writer censured Richard the rich duke of Cornwal, suing to be emperour, for his profuse spending, *qui effudit pecuniam ante pedes principum electorum sicut aquam*, that scattered money like water ; I do censure them. *Stulta Anglia*, (saith he) *quæ tot denariis sponte est privata ; stulti principes Alemaniæ, qui nobile jus suum pro pecuniâ vendiderunt*. Spend-thrifts, bribers, and bribe-takers, are fools ; and so are [6] all they that cannot keep, disburse, or spend, their moneys well.

---

[1] Heliodorus Carthaginiensis ad extremum orbis sarcophago testamento me hîc jussi condier, ut viderem an quis insanior ad me visendum usque ad hæc loca penetraret. Ortelius, in Gad. [2] If it be his work ; which Gasper Veretus suspects. [3] Livy. Ingentes virtutes ; ingentia vitia. [4] Hor. Quisquis ambitione malâ aut argenti pallet amore ; Quisquis luxuriâ, tristique superstitione. Per. [5] Chronica Slavonica, ad annum 1257, de cujus pecuniâ jam incredibilia dixerunt. [6] A fool and his money are soon parted.

DEMOCRITUS TO THE READER. 107

I might say the like of angry, peevish, envious, ambitious (*¹Anticyras melior sorbere meracas*), Epicures, atheists, schismaticks, hereticks: *hi omnes habent imaginationem læsam* (saith Nymannus); *and their madness shall be evident*, 2 Tim. 3. 9. ²Fabatus, an Italian, holds sea-faring men all mad; *the ship is mad, for it never stands still; the mariners are mad, to expose themselves to such imminent dangers: the waters are raging mad, in perpetual motion : the winds are as mad as the rest: they know not whence they come, whither they would go; and those men are maddest of all that go to sea: for one fool at home, they find forty abroad.* He was a mad man that said it; and thou, peradventure, as mad to read it. ³Felix Platerus is of opinion all alchymists are mad, out of their wits; ⁴Athenæus saith as much of fiddlers, *et Musarum luscinias* ⁵, musicians; *omnes tibicines insaniunt; ubi semel efflant, avolat illico mens;* in comes musick at one ear; out goes wit at another. Proud and vain glorious persons are certainly mad; and so are ⁶ lascivious; I can feel their pulses beat hither; horn mad some of them, to let others lye with their wives, and wink at it.

To insist ⁷ in all particulars, were an Herculean task, to ⁸ reckon up ⁹ *insanas substructiones, insanos labores, insanum luxum,* mad labours, mad books, endeavours, carriages, gross ignorance, ridiculous actions, absurd gestures, *insanam gulam, insaniam villarum, insana jurgia,* as Tully terms them, madness of villages, stupend structures, as those Ægyptian pyramids, labyrinths and Sphinges, which a company of crowned asses, *ad ostentationem opum,* vainly built, when neither the architect nor king that made them, or to what use and purpose, are yet known. To insist in their hypocrisie, inconstancy, blindness, rashness, *dementem temeritatem,* fraud, cozenage, malice, anger, impudence, ingratitude, ambition, gross superstition, ¹⁰ *tempora infecta et adulatione sordida,* as in Tiberius times, such base flattery, stupend, parasitical fawning and colloguing, &c. brawls, conflicts, desires, contentions, it would ask an expert Vesalius to anatomize every member. Shall I say? Jupiter himself, Apollo, Mars, &c. doted: and monster-conquering Hercules, that subdued the world, and helped others, could not relieve himself in this : but mad he was at last. And

---

¹ Orat. de imag.—Ambitiosus et audax naviget Anticyras.   ² Navis stulta, quæ continuo movetur ; nautæ stulti, qui se periculis exponunt; aqua insana, quæ sic fremit, &c. aër jactatur, &c. qui mari se committit, stolidum unum terrâ fugiens, 40 mari invenit. Gasper Ens. Moros.   ³ Cap. de alien. mentis.   ⁴ Deipnosophist. lib. 8.   ⁵ Tibicines mente capti. Erasm. Chil. 4. cen. 7.   ⁶ Prov. 30. Insana libido.—Hic, rogo, non furor est ? non est hæc mentula demens ? Mart. ep. 74. l. 3.   ⁷ Mille puellarum et puerorum mille furores.   ⁸ Uter est insanior horum ? Hor. Ovid. Virg. Plin.   ⁹ Plin. lib. 36.   ¹⁰ Tacitus, 3 Annal.

108   DEMOCRITUS TO THE READER.

where shall a man walk, converse with whom, in what province,
city, and not meet with Signior Deliro, or Hercules Furens,
Mænades, and Corybantes? Their speeches say no less. [1] *E
fungis nati homines ;* or else they fetched their pedigree from
those that were struck by Sampson with the jaw-bone of an
ass, or from Deucalion and Pyrrha's stones ; for *durum genus
sumus,* [2] *marmorei sumus;* we are stony-hearted, and savour
too much of the stock, as if they had all heard that inchanted
horn of Astolpho (that English duke in Ariosto), which never
sounded but all its auditors were mad, and for fear ready
to make away themselves ; [3] or landed in the mad haven in
the Euxine sea of *Daphnis insana,* which had a secret quality to dementate; they are a company of giddy-heads, afternoon men; it is midsomer moon still, and the dog-dayes
last all the year long : they are all mad.   Whom shall I then
except? Ulricus Huttenus [4] *Nemo ; nam Nemo omnibus horis
sapit ; Nemo nascitur sine vitiis ; crimine Nemo caret ; Nemo sorte suâ vivit contentus ; Nemo in amore sapit ; Nemo
bonus ; Nemo sapiens ; Nemo est ex omni parte beatus, &c.*
and therefore Nicholas Nemo, or Monsieur Nobody, shall go
free : *Quid valeat nemo, nemo referre potest.*   But whom
shall I except in the second place? such as are silent : *vir sapit, qui pauca loquitur ;* [5] no better way to avoid folly and
madness, than by taciturnity.   Whom in a third; all senators, magistrates; for all fortunate men are wise, and con-
querours valiant, and so are all great men ; *non est bonum
ludere cum diis ;* they are wise by authority, good by their
office and place ; *his licet impune pessimos esse,* (some say) we
must not speak of them; neither is it fit; *per me sint omnia
protinus alba;* I will not think amiss of them.   Whom next?
Stoicks ? *Sapiens Stoicus;* and he alone is subject to no perturbations, (as [6] Plutarch scoffs at him) *he is not vexed with
torments, or burnt with fire, foiled by his adversary, sold of
his enemy.   Though he be wrinkled, sand-blind, toothless,
and deformed ; yet he is most beautiful, and like a god, a
king in conceit, though not worth a groat.   He never dotes,
never mad, never sad, drunk ; because vertue cannot be taken*

---

[1] Ovid. 7. Met. E fungis nati homines, ut olim Corinthi primævi illius loci
accolæ, quia stolidi et fatui fungis nati dicebantur.   Idem et alibi dicas.
[2] Famian.   Strada, de bajulis, de marmore semisculptis.   [3] Arrianus,
periplo maris Euxini, portûs ejus meminit, et Gillius, l. 3. de Bosphor. Thracio.
Et laurus insana, quæ, allata in convivium, convivas omnes insaniâ affecit.
Guliel. Stucchius, comment. &c.   [4] Lepidum poëma, sic inscrip-
tum.   [5] Stultitiam dissimulare non potes, nisi taciturnitate.   [6] Ex-
tortus, non cruciatur ; ambustus, non læditur; prostratus in luctâ, non vincitur ;
non fit captivus, ab hoste venundatus.   Et si rugosus, senex, edentulus, luscus,
deformis, formosus tamen, et deo similis, felix, dives, rex, nullius egens, etsi
denario non sit dignus.

DEMOCRITUS TO THE READER.   109

away (as [1] Zeno holds) *by reason of strong apprehension :* but
he was mad to say so. [2] *Anticyræ cœlo huic est opus, aut
dolabrá :* he had need to be bored, and so had all his fellows,
as wise as they would seem to be.   Chrysippus himself liberally grants them to be fools as well as others, at certain times,
upon some occasions : *amitti virtutem ait per ebrietatem,
aut atribilarium morbum :* it may be lost by drunkenness or
melancholy; he may be sometimes crazed as well as the rest :
[3] *ad summam, sapiens, nisi quum pituita molesta.*   I should
here except some cynicks, Menippus, Diogenes, that Theban
Crates, or, to descend to these times, that omniscious, only
wise fraternity [4] of the Rosie Cross, those great theologues,
politicians, philosophers, physicians, philologers, artists, &c.
of whom S. Bridget, Albas Joacchimus, Leicenbergius, and
such divine spirits, have prophesied, and made promise to the
world, if at least there be any such, (Hen. [5] Neuhusius makes
a doubt of it, [6] Valentinus Andreas, and others) or an Elias Artifex their Theophrastian master; whom though Libavius and
many deride and carp at, yet some will have to be *the* [7] *renewer
of all arts and sciences,* reformer of the world, and now
living ; for so Johannes Montanus Strigoniensis (that great
patron of Paracelsus) contends, and certainly avers [8] *a most
divine man,* and the quintessence of wisdom, wheresoever he
is : for he, his fraternity, friends, &c. are all [9] *betrothed to
wisdom,* if we may believe their disciples and followers.   I
must needs except Lipsius and the pope, and expunge their
name out of the catalogue of fools ; for, besides that parasitical
testimony of Dousa,

> A sole exoriente, Mæotidas usque paludes,
>   Nemo est, qui Justo se æquiparare queat—

Lipsius saith of himself, that he was [10] *humani generis quidam
pædagogus voce et stylo,* a grand signior, a master, a tutor
of us all ; and for thirteen years, he brags, how he sowed
wisdom in the Low Countreys, (as Ammonius the philosopher
sometimes did in Alexandria) [11] *cum humanitate literas, et sapientiam cum prudentiá: antistes sapientiæ,* he shall be *sapientum octavus.*   The pope is more than a man, as [12] his parrots
often make him—a demi-god ; and besides his holiness cannot
err, *in cathedrá* belike : and yet some of them have been

---

[1] Illum contendunt non injuriâ affici, non insaniâ, non inebriari, quia virtus
non eripitur ob constantes comprehensiones. Lips. Phys. Stoic. lib. 3. diffi. 18.
[2] Tarreus Hebus, epig. 102. l. 8.   [3] Hor.   [4] Fratres sanct. Roseæ Crucis.
[5] An sint, quales sint, unde nomen illud asciverint.   [6] Turri Babel.
[7] Omnium artium et scientiarum instaurator.   [8] Divinus ille vir, auctor
notarum in ep. Rog. Bacon. ed. Hambur. 1608.   [9] Sapientiæ desponsati.
[10] Solus hic est sapiens, alii volitant velut umbræ.   [11] In ep. ad Balthas.
Moretum.   [12] Rejectiunculæ ad Patavum. Felinus cum reliquis.

110   DEMOCRITUS TO THE READER.

magicians, hereticks, atheists, children ; and, as Platina saith of John 22, *Etsi vir literatus, multa stoliditatem et levitatem præ se ferentia egit, stolidi et socordis vir ingenii;* a scholar sufficient; yet many things he did foolishly. Lightly, I can say no more in particular ; but in general terms to the rest, they are all mad, their wits are evaporated, and (as Ariosto feigns, l. 34) kept in jars above the moon.

> Some lose their wits with love, some with ambition,
> Some, following [1]lords and men of high condition.
> Some, in fair jewels rich and costly set,
> Others in poetry, their wits forget.
> Another thinks to be an alchymist,
> Till all be spent, and that his number's mist.

Convict fools they are, mad men upon record ; and, I am afraid, past cure, many of them; [2] *crepant inguina;* the symptomes are manifest; they are all of Gotam parish :

> [3] Quum furor haud dubius, quum sit manifesta phrenesis,

what remains then [4] but to send for *lorarios,* those officers to carry them all together for company to Bedlam, and set Rabelais to be their physician.

If any man shall ask in the mean time, who I am, that so boldly censure others, *tu nullane habes vitia?* Have I no faults? [5] Yes, more than thou hast, whatsoever thou art. *Nos numerus sumus:* I confess it again, I am as foolish, as mad as any one.

> [6] Insanus vobis videor : non deprecor ipse,
> Quo minus insanus———

I do not deny it; *demens de populo dematur.* My comfort is, I have more fellows, and those of excellent note. And though I be not so right or so discreet as I should be, yet not so mad, so bad neither, as thou perhaps takest me to be.

To conclude, this being granted, that all the world is melancholy, or mad, dotes, and every member of it, I have ended my task, and sufficiently illustrated that which I took upon me to demonstrate at first. At this present I have no more to say. *His sanam mentem Democritus;* I can but wish my self and them a good physician, and all of us a better mind.

---

[1] Magnum virum sequi est sapere, *some think; others* desipere.   Catul.
[2] Plaut. Menæch.   [3] In Sat. 14.   [4] Or to send for a cook to the Anticyræ, to make hellebor pottage, settle-brain pottage.   [5] Aliquantulum tamen inde me solabor, quod unà cum multis et sapientibus et celeberrimis viris ipse insipiens sim; quod de se, Menippus Luciani in Necyomantiâ.   [6] Petronius, in Catalect.

2

DEMOCRITUS TO THE READER. 111

And although, for the abovenamed reasons, I had a just cause to undertake this subject, to point at these particular species of dotage, that so men might acknowledge their imperfections, and seek to reform what is amiss; yet I have a more serious intent at this time; and—to omit all impertinent digressions—to say no more of such as are improperly melancholy, or metaphorically mad, lightly mad, or in disposition, as stupid, angry, drunken, silly, sottish, sullen, proud, vainglorious, ridiculous, beastly, pievish, obstinate, impudent, extravagant, dry, doting, dull, desperate, harebrain'd, &c. mad, frantick, foolish, heteroclites, which no new [1] hospital can hold, no physick help—my purpose and endeavour is, in the following discourse to anatomize this humour of melancholy, through all his parts and species, as it is an habit, or an ordinary disease, and that philosophically, medicinally—to shew the causes, symptomes, and several cures of it, that it may be the better avoided; moved thereunto for the generality of it, and to do good, it being a disease so frequent, as [2] Mercurialis observes, *in these our dayes; so often happening,* saith [3] Laurentius, *in our miserable times,* as few there are that feel not the smart of it. Of the same mind is Ælian Montaltus, [4] Melancthon, and others; [5] Julius Cæsar Claudinus calls it the *fountain of all other diseases, and so common in this crazed age of ours, that scarce one of a thousand is free from it;* and that splenetick hypochondriacal wind especially, which proceeds from the spleen and short ribs. Being then it is a disease so grievous, so common, I know not wherein to do a more general service, and spend my time better, than to prescribe means how to prevent and cure so universal a malady, an epidemical disease, that so often, so much, crucifies the body and mind.

If I have over-shot my self in this which hath been hitherto said, or that it is (which I am sure some will object) too phantastical, *too light and comical for a divine, too satyrical for one of my profession,* I will presume to answer with [6] Erasmus, in like case, 'Tis not I, but Democritus: *Democritus dixit :* you must consider what it is to speak in ones own or anothers person, an assumed habit and name; a difference betwixt him that affects or acts a princes, a philosophers, a magistrates, a fools part, and him that is so indeed; and what

---

[1] That, I mean, of Andr. Vale. Apolog. mancip. l. 1. et 26. Apol. [2] Hæc affectio nostris temporibus frequentissima. [3] Cap. 15. de Mel. [4] De animâ. Nostro hoc sæculo morbus frequentissimus. [5] Consult. 98. Adeo nostris temporibus frequenter ingruit, ut nullus fere ab ejus labe immunis reperiatur, et omnium fere morborum occasio existat. [6] Mor. Encom. Si quis calumnietur levius esse quam decet theologum, aut mordacius quam deceat Christianum.

DEMOCRITUS TO THE READER.

liberty those old satyrists have had: it is a cento collected from others: not I, but they, that say it.

> [1]Dixero si quid forte jocosius, hoc mihi juris
> Cum veniâ dabis————

Take heed you mistake me not. If I do a little forget my self, I hope you will pardon it. And to say truth, why should any man be offended, or take exceptions at it?

> ————— Licuit, semperque licebit,
> Parcere personis, dicere de vitiis.

> It lawful was of old, and still will be,
> To speak of vice, but let the name go free.

I hate their vices, not their persons. If any be displeased or take ought unto himself, let him not expostulate or cavil with him that said it (so did [2] Erasmus excuse himself to Dorpius, *si parva licet componere magnis;* and so do I: *but let him be angry with himself, that so betrayed and opened his own faults in applying it to himself.* [3] *If he be guilty and deserve it, let him amend, whosoever he is, and not be angry. He that hateth correction is a fool,* Prov. 12. 1. If he be not guilty, it concerns him not; it is not my freeness of speech, but a guilty conscience, a gauled back of his own, that makes him winch.

> Suspicione si quis errabit suâ,
> Et rapiet ad se, quod erit commune omnium,
> Stulte nudabit animi conscientiam.

I deny not, this, which I have said, savours a little of Democritus. [4] *Quamvis ridentem, dicere verum quid vetat?* one may speak in jest, and yet speak truth. It is somewhat tart, I grant it: *acriora orexim excitant embammata,* as he said; sharp sauces increase appetite;

> [5] Nec cibus ipse juvat, morsu fraudatus aceti.

Object then and cavil what thou wilt, I ward all with [6] Democritus buckler: his medicine shall salve it; strike where thou wilt, and when: *Democritus dixit;* Democritus will answer it. It was written by an idle fellow, at idle times, about our Saturnalian or Dionysian feast, when, as he said, *nullum libertati periculum est,* servants in old Rome had liberty to say and do what them list. When our countrey-men sacrificed

---

[1] Hor. Sat. 4. l. 1.   [2] Epi. ad Dorpium de Moriâ. Si quispiam offendatur, et sibi vindicet, non habet quod expostulet cum eo qui scripsit; ipse, si volet, secum agat injuriam, utpote sui proditor, qui declaravit hoc ad se proprie pertinere. [3] Si quis se læsum clamabit, aut conscientiam prodit suam, aut certe metum. Phæd. l. 3. Æsop. Fab.   [4] Hor.   [5] Mart. l. 7. 22.   [6] Ut lubet, feriat: abstergam hos ictus Democriti pharmaco.

DEMOCRITUS TO THE READER.

113

to their goddess [1] Vacuna, and sat tipling by their Vacunal fires, I writ this, and published this. Ουτις ελεγεν· it is *neminis nihil.* The time, place, persons, and all circumstances, apologize for me; and why may I not then be idle with others? speak my mind freely? If you deny me this liberty, upon these presumptions I will take it: I say again, I will take it.

> [2] Si quis est, qui dictum in se inclementius
> Existimarit esse, sic existimet.

If any man take exceptions, let him turn the buckle of his girdle; I care not. I owe thee nothing, reader: I look for no favour at thy hands; I am independent; I fear not.

No, I recant; I will not; I care, I fear; I confess my fault, acknowledge a great offence;

> ————motos præstat componere fluctus :

I have overshot my self; I have spoken foolishly, rashly, unadvisedly, absurdly; I have anatomized mine own folly. And now, methinks, upon a sudden I am awaked as it were out of a dream; I have had a raving fit, a phantastical fit, ranged up and down, in and out; I have insulted over most kind of men, abused some, offended others, wronged my self; and now, being recovered, and perceiving mine error, cry with [3] Orlando, *Solvite me.* Pardon *(O boni!)* that which is past; and I will make you amends in that which is to come: I promise you a more sober discourse in my following treatise.

If, through weakness, folly, passion, [4] discontent, ignorance, I have said amiss, let it be forgotten and forgiven. I acknowledge that of [5] Tacitus to be true, *Asperæ facetiæ, ubi nimis ex vero traxêre, acrem sui memoriam relinquunt :* a bitter jeast leaves a sting behind it; and as an honourable man observes, [6] *They fear a satyrists wit, he their memories.* I may justly suspect the worst; and, though I hope I have wronged no man, yet, in Medeas words, I will crave pardon,

> —— Illud jam voce extremâ peto,
> Ne, si qua noster dubius effudit dolor,
> Maneant in animo verba ; sed melior tibi
> Memoria nostri subeat ; hæc iræ data
> Obliterentur————

---

[1] Rusticorum dea præesse vacantibus et otiosis putabatur, cui post labores agricola sacrificabat. Plin. l. 3. c. 12. Ovid. l. 6. Fast. Jam quoque cum fiunt antiquæ sacra Vacunæ, Ante Vacunales stantque sedentque focos. Rosinus.   [2] Ter. prol. Eunuch.   [3] Ariost. l. 39. st. 58.   [4] Ut enim ex studiis gaudium, sic studia ex hilaritate proveniunt. Plinius Maximo suo, ep. lib. 8.   [5] Annal. 15. [6] Sir Francis Bacon in his Essayes, now Viscount S. Albanes.

VOL. I.   I

DEMOCRITUS TO THE READER.

And, in my last words, this I do desire,
That what in passion I have said, or ire,
May be forgotten, and a better mind
Be had of us, hereafter as you find.

I earnestly request every private man, as Scaliger did Cardan, not to take offence. I will conclude in his lines, *Si me cognitum haberes, non solum donares nobis has facetias nostras, sed etiam indignum duceres, tam humanum animum, lene ingenium, vel minimam suspicionem deprecari oportere.* If thou knewest my [1] modesty and simplicity, thou wouldst easily pardon and forgive what is here amiss, or by thee misconceived. If hereafter, anatomizing this surly humour, my hand slip, and, as an unskilful prentice, I launch too deep, and cut through skin and all at unawares, make it smart, or cut awry, [2] pardon a rude hand, an unskilful knife; 'tis a most difficult thing to keep an even tone, a perpetual tenor, and not sometimes to lash out; *difficile est satyram non scribere;* there be so many objects to divert, inward perturbations to molest; and the very best may sometimes err; *aliquando bonus dormitat Homerus:* it is impossible not in so much to overshoot:

——— opere in longo fas est obrepere somnum.

But what needs all this? I hope there will no such cause of offence be given; if there be,

[3] Nemo aliquid recognoscat : nos mentimur omnia.

I'le deny all (my last refuge), recant all, renounce all I have said, if any man except, and with as much facility excuse, as he can accuse: but I presume of thy good favour, and gracious acceptance, gentle reader. Out of an assured hope and confidence thereof, I will begin.

---

[1] Quod Probus Persii βιογραφος virginali verecundia Persium fuisse dicit, ego, &c.   [2] Quas aut incuria fudit, aut humana parum cavit natura. Hor.   [3] Prol. Quer. Plaut.

Lectori male feriato.

TU vero cavesis, edico, quisquis es, ne temere sugilles authorem hujusce operis, aut cavillator irrideas. Imo ne vel ex aliorum censurâ tacite obloquaris, (vis dicam verbo?) nequid nasutulus inepte improbes, aut falso fingas. Nam si talis reverâ sit, qualem præ se fert, Junior Democritus, *seniori* Democrito *saltem affinis, aut ejus genium vel tantillum sapiat; actum de te; censorem æque ac delatorem* [1] *aget e contra* (petulanti splene cum sit); *sufflabit te in jocos, comminuet in sales, addo etiam, et* deo Risui *te sacrificabit.*

Iterum moneo, ne quid cavillere, ne (dum Democritum Juniorem *conviciis infames, aut ignominiose vituperes, de te non male sentientem) tu idem audias ab amico cordato, quod olim vulgus* Abderitanum *ab* [2] Hippocrate, *concivem bene meritum et popularem suum* Democritum *pro insano habens;* Nec tu, Democrite, sapis; stulti autem et insani Abderitæ.

[3] Abderitanæ pectora plebis habes.

Hæc te paucis admonitum volo, male feriate Lector. Abi.

---

[1] Si me commôrit, melius non tangere, clamo. Hor. [2] Hippoc. epist. Damageto. Accersitus sum, ut Democritum, tamquam insanum, curarem : sed postquam conveni, non, per Jovem, desipientiæ negotium, sed rerum omnium receptaculum deprehendi; ejusque ingenium demiratus sum. Abderitanos vero tamquam non sanos accusavi, veratri potione ipsos potius eguisse dicens. [3] Mart.

HERACLITE, fleas! misero sic convenit ævo :
  Nil nisi turpe vides, nil nisi triste vides.
Ride etiam, quantumque lubet, Democrite, ride :
  Non nisi vana vides, non nisi stulta vides.
Is fletu, hic risu, modo gaudeat ; unus utrique
  Sit licet usque labor, sit licet usque dolor.
Nunc opus est (nam totus, eheu! jam desipit orbis)
  Mille Heraclitis, milleque Democritis.
Nunc opus est (tanta est insania) transeat omnis
  Mundus in Anticyras, gramen in Helleborum.

THE

SYNOPSIS

OF THE

FIRST PARTITION.

In diseases, consider, *Sect.* 1. *Mem.* 1.

Their Causes *Subs.* 1.
- Impulsive; — Sin, concupiscence, &c.
- Instrumental; — Intemperance, all second causes, &c.

Or

Definition, Number, Division. *Subs.* 2.

Of the body 300, which are
- Epidemical, as Plague, Plica, &c. or
- Particular, as Gout, Dropsie, &c.
- In disposition: as all purturbations, evil affections, &c.

or

Of the head or mind. *Subs.* 3.

Or — Dotage.

Habits, as *Subs.* 4.
- Dotage.
- Phrensie.
- Madness.
- Ecstasie.
- Lycanthropia.
- Chorus sancti Viti.
- Hydrophobia.
- Possession or obsession of Devils.
- Melancholy. *See* ♈.

♈ Melancholy: in which consider

Its Æquivocations, in Disposition, Improper, &c. *Subs.* 5.

Memb. 2. To its explication, a digression of anatomy, in which observe parts of *Subs.* 1.

Body hath parts *Subs.* 1.
- contained, as
  - Humours, Blood, Phlegm, Choler, Melancholy.
  - Spirits; vital, natural, animal.
- or
- containing
  - Similar; spermatical, or flesh, bones, nerves, &c.
  - Dissimilar; brain, heart, liver, &c. *Subs.* 4.

Or

Soul and his faculties, as
- Vegetal. *Subs.* 5.
- Sensible. *Subs.* 6, 7, 8.
- Rational. *Subs.* 9, 10, 11.

Memb. 3. Its definition, name, difference, *Subs.* 1.
The part and parties affected, affection, &c. *Subs.* 2.
The matter of melancholy, natural, unnatural, &c. *Subs.* 4.

Species, or kinds, which are

Proper, to parts, as
- Of the head alone, Hypochondriacal, or windy melancholy. Of the whole body,
  - with their several causes, symptomes, prognosticks, cures.

Or

Indefinite; as Love-melancholy, the subject of the third Partition.

Its causes in general. *Sect.* 2. A.
Its Symptomes or signs. *Sect.* 3. B.
Its Prognosticks or indications. *Sect.* 4. 4.
Its Cures; the subject of the second Partition.

SYNOPSIS OF THE FIRST PARTITION.

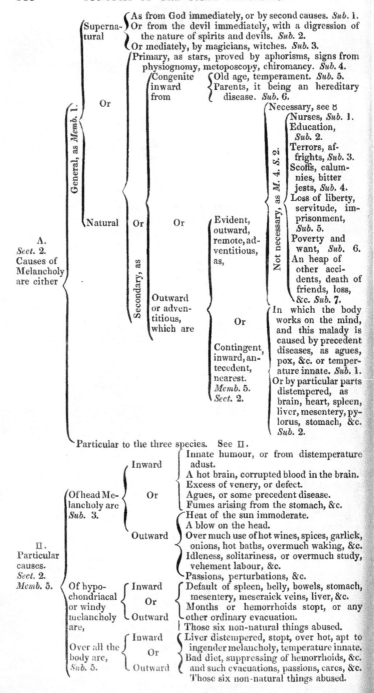

SYNOPSIS OF THE FIRST PARTITION.   119

Bread; coarse and black, &c.
Drink; thick, thin, sowre, &c.
Water unclean, milk, oyl, vinegar, wine, spices, &c.

Substance

Flesh
Parts; heads, feet, entrails, fat, bacon, blood, &c.
Kinds { Bief, pork, venison, hares, goats, pigeons, peacocks, fen-fowl, &c.

Herbs, Fish, &c.
Of fish; all shell-fish, hard and slimy fish, &c.
Of herbs; pulse, cabbage, mellons, garlick, onions, &c.
All roots, raw fruits, hard and windy meats.

Diet offending in Sub. 3.

Quality, as in { Preparing, dressing, sharp sauces, salt meats, indurate, sowced, fryed, broiled, or made-dishes, &c.

Quantity { Disorder in eating, immoderate eating, or at unseasonable times, &c. Subs. 2.
Custom; delight, appetite, altered, &c. Subs. 3.

Retention and evacuation Subs. 4. { Costiveness, hot baths, sweating, issues stopped, Venus in excess, or in defect, phlebotomy, purging, &c.

Air; hot, cold, tempestuous, dark, thick, foggy, moorish, &c. Subs. 5.

Exercise, Sub. 6. { Unseasonable, excessive, or defective, of body or minde, solitariness, idleness, a life out of action, &c.

Sleep and waking, unseasonable, inordinate, over much, over little, &c. Sub. 7.

8
Necessary causes, as those six non-natural things, which are, Sect. 2. Memb. 5.

Mem. 3. Sect. 2. Passions and perturbations of the mind, Subs. 2. With a digression of the force of imagination. Sub. 2. and division of passions into Sub. 3.

Irascible

or

concupiscible.

Sorrow, cause and symptome, Sub.4. Fear, cause and symptome, Sub.5. Shame, repulse, disgrace, &c. Sub. 6. Envy and malice, Sub. 7. Emulation, hatred, faction, desire of revenge, Sub. 8. Anger a cause, Sub. 9. Discontents, cares, miseries, &c. Sub. 10.

Vehement desires, ambition, Sub. 11. Covetousness, φιλαργυριαν, Sub.12. Love of pleasures, gaming in excess, &c. Sub 13. Desire of praise, pride, vain-glory, &c. Sub. 14. Love of learning, study in excess, with a digression of the misery of scholars, and why the Muses are melancholy, Sub. 15.

SYNOPSIS OF THE FIRST PARTITION.

B. Symptomes of melancholy are either Sect. 3.

General, as of Memb. 1. — Body, as ill digestion, crudity, wind, dry brains, hard belly, thick blood, much waking, heaviness and palpitation of heart, leaping in many places, &c. *Sub.* 1.

or

Mind **Or**

Common to all or most, — Fear and sorrow without a just cause, suspicion, jealousie, discontent, solitariness, irksomeness, continual cogitations, restless thoughts, vain imaginations, &c. *Subs.* 2.

Particular to private persons, according to *Sub.* 3. 4. **Or**

Celestial influences, as ♄ ♃ ♂, &c. parts of the body, heart, brain, liver, spleen, stomach, &c.

Humours
- Sanguine are merry still, laughing, pleasant, meditating on playes, women, musick, &c.
- Phlegmatick, slothful, dull, heavy, &c.
- Cholerick, furious, impatient, subject to hear and see strange apparitions, &c.
- Black, solitary, sad; they think they are bewitcht, dead, &c.

Or mixt of these four humours adust, or not adust, infinitely varied.

Their several customs, conditions, inclinations, discipline, &c. — Ambitious thinks himself a king, a lord; covetous runs on his money; lascivious on his mistris; religious hath revelations, visions, is a prophet, or troubled in mind; a scholar on his book, &c.

Continuance of time as the humor is intended or remitted, &c.
- Pleasant at first, hardly discerned; afterwards harsh and intolerable, if inveterate.
- Hence some make three degrees,
  1. *Falsa cogitatio.*
  2. *Cogitata loqui.*
  3. *Exsequi loqutum.*
- By fits, or continuate, as the object varies, pleasing or displeasing.

Simple, or as it is mixt with other diseases, apoplexies, gout, *caninus appetitus*, &c. so the symptomes are various.

SYNOPSIS OF THE FIRST PARTITION. 121

Particular symptomes to the three distinct species. Sect. 3. Mem. 2.

Head melancholy. Sub. 1.

In body { Head-ach, binding, heaviness, vertigo, lightness, singing of the ears, much waking, fixed eyes, high colour, red eyes, hard belly, dry body; no great sign of melancholy in the other parts.

Or

In mind. { Continual fear, sorrow, suspicion, discontent, superfluous cares, solicitude, anxiety, perpetual cogitation of such toyes they are possessed with, thoughts like dreams, &c.

Hypochondriacal or windy melancholy. Sub. 2.

In body { Wind, rumbling in the guts, belly-ake, heat in the bowels, convulsions, crudities, short wind, sowr and sharp belchings, cold sweat, pain in the left side, suffocation, palpitation, heaviness of the heart, singing in the ears, much spittle, and moist, &c.

Or

In mind. { Fearful, sad, suspicious, discontent, anxiety, &c. Lascivious by reason of much wind, troublesome dreams, affected by fits, &c.

Over all the body. Sub. 3.

In body { Black, most part lean, broad veins, gross, thick blood, their hemorrhoids commonly stopped, &c.

Or

In mind. { Fearful, sad, solitary, hate light, averse from company, fearful dreams, &c.

Symptomes of nuns, maids, and widows melancholy, in body and mind, &c.

A reason of these symptomes. Memb. 3. { Why they are so fearful, sad, suspicious without a cause, why solitary, why melancholy men are witty, why they suppose they hear and see strange voices, visions, apparitions.

Why they prophesie, and speak strange languages; whence comes their crudity, rumbling, convulsions, cold sweat, heaviness of heart, palpitation, cardiaca, fearful dreams, much waking, prodigious phantasies.

C. Prognosticks of melancholy. Sect. 4.

Tending to good, as { Morphew, scabs, itch, breaking out, &c.
Black jaundise.
If the hemorrhoids voluntarily open.
If varices appear.

Tending to evil, as { Leanness, dryness, hollow-eyed, &c.
Inveterate melancholy is incurable.
If cold, it degenerates often into epilepsie, apoplexy, dotage, or into blindness.
If hot, into madness, despair, and violent death.

Corollaries and questions. { The grievousness of this above all other diseases.
The diseases of the mind are more grievous than those of the body.
Whether it be lawful, in this case of melancholy, for a man to offer violence to himself. *Neg.*
How a melancholy or mad man, offering violence to himself, is to be censured.

THE

FIRST PARTITION.

THE FIRST {
SECTION.
MEMBER.
SUBSECTION.
}

Man's Excellency, Fall, Miseries, Infirmities; The causes of them.

Man's Excellency.]   MAN, the most excellent and noble creature of the world, *the principal and mighty work of God, wonder of nature,* as Zoroaster calls him; *audacis naturæ miraculum, the [1]marvail of marvails,* as Plato; *the [2] abridgement and epitome of the world,* as Pliny; *microcosmus,* a little world, a model of the world, [3]soveragn lord of the earth, viceroy of the world, sole commander and governour of all the creatures in it; to whose empire they are subject in particular, and yield obedience; far surpassing all the rest, not in body only, but in soul; [4]*imaginis imago,* [5]created to Gods own [6]*image* to that immortal and incorporeal substance, with all the faculties and powers belonging unto it; was at first pure, divine, perfect, happy, [7]*created after God in true holiness and righteousness; Deo congruens,* free from all manner of infirmities, and put in Paradise, to know God, to praise and glorifie him, to do his will,

> Ut dîs consimiles parturiat deos,

(as an old poet saith) to propagate the church.

Mans fall and misery.]   But this most noble creature, *Heu tristis, et lacrymosa commutatio!* ([8] one exclaims) O pitiful change! is fallen from that he was, and forfeited his

---

[1] Magnum miraculum.   [2] Mundi epitome, naturæ deliciæ.   [3] Finis rerum omnium, cui sublunaria serviunt.   Scalig. exercit. 365, sec. 3. Vales. de sacr. Phil. c. 5.   [4] Ut in numismate Cæsaris imago, sic in homine Dei.   [5] Gen. 1.   [6] Imago mundi in corpore; Dei in animâ.   Exemplumque Dei quisque est in imagine parvâ.   [7] Eph. 4. 24.   [8] Palanterius.

124   *Diseases in General.*   [Part. 1. Sec. 1.

estate, become *miserabilis homuncio,* a castaway, a caitiff, one
of the most miserable creatures of the world, if he be considered in his own nature, an unregenerate man, and so much
obscured by his fall, that (some few reliques excepted) he is
inferior to a beast : [1] *man in honour that understandeth not, is
like unto beasts that perish;* so David esteems him : a monster
by stupend metamorphosis, [2] *a fox, a dog, a hog ;* what not ?
Quantum mutatus ab illo! How much altered from that he was;
before blessed and happy, now miserable and accursed; [3] *he
must eat his meat in sorrow,* subject to death and all manner of
infirmities, all kinds of calamities.

A description of melancholy.] *Great travel is created
for all men, and an heavy yoke on the sons of Adam, from
the day that they go out of their mothers womb, unto that
day they return to the mother of all things; namely, their
thoughts, and fear of their hearts, and their imagination
of things they wait for, and the day of death. From him
that sitteth in the glorious throne, to him that sitteth beneath in the earth and ashes—from him that is cloathed in
blue silk, and weareth a crown, to him that is cloathed in
simple linnen—wrath, envy, trouble, and unquietness, and
fear of death, and rigour and strife, and such things, come
to both man and beast, but sevenfold to the ungodly* [4]. All this
befalls him in this life, and peradventure eternal misery in the
life to come.

Impulsive cause of mans misery and infirmities.] The
impulsive cause of these miseries in man, this privation or
destruction of Gods image, the cause of death and diseases,
of all temporal and eternal punishments, was the sin of our
first parent Adam, [5] in eating of the forbidden fruit, by the
devils instigation and allurement—his disobedience, pride, ambition, intemperance, incredulity, curiosity ; from whence proceeded original sin, and that general corruption of mankind—
as from a fountain, flowed all bad inclinations, and actual transgressions, which cause our several calamities, inflicted upon us
for our sins. And this, belike, is that which our fabulous poets
have shadowed unto us in the tale of [6] Pandoras box, which, being opened through her curiosity, filled the world full of all manner of diseases. It is not curiosity alone, but those other crying sins of ours, which pull these several plagues and miseries
upon our heads. For *ubi peccatum, ibi procella,* as [7] Chrysostom well observes. [8] *Fools by reason of their transgres-*

---

[1] Ps. 49. 20.   [2] Lasciviâ superat equum, impudentiâ canem, astu vulpem, furore leonem. Chrys. 23. Gen.   [3] Gen. 3. 17.   [4] Ecclus. 40. 1,
2, 3, 4, 5. 8.   [5] Gen. 3. 16.   [6] Illa cadens tegmen manibus decussit,
et unâ Perniciem immisit miseris mortalibus atram. Hesiod. 1. oper.   [7] Hom.
5, ad pop. Antioch.   [8] Psal. 107. 17.

Mem. 1. Subs. 1.] *Diseases in General.* **125**

sion, and because of their iniquities, are afflicted. [1] *Fear cometh like sudden desolation, and destruction like a whirlewinde, affliction and anguish,* because they did not fear God.

Are you shaken with wars? [2] (as Cyprian well urgeth to Demetrius,) *are you molested with dearth and famine? is your health crushed with raging diseases? is mankind generally tormented with epidemical maladies? 'tis all for your sins,* Hag. 1. 9, 10. Amos 1. Jer. 7. God is angry, punisheth, and threateneth, because of their obstinacy and stubbornness, they will not turn unto him. [3] *If the earth be barren then for want of rain; if, dry and squalid, it yield no fruit; if your fountains be dried up, your wine, corn, and oyle blasted; if the air be corrupted and men troubled with diseases, 'tis by reason of their sins,* which (like the blood of Abel) cry loud to heaven for vengeance, Lam. 5. 15. *That we have sinned, therefore our hearts are heavy,* Isa. 59. 11, 12. *We roar like bears, and mourn like doves, and want health, &c. for our sins and trespasses.* But this we cannot endure to hear, or to take notice of. Jer. 2. 30. *We are smitten in vain, and receive no correction;* and, cap. 5. 3. *Thou hast stricken them; but they have not sorrowed; they have refused to receive correction; they have not returned. Pestilence he hath sent; but they have not turned to him,* Amos 4. [4] Herod could not abide John Baptist, nor [5] Domitian endure Apollonius to tell the causes of the plague at Ephesus, his injustice, incest, adultery, and the like.

To punish therefore this blindness and obstinacy of ours, as a concomitant cause and principal agent, is God's just judgement, in bringing these calamities upon us, to chastise us, (I say) for our sins, and to satisfie Gods wrath: for the law requires obedience or punishment, as you may read at large, Deut. 28. 15. *If they will not obey the Lord, and keep his commandments and ordinances, then all these curses shall come upon them.* [6] *Cursed in the town, and in the field, &c.* [7] *Cursed in the fruit of the body, &c.* [8] *The Lord shall send thee trouble and shame, because of thy wickedness.* And a little after, [9] *The Lord shall smite thee with the botch of Ægypt, and with emrods, and scab, and itch; and thou canst not be healed;* [10] *with madness, blindness, and astonishing*

---

[1] Prov. i. 27.   [2] Quod autem crebrius bella concutiant, quod sterilitas et fames solicitudinem cumulent, quod sævientibus morbis valetudo frangitur, quod humanum genus luis populatione vastatur; ob peccatum omnia. Cypr.   [3] Si raro desuper pluvia descendat, si terra situ pulveris squaleat, si vix jejunas et pallidas herbas sterilis gleba producat, si turbo vineam debilitet, &c. Cypr.   [4] Mat. 14. 3.   [5] Philostratus, lib. 8. vit. Apollonii. Injustitiam ejus, et sceleratas nuptias, et cætera quæ præter rationem fecerat, morborum caussas dixit.   [6] 16.   [7] 18.   [8] 20.   [9] Vers. 17.   [10] 28. Deus, quos diligit, castigat.

126   *Diseases in General.*   [Part. 1. Sec. 1.

of heart. This Paul seconds, Rom. 2. 9. *Tribulation and anguish on the soul of every man that doth evil.* Or else these chastisements are inflicted upon us for our humiliation, to exercise and try our patience here in this life, to bring us home, to make us to know God and our selves, to inform and teach us wisdom. [1] *Therefore is my people gone into captivity, because they had no knowledge; therefore is the wrath of the Lord kindled against his people, and he hath stretched out his hand upon them.* He is desirous of our salvation, [2] *nostræ salutis avidus,* saith Lemnius, and for that cause pulls us by the ear many times, to put us in mind of our duties, *that they which erred might have* [3] *understanding,* (as Isay speaks, 29. 24.) *and so to be reformed.* I *am afflicted and at the point of death,* so David confesseth of himself, Psal. 88. 15. v. 9. *Mine eyes are sorrowful through mine affliction:* and that made him turn unto God. Great Alexander, in the midst of all his prosperity, by a company of parasites deified, and now made a god, when he saw one of his wounds bleed, remembered that he was but a man, and remitted of his pride. *In morbo recolligit se animus,* as [4] Pliny well perceived: *in sickness the mind reflects upon it self, with judgement surveys it self, and abhors its former courses;* insomuch that he concludes to his friend Maximus, [5] *that it were the period of all philosophy, if we could so continue, sound, or perform but a part of that which we promised to do, being sick.* Who so *is wise then, will consider these things,* as David did, (Psal. 144. verse last) and, whatsoever fortune befall him, make use of it—if he be in sorrow, need, sickness, or any other adversity, seriously to recount with himself, why this or that malady, misery, this or that incurable disease, is inflicted upon him; it may be for his good; [6] *sic expedit,* as Peter said of his daughters ague. Bodily sickness is for his souls health; *periisset, nisi periisset;* had he not been visited, he had utterly perished; for [7] *the Lord correcteth him whom he loveth, even as a father doth his child in whom he delighteth.* If he be safe and sound on the other side, and free from all manner of infirmity; [8] *et cui*

Gratia, forma, valetudo contingat abunde,
Et mundus victus, non deficiente crumenâ—

[1] Isa. 5. 13. vers. 15.   [2] Nostræ salutis avidus, continenter aures vellicat, ac calamitate subinde nos exercet. Levinus Lemn. l. 2. c. 29. de occult. nat. mir.
[3] Vexatio dat intellectum. Esay 28. 19.   [4] Lib. 7. Cum judicio, mores et facta recognoscit, et se intuetur.—Dum fero languorem, fero religionis amorem: Expers languoris, non sum memor hujus amoris.   [5] Summam esse totius philosophiæ, ut tales esse sani perseveremus, quales nos futuros esse infirmi profitemur.   [6] Petrarch.   [7] Prov. 3. 12.   [8] Hor. Epist. lib. 1. 4.

Mem. 1. Subs. 1.]   *Diseases in General.*   127

> And that he have grace, beauty, favour, health,
> A cleanly diet, and abound in wealth—

yet, in the midst of his prosperity, let him remember that caveat of Moses, [1] *beware that he do not forget the Lord his God;* that he be not puffed up, but acknowledge them to be his good gifts and benefits, and [2] *the more he hath, to be more thankful,* (as Agapetianus adviseth) and use them aright.

Instrumental causes of our infirmities.] Now the instrumental causes of these our infirmities are as diverse, as the infirmities themselves. Stars, heavens, elements, &c. and all those creatures which God hath made, are armed against sinners. They were indeed once good in themselves; and that they are now, many of them, pernicious unto us, is not in their nature, but our corruption which hath caused it. For, from the fall of our first parent Adam, they have been changed, the earth accursed, the influence of stars altered; the four elements, beasts, birds, plants, are now ready to offend us. *The principal things for the use of man are water, fire, iron, salt, meal, wheat, honey, milk, oile, wine, clothing, good to the godly, to the sinners turned to evil,* Ecclus. 39. 26. *Fire, and hail, and famine, and dearth, all these are created for vengeance,* Ecclus. 39. 29. The heavens threaten us with their comets, stars, planets, with their great conjunctions, eclipses, oppositions, quartiles, and such unfriendly aspects; the air with his meteors, thunder and lightning, intemperate heat and cold, mighty winds, tempests, unseasonable weather; from which proceed dearth, famine, plague, and all sorts of epidemical diseases, consuming infinite myriads of men. At Cayro in Ægypt, every third year, (as it is related by [3] Boterus, and others) 300,000 dye of the plague; and 200,000 in Constantinople, every fifth or seventh at the utmost. How doth the earth terrifie and oppress us with terrible earthquakes, which are most frequent in [4] China, Japan, and those eastern climes, swallowing up sometimes six cities at once! How doth the water rage with his inundations, irruptions, flinging down towns, cities, villages, bridges, &c. besides shipwracks; whole islands are sometimes suddenly over-whelmed with all their inhabitants, as in [5] Zealand, Holland, and many parts of the continent drowned, as the [6] lake Erne in Ireland! [7] *Nihilque præter arcium cada-*

---

[1] Deut. 8. 11. Qui stat, videat ne cadat.   [2] Quanto majoribus beneficiis a Deo cumulatur, tanto obligatiorem se debitorem fateri.   [3] Boterus de Inst. Urbium.   [4] Lege hist. relationem Lod. Frois de rebus Japonicis ad annum 1596.   [5] Guicciard. descript. Belg. an. 1421.   [6] Giraldus Cambrens. [7] Janus Dousa, ep. lib. 1. car. 10.

vera patenti cernimus freto. In the fenns of Freesland, 1230, by reason of tempests, [1] the sea drowned *multa hominum millia, et jumenta sine numero,* all the country almost, men and cattle in it. How doth the fire rage, that merciless element, consuming in an instant whole cities! What town, of any antiquity or note, hath not been once, again and again, by the fury of this merciless element, defaced, ruinated, and left desolate? In a word,

[2] Ignis pepercit ? unda mergit ; aëris
Vis pestilentis æquori ereptum necat ;
Bello superstes, tabidus morbo perit.

Whom fire spares, sea doth drown ; whom sea,
Pestilent ayre doth send to clay ;
Whom war scapes, sickness takes away.

To descend to more particulars, how many creatures are at deadly feud with men ! Lions, wolves, bears, &c. some with hoofs, horns, tusks, teeth, nails : how many noxious serpents and venemous creatures, ready to offend us with sting, breath, sight, or quite kill us ! How many pernicious fishes, plants, gums, fruits, seeds, flowers, &c. could I reckon up on a sudden, which by their very smell, many of them, touch, taste, cause some grievous malady, if not death it self ! Some make mention of a thousand several poysons : but these are but trifles in respect. [3] The greatest enemy to man is man, who, by the devils instigation, is still ready to do mischief—his own executioner, a wolf, a devil to himself and others. We are all brethren in Christ, or at least should be—members of one body, servants of one Lord ; and yet no fiend can so torment, insult over, tyrannize, vex, as one man doth another. Let me not fall, therefore, (saith David, when wars, plague, famine, were offered) into the hands of men, merciless and wicked men :

[4] ———Vix sunt homines hoc nomine digni ;
Quamque lupi, sævæ plus feritatis habent.

We can, most part, foresee these epidemical diseases, and, likely, avoid them. Dearths, tempests, plagues, our astrologers foretell us : earth-quakes, inundations, ruines of houses, consuming fires, come by little and little, or make some noise beforehand ; but the knaveries, impostures, injuries, and villanies of men no art can avoid. We can keep our professed enemies from our cities, by gates, walls and towers, defend our selves

[1] Munster. l. 3. Cos. cap. 462.   [2] Buchanan. Baptist.   [3] Homo homini lupus ; homo homini dæmon.   [4] Ovid. de Trist. l. 5. Eleg. 7.

Mem. 1. Subs. 1.] *Diseases in General.*

from thieves and robbers by watchfulness and weapons: but this malice of men, and their pernicious endeavours, no caution can divert, no vigilancy foresee, we have so many secret plots and devices to mischief one another: sometimes by the devils help, as magicians, [1] witches; sometimes by impostures, mixtures, poysons, stratagems, single combats, wars, (we hack and hew, as if we were *ad internecionem nati,* like Cadmus souldiers born to consume one another:—'tis an ordinary thing to read of an hundred and two hundred thousand men slain in a battle) besides all manner of tortures, brasen bulls, racks, wheels, strappadoes, guns, engines, &c. [2] *Ad unum corpus humanum supplicia plura, quam membra :* we have invented more torturing instruments, than there be several members in a mans body, as Cyprian well observes. To come nearer yet, our own parents, by their offences, indiscretion, and intemperance, are our mortal enemies. [3] *The fathers have eaten sowr grapes ; and the childrens teeth are set on edge.* They cause our grief many times, and put upon us hereditary diseases, inevitable infirmities : they torment us; and we are ready to injure our posterity,

———— [4] mox daturi progeniem vitiosiorem ;

and the latter end of the world, as [5] Paul foretold, is still like to be worst. We are thus bad by nature, bad by kind, but far worse by art, every man the greatest enemy unto himself. We study many times to undo our selves, abusing those good gifts which God hath bestowed upon us, health, wealth, strength, wit, learning, art, memory, to our own destruction: [6] *Perditio tua ex te.* As [7] Judas Maccabæus killed Apollonius with his own weapons, we arm ourselves to our own overthrows: and use reason, art, judgement, all that should help us, as so many instruments to undo us. Hector gave Ajax a sword, which, so long as he fought against enemies, served for his help and defence ; but after he began to hurt harmless creatures with it, turned to his own hurtless bowels. Those excellent means, God hath bestowed on us, well imployed, cannot but much avail us: but, if otherwise perverted, they ruine and confound us; and so, by reason of our indiscretion and weakness, they commonly do: we have too many instances. This S. Austin acknowledgeth of himself in his humble Confessions ; *promptness of wit, memory, eloquence, they were Gods good gifts; but he did not use them to his glory.* If you will particularly know how, and by what

[1] Miscent aconita novercæ. [2] Lib. 2. Epist. 2. ad Donatum. [3] Ezech. 18. 2. [4] Hor. l. 3. Od. 6. [5] 2 Tim. 3. 2. [6] Ezech. 18. 31. [7] 1 Macc. 3. 12.

VOL. 1.

130 *Def. Num. Div. of Diseases.* [Part. 1. Sec. 1.

means, consult physicians; and they will tell you, that it is in offending some of those six non-natural things, of which I shall after [1] dilate more at large : they are the causes of our infirmities, our surfeiting, and drunkenness, our immoderate insatiable lust, and prodigious riot. *Plures crapula, quam gladius,* is a true saying—the board consumes more than the sword. Our intemperance it is, that pulls so many several incurable diseases upon our heads, [2] that hastens old age, perverts our temperature, and brings upon us sudden death. And, last of all, that which crucifies us most, is our own folly, madness, *(quos Jupiter perdit, dementat ;* by substraction of his assisting grace, God permits it) weakness, want of government, our facility, and proneness in yielding to several lusts, in giving way to every passion and perturbation of the mind; by which means we metamorphose our selves, and degenerate into beasts ; all which that prince of [3] poets observed of Agamemnon, that, when he was well pleased, and could moderate his passion, he was—*os oculosque Jovi par*—like Jupiter in feature, Mars in valour, Pallas in wisdom, another God; but, when he became angry, he was a lyon, a tiger, a dog, &c. there appeared no sign or likeness of Jupiter in him : so we, as long as we are ruled by reason, correct our inordinate appetite, and conform our selves to Gods word, are as so many living saints : but, if we give reins to lust, anger, ambition, pride, and follow our own wayes, we degenerate into beasts, transform our selves, overthrow our constitutions, [4] provoke God to anger, and heap upon us this of melancholy, and all kinds of incurable diseases, as a just and deserved punishment of our sins.

SUBSECT. II.

THE ⎰ DEFINITION ⎱
  ⎱ NUMBER ⎰ OF DISEASES.
  ⎰ DIVISION ⎱

WHAT a disease is, almost every physician defines. [5] Fernelius calleth it an *affection of the body contrary to nature—* [6] Fuchsius and Crato, *an hindrance, hurt, or alteration of any action of the body, or part of it—*[7] Tholosanus, *a dissolution of that league which is between body and soul, and a pertur-*

---

[1] Part 1. Sect. 2. Memb. 2.   [2] Nequitia est, quæ te non sinit esse senem. [3] Homer. Iliad.   [4] Intemperantia, luxus, ingluvies, et infinita hujusmodi flagitia, quæ divinas pœnas merentur. Crato.   [5] Fern. Path. l. 1. c. 1. Morbus est affectus contra naturam corpori insidens.   [6] Fuchs. Instit. l. 3. Sect. 1. c. 3. a quo primum vitiatur actio.   [7] Dissolutio fœderis in corpore, ut sanitas est consummatio.

Mem. 1. Subs. 2.] *Def. Num. Div. of Diseases.* 131

bation of it ; as health the perfection, and makes to the preservation of it—[1] Labeo in Agellius, *an ill habit of the body, opposite to nature, hindering the use of it*—others otherwise, all
to this effect.

Number of diseases.] How many diseases there are, is a
question not yet determined. [2] Pliny reckons up 300, from
the crown of the head, to the sole of the foot: elsewhere he
saith *morborum infinita multitudo*, their number is infinite.
Howsoever it was in those times, it boots not; in our dayes, I
am sure the number is much augmented :

> ——[3]macies, et nova febrium
> Terris incubuit cohors :

for, besides many epidemical diseases unheard of, and altogether unknown to Galen and Hippocrates, as *scorbutum,
small pox, plica, sweating sickness, morbus Gallicus, &c.* we
have many proper and peculiar almost to every part.

No man free from some disease or other.] No man
amongst us so sound, of so good a constitution, that hath not
some impediment of body or mind. *Quisque suos patimur
manes ;* we have all our infirmities, first or last, more or less.
There will be, peradventure, in an age, or one of a thousand,
like Zenophilus the musician in [4] Pliny, that may happily live
105 years without any manner of impediment; a Pollio
Romulus, that can preserve himself [5] *with wine and oyle;* a
man as fortunate as Q. Metellus, of whom Valerius so much
braggs ; a man as healthful as Otto Herwardus, a senator of
Ausborrow in Germany, (whom [6] Leovitius the astrologer
brings in for an example and instance of certainty in his art)
who, because he had the significatours in his geniture fortunate, and free from the hostile aspects of Saturn and Mars,
being a very old man, [7] *could not remember that ever he was
sick.* [8] Paracelsus may bragg, that he could make a man live
400 years or more, if he might bring him up from his infancy,
and diet him as he list; and some physicians hold, that there is
no certain period of mans life, but it may still, by temperance
and physick, be prolonged. We find in the mean time, by
common experience, that no man can escape, but that of
[9] Hesiod is true :

> Πλειη μεν γαρ γαια κακων, πλειη δε θαλασσα·
> Νουσοι δ' ανθρωποισιν εφ' ημερῃ, ηδ' επι νυκτι,
> Αυτοματοι φοιτωσι ——

---

[1] Lib. 4. cap. 2. Morbus est habitus contra naturam, qui usum ejus, &c.
[2] Cap. 11. lib. 7. [3] Horat. [4] Cap. 50. lib. 7. Centum et quinque vixit
annos sine ullo incommodo. [5] Intus mulso, foras oleo. [6] Exemplis
genitur. præfixis Ephemer. cap. de infirmitat. [7] Qui, quoad pueritiæ ulti-
mam memoriam recordari potest, non meminit se ægrotum decubuisse. [8] Lib.
de vitâ longâ. [9] Oper. et dies.

K 2

132   *Div. of the Diseases of the Head.* [Part. 1. Sec. 1.

Th' earth's full of maladies, and full the sea,
Which set upon us both by night and day.

Division of diseases.] If you require a more exact division
of these ordinary diseases which are incident to men, I refer
you to physicians: [1] they will tell you of *acute* and *chronick*,
first and *secundary, lethales, salutares, errant, fixed, simple,
compound, connexed* or *consequent,* belonging to *parts* or the
whole, in *habit* or in *disposition, &c.* My division at this
time (as most befitting my purpose) shall be into those of the
body and mind. For them of the body, (a brief catalogue of
which Fuchsius hath made, *Institut. lib. 3. sec. 1. cap.* 11.)
I refer you to the voluminous tomes of Galen, Aretæus,
Rhasis, Avicenna, Alexander, Paulus, Aëtius, Cordonerius;
and those exact neotericks, Savanarola, Cappivaccius, Donatus,
Altomarus, Hercules de Saxoniâ, Mercurialis, Victorius Faventinus, Wecker, Piso, &c. that have methodically and elabo-
rately written of them all. Those of the mind and head I will
briefly handle, and apart.

SUBSECT. III.

Division of the Diseases of the Head.

THESE diseases of the mind, forasmuch as they have their
chief seat and organs in the head, are commonly repeated
amongst the diseases of the head, which are divers, and vary
much according to their site: for in the head, as there be
several parts, so there be divers grievances, which, according
to that division of [2] Heurnius, (which he takes out of Arculanus) are inward or outward (to omit all others which pertain to eyes and ears, nostrils, gums, teeth, mouth, palate,
tongue, wesel, chops, face, &c.) belonging properly to the
brain, as baldness, falling of hair, furfair, lice, &c. [3] Inward
belonging to the skins next to the brain, called *dura* and *pia
mater,* as all head aches, &c. or to the ventricles, caules,
kells, tunicles, creeks, and parts of it, and their passions,
as *caros, vertigo, incubus, apoplexie, falling-sickness.* The
diseases of the *nerves; crampes, stupor, convulsion, tremor,
palsie;* or belonging to the excrements of the brain, *catarrhes, sneezing, rheumes, distillations;* or else those that

---

[1] See Fernelius, Path. lib. 1. cap. 9, 10, 11, 12. Fuchsius, instit. l. 3. sect. 1.
c. 7. Wecker. Synt.   [2] Præfat. de morbis capitis. In capite ut variæ
habitant partes, ita variæ querelæ ibi eveniunt.   [3] Of which read Heurnius,
Montaltus, Hildesheim, Quercetan, Jason Pratensis, &c.

Mem. 1. Subs. 4.] *Diseases of the Mind.* 133

pertain to the substance of the brain it self, in which are conceived, *phrensie, lethargie, melancholy, madness, weak memory, sopor,* or *coma vigilia* and *vigil coma.* Out of these again I will single such as properly belong to the *phantasie,* or *imagination,* or *reason* it self, which [1] Laurentius calls the diseases of the mind; and Hildesheim, *morbos imaginationis, aut rationis læsæ,* which are three or four in number, *phrensie, madness, melancholy, dotage* and their kinds, as *hydrophobia, lycanthropia, chorus sancti Viti, morbi dæmoniaci;* which I will briefly touch and point at, insisting especially in this of *melancholy,* as more eminent than the rest, and that through all his kinds, causes, symptomes, prognosticks, cures; as Lonicerus hath done *de Apoplexiâ,* and many other of such particular diseases. Not that I find fault with those which have written of this subject before, as Jason Pratensis, Laurentius Montaltus, T. Bright, &c. they have done very well in their several kinds and methods : yet that which one omits, another may haply see ; that which one contracts, another may inlarge. To conclude with [2] Scribanius, *that which they had neglected, or perfunctorily handled, we may more thoroughly examine; that which is obscurely delivered in them, may be perspicuously dilated and amplified by us,* and so made more familiar and easie for every mans capacity, and the common good ; which is the chief end of my discourse.

SUBSECT. IV.

Dotage, Phrensie, Madness, Hydrophobia, Lycanthropia, Chorus sancti Viti, Extasis.

Delirium, dotage.] Dotage, fatuity, or folly, is a common name to all the following species, as some will have it. [3] Laurentius and [4] Altomarus comprehended *madness, melancholy,* and the rest, under this name, and call it the *summum genus* of them all. If it be distinguished from them, it is *natural* or *ingenite,* which comes by some defect of the organs, and over-moist brain, as we see in our common fools; and is for the most part intended or remitted in particular men, and thereupon some are wiser than other; or else it is acquisite, an appendix or symptome of some other disease, which comes or goes ; or, if it continue, a sign of *melancholy* it self.

---

[1] Cap. 2. de melanchol.   [2] Cap. 2. de Physiologiâ sagarum. Quod alii minus recte fortasse dixerint, nos examinare, melius dijudicare, corrigere, studeamus.   [3] Cap. 4. de mel.   [4] Art. med. c. 7.

134   *Diseases of the Mind.*   [Part. 1. Sec. 1.

Phrensie.] *Phrenitis* (which the Greeks derive from the
word φρην) is a disease of the miud, with a continual madness
or dotage, which hath an acute fever annexed, or else an inflammation of the brain, or the membranes or kells of it, with
an acute fever, which causeth madness and dotage. It differs
from *melancholy* and *madness*, because their dotage is without
an ague : this continual, with waking, or memory decayed, &c.
Melancholy is most part silent, this clamorous ; and many
such like differences are assigned by physicians.

Madness.] *Madness, phrensie,* and *melancholy,* are confounded by Celsus, and many writers ; others leave out *phrensie,*
and make *madness* and *melancholy* but one disease ; which
[1] Jason Pratensis especially labours, and that they differ only
secundum majus or *minus,* in quantity alone, the one being a
degree to the other, and both proceeding from one cause. They
differ *intenso et remisso gradu,* saith [2] Gordonius, as the humour is intended or remitted. Of the same mind is [3] Aretæus,
Alexander Tertullianus, Guianerius, Savanarola, Heurnius ;
and Galen himself writes promiscuously of them both, by reason of their affinity : but most of our neotericks do handle them
apart, whom I will follow in this treatise. *Madness* is therefore defined to be a vehement *dotage ;* or raving without a
fever, far more violent than *melancholy,* full of anger and cla-
mour, horrible looks, actions, gestures, troubling the patients
with far greater vehemency both of body and mind, without all
fear and sorrow, with such impetuous force and boldness, that
sometimes three or four men cannot hold them ; differing only
in this from *phrensie,* that it is without a fever, and their
memory is, most part, better.   It hath the same causes as the
other, as choler adust, and blood incensed, brains inflamed, &c.
[4] Fracastorius adds, *a due time and full age* to this definition,
to distinguish it from children, and will have it *confirmed im-
potency,* to separate it from *such as accidently come and go
again, as by taking henbane, nightshade, wine, &c.* Of
this fury there be divers kinds ; [5] *ecstasie,* which is familiar
with some persons, as Cardan saith of himself, he could be in
one when he list ; in which the Indian priests deliver their
oracles, and the witches in Lapland (as Olaus Magnus writeth,
l. 3. cap. 18. *extasi omnia prædicere)* answer all questions

---

[1] Plerique medici uno complexu perstringunt hos duos morbos, quod ex eâdem
caussâ oriantur, quodque magnitudine et modo solum distent, et alter gradus ad
alterum existat. Jason Pratens.   [2] Lib. Med.   [3] Pars maniæ mihi videtur.   [4] Insanus est, qui ætate debitâ, et tempore debito, per se, non mo-
mentaneam et fugacem, ut vini, solani, hyoscyami, sed confirmatam habet impo-
tentiam bene operandi circa intellectum. l. 2. de intellectione.   [5] Of which
read Felix Plater, cap. 3. de mentis alienatione.

Mem. 1. Subs. 4.]   *Diseases of the mind.*   135

in an extasis you will ask; what your friends do, where they are, how they fare, &c.   The other *species* of this fury are *enthusiasms, revelations,* and *visions,* so often mentioned by Gregory and Beda in their works; obsession or possession of devils, *Sibylline prophets,* and poetical *Furies;* such as come by eating noxious herbs, tarantulas stinging, &c. which some reduce to this.   The most known are these, *lycanthropia, hydrophobia, chorus sancti Viti.*

Lycanthropia.]   *Lycanthropia,* which Avicenna calls *cucubuth,* others, *lupinam insaniam,* or wolf-madness, when men run howling about graves and fields in the night, and will not be perswaded but that they are wolves, or some such beasts— [1]Aëtius and [2]Paulus call it a kind of *melancholy;* but I should rather refer it to *madness,* as most do. Some make a doubt of it, whether there be any such disease.   [3]Donat. ab Altomari saith, that he saw two of them in his time: [4]Wierus tells a story of such a one at Padua, 1541, that would not believe to the contrary, but that he was a wolf. He hath another instance of a Spaniard who thought himself a bear.   [5]Forestus confirms as much by many examples; one, amongst the rest, of which he was an eye witness, at Alcmaer in Holland—a poor husbandman that still hunted about graves, and kept in churchyards, of a pale, black, ugly, and fearful look.   Such, belike, or little better, were king Prœtus [6]daughters, that thought themselves kine; and Nebuchadnezzar, in Daniel, as some interpreters hold, was only troubled with this kind of madness. This disease perhaps gave occasion to that bold assertion of [7]Pliny, *some men were turned into wolves in his time, and from wolves to men again;* and to that fable of Pausanias, of a man that was ten years a wolf, and afterwards turned to his former shape: to [8]Ovids tale of Lycaon, &c. He that is desirous to hear of this disease, or more examples, let him read Austin in his eighteenth book *de Civitate Dei, cap. 5*; *Mizaldus, cent. 5. 77*; *Sckenkius, lib. 1. Hildesheim, spicil. 2. de Maniâ; Forestus, lib. 10. de Morbis Cerebri; Olaus Magnus; Vincentius Bellavicensis, spec. met. lib. 31. c. 122; Pierius, Bodine, Zuinger, Zeilgur, Peucer, Wierus, Spranger, &c.* This malady, saith Avicenna, troubleth men most in February, and is now a dayes frequent in Bohemia and Hungary, according to [9]Heurnius.   Schernitzius will have it common in Livonia.   They lye hid, most part all day, and go abroad in the

[1] Lib. 6, cap. 11.   [2] Lib. 3. cap. 16.   [3] Cap. 9. Art. med.   [4] De præstig. Dæmonum. l. 3. cap. 21.   [5] Observat. lib. 10. de morbis cerebri, c. 15. [6] Hippocrates, lib. de insaniâ.   [7] Lib. 8. cap. 22. Homines interdum lupos fieri; et contra.   [8] Met. l. 1.   [9] Cap. de Man.

136 *Diseases of the Mind.* [Part. 1. Sec. 1.

night, barking, howling, at graves and deserts ; [1] *they have usually hollow eyes, scabbed legs and thighs, very dry and pale,* [2] saith Altomarus : he gives a reason there of all the symptomes, and sets down a brief cure of them.

Hydrophobia is a kind of madness, well known in every village, which comes by the biting of a mad dog, or scratching (saith [3] Aurelianus), touching, or smelling alone sometimes (as [4] Sckenkius proves), and is incident to many other creatures as well as men ; so called, because the parties affected cannot endure the sight of water, or any liquor, supposing still they see a mad dog in it. And (which is more wonderful) though they be very dry, (as in this malady they are) they will rather dye than drink. [5] Cœlius Aurelianus, an ancient writer, makes a doubt whether this hydrophobia be a passion of the body or the mind. The part affected is the brain : the cause, poyson that comes from the mad dog, which is so hot and dry, that it consumes all the moisture in the body. [6] Hildesheim relates of some that dyed so mad, and, being cut up, had no water, scarce blood, or any moisture left in them. To such as are so affected, the fear of water begins at fourteen dayes after they are bitten, to some again not till forty or sixty dayes after : commonly, saith Heurnius, they begin to rave, flye water, and glasses, to look red, and swell in the face, about twenty dayes after, (if some remedy be not taken in the mean time), to lye awake, to be pensive, sad, to see strange visions, to bark and howl, to fall into a swoun, and oftentimes fits of the falling sickness. [7] Some say, little things like whelps will be seen in their urines. If any of these signs appear, they are past recovery. Many times these symptomes will not appear till six or seven moneths after, saith [8] Codronchus : and sometimes not till seven or eight years, as Guianerius ; twelve, as Albertus ; six or eight moneths after, as Galen holds. Baldus the great lawyer dyed of it : an Augustin frier, and a woman in Delph, that were [9] Forestus patients, were miserably consumed with it. The common cure in the countrey (for such at least as dwell near the sea side) is to duck them over head and ears in sea water ; some use charms ; every good wife can prescribe medicines. But the best cure to be had in such cases, is from the most approved physicians. They that will read of them, may consult with Dioscorides, *lib.* 6. *cap.* 37. Heurnius, Hildesheim, Cappivaccius, Forestus, Sckenkius, and, before all others, Codronchus an Italian, who hath lately written two exquisite books of this subject.

[1] Ulcerata crura ; sitis ipsis adest immodica ; pallidi ; lingua sicca.   [2] Cap. 9. art. Hydrophobia.   [3] Lib. 3. cap. 9.   [4] Lib. 7. de Venenis.   [5] Lib. 3. cap. 13. de morbis acutis.   [6] Spicil. 2.   [7] Sckenkius. 7. lib. de Venenis.   [8] Lib. de Hydrophobiâ.   [9] Observat. lib. 10. 25.

Mem. 1. Subs. 4.] *Diseases of the Mind.* 137

Chorus sancti Viti.] *Chorus sancti Viti*, or S. Vitus dance;
the lascivious dance [1] Paracelsus calls it, because they that are
taken with it, can do nothing but dance till they be dead, or
cured. It is so called, for that the parties so troubled were
wont to go to S. Vitus for help; and, after they had danced
there a while, they were [2] certainly freed. 'Tis strange to hear
how long they will dance, and in what manner, over stools, forms,
tables: even great-bellied women sometimes (and yet never hurt
their children) will dance so long that they can stir neither hand
nor foot, but seem to be quite dead. One in red cloaths they
cannot abide. Musick, above all things, they love; and therefore magistrates in Germany will hire musicians to play to
them, and some lusty sturdy companions to dance with them.
This disease hath been very common in Germany, as appears
by those relations of [3] Sckenkius, and Paracelsus in his book of
Madness, who brags how many several persons he hath cured
of it. Felix Platerus *(de Mentis Alienat. cap. 3.)* reports of a
woman in Basil whom he saw, that danced a whole moneth
together. The Arabians call it a kind of *palsie.* Bodine, in
his fifth book *de Repub. cap.* 1. speaks of this infirmity; Monavius, in his last epistle to Scoltizius, and in another to Dudi-
thus, where you may read more of it.

The last kind of madness or melancholy is that demoniacal
(if I may so call it) obsession or possession of devils, which
Platerus and others would have to be præternatural: stupend
things are said of them, their actions, gestures, *contortions*,
fasting, prophesying, speaking languages they were never
taught, &c. many strange stories are related of them, which
because some will not allow, (for Deacon and Darrel have
written large volumes on this subject *pro et con.)* I voluntarily omit.

[4] Fuchsius, *Institut. lib. 3. sec. 1. cap.* 11, Felix Plater, [5] Laurentius, add to these another *fury* that proceeds from *love*, and
another from *study*, another divine or *religious fury ;* but these
more properly belong to *melancholy ;* of all which I will speak
[6] apart, intending to write a whole book of them.

[1] Lascivam choream. To. 4. de morbis amentium. Tract. 1. [2] Eventu,
ut plurimum, rem ipsam comprobante. [3] Lib. 1. cap. de Maniâ. [4] Cap.
3. de mentis alienat. [5] Cap. 4. de mel. [6] PART 3.

138   *Melancholy in Disposition.*   [Part. 1. Sec. 1.

SUBSECT. V.

Melancholy in Disposition, improperly so called.
Æquivocations.

MELANCHOLY, the subject of our present discourse, is
either in disposition, or habit.   In disposition is that transitory
melancholy which comes and goes upon every small occasion of
sorrow, need, sickness, trouble, fear, grief, passion, or perturbation of the mind, any manner of care, discontent, or thought,
which causeth anguish, dulness, heaviness and vexation of spirit,
any wayes opposite to pleasure, mirth, joy, delight, causing
frowardness in us, or a dislike.   In which equivocal and improper sense, we call him melancholy, that is dull, sad, sowr, lumpish, ill-disposed, solitary, any way moved, or displeased.   And
from these melancholy dispositions [1] no man living is free, no
Stoick, none so wise, none so happy, none so patient, so
generous, so godly, so divine, that can vindicate himself: so well
composed, but more or less, sometime or other, he feels the
smart of it.   Melancholy in this sense, is the character of mortality.   [2] *Man, that is born of a woman, is of short continuance,*
and full of trouble. Zeno, Cato, Socrates himself—whom [3] Ælian
so highly commends for a moderate temper, that *nothing could*
disturb him; but, going out, and coming in, still Socrates kept the
same serenity of countenance, what misery soever befel him—
(if we may believe Plato his disciple) was much tormented with
it.   Q. Metellus, in whom [4] Valerius gives instance of all happiness, *the most fortunate man then living, born in that most*
flourishing city of Rome, of noble parentage, a proper man of
person, well qualified, healthful, rich, honourable, a senator, a
consul, happy in his wife, happy in his children, &c. yet this man
was not void of melancholy: he had his share of sorrow. [5] Polycrates Samius, that flung his ring into the sea, because he would
participate of discontent with others, and had it miraculously
restored to him again shortly after by a fish taken as he angled,
was not free from melancholy dispositions.   No man can cure

---

[1] De quo homine securitas? de quo certum gaudium?   Quocunque se con-
vertit, in terrenis rebus amaritudinem animi inveniet.   Aug. in Psal. 8. 5.
[2] Job 1. 14.   [3] Omni tempore Socratem eodem vultu videri, sive domum
rediret, sive domo egrederetur.   [4] Lib. 7. cap. 1.   Natus in florentissimâ
totius orbis civitate, nobilissimis parentibus, corporis vires habuit, et rarissimas
animi dotes, uxorem conspicuam, pudicam, felices liberos, consulare decus, sequentes triumphos, &c.   [5] Ælian.

Mem. 1. Subs. 5.] *Melancholy in Disposition.* 139

himself: the very gods had bitter pangs, and frequent passions, as their own [1] poets put upon them. In general [2] *as the heaven, so is our life, sometimes fair, sometimes overcast, tempestuous, and serene ; as in a rose, flowers and prickles ; in the year it self, a temperate summer sometimes, a hard winter, a drowth, and then again pleasant showers ; so is our life intermixt with joyes, hopes, fears, sorrows, calumnies : Invicem cedunt dolor et voluptas :* there is a succession of pleasure and pain.

> ————————[3] medio de fonte leporum
> Surgit amari aliquid, quod in ipsis floribus angat.

Even in the midst of laughing there is sorrow (as [4] Solomon holds) : even in the midst of all our feasting and jollity, (as [5] Austin infers in his Com. on Psal. 41) there is grief and discontent. *Inter delicias, semper aliquid sævi nos strangulat :* for a pint of honey, thou shalt here likely find a gallon of gaul; for a dram of pleasure, a pound of pain; for an inch of mirth, an ell of moan: as ivy doth an oak, these miseries encompass our life: and, 'tis most absurd and ridiculous for any mortal man to look for a perpetual tenour of happiness in his life. Nothing so prosperous and pleasant, but it hath [6] some bitterness in it, some complaining, some grudging; 'tis all γλυκυπικρον, a mixt passion, and, like a chequer table, black and white: men, families, cities, have their falls and wanes, now trines, sextiles, then quartiles and oppositions. We are not here, as those angels, celestial powers and bodies, sun and moon, to finish our course without all offence, with such constancy, to continue for so many ages; but subject to infirmities, miseries, interrupt, tossed and tumbled up and down, carried about with every small blast, often molested and disquieted upon each slender occasion, [7] uncertain, brittle; and so is all that we trust unto. [8] *And he that knows not this, and is not armed to endure it, is not fit to live in*

---

[1] Homer. Iliad. [2] Lipsius, cent. 3. ep. 45. Ut cœlum, sic nos homines sumus: illud ex intervallo nubibus obducitur et obscuratur. In rosario flores spinis intermixti. Vita similis aëri ; udum modo, sudum, tempestas, serenitas : ita vices rerum sunt, præmia gaudiis, et sequaces curæ. [3] Lucretius, l. 4. 1124. [4] Prov. 14. 3. Extremum gaudii luctus occupat. [5] Natalitia inquit celebrantur ; nuptiæ hîc sunt ; at ibi quid celebratur, quod non dolet, quod non transit ? [6] Apuleius, 4 florid. Nihil quidquid homini tam prosperum divinitus datum, quin ei admixtum sit aliquid difficultatis, ut etiam amplissimâ quâquâ lætitiâ, subsit quæpiam vel parva querimonia, conjugatione quâdam mellis et fellis. [7] Caduca nimirum et fragilia, et puerilibus consentanea crepundiis, sunt ista quæ vires et opes humanæ vocantur : affluunt subito ; repente dilabuntur ; nullo in loco, nullâ in personâ, stabilibus nixa radicibus consistunt; sed incertissimo flatu fortunæ, quos in sublime extulerunt, improviso recursu destitutos in profundo miseriarum valle miserabiliter immergunt. Valerius, l. 6. c. 9. [8] Huic seculo parum aptus es ; aut potius omnium nostrorum conditionem ignoras, quibus reciproco quodam nexu, &c. Lorchanus Gallobelgicus, lib. 3. ad annum 1598.

140   *Melancholy in Disposition.*   [Part. 1. Sec. 1.

this world (as one condoles our time); *he knows not the condition of it, where, with a reciprocal tye, pleasure and pain are still united, and succeed one another in a ring.   Exi e mundo ;* get thee gone hence, if thou canst not brook it : there is no way to avoid it, but to arm thy self with patience, with magnanimity, to [1]oppose thy self unto it, to suffer affliction as a good souldier of Christ, as [2]Paul adviseth, constantly to bear it. But forasmuch as so few can embrace this good counsel of his, or use it aright, but rather, as so many bruit beasts, give way to their passion, voluntarily subject and precipitate themselves into a labyrinth of cares, woes, miseries, and suffer their souls to be overcome by them, cannot arm themselves with that patience as they ought to do, it falleth out oftentimes that these *dispositions* become *habits*, and *many effects contemned* (as [3]Seneca notes) *make a disease.   Even as one distillation, not yet grown to custome, makes a cough, but continual and inveterate causeth a consumption of the lungs;* so do these our melancholy provocations ; and, according as the humour it self is intended or remitted in men, as their temperature of body or rational soul is better able to make resistance, so are they more or less affected : for that which is but a flea-biting to one causeth unsufferable torment to another; and which one by his singular moderation and well composed carriage can happily overcome, a second is no whit able to sustain; but, upon every small occasion of mis-conceived abuse, injury, grief, disgrace, loss, cross, rumour, &c. (if solitary, or idle) yields so far to passion, that his complexion is altered, his digestion hindred, his sleep gone, his spirits obscured, and his heart heavy, his hypocondries mis-affected ; wind, crudity, on a sudden overtake him, and he himself overcome with *melancholy.*   As it is with a man imprisoned for debt, if once in the gaol, every creditor will bring his action against him, and there likely hold him—if any discontent seise upon a patient, in an instant all other perturbations (for, *quâ data porta, ruunt)* will set upon him; and then, like a lame dog or broken-winged goose, he droops, and pines away, and is brought at last to that ill habit or malady of melancholy it self: so that, as the philosophers make [4]eight degrees of heat and cold, we may make eighty eight of *melancholy,* as the parts affected are diversely seised with it, or have been plunged more or less into this infernal gulf, or waded deeper into it.   But all these *melancholy* fits, howso-

---

[1] Horsum omnia studia dirigi debent, ut humana fortiter feramus.   [2] 2 Tim. 2. 3.   [3] Epist. 75. l. 10.   Affectus frequentes contemptique morbum faciunt. Destillatio una, nec adhuc in morem adducta, tussim facit ; assidua et vetus, phthisim.   [4] Calidum ad octo : frigidum ad octo.   Una hirundo non facit æstatem.

Mem. 2. Subs. 1.] *Digression of Anatomy.* 141

ever pleasing at first, or displeasing, violent and tyrannizing over those whom they seise on for the time—yet these fits, I say, or men affected, are but improperly so called, because they continue not, but come and go, as by some objects they are moved. This *melancholy,* of which we are to treat, is an habit, *morbus sonticus,* or *chronicus,* a chronick or continuate disease, a settled humour, as [1] Aurelianus and [2] others call it, not errant, but fixed: and as it was long increasing, so, now being (pleasant or painful) grown to an habit, it will hardly be removed.

SECT. I.—MEMB. II.

SUBSECT. I.

Digression of Anatomy.

BEFORE I proceed to define the disease of *melancholy,* what it is, or to discourse farther of it, I hold it not impertinent to make a brief digression of the anatomy of the body and faculties of the soul, for the better understanding of that which is to follow: because many hard words will often occur, as *myrache, hypochondries, hæmorrhoids, &c. imagination, reason, humours, spirits, vital, natural, animal, nerves, veins, arteries, chylus, pituita;* which of the vulgar will not so easily be perceived, what they are, how cited, and to what end they serve. And, beside, it may peradventure give occasion to some men to examine more accurately, search farther into this most excellent subject, (and thereupon, with that royal [3] prophet, to praise God ; *for a man is fearfully and wonderfully made, and curiously wrought*) that have time and leisure enough, and are sufficiently informed in all other worldly businesses, as to make a good bargain, buy and sell, to keep and make choice of a fair hauk, hound, horse, &c. but, for such matters as concern the knowledge of themselves, they are wholly ignorant and careless ; they know not what this body and soul are, how combined, of what parts and faculties they consist, or how a man differs from a dog. And what can be more ignominious and filthy (as [4] Melancthon well inveighs) *than for a man not to know the structure and composition of his own body? especially since the knowledge of it tends so much to the preservation of his health, and information of his manners.* To stir them up therefore to this study, to peruse those elaborate works of

---

[1] Lib. 1. c. 6.   [2] Fuchsius, l. 3. sec. cap. 7. Hildesheim, fol. 130.
[3] Psal. 39. 13.   [4] De animâ. Turpe enim est homini ignorare sui corporis (ut ita dicam) ædificium, præsertim cum ad valetudinem et mores hæc cognitio plurimum conducat.

142   *Division of the Body.*   [Part. 1. Sec. 1.

[1] Galen, Bauhinus, Plater, Vesalius, Falopius, Laurentius, Remelinus, &c. which have written copiously in *Latin*—or that which some of our industrious countrey-men have done in our mother tongue, not long since, as that translation of [2] Columbus, and [3] Microcosmographia, in thirteen books—I have made this brief digression. Also because [4] Wecker, [5] Melancthon, [6] Fernelius, [7] Fuchsius, and those tedious tracts *de Animâ* (which have more compendiously handled and written of this matter) are not at all times ready to be had—to give them some small taste or notice of the rest, let this epitome suffice.

SUBSECT. II.

Division of the Body. Humours. Spirits.

OF the parts of the Body there be many divisions: the most approved is that of [8] Laurentius, out of Hippocrates, which is into parts *contained*, or *containing. Contained* are either *humours* or *spirits.*

Humours.] A humour is a liquid or fluent part of the body, comprehended in it, for the preservation of it, and is either innate or born with us, or adventitious and acquisite. The radical or innate is daily supplyed by nourishment, which some call *cambium*, and make those secundary humours of *ros* and *gluten* to maintain it; or acquisite, to maintain these four first primary humours, coming and proceeding from the first concoction in the liver, by which means *chylus* is excluded. Some divide them into profitable, and excrementitious. But [9] Crato (out of Hippocrates) will have all four to be juyce, and not excrements, without which no living creature can be sustained; which four, though they be comprehended in the mass of blood, yet they have their several affections, by which they are distinguished from one another, and from those adventitious, *peccant or* [10] *diseased humours*, as Malancthon calls them.

Blood.] Blood is a hot, sweet, temperate, red humour prepared in the *mesaraicke* veins, and made of the most temperate parts of the *chylus* in the liver, whose office is to nourish the whole body, to give it strength and colour, being dispersed, by the veins, through every part of it. And from it

---

[1] De usu part. [2] History of man. [3] D. Crooke. [4] In Syntaxi. [5] De animâ. [6] Instit. lib. 1. [7] Physiol. l. 1, 2. [8] Anat. l. 1. c. 18. [9] In Micro. Succos, sine quibus animal sustentari non potest. [10] Morbosos humores.

spirits are first begotten in the heart, which afterwards, by the *arteries*, are communicated to the other parts.

Pituita, or phlegm, is a cold and moist humour, begotten of the colder part of the *chylus* (or white juyce coming out of the meat digested in the stomach) in the liver; his office is to nourish and moisten the members of the body, which, as the tongue, are moved, that they be not over-dry.

Choler is hot and dry, bitter, begotten of the hotter parts of the *chylus*, and gathered to the gall : it helps the natural heat and senses, and serves to the expelling of excrements.

Melancholy.] *Melancholy*, cold and dry, thick, black, and sowr, begotten of the more fæculent part of nourishment, and purged from the spleen, is a bridle to the other two hot humours, *blood* and *choler*, preserving them in the blood, and nourishing the bones. These four humours have some analogy with the four elements, and to the four ages in man.

Serum, Sweat, Tears.] To these humours you may add *serum*, which is the matter of urine, and those excrementitious humours of the third concoction, sweat and tears.

Spirits.] Spirit is a most subtile vapour, which is expressed from the *blood*, and the instrument of the soul, to perform all his actions; a common tye or *medium* betwixt the body and the soul, as some will have it; or (as [1] Paracelsus) a fourth soul of itself. Melancthon holds the fountain of these spirits to be the *heart;* begotten there, and afterward conveyed to the brain, they take another nature to them. Of these spirits there be three kinds, according to the three principal parts, *brain, heart, liver; natural, vital, animal.* The *natural* are begotten in the *liver*, and thence dispersed through the veins, to perform those natural actions. The *vital spirits* are made in the heart of the *natural*, which, by the arteries, are transported to all the other parts: if these *spirits* cease, then life ceaseth, as in a *syncope* or swouning. The *animal spirits*, formed of the *vital*, brought up to the brain, and diffused by the nerves, to the subordinate members, give sense and motion to them all.

SUBSECT. III.

Similar Parts.

Similar Parts.] Containing parts, by reason of their more solid substance, or either *homogeneal* or *heterogeneal, similar* or *dissimilar;* (so Aristotle divides them, *lib.* 1. *cap.* 1. *de Hist. Animal.* Laurentius, *cap.* 20. *lib.* 1.) *Similar*, or *homogeneal*, are such as, if they be divided, are still severed into

---

[1] Spiritalis anima.

144 *Similar Parts.* [Part. 1. Sec. 1.

parts of the same nature, as water into water. Of these some be *spermatical*, some *fleshy*, or carnal. [1]*Spermatical* are such as are immediately begotten of the seed, which are *bones, gristles, ligaments, membranes, nerves, arteries, veins, skins, fibres or strings, fat.*

Bones.] The bones are dry and hard, begotten of the thickest of the seed, to strengthen and sustain other parts; some say there be three hundred and four, some three hundred and seven, or three hundred and thirteen, in mans body. They have no nerves in them, and are therefore without sense.

A *gristle* is a substance softer than bone, and harder than the rest, flexible, and serves to maintain the parts of motion.

Ligaments are they that tye the bones together, and other parts to the bones, with their subserving tendons. *Membranes* office is to cover the rest.

Nerves, or sinews, are membranes without, and full of marrow within: they proceed from the brain, and carry the animal spirits for sense and motion. Of these some be harder, some softer: the softer serve the senses; and there be seven pair of them. The first be the optick *nerves*, by which we see; the second move the eyes; the third pair serve for the tongue to taste; the fourth pair for the taste in the palat; the fifth belong to the ears; the sixth pair is most ample, and runs almost over all the bowels; the seventh pair moves the tongue. The harder sinews serve for the motion of the inner parts, proceeding from the marrow in the back, of whom there be thirty combinations—seven of the neck, twelve of the breast, &c.

Arteries.] *Arteries* are long and hollow, with a double skin to convey the vital spirits; to discern which the better, they say that Vesalius the anatomist was wont to cut up men alive. [2] They arise in the left side of the heart, and are principally two, from which the rest are derived, *aorta*, and *venosa*. *Aorta* is the root of all the other, which serves the whole body; the other goes to the lungs, to fetch ayr to refrigerate the heart.

Veins.] Veins are hollow and round like pipes; arising from the liver, carrying blood and natural spirits, they feed all the parts. Of these there be two chief, *vena porta*, and *vena cava*, from which the rest are corrivated. That *vena porta* is a vein, coming from the concave of the liver, and receiving those mesaraical veins, by whom he takes the *chylus* from the stomach and guts, and conveys it to the liver. The other derives blood from the liver, to nourish all other dispersed members. The branches of that *vena porta* are the *mesaraical* and *hæmorrhoids*. The branches of the *cava* are *inward* or *out-*

---

[1] Laurentius, c. 20. 1. 1. Anat.   [2] In these they observe the beating of the pulse.

Mem. 2. Subs. 4.]   *Anatomy of the Body.*   145

ward—inward—seminal or *emulgent—outward,* in the head, arms, feet, &c. and have several names.

Fibræ, Fat, Flesh.] *Fibræ* are strings, white and solid, dispersed through the whole member, and right, oblique, transverse, all which have their several uses. *Fat* is a similar part, moist, without blood, composed of the most thick and unctuous matter of the blood. The [1] skin covers the rest, and hath *cuticulam,* or a little skin under it. *Flesh* is soft and ruddy, composed of the congealing of blood, &c.

SUBSECT. IV.

Dissimilar parts.

Dissimilar parts are those which we call *organical,* or *instrumental;* and they be *inward,* or *outward.* The chiefest outward parts are situate forward or backward. *Forward,* the crown and foretop of the head, skull, face, forehead, temples, chin, eyes, ears, nose, &c. neck, breast, chest, upper and lower part of the belly, hypochondries, navel, groyn, flank, &c. *Backward,* the hinder part of the head, back, shoulders, sides, loyns, hip-bones, *os sacrum,* buttocks, &c. Or joynts, arms, hands, feet, leggs, thighs, knees, &c. Or common to both, which because they are obvious and well known, I have carelessly repeated, *eaque præcipua et grandiora tantum: quod reliquum, ex libris de animâ, qui volet, accipiat.*

Inward organical parts, which cannot be seen, are divers in number, and have several names, functions, and divisions; but that of [2] Laurentius is most notable, into *noble,* or *ignoble* parts. Of the *noble* there be three principal parts, to which all the rest belong, and whom they serve—*brain, heart, liver;* according to whose site, three regions, or a threefold division is made of the whole body; as, first, of the *head,* in which the animal organs are contained, and brain it self, which by his nerves gives sense and motion to the rest, and is (as it were) a privy counsellour, and chancellour, to the *heart.* The second region is the chest, or middle *belly,* in which the heart as king keeps his court, and by his arteries communicates life to the whole body. The third region is the lower *belly,* in which the liver resides as a legate *a latere,* with the rest of those natural organs, serving for concoction, nourishment, expelling of excre-

---

[1] Cujus est pars similaris a vi cutificâ ut interiora muniat. Capivac. Anat. pag. 252.   [2] Anat. lib. 1. c. 19. Celebris est et pervulgata partium divisio in principes et ignobiles partes.

VOL. I.   L

146   *Anatomy of the Body.*   [Part. 1. Sec. 1.

ments. This lower region is distinguished from the upper by
the *midriff*, or *diaphragma*, and is subdivided again by [1] some
into three concavities, or regions, upper, middle, and lower—
the upper, of the hypochondries, in whose right side is the
liver, the left the *spleen* (from which is denominated hypochondriacal melancholy)—the second, of the navel and flanks,
divided from the first by the *rim*—the last, of the water-
course, which is again subdivided into three other parts. The
Arabians make two parts of this region, *epigastrium*, and *hypo-
gastrium*; upper, or lower. *Epigastrium* they call *mirach*,
from whence comes *mirachialis melancholia*, sometimes mentioned of them. Of these several regions I will treat in brief
apart; and, first, of the third region, in which the natural
organs are contained.

The lower region. Natural Organs.] But you that are
readers, in the mean time, *suppose you were now brought
into some sacred temple or majestical palace,* (as [2] Melancthon saith) *to behold not the matter only, but the singular
art, workmanship, and counsel of this our great Creator.
And 'tis a pleasant and profitable speculation, if it be considered aright.* The parts of this *region*, which present themselves to your consideration and view, are such as serve to *nutrition* or *generation.* Those of *nutrition* serve to the first or
second concoction, as the *œsophagus* or gullet, which brings
meat and drink into the *stomach.* The *ventricle* or stomach,
which is seated in the midst of that part of the belly beneath
the *midriff*, the kitchen (as it were) of the first concoction, and
which turns our meat into *chylus.* It hath two mouths, one
above, another beneath. The upper is sometimes taken for the
stomach it self: the lower and nether door (as Wecker calls it)
is named *pylorus.* This stomach is sustained by a large kell or
kaull, called *omentum ;* which some will have the same with
peritonæum, or rim of the belly. From the *stomach* to the very
fundament, are produced the *guts* or *intestina,* which serve a
little to alter and distribute the *chylus,* and convey away the
excrements. They are divided into small and great, by reason
of their site and substance, slender or thicker: the slender is
duodenum, or whole gut, which is next to the stomach, some
twelve inches long (saith [3] Fuchsius). *Jejunum*, or empty gut,
continuate to the other, which hath many *mesaraick veins*
annexed to it, which take part of the *chylus* to the liver from
it. *Ilion*, the third, which consists of many crinkles, which
serves with the rest to receive, keep, and distribute the *chylus*

---

[1] D. Crooke, out of Galen and others.   [2] Vos vero veluti in templum ac sa-
crarium quoddam vos duci putetis, &c. Suavis et utilis cognitio.   [3] Lib. 1.
cap. 12. sect. 5.

Mem. 2. Subs. 4.]   *Anatomy of the Body.*   147

from the *stomach*. The thick guts are three, the *blind gut*,
colon, and *right gut*. The *blind* is a thick and short gut,
having one mouth in which the *ilion* and *colon* meet : it receives
the excrements, and conveys them to the *colon*. This *colon*
hath many windings, that the excrements pass not away too
fast: the *right gut* is straight, and conveys the excrements to
the *fundament*, whose lower part is bound up with certain
muscles, called *sphincteres*, that the excrements may be the
better contained, until such time a man be willing to go to the
stool. In the midst of these guts is situated the *mesenterium*
or *midriff*, composed of many veins, arteries, and much fat,
serving chiefly to sustain the guts. All these parts serve the
first concoction. To the second, which is busied either in re-
fining the good nourishment, or expelling the bad, is chiefly
belonging the liver, like in colour to congealed blood, the shop
of blood, situate in the right *hypochondry*, in figure like to an
half moon ; *generosum membrum*, Melancthon stiles it ; a generous part : it serves to turn the *chylus* to blood, for the nourishment of the body. The excrements of it are either *cholerick* or *watery*, which the other subordinate parts convey. The
gall, placed in the concave of the *liver*, extracts *choler* to it:
the *spleen*, *melancholy ;* which is situate on the left side, over
against the *liver*, a spungy matter that draws this black *choler*
to it by a secret vertue, and feeds upon it, conveying the rest
to the bottom of the stomach, to stir up appetite, or else to
the guts as an excrement. That watery matter the two kid-
neys expurgate by those emulgent veins, and *ureters*. The
emulgent draw this superfluous moisture from the blood; the
two *ureters* convey it to the *bladder*, which, by reason of his
site in the lower belly, is apt to receive it, having two parts,
neck and bottom: the bottom holds the water ; the neck is
constringed with a muscle, which, as a porter, keeps the water
from running out against our will.

Members of generation are common to both sexes, or peculiar to one ; which, because they are impertinent to my purpose, I do voluntarily omit.

Middle region.] Next in order is the *middle region*, or
chest, which comprehends the vital faculties and parts; which
(as I have said) is separated from the lower belly by the *diaphragma* or *midriff*, which is a skin consisting of many nerves,
membranes ; and, amongst other uses it hath, is the instrument of laughing. There is also a certain thin membrane, full
of sinews, which covereth the whole chest within, and is called
pleura, the seat of the disease called *pleurisie*, when it is inflamed. Some add a third skin, which is termed *mediastinus*,
which divides the chest into two parts, right and left. Of this
region the principal part is the *heart*, which is the seat and

L 2

148   *Anatomy of the Body.*   [Part. 1. Sec. 1.

fountain of life, of heat, of spirits, of pulse, and respiration :
the sun of our body, the king and sole commander of it : the
seat and organ of all passions and affections; *(primum vivens,
ultimum moriens:* it lives first, and dies last in all creatures) of
a pyramidical form, and not much unlike to a pine-apple; [1] a
part worthy of admiration, that can yield such variety of affections, by whose motion it is dilated or contracted, to stir and
command the humours in the body; as, in sorrow, melancholy ;
in anger, choler ; in joy, to send the blood outwardly ; in sorrow,
to call it in ; moving the humours, as horses do a· chariot.
This *heart,* though it be one sole member, yet it may be divided
into two creeks, *right* and *left.* The *right* is like the moon increasing, bigger than the other part, and receives blood from
vena cava, distributing some of it to the *lungs,* to nourish
them, the rest to the left side, to ingender spirits. *The left
creek* hath the form of a *cone,* and is the seat of life, which
(as a torch doth oyl) draws blood unto it, begetting of it spirits
and fire; and, as fire in a torch, so are spirits in the blood ;
and, by that great *artery* called *aorta,* it sends vital spirits over
the body, and takes aire from the lungs, by that *artery* which
is called *venosa;* so that both creeks have their vessels ; the
right two veins; the left two arteries, besides those two
common anfractuous ears, which serve them both ; the one to
hold blood, the other aire, for several uses. The *lungs* is a
thin spungy part, like an oxe hoof, (saith [2] Fernelius) the
town-clark or cryer ([3] one terms it), the instrument of voice,
as an orator to a king; annexed to the heart, to express his
thoughts by voice. That it is the instrument of voice is manifest, in that no creature can speak or utter any voice, which
wanteth these lights. It is, besides, the instrument of respiration, or breathing; and its office is to cool the *heart,* by sending aire unto it by the *venosal artery,* which vein comes to the
lungs by that *aspera arteria,* which consists of many gristles,
membranes, nerves, taking in aire at the nose and mouth,
and, by it likewise, exhales the fumes of the *heart.*

In the upper *region* serving the animal faculties, the chief
organ is the *brain,* which is a soft, marrowish, and white substance, ingendred of the purest part of seed and spirits, included by many skins, and seated within the skull or brain-pan;
and it is the most noble organ under heaven, the dwelling-house
and seat of the soul, the habitation of wisdom, memory, judge-

---

[1] Hæc res est præcipue digna admiratione, quod tantâ affectuum varietate
cietur cor, quod omnes res tristes et lætæ statim corda feriunt et movent.
[2] Physio. l. 1. c. 8.   [3] Ut orator regi, sic pulmo, vocis instrumentum, annec-
titur cordi, &c. Melancth.

Mem. 2. Subs. 5.] *Anatomy of the Soul.* 149

ment, reason, and in which man is most like unto God: and therefore nature hath covered it with a skull of hard bone, and two skins or membranes, whereof the one is called *dura mater,* or *meninx,* the other *pia mater.* The *dura mater* is next to the skull, above the other, which includes and protects the brain. When this is taken away, the *pia mater* is to be seen, a thin membrane, the next and immediate cover of the brain, and not covering only, but entering into it. The *brain* it self is divided into two parts, the *fore* and *hinder part.* The *fore part* is much bigger than the other, which is called the *little brain* in respect of it. This *fore part* hath many concavities, distinguished by certain ventricles, which are the receptacles of the spirits, brought hither by the arteries from the heart, and are there refined to a more heavenly nature, to perform the actions of the soul. Of these ventricles there be three, *right, left,* and *middle.* The *right* and *left* answer to their site, and beget animal spirits; if they be any way hurt, sense and motion ceaseth. These ventricles, moreover, are held to be the seat of the common sense. The *middle ventricle* is a common concourse and cavity of them both, and hath two passages; the one to receive *pituita;* and the other extends it self to the fourth creek: in this they place *imagination* and *cogitation;* and so the three ventricles of the fore part of the *brain* are used. The fourth creek, behind the head, is common to the *cerebel* or little brain, and marrow of the back-bone, the least and most solid of all the rest, which receives the animal spirits from the other ventricles, and conveys them to the marrow in the back, and is the place where they say the memory is seated.

SUBSECT. V.

Of the Soul and her Faculties.

ACCORDING to [1] Aristotle, the soul is defined to be εντελε-χεια, *perfectio et actus primus corporis organici, vitam habentis in potentiá*—the perfection or first act of an organical body, having power of life; which most [2] philosophers approve. But many doubts arise about the *essence, subject, seat, distinction,* and subordinate faculties, of it. For the essence and particular knowledge, of all other things it is most hard (be it of man or beast) to discern, as [3] Aristotle himself, [4] Tully, [5] Picus Mirandula, [6] Tolet, and other neoterick philosophers,

---

[1] De anim. c. 1. [2] Scalig. exerc. 307. Tolet. in lib. de animâ, cap. 1, &c.
[3] De animâ, cap. 1. [4] Tuscul. quæst. [5] Lib. 6. Doct. Val. Gentil.
c. 13. pag. 1216. [6] Aristot.

150   *Anatomy of the Soul.*   [Part. 1. Sec. 1.

confess. [1] *We can understand all things by her; but, what she is, we cannot apprehend.* Some therefore make one *soul*, divided into three principal faculties; others, three distinct *souls;* (which question of late hath been much controverted by Picolomineus, and Zabarel) [2] Paracelsus will have four *souls*, adding to the three granted faculties, a *spiritual soul;* (which opinion of his, Campanella, in his book *de* [3] *Sensu rerum*, much labours to demonstrate and prove, because carkasses bleed at the sight of the murderer; with many such arguments:) and [4] some, again, one soul of all creatures whatsoever, differing only in organs; and that beasts have reason as well as men, though, for some defect of organs, not in such measure. Others make a doubt, whether it be all in all, and all in every part; which is amply discussed in Zabarel among the rest. The [5] common division of the *soul* is into three principal faculties, *vegetal, sensitive,* and *rational*, which make three distinct kind of living creatures—*vegetal* plants, *sensible* beasts, *rational* men. How these three principal faculties are distinguished and connected, *humano ingenio inaccessum videtur*, is beyond humane capacity, as [6] Taurellus, Philip, Flavius, and others, suppose. The inferiour may be alone; but the superiour cannot subsist without the other; so *sensible* includes *vegetal, rational,* both which are contained in it, (saith Aristotle) *ut trigonus in tetragono*, as a triangle in a quadrangle.

Vegetal soul.] *Vegetal*, the first of the three distinct faculties, is defined to be *a substantial act of an organical body, by which it is nourished, augmented, and begets another like unto it self:* in which definition, three several operations are specified, *altrix, auctrix, procreatrix.* The first is [7] nutrition, whose object is nourishment, meat, drink, and the like; his organ the liver, in sensible creatures; in plants, the root or sap. His office is to turn the nutriment into the substance of the body nourished, which he performs by natural heat. This nutritive operation hath four other subordinate functions or powers belonging to it—*attraction, retention, digestion, expulsion.*

Attraction.] [8] *Attraction* is a ministering faculty, which (as a loadstone doth iron) draws meat into the stomach, or as a lamp doth oyle; and this attractive power is very necessary in plants, which suck up moisture by the root, as another mouth, into the sap, as a like stomach.

---

[1] Animâ quæque intelligimus; et tamen, quæ sit ipsa, intelligere non valemus. [2] Spiritualem animam a reliquis distinctam tuetur, etiam in cadavere inhærentem post mortem per aliquot menses. [3] Lib. 3. cap. 31. [4] Cœlius, lib. 2. c. 31. Plutarch. in Grillo. Lips. cen. 1. ep. 50. Jossius de Risu et Fletu, Averroes, Campanella, &c. [5] Philip. de Animâ, ca. 1. Cœlius, 20. antiq. cap. 3. Plutarch. de placit. Philos. [6] De vit. et mort. part. 2. c. 3. prop. 1. de vit. et mort. 2. c. 22. [7] Nutritio est alimenti transmutatio, viro naturalis. Scal. exerc. 101. sect. 17. [8] See more of attraction in Scal. exerc. 343.

Retention.] *Retention* keeps it, being attracted unto the stomach, until such time it be concocted; for, if it should pass away straight, the body could not be nourished.

Digestion.] *Digestion* is performed by natural heat; for, as the flame of a torch consumes oyle, wax, tallow, so doth it alter and digest the nutritive matter. Indigestion is opposite unto it, for want of natural heat. Of this *digestion* there be three differences, *maturation, elixation, assation.*

Maturation.] *Maturation* is especially observed in the fruits of trees, which are then said to be ripe, when the seeds are fit to be sown again. *Crudity* is opposed to it, which gluttons, Epicures, and idle persons are most subject unto, that use no exercise to stir up natural heat, or else choke it, as too much wood puts out a fire.

Elixation.] *Elixation* is the seething of meat in the stomach, by the said natural heat, as meat is boyled in a pot; to which corruption or putrefaction is opposite.

Assation.] *Assation* is a concoction of the inward moisture by heat; his opposite his *semiustulation.*

Order of concoction four-fold.] Besides these three several operations of *digestion*, there is a fourfold order of concoction; *mastication*, or chewing in the mouth; *chylification* of this so chewed meat in the stomach; the third is in the *liver*, to turn this *chylus* into blood, called *sanguification;* the last is *assimulation*, which is in every part.

Expulsion.] *Expulsion* is a power of *nutrition*, by which it expells all superfluous excrements and reliques of meat and drink, by the guts, bladder, pores; as by purging, vomiting, spitting, sweating, urine, hairs, nails, &c.

Augmentation.] As this *nutritive faculty* serves to nourish the body, so doth the *augmenting faculty* (the second operation or power of the *vegetal faculty*) to the increasing of it in quantity, according to all dimensions, long, broad, thick, and to make it grow till it come to his due proportion and perfect shape; which hath his period of augmentation, as of consumption, and that most certain, as the poet observes:

Stat sua cuique dies; breve et irreparabile tempus
Omnibus est vitæ——

A term of life is set to every man,
Which is but short; and pass it no one can.

Generation.] The last of these *vegetal faculties* is *generation*, which begets another by means of seed, like unto it self, to the perpetual preservation of the *species*. To this faculty they ascribe three subordinate operations; the first to turn nourishment into seed, &c.

152 *Anatomy of the Soul.* [Part. 1. Sec. 1.

Life and death concomitants of the vegetal faculties.] Necessary concomitants or affections of this *vegetal faculty* are life, and his privation, death. To the preservation of life the natural heat is most requisite, though siccity and humidity, and those first qualities, be not excluded. This heat is likewise in plants, as appears by their increasing, fructifying, &c. though not so easily perceived. In all bodies it must have radical [1] moisture to preserve it, that it be not consumed; (to which preservation our clime, countrey, temperature, and the good or bad use of those six non-natural things, avail much) for, as this natural heat and moisture decayes, so doth our life it self: and, if not prevented before by some violent accident, or interrupted through our own default, is in the end dryed up by old age, and extinguished by death for want of matter, as a lamp, for defect of oyl to maintain it.

SUBSECT. VI.

Of the sensible Soul.

NEXT in order is the *sensible faculty*, which is as far beyond the other in dignity, as a beast is preferred to a plant, having those vegetal powers included in it. 'Tis defined an *act of an organical body, by which it lives, hath sense, appetite, judgement, breath, and motion.* His object, in general, is a sensible or passible quality, because the sense is affected with it. The general organ is the brain, from which principally the sensible operations are derived. The *sensible soul* is divided into two parts, *apprehending* or *moving.* By the *apprehensive* power, we perceive the species of sensible things, present or absent, and retain them as wax doth the print of a seal. By the moving, the body is outwardly carried from one place to another, or inwardly moved by spirits and pulse. The *apprehensive* faculty is subdivided into two parts, *inward* or *outward—outward*, as the five senses, of *touching, hearing, seeing, smelling, tasting;* to which you may add Scaligers sixth sense of *titillation*, if you please, or that of *speech*, which is the sixth external sense, according to Lullius. *Inward* are three, *common sense, phantasie, memory.* Those five outward senses have their object in outward things only, and such as are present, as the eye sees no colour except it be at hand, the ear sound. Three of these senses are of commodity, *hearing, sight,* and *smell;*

---

[1] Vita consistit in calido et humido.

two of necessity, *touch* and *taste*, without which we cannot live. Besides, the *sensitive* power is *active* or *passive*—*active* as, in sight, the eye sees the colour; *passive*, when it is hurt by his object, as the eye by the sun beams, (according to that axiom *visibile forte destruit sensum*) or if the object be not pleasing, as a bad sound to the ear, a stinking smell to the nose, &c.

Sight.] Of these five senses, *sight* is held to be most precious, and the best, and that by reason of his object; it sees the whole body at once ; by it we learn, and discern all things —a sense most excellent for use. To the *sight* three things are required ; the *object*, the *organ*, and the *medium*. The *object* in general is *visible*, or that which is to be seen, as colours, and all shining bodies. The *medium* is the illumination of the aire, which comes from [1] light, commonly called *diaphanum;* for, in dark, we cannot see. The *organ* is the eye, and chiefly the apple of it, which, by those optick nerves concuring both in one, conveys the sight to the common sense. Betwixt the organ and the object, a true distance is required, that it be not too near, or too far off. Many excellent questions appertain to this sense, discussed by philosophers ; as, whether this sight be caused *intra mittendo, vel extra mittendo, &c.* by receiving in the visible species, or sending of them out; which [2] Plato, [3] Plutarch, [4] Macrobius, [5] Lactantius, and others, dispute. And, besides, it is the subject of the *perspectives,* of which Alhazen the Arabian, Vitellio, Roger Bacon, Baptista Porta, Guidus Ubaldus, Aquilonius, &c. have written whole volumes.

Hearing.] Hearing, a most excellent outward sense, *by which we learn and get knowledge.* His object is sound, or that which is heard ; the *medium*, aire ; *organ*, the ear. To the sound, which is a collision of the aire, three things are required ; a body to strike, as the hand of a musician ; the body strucken, which must be solid and able to resist; as a bell, lute-string : not wooll, or spunge; the *medium*, the aire, which is *inward* or *outward ;* the outward, being struck or collided by a solid body, still strikes the next air, until it come to that inward natural aire, which, as an exquisite organ, is contained in a little skin formed like a drum-head, and, struck upon by certain small instruments like drum-sticks, conveys the sound, by a pair of nerves appropriated to that use, to the *common sense,* as to a judge of sounds. There is great variety and much delight in them; for the knowledge of which consult with Boëthius, and other musicians.

---

[1] Lumen est actus perspicui. Lumen a luce provenit; lux est in corpore lucido.
[2] In Phædon.　　　[3] Satur. 7. c. 14.　　　[4] Lac. cap. 8. de opif. Dei, 1.
[5] De pract. Philos. 4.

154   *Anatomy of the Soul.*   [Part. 1. Sec. 1.

Smelling.] Smelling is an *outward sense, which apprehends by the nostrils, drawing in aire;* and, of all the rest, it is the weakest sense in men. The organ in the nose, or two small hollow pieces of flesh a little above it: the *medium* the aire to men, as water to fish : the *object, smell,* arising from a mixt body resolved, which whether it be a quality, fume, vapour, or exhalation, I will not now dispute, or of their differences, and how they are caused. This sense is an organ of health, as sight and hearing (saith [1] Agellius) are of discipline; and that by avoiding bad smells, as by choosing good, which do as much alter and affect the body many times, as *diet* it self.

Taste.] *Taste,* a necessary sense, *which perceives all savours by the tongue and palate, and that by means of a thin spittle, or watery juice.* His *organ* is the *tongue* with his tasting nerves; the *medium,* a watery juice; the *object, taste,* or savour, which is a quality in the juice, arising from the mixture of things tasted. Some make eight species or kinds of savour, bitter, sweet, sharp, salt, &c. all which sick men (as in an ague) cannot discern, by reason of their organs misaffected.

Touching.] *Touch,* the last of the senses, and most ignoble, yet of as great necessity as the other, and of as much pleasure. This sense is exquisite in men, and, by his nerves dispersed all over the body, perceives any tactile quality. His *organ,* the *nerves;* his *object,* those first qualities, hot, dry, moist, cold; and those that follow them, hard, soft, thick, thin, &c. Many delightsome questions are moved by philosophers about these five senses, their organs, objects, mediums, which for brevity I omit.

SUBSECT. VII.

Of the Inward Senses.

Common sense.] *Inner senses* are three in number, so called, because they be within the brain-pan, as *common sense, phantasie, memory.* Their objects are not only things present, but they perceive the sensible species of things *to come, past, absent,* such as were before in the sense. *This common sense* is the judge or moderator of the rest, by whom we discern all differences of objects; for by mine eye I do not know that I see, or by mine ear that I hear, but by my *common sense,* who judgeth of sounds and colours: they are but the organs to bring the species to be censured; so that all their objects are his, and all their offices are his. The forepart of the brain is his organ or seat.

[1] Lib. 19. cap. 2.

Phantasie.] *Phantasie*, or imagination, which some call *æstimative*, or *cogitative*, (confirmed, saith [1] Fernelius, by frequent meditation) is an inner sense, which doth more fully examine the species perceived by *common sense*, of things present or absent, and keeps them longer, recalling them to mind again, or making new of his own. In time of sleep, this faculty is free, and many times conceives strange, stupend, absurd shapes, as in sick men we commonly observe. His *organ* is the middle cell of the brain ; his *objects*, all the species communicated to him by the *common sense*, by comparison of which, he feigns infinite other unto himself. In *melancholy* men, this faculty is most powerful and strong, and often hurts, producing many monstrous and prodigious things, especially if it be stirred up by some terrible object, presented to it from *common sense* or *memory*. In poets and painters, *imagination* forcibly works, as appears by their several fictions, anticks, images, as Ovid's house of Sleep, Psyches palace in Apuleius, &c. In men it is subject and governed by *reason*, or at least should be; but, in brutes, it hath no superiour, and is *ratio brutorum*, all the reason they have.

Memory.] *Memory* layes up all the species which the senses have brought in, and records them as a good *register*, that they may be forth-coming when they are called for by *phantasie* and *reason*. His object is the same with *phantasie ;* his seat and *organ*, the back part of the brain.

Affections of the senses, sleep and waking.] The affections of these senses are *sleep* and *waking*, common to all sensible creatures. *Sleep is a rest or binding of the outward senses, and of the common sense, for the preservation of body and soul* (as [2] Scaliger defines it) ; for, when the common sense resteth, the outward senses rest also. The phantasie alone is free, and his commander, reason; as appears by those imaginary dreams, which are of divers kinds, *natural*, *divine*, *dæmoniacal*, *&c.* which vary according to humours, diet, actions, objects, &c. of which, Artemidorus, Cardanus, and Sambucus, with their several interpretators, have written great volumes. This ligation of senses proceeds from an inhibition of spirits, the way being stopped by which they should come ; this stopping is caused of vapours arising out of the stomach, filling the nerves, by which the spirits should be conveyed. When these vapours are spent, the passage is open, and the spirits perform their accustomed duties ; so that *waking is the action and motion of the senses, which the spirits, dispersed over all parts, cause.*

---

[1] Phys. l. 5. c. 8.   [2] Exercit. 280.

156   *Anatomy of the Soul.*   [Part. 1. Sec. 1.

SUBSECT. VIII.

Of the Moving Faculty.

Appetite.] THIS *moving faculty* is the other power of the *sensitive soul*, which causeth all those *inward and outward animal motions in the body*. It is divided into two faculties, the power of *appetite* and of *moving from place to place*. This of appetite is threefold, (so some will have it) *natural*, as it signifies any such inclination, as of a stone to fall downward, and such actions as *retention, expulsion*, which depend not of sense, but are *vegetal*, as the appetite of meat and drink, hunger and thirst. *Sensitive* is common to men and brutes. *Voluntary;* the third, or intellective, which commands the other two in men, and is a curb unto them, or at least should be (but for the most part is captivated and over-ruled by them: and men are led like beasts by sense, giving reins to their concupiscence and several lusts); for by this appetite the soul is led or inclined to follow that good which the senses shall approve, or avoid that which they hold evil. His object being good or evil, the one he embraceth, the other he rejecteth—according to that aphorism, *omnia appetunt bonum*, all things seek their own good, or at least seeming good. This power is inseparable from sense; for, where sense is, there is likewise pleasure and pain. His *organ* is the same with the *common sense*, and is divided into two powers, or inclinations, *concupiscible* or *irascible*, or (as [1] one translates it) *coveting, anger-invading*, or impugning. *Concupiscible* covets always pleasant and delightsome things, and abhorrs that which is distasteful, harsh, and unpleasant. *Irascible,* [2] *quasi aversans per iram et odium*, as avoiding it with anger and indignation. All affections and perturbations arise out of these two fountains, which although the Stoicks make light of, we hold natural, and not to be resisted. The good affections are caused by some object of the same nature ; and, if present, they procure joy, which dilates the heart, and preserves the body: if absent, they cause hope, love, desire, and concupiscence. The bad are *simple* or *mixt; simple*, for some bad object present, as sorrow, which contracts the heart, macerates the soul, subverts the good estate of the body, hindering all the operations of it, causing melancholy, and many times death itself; or future, as fear. Out of these two, arise those mixt affections and passions of anger, which is a desire of revenge—hatred, which is inveterate anger—zeal,

---

[1] T. W. Jesuit, in his Passions of the Mind.   [2] Velcurio.

which is offended with him who hurts that he loves—and επιχαιρεκακια, a compound affection of joy and hate, when we rejoyce at other mens mischief, and are grieved at their prosperity—pride, self-love, emulation, envy, shame, &c. of which elsewhere.

Moving from place to place, is a faculty necessarily following the other : for in vain were it otherwise to desire and to abhor, if we had not likewise power to prosecute or eschew, by moving the body from place to place. By this faculty therefore we locally move the body, or any part of it, and go from one place to another : to the better performance of which, three things are requisite—that which moves; by what it moves ; that which is moved. That which moves is either the efficient cause, or end. The end is the object, which is desired or eschewed, as in a dog to catch a hare, &c. The efficient cause in man is *reason,* or his subordinate phantasie, which apprehends good or bad objects; in brutes, *imagination* alone, which moves the *appetite,* the *appetite* this faculty, which, by an admirable league of nature, and by mediation of the spirit, commands the organ by which it moves : and that consists of nerves, muscles, cords, dispersed through the whole body, contracted and relaxed as the spirits will, which move the muscles, or [1] nerves in the midst of them, and draw the cord, and so, *per consequens,* the joynt, to the place intended. That which is moved is the body or some member apt to move. The motion of the body is divers, as going, running, leaping, dancing, sitting, and such like, referred to the predicament of *situs.* Worms creep, birds fly, fishes swim : and so of parts, the chief of which is *respiration* or breathing, and is thus performed : the outward aire is drawn in by the *vocal artery,* and sent by mediation of the *midriff* to the lungs, which, dilating themselves as a pair of bellows, reciprocally fetch it in, and send it out to the heart to cool it; and from thence, now being hot, convey it again, still taking in fresh. Such a like motion is that of the *pulse,* of which, because many have written whole books, I will say nothing.

SUBSECT. IX.

Of the Rational Soul.

In the precedent subsections, I have anatomized those inferior faculties of the soul ; the *rational* remaineth, a *pleasant, but a doubtful subject* (as [2] one terms it), and with the like

---

[1] Nervi a spiritu moventur, spiritus ab animâ. Melanct.   [2] Velcurio. Jucundum et anceps subjectum.

158   *Anatomy of the Soul.*   [Part. 1. Sec. 1.

brevity to be discussed. Many erroneous opinions are about
the essence and original of it; whether it be fire, as Zeno held;
harmony, as Aristoxenus ; number, as Xenocrates; whether it
be organical, or inorganical ; seated in the brain, heart, or
blood; mortal, or immortal: how it comes into the body.
Some hold that it is *ex traduce*, as *Phil.* 1. *de Animâ, Tertullian, Lactantius de opific. Dei, cap.* 19. *Hugo, lib. de Spiritu
et Animâ, Vincentius Bellavic. spec. natural. lib.* 23. *cap.* 2. *et*
11. Hippocrates, Avicenna, and many [1] late writers; that one
man begets another, body and soul ; or, as a candle from a
candle, to be produced from the seed : otherwise, say they, a
man begets but half a man, and is worse than a beast, that
begets both matter and form ; and, besides, the three faculties
of the soul must be together infused ; which is most absurd, as
they hold, because in beasts they are begot (the two inferiour I
mean), and may not be well separated in men. [2] Galen supposeth the soul *crasin esse*, to be the temperature it self; Trismegistus, Musæus, Orpheus, Homer, Pindarus, Pherecydes
Syrus, Epictetus, with the Chaldees and Ægyptians, affirmed
the soul to be immortal, as did those Britan [3] Druides of old.
The [4]Pythagoreans defend *metempsychosis and palingenesia—*
that souls go from one body to another, *epotâ prius Lethes
undâ*, as men into wolves, bears, dogs, hogs, as they were inclined in their lives, or participated in conditions :

——————————————————————[5] inque ferinas
Possumus ire domos, pecudumque in pectora condi.

[6] Lucians cock was first Euphorbus, a captain :

Ille ego, (nam memini) Trojani tempore belli,
Panthoïdes Euphorbus eram,

a horse, a man, a spunge. [7] Julian the Apostate thought Alexanders soul was descended into his body : Plato, in Timæo, and
in his Phædon, (for ought I can perceive) differs not much from
this opinion, that it was from God at first, and knew all : but,
being inclosed in the body, it forgets, and learns anew, which
he calls *reminiscentia*, or *recalling ;* and that it was put into
the body for a punishment, and thence it goes into a beasts, or
mans, (as appears by his pleasant fiction *de sortitione animarum, lib.* 10. *de rep.)* and, after [8] ten thousand years, is to return into the former body again:

---

[1] Goclenius, in ψυχολ. pag. 302.   Bright, in Phys. Scrib. l. 1. David Crusius,
Melancthon, Hippius Hernius, Levinus Lemnius, &c.   [2] Lib. an mores sequantur, &c.   [3] Cæsar. 6. com.   [4] Read Æneas Gazeus dial. of the immortality of the soul·   [5] Ovid. Met. 15.   [6] In Gallo. Idem.   [7] Nicephorus, hist. l. 10. c. 35.   [8] Phæd.

Mem. 2. Subs. 9.] *Anatomy of the Soul.* 159

——————[1] post varios annos, per mille figuras,
Rursus ad humanæ fertur primordia vitæ.

Others deny the immortality of it, which Pomponatus of Padua
decided out of Aristotle not long since, *Plinius Avunculus,
cap. 7. lib. 2. et lib. 7. cap. 55. Seneca, lib. 7. epist. ad Luci-
lium, epist. 55. Dicæarchus, in Tull. Tusc. Epicurus, Aratus,
Hippocrates, Galen, Lucretius, lib.* 1.

(Præterea gigni pariter cum corpore, et unà
Crescere sentimus, pariterque senescere, mentem)

Averroes, and I know not how many neotericks. [2] *This question of the immortality of the soul is diversely and wonderfully
impugned and disputed, especially amongst the Italians of late,*
saith Jab. Colerus, *lib. de immort. animæ, cap.* 1. The Popes
themselves have doubted of it. Leo Decimus, that Epicurean
Pope, as [3]some record of him, caused this question to be discussed *pro* and *con* before him, and concluded at last, as a prophane and atheistical moderator, with that verse of Cornelius
Gallus,

Et redit in nihilum, quod fuit ante nihil;

it began of nothing, and in nothing it ends. Zeno and his
Stoicks (as [4] Austin quotes him) supposed the soul so long to
continue, till the body was fully putrified, and resolved into
materia prima ; but, after that, *in fumos evanescere,* to be extinguished and vanish ; and in the mean time whilst the body
was consuming, it wandered all abroad, *et e longinquo multa an-
nunciare,* and (as that Clazomenian Hermotimus averred) saw
pretty visions, and suffered I know not what.

[5] Errant exsangues sine corpore et ossibus umbræ.

Others grant the immortality thereof; but they make many fabulous fictions in the mean time of it, after the departure from
the body—like Platos Elysian fields, and the Turkie paradise.
The souls of good men they deified ; the bad (saith [6] Austin)
became devils, as they supposed ; with many such absurd tenents, which he hath confuted. Hierom, Austin, and other
fathers of the church, hold that the soul is immortal, created
of nothing, and so infused into the child or *embrio* in his
mothers womb, six months after the [7] conception ; not as
those of brutes, which are *ex traduce,* and, dying with them,

---

[1] Claudian. lib. 1. de rapt. Proserp.   [2] Hæc quæstio multos per annos
varie ac mirabiliter impugnata, &c.   [3] Colerus, ibid.   [4] De eccles. dog.
cap. 16.   [5] Ovid. 4. Met.   [6] Bonorum lares, malorum vero larvas et
lemures.   [7] Some say at three days, some six weeks, others otherwise.

160 *Anatomy of the Soul.* [Part. 1. Sec. 1.

vanish into nothing—to whose divine treatises, and to the Scriptures themselves, I rejourn all such atheistical spirits, as Tully did Atticus, doubting of this point, to Platos Phædon: or, if they desire philosophical proofs and demonstrations, I refer them to *Niphus, Nic. Faventinus* Tracts of this subject, to *Franc.* and *John Picus in digress. sup. 3. de Animâ, Tholosanus, Eugubinus,* to *Soto, Canas, Thomas, Peresius, Dandinus, Colerus,* to that elaborate Tract in Zanchius, to Tolets Sixty Reasons, and Lessius Twenty-two Arguments, to prove the immortality of the soul. Campanella, *lib. de sensu rerum,* is large in the same discourse, Albertinus the Schoolman, Jacob. Nactantus, *tom. 2. op.* handleth it in four questions—Antony Brunus, Aonius Palearius, Marinus Marcennus, with many others. This *reasonable soul,* which Austin calls a spiritual substance moving it self, is defined by philosophers to be *the first substantial act of a natural, humane, organical body, by which a man lives, perceives, and understands, freely doing all things, and with election:* out of which definition we may gather, that this *rational soul* includes the powers, and performs the duties, of the two other, which are contained in it; and all three faculties make one soul, which is inorganical of it self (although it be in all parts), and incorporeal, using their organs and working by them. It is divided into two chief parts, differing in office only, not in essence—the *understanding,* which is the *rational* power *apprehending;* the *will,* which is the *rational* power *moving;* to which two, all the other rational powers are subject and reduced.

SUBSECT. X.

Of the Understanding.

Understanding is a power of the soul, [1] *by which we perceive, know, remember, and judge, as well singulars as universals, having certain innate notices or beginnings of arts, a reflecting action, by which it judgeth of his own doings, and examines them.* Out of this definition, (besides his chief office, which is to apprehend, judge all that he performs, without the help of any instruments or organs) three differences appear betwixt a man and a beast: as first, the sense only comprehends *singularities,* the understanding *universalities:* secondly, the sense hath no innate notions: thirdly, brutes cannot reflect upon themselves. Bees indeed make neat

---

[1] Melanct.

Mem. 2. Subs. 10.] *Anatomy of the Soul.* 161

and curious works, and many other creatures besides; but
when they have done, they cannot judge of them.   His object
is God, *Ens,* all nature, and whatsoever is to be understood :
which successively it apprehends.   The object first moving the
understanding, is some sensible thing; after, by discoursing,
the mind finds out the corporeal substance, and from thence
the spiritual.   His actions (some say) are *apprehension, composition, division, discoursing, reasoning, memory* (which some
include in *invention*), and *judgement.*   The common divisions
are of the understanding, *agent,* and *patient; speculative,* and
practick; in *habit,* or in *act; simple,* or *compound.*   The *agent*
is that which is called the *wit* of man, *acumen* or subtilty,
sharpness of invention, when he doth invent of himself without
a teacher, or learns anew—which abstracts those intelligible
species from the phantasie, and transferrs them to the passive
understanding, [1] *because there is nothing in the understanding,
which was not first in the sense.*   That which the imagination
hath taken from the sense, this agent judgeth of, whether it be
true or false; and, being so judged, he commits it to the *passible* to be kept.   The *agent* is a doctor or teacher; the *passive,*
a scholar; and his office is to keep and farther judge of such
things as are committed to his charge; as a bare and rased
table at first, capable of all forms and notions.   Now these notions are twofold, *actions* or *habits;* actions, by which we take
notions of, and perceive things: *habits,* which are durable lights
and notions, which we may use when we will.   [2] Some reckon
up eight kinds of them, *sense, experience, intelligence, faith,
suspicion, errour, opinion, science;* to which are added *art, prudency, wisdom;* as also [3] *synteresis, dictamen rationis, conscience;*
so that, in all, there be fourteen species of the *understanding,*
of which some are *innate,* as the three last mentioned ; the
other are gotten by doctrine, learning, and use.   Plato will
have all to be innate : Aristotle reckons up but five intellectual
habits: two *practick,* as *prudency,* whose end is to practise, to
fabricate ; *wisdom,* to comprehend the use and experiments of
all notions and habits whatsoever : which division of Aristotle
(if it be considered aright) is all one with the precedent : for,
three being innate, and five acquisite, the rest are improper,
imperfect, and, in a more strict examination, excluded.   Of all
these I should more amply dilate, but my subject will not
permit.   Three of them I will only point at, as more necessary
to my following discourse.

Synteresis, or the purer part of the conscience, is an innate

---

[1] Nihil in intellectu, quod non prius fuerat in sensu.   [2] Velcurio.
[3] The pure part of the conscience.

VOL. I.   M

162   *Anatomy of the Soul.*   [Part. 1. Sec. 1.

habit, and doth signifie *a conservation of the knowledge of the
law of God and Nature, to know good or evil:* and (as our
divines hold) it is rather in the *understanding,* than in the *will.*
This makes the *major* proposition in a practick *syllogism.*
The *dictamen rationis* is that which doth admonish us to do
good or evil, and is the *minor* in the *syllogism.* The conscience is that which approves good or evil, justifying or condemning our actions, and is the conclusion of the *syllogism;* as
in that familiar example of Regulus the Roman, taken prisoner
by the Carthaginians, and suffered to go to Rome, on that
condition he should return again, or pay so much for his ransom. The *synteresis* proposeth the question ; his word, oath,
promise, is to be religiously kept, although to his enemy, and
that by the law of nature—[1] *do not that to another, which thou
wouldest not have done to thy self. Dictamen* applies it to him,
and dictates this or the like: Regulus, thou wouldst not
another man should falsifie his oath, or break promise with
thee : *conscience* concludes, Therefore, Regulus, thou dost well
to perform thy promise, and oughtest to keep thine oath.
More of this, in *Religious Melancholy.*

SUBSECT. XI.

Of the Will.

Will is the other power of the *rational soul,* [2] *which covets
or avoids such things as have been before judged and apprehended by the understanding.* If good, it approves; if evil,
it abhors it: so that his object is either good or evil. Aristotle
calls this our *rational appetite;* for as, in the *sensitive,* we are
moved to good or bad by our *appetite,* ruled and directed by
sense ; so, in this, we are carried by *reason.* Besides, the
sensitive appetite hath a particular object, good or bad ; this,
an universal, immaterial : that respects only things delectable
and pleasant : this, honest. Again, they differ in liberty. The
sensual appetite seeing an object, if it be a convenient good,
cannot but desire it; if evil, avoid it : but this is free in his
essence, [3] *much now depraved, obscured, and faln from his first
perfection, yet, in some of his operations, still free,* as to go,
walk, move at his pleasure, and to choose whether it will do, or
not do, steal, or not steal. Otherwise in vain were laws, de-

---

[1] Quod tibi fieri non vis, alteri ne feceris.   [2] Res ab intellectu monstratas re-
cipit, vel rejicit ; approbat, vel improbat. Philip.—Ignoti nulla cupido.   [3] Melancthon. Operationes plerumque feræ, etsi libera sit illa in essentiâ suâ.

Mem. 2. Subs. 11.]   *Of the Will.*   163

liberations, exhortations, counsels, precepts, rewards, promises, threats, and punishments: and God should be the author of sin. But, in [1] spiritual things, we will no good; prone to evil, (except we be regenerate, and led by the Spirit,) we are egged on by our natural concupiscence, and there is αταξια, a confusion in our powers; [2] *our whole will is averse from God and his law,* not in natural things only, as to eat and drink, lust, to which we are led headlong by our temperature and inordinate appetite :

> [3] Nec nos obniti contra, nec tendere tantum,
> Sufficimus,———

we cannot resist; our concupiscence is originally bad, our heart evil; the seat of our affections captivates and enforceth our will : so that, in voluntary things, we are averse from God and goodness, bad by nature, by [4] ignorance worse; by art, discipline, custome, we get many bad habits, suffering them to domineer and tyrannize over us ; and the devil is still ready at hand with his evil suggestions, to tempt our depraved will to some ill disposed action, to precipitate us to destruction, except our *will* be swayed and counterpoised again with some divine precepts, and good motions of the Spirit, which many times restrain, hinder, and check us, when we are in the full career of our dissolute courses. So David corrected himself when he had Saul at a vantage. Revenge and malice were as two violent oppugners on the one side ; but honesty, religion, fear of God, with-held him on the other.

The actions of the *will* are *velle* and *nolle,* to will and nill, (which two words comprehend all; and they are good or bad, accordingly as they are directed) and some of them freely performed by himself; although the *Stoicks* absolutely deny it, and will have all things inevitably done by *destiny,* imposing a fatal necessity upon us, which we may not resist : yet we say that our will is free in respect of us, and things contingent, howsoever, in respect of Gods determinate counsel, they are inevitable and necessary. Some other actions of the *will* are performed by the inferiour powers, which obey him, as the *sensitive* and *moving appetite ;* as to open our eyes, to go hither and thither, not to touch a book, to speak fair or foul : but this appetite is many times rebellious in us, and will not be contained within the lists of sobriety and temperance. It was (as I said) once well agreeing with reason ; and there was an ex-

---

[1] In civilibus libera, sed non in spiritualibus. Osiander.   [2] Tota voluntas aversa a Deo. Omnis homo mendax.   [3] Virg.   [4] Vel propter ignorantiam, quod bonis studiis non sit instructa mens, ut debuit, aut divinis præceptis exculta.

M 2

164 *Of the Will.* [Part. 1. Sec. 1.

cellent consent and harmony betwixt them: but that is now dissolved, they often jar; *reason* is overborne by *passion*,

(Fertur equis auriga; neque audit currus habenas)

as so many wild horses run away with a chariot, and will not be curbed. We know many times what is good, but will not do it, as she said,

——[1] Trahit invitam nova vis; aliudque cupido,
Mens aliud, suadet:

lust counsels one thing, reason another; there is a new reluctancy in men.

[2] Odi: nec possum, cupiens, non esse, quod odi.

We cannot resist; but, as Phædra confessed to her nurse, [3] *quæ loqueris, vera sunt; sed furor suggerit sequi pejora:* she said well and true (she did acknowledge it); but head-strong passion and fury made her to do that which was opposite. So David knew the filthiness of his fact, what a loathsome, foul, crying sin adultery was; yet, notwithstanding, he would commit murther, and take away another mans wife—enforced, against reason, religion, to follow his appetite.

Those *natural* and *vegetal* powers are not commanded by *will* at all; for *who can add one cubit to his stature?* These other may, but are not: and thence come all those head-strong passions, violent perturbations of the mind, and many times vitious habits, customs, feral diseases, because we give so much way to our *appetite*, and follow our inclination, like so many beasts. The principal *habits* are two in number, *vertue* and *vice*, whose peculiar definitions, descriptions, differences, and kinds, are handled at large in the *ethicks*, and are indeed the subject of *moral philosophy*.

MEMB. III.

SUBSECT. I.

Definition of Melancholy, Name, Difference.

HAVING thus briefly anatomized the body and soul of man, as a preparative to the rest—I may now freely proceed to treat of my intended object, to most mens capacity: and, after many ambages, perspicuously define what this *melancholy* is, shew his *name*, and *differences*. The *name* is imposed from

---

[1] Medea, Ovid.   [2] Ovid.   [3] Seneca, Hipp.

Mem. 3. Subs. 1.]   *Definition of Melancholy.*   165

the matter, and disease denominated from the material cause, (as Bruel observes) Μελαγχολια, *quasi* Μελαινα χολη, from black choler. And, whether it be a cause or an effect, a disease, or symptome, let Donatus Altomarus, and Salvianus, decide; I will not contend about it. It hath several descriptions, notations, and definitions. [1]Fracastorius, in his second book of intellect, calls those *melancholy, whom abundance of that same depraved humour of black choler hath so misaffected, that they become mad thence, and dote in most things, or in all, belonging to election, will, or other manifest operations of the understanding.* [2]Melanelius out of Galen, Ruffus, Aëtius, describe it to be *a bad and pievish disease, which makes men degenerate into beasts;* Galen, *a privation or infection of the middle cell of the head, &c.* defining it from the part affected; which [3]Hercules de Saxoniâ approves, *lib.* 1. *cap.* 16. calling it *a deprivation of the principal function:* Fuchsius, *lib.* 1. *cap.* 23. Arnoldus Breviar. *lib.* 1. *cap.* 18. Guianerius, and others. *By reason of black choler,* Paulus adds. Halyabbas simply calls it a *commotion of the mind;* Aretæus, [4]*a perpetual anguish of the soul, fastned on one thing, without an ague;* which definition of his, Mercurialis (*de affect. cap. lib.* 1. *cap.* 10.) taxeth; but Ælianus Montaltus, defends, (*lib. de morb. cap.* 1. *de Melan.*) for sufficient and good. The common sort define it to be *a kind of dotage without a fever, having, for his ordinary companions, fear and sadness, without any apparent occasion.* So doth Laurentius, *cap.* 4. Piso, *lib.* 1. *cap.* 43. Donatus Altomarus, *cap.* 7. *art. medic.* Jacchinus, *in com. in lib.* 9. Rhasis ad Almansor, *cap.* 15. Valesius, *exerc.* 17. Fuchsius, *institut.* 3. *sec.* 1. *c.* 11. *&c.* which common definition, howsoever approved by most, [5]Hercules de Saxoniâ will not allow of, nor David Crusius, *Theat. morb. Herm. lib.* 2. *cap.* 6: he holds it unsufficient, [6]*as rather shewing what it is not, than what it is;* as omitting the specifical difference, the phantasie and brain: but I descend to particulars. The *summum genus* is *dotage,* or *anguish of the mind,* saith Aretæus;—*of a principal part,* Hercules de Saxoniâ adds, to distinguish it from cramp and palsie, and such diseases as belong to the outward sense and motions; *" depraved,"* [7] to distinguish it from folly and madness, (which Montaltus makes *angor animi* to separate) in which those functions are not depraved, but rather abolished; *" without an*

[1] Melancholicos vocamus, quos exsuperantia vel pravitas melancholiæ ita male habet, ut inde insaniant vel in omnibus, vel in pluribus, iisque manifestis, sive ad rectam rationem, voluntatem, pertinent, vel electionem, vel intellectûs operationes.
[2] Pessimum et pertinacissimum morbum, qui homines in bruta degenerare cogit.
[3] Panth. Med.   [4] Angor animi in unâ contentione defixus, absque febre.
[5] Cap. 16. l. 1.   [6] Eorum definitio, morbus quid non sit, potius quám quid sit, explicat.   [7] Animæ functiones imminuuntur in fatuitate, tolluntur in maniâ, depravantur solum in melancholiâ. Herc. de Sax. cap. 1. tract. de Melanch.

166   *Of the Parts affected, &c.*   [Part. 1. Sec. 1.

ague" is added by all, to sever it from *phrensie,* and that *melancholy* which is in a pestilent fever. "*Fear* and *sorrow*" make it differ from *madness* : "*without a cause*" is lastly inserted, to specifie it from all other ordinary passions of "*fear and sorrow.*" We properly call that *dotage,* as [1] Laurentius interprets it, *when some one principal faculty of the mind, as imagination or reason, is corrupted, as all melancholy persons have.* It is without a fever, because the humour is, most part, cold and dry, contrary to putrefaction. *Fear* and *sorrow* are the true characters and inseparable companions of most *melancholy,* not all, as Her. de Saxoniâ (*Tract. posthumo de Melancholiâ, cap. 2.*) well excepts ; for, to some, it is most pleasant, as to such as laugh most part ; some are bold again, and free from all manner of fear and grief, as hereafter shall be declared.

SUBSECT. II.

Of the parts affected.   Affection.   Parties affected.

SOME difference I find amongst writers, about the principal part affected in this disease, whether it be the *brain* or *heart,* or some other member. Most are of opinion that it is the *brain;* for, being a kind of *dotage,* it cannot otherwise be, but that the *brain* must be affected, as a similar part, be it by [2] *consent* or *essence,* not in his ventricles, or any obstructions in them, (for then it would be an apoplexie, or epilepsie, as [3] Laurentius well observes) but in a cold dry distemperature of it in his substance, which is corrupt and become too cold, or too dry, or else too hot, as in madmen, and such as are inclined to it : and this [4] Hippocrates confirms, Galen, Arabians, and most of our new writers. Marcus de Oddis (in a consultation of his, quoted by [5] Hildesheim), and five others there cited, are of the contrary part, because fear and sorrow, which are passions, be seated in the heart. But this objection is sufficiently answered by [6] Montaltus, who doth not deny that the heart is affected (as [7] Melanelius proves out of Galen) by reason of his vicinity, and so is the *midriff* and many other parts. They do *compati,* and have a fellow-feeling by the law of nature : but, for as much as this malady is caused by precedent *imagination,* with the *appetite,* to whom spirits obey, and are subject to those

---

[1] Cap. 4. de mel.   [2] Per consensum, sive per essentiam.   [3] Cap. 4. de mel.   [4] Sec. 7. de mor. vulgar. lib. 6.   [5] Spicil. de melancholiâ. [6] Cap. 3. de mel. Pars affecta cerebrum, sive per consensum sive per cerebrum contingat, et procerum auctoritate et ratione stabilitur.   [7] Lib. de mel. Cor vero, vicinitatis ratione, unà afficitur, ac septum transversum, ac stomachus, cum dorsali spinâ, &c.

Mem. 3. Subs. 2.] *Of the Parts affected, &c.* 167

principal parts; the *brain* must needs primarily be mis-affected, as the seat of *reason :* and then the *heart* as the seat of *affection.* [1] Capivaccius and Mercurialis have copiously discussed this question; and both conclude the subject is the inner *brain,* and from thence it is communicated to the *heart,* and other inferiour parts, which sympathize and are much troubled, especially when it comes by consent, and is caused by reason of the *stomach,* or *myrache* (as the Arabians term it), or whole body, liver, or [2] spleen, which are seldom free, *pylorus, mesaraick veins, &c.* For our body is like a clock; if one wheel be amiss, all the rest are disordered; the whole fabrick suffers: with such admirable art and harmony is a man composed, such excellent proportion, as Lodovicus Vives, in his *Fable of man,* hath elegantly declared.

As many doubts almost arise about the [3] *affection,* whether it be *imagination* or *reason* alone, or both, Hercules de Saxoniâ proves it out of Galen, Aëtius, and Altomarus, that the sole fault is in [4] *imagination :* Bruel is of the same mind : Montaltus (in his *2 cap.* of *Melancholy)* confutes this tenet of theirs, and illustrates the contrary by many examples, as of him that thought himself a shell-fish: of a nun, and of a desperate monk that would not be perswaded but that he was damned. *Reason* was in fault (as well as *imagination),* which did not correct this error. They make away themselves oftentimes, and suppose many absurd and ridiculous things. Why doth not *reason* detect the fallacy, settle, and perswade, if she be free? [5] Avicenna therefore holds both corrupt : to whom most Arabians subscribe. The same is maintained by [6] Aretæus, Gorgonius, [7] Guianerius, &c. To end the controversie, no man doubts of *imagination,* but that it is hurt and misaffected here. For the other, I determine (with [8] Albertinus Bottonus, a doctor of Padua) that it is first in *imagination, and afterwards in reason, if the disease be inveterate, or as it is more or less of continuance ;* but by accident, as [9] Herc. de Saxoniâ adds : *faith, opinion, discourse, ratiocination, are all accidentally depraved by the default of imagination.*

Parties affected.] To the part affected, I may here add the parties, which shall be more opportunely spoken of elsewhere,

---

[1] Lib. 1. cap. 10. Subjectum est cerebrum interius.   [2] Raro quisquam tumorem effugit lienis, qui hoc morbo afficitur. Piso. Quis affectus.   [3] See Donat. ab Altomar.   [4] Facultas imaginandi, non cogitandi, nec memorandi, læsa hîc.   [5] Lib. 3. Fen. 1. Tract. 4. cap. 8.   [6] Lib. 3. cap. 5.   [7] Lib. Med. cap. 19. part. 2. Tract. 15. cap. 2.   [8] Hildesheim, spicil. 2. de Melanc. fol. 207, et fol. 127. Quandoque etiam rationalis si affectus inveteratus sit. [9] Lib. posthumo de Melanc. edit. 1620. Depravatur fides, discursus, opinio, &c. per vitium imaginationis, ex accidenti.

168   *Of the Parts affected, &c.*   [Part. 1. Sec. 1.

now only signified. Such as have the *Moon, Saturn, Mercury* mis-affected in their genitures—such as live in over-cold, or over-hot climes—such as are born of *melancholy* parents, as offend in those six non-natural things, are black, or of an high sanguine complexion, [1] that have little heads, that have a hot heart, moist brain, hot liver and cold stomach, have been long sick—such as are solitary by nature, great students, given to much contemplation, lead a life out of action—are most subject to *melancholy*. Of sexes, both, but men more often; yet [2] women mis-affected are far more violent, and grievously troubled. Of seasons of the year, the *autumn* is most melancholy. Of peculiar times, old age, from which natural melancholy is almost an inseparable accident; but this artificial malady is more frequent in such as are of a [3] middle age. Some assign forty years; Gariopontus, 30; Jubertus excepts neither young nor old from this adventitious. [4] Daniel Sennertus involves all of all sorts, out of common experience ; *in omnibus omnino corporibus cujuscunque constitutionis, dominatur.* Aëtius and Aretæus ascribe into the number *not only* [5] *discontented, passionate, and miserable persons, swarthy, black, but such as are most merry and pleasant, scoffers, and high coloured. Generally,* [6] saith Rhasis, [7] *the finest wits, and most generous spirits, are, before other, obnoxious to it.* I cannot except any complexion, any condition, sex, or age, but [8] fools and *Stoicks,* which (according to [9] Synesius) are never troubled with any manner of passion, but (as Anacreons *cicada, sine sanguine et dolore) similes fere diis sunt.* Erasmus vindicates fools from this melancholy catalogue, because they have most part moist brains and light hearts ; [10] *they are free from ambition, envy, shame, and fear ; they are neither troubled in conscience, nor macerated with cares, to which our whole life is most subject.*

---

[1] Qui parvum caput habent, insensati plerique sunt. Arist. in physiognomiâ. [2] Aretæus, lib. 3. c. 5.   [3] Qui prope statum sunt. Aret. Mediis convenit ætatibus. Piso.   [4] De quartano.   [5] Pronus ad melancholiam non tam mœstus, sed et hilares, jocosi, cachinnantes, irrisores, et qui plerumque prærubri sunt.   [6] Lib. 1. part. 2. cap. 11.   [7] Qui sunt subtilis ingenii, et multæ perspicacitatis, de facili incidunt in melancholiam. lib. 1. con. tract. 9.   [8] Nunquam sanitate mentis excidit, aut dolore capitur. Erasm.   [9] In laud. calvit. [10] Vacant conscientiæ carnificinâ, nec pudefiunt, nec verentur, nec dilacerantur millibus curarum, quibus tota vita obnoxia est.

SUBSECT. III.

Of the matter of Melancholy.

Of the matter of *melancholy*, there is much question betwixt Avicen and Galen, as you may read in [1] Cardans Contradictions. [2] Valesius controversies, Montanus, Prosper Calenus, Capivaccius, [3] Bright, [4] Ficinus, that have written either whole tracts, or copiously of it, in their several treatises of this subject. [5] *What this humour is, or whence it proceeds, how it is ingendred in the body, neither Galen, nor any old writer, hath sufficiently discussed, as Jacchinus thinks :* the neotericks cannot agree. Montanus, in his Consultations, holds *melancholy* to be *material* or *immaterial;* and so doth Arculanus. The *material* is one of the four humours before mentioned, and natural : the *immaterial* or adventitious, acquisite, redundant, unnatural, artificial, which [6] Hercules de Saxoniâ will have reside in the spirits alone, and to proceed from an *hot, cold, dry, moist distemperature, which, without matter, alters the brain and functions of it.* Paracelsus wholly rejects and derides this division of four humours and complexions ; but our Galenists generally approve of it, subscribing to this opinion of Montanus.

This material *melancholy* is either simple or *mixt*—offending in *quantity* or *quality*, varying according to his place, where it setleth, as brain, spleen, mesaraick veins, heart, womb, and stomach—or differing according to the mixture of those natural humours amongst themselves, or four unnatural adust humours, as they are diversly tempered and mingled. If natural *melancholy* abound in the body, which is cold and dry, *so that it be more* [7] *than the body is well able to bear, it must needs be distempered* (saith Faventius) *and diseased :* and so the other, if it be depraved, whether it arise from that other *melancholy* of *choler* adust, or from *blood*, produceth the like effects, and is, as Montaltus contends, if it come by adustion of humours, most part hot and dry. Some difference I find, whether this *melancholy* matter may be ingendred of all four humours, about the colour and temper of it. Galen holds it

---

[1] Lib. 1. tract 3. contradic. 18.   [2] Lib. 1. cont. 21.   [3] Bright, cap. 16. [4] Lib. 1. cap. 6. de sanit. tuendâ.   [5] Quisve aut qualis sit humor, aut quæ istius differentiæ, et quomodo gignatur in corpore, scrutandum ; hac enim in re multi veterum laboraverunt ; nec facile accipere ex Galeno sententiam, ob loquendi varietatem. Leon. Jac. com. in 9. Rhasis, cap. 15. cap. 16. in 9. Rhasis. [6] Tract. posthum. de Melan. edit. Venetiis, 1620. cap. 7. et 8. Ab intemperie calidâ, humidâ, &c.   [7] Secundum magis aut minus : si in corpore fuerit ad intemperiem, plusquam corpus salubriter ferre poterit ; inde corpus morbosum efficitur.

170   *Matter of Melancholy.*   [Part. 1. Sec. 1.

may be ingendred of three alone, excluding *flegm*, or *pituita*;
whose true assertion [1] Valesius and Menardus stifly maintain:
and so doth [2] Fuchsius, Montaltus, [3] Montanus. How (say
they) can white become black? But Hercules de Saxoniâ *(l.
post. de mela. c.* 8,) and [4] Cardan are of the opposite part (it
may be ingendred of flegm, *etsi raro contingat*, though it seldom
come to pass); so is [5] Guianerius, and Laurentius (*c.* 1), with
Melancthon (in his book *de Animâ*, and chapter of humours;
he calls it *asininam*, dull, swinish *melancholy*, and saith that he
was an eye-witness of it); so is [6] Wecker. From *melancholy*
adust ariseth one kind, from *choler* another, which is most
bruitish; another from *flegm*, which is dull; and the last from
blood, which is best. Of these, some are cold and dry, others
hot and dry, [7] varying according to their mixtures, as they are
intended and remitted. And indeed, as Rhodericus a Fons.
(cons. 12. *l.)* determines, ichorous, and those serous matters,
being thickned, become flegm; and flegm degenerates into
choler; choler adust becomes *æruginosa melancholia*, as vinegar
out of purest wine putrified, or by exhalation of purer spirits,
is so made, and becomes sowr and sharp: and, from the sharpness of this humour, proceed much waking, troublesome thoughts
and dreams, &c. so that I conclude as before. If the humour
be cold, it 'is (saith [8] Faventinus) *a cause of dotage, and produceth milder symptomes : if hot, they are rash, raving mad,
or inclining to it.* If the brain be hot, the animal spirits are
hot, much madness follows, with violent actions: if cold, fatuity
and sottishness ([9] Capivaccius). [10] *The colour of this mixture
varies likewise according to the mixture, be it hot or cold;* 'tis
sometimes black, sometimes not (Altomarus). The same [11] Melanelius proves out of Galen: and Hippocrates, in his book of
Melancholy (if at least it be his) giving instance in a burning
coal, *which, when it is hot, shines ; when it is cold, looks black ;
and so doth the humour.* This diversity of melancholy matter
produceth diversity of effects. If it be within the [12] body, and
not putrified, it causeth black jaundise; if putrified, a quartan
ague: if it break out to the skin, leprosie: if to parts several
maladies, as scurvy, &c. If it trouble the mind, as it is diversly mixt, it produceth several kinds of madness and dotage;
of which in their place.

[1] Lib. 1. controvers. cap. 21.   [2] Lib. 1. sect. 4. c. 4.   [3] Concil. 26.
[4] Lib. 2. contradic. cap. 11.   [5] De feb. tract. diff. 2. c. 1. Non est negandum ex
hâc fieri melancholicos.   [6] I In Syntax.   [7] Varie aduritur et miscetur, unde
variæ amentium species. Melanct.   [8] Humor frigidus delirii caussa ; furoris
calidus, &c.   [9] Lib. 1. cap. 10. de affect. cap.   [10] Nigrescit hic humor, aliquando supercalefactus, aliquando superfrigefactus. cap. 7.   [11] Humor hic
niger aliquando præter modum calefactus, et alias refrigeratus evadit : nam re-
centibus carbonibus ei quid simile accidit, qui, durante flammâ, pellucidissime
candent, eâ exstinctâ prorsus nigrescunt. Hippocrates.   [12] Guianerius,
diff. 2. cap. 7.

SUBSECT. IV.

Of the species or kinds of Melancholy.

WHEN the matter is divers and confused, how should it otherwise be, but that the species should be divers and confused ? Many new and old writers have spoken confusedly of it, confounding *melancholy* and *madness*, as [1] Heurnius, Guianerius, Gordonius, Sallustius Salvianus, Jason Pratensis, Savanarola, that will have *madness* no other than *melancholy* in extent, differing (as I have said) in degrees. Some make two distinct species, as Ruffus Ephesius an old writer, Constantinus, Africanus, Aretæus, [2] Aurelianus, [3] Paulus Ægineta : others acknowledge a multitude of kinds, and leave them indefinite, as Aëtius (in his *Tetrabiblos*), [4] Avicenna *(lib.* 3. *Fen.* 1. *Tract.* 4. *cap.* 18), Arculanus *(cap.* 16. *in* 9), Rhasis, Montanus *(med. part* 1.) [5] *If natural melancholy be adust, it maketh one kind; if blood, another; if choler, a third, differing from the first; and so many several opinions there are about the kinds, as there be men themselves.* [6] Hercules de Saxoniâ sets down two kinds, *material and immaterial: one from spirits alone, the other from humours and spirits.* Savanarola *(Rub.* 11. *Tract.* 6. *cap.* 1. *de ægritud. capitis)* will have the kinds to be infinite; one from the *myrache*, called *myrachialis* of the Arabians; another *stomachalis* from the *stomach ;* another from the *liver, heart, womb, hæmorrhoids ;* [7] *one beginning, another consummate.* Melancthon seconds him ; [8] *as the humour is diversly adust and mixt, so are the species divers.* But what these men speak of species, I think ought to be understood of symptomes; and so doth [9] Arculanus interpret himself: infinite species, *id est,* symptomes: and, in that sense, (as Jo. Gorrhæus acknowledgeth in his medicinal definitions) the species are infinite : but they may be reduced to three kinds, by reason of their seat—*head, body, and hypochondries.* This threefold division is approved by Hippocrates in his book of Melancholy, (if it be his, which some suspect) by Galen *(lib.* 3. *de loc. affectis, cap.* 6*)*, by Alexander *(lib.* 1. *cap.* 16*)*, *Rhasis (lib.* 1. *Continent. Tract.* 9. *lib.* 1. *cap.* 16), Avicenna, and most of our

---

[1] Non est mania, nisi extensa melancholia.   [2] Cap. 6. lib. 1.   [3] 2 Ser. 2. cap. 9. Morbus hic est omnifarius.   [4] Species indefinitæ sunt.   [5] Si aduratur naturalis melancholia, alia sit species; si sanguis, alia ; si flava bilis, alia, diversa a primis. Maxima est inter has differentia ; et tot doctorum sententiæ, quot ipsi numero sunt.   [6] Tract. de mel. cap. 7.   [7] Quædam incipiens, quædam consummata.   [8] Cap. de humor. lib. de animâ. Varie aduritur et miscetur ipsa melancholia ; unde variæ amentium species.   [9] Cap. 16. in 9. Rhasis.

172   *Species of Melancholy.*   [Part. 1. Sec. 1.

new writers. Th. Erastus makes two kinds; one perpetual, which is *head melancholy ;* the other interrupt, which comes and goes by fits, which he subdivides into the other two kinds, so that all comes to the same pass. Some again make four or five kinds with Rodericus a Castro *(de morbis mulier.* lib. 2. *c. 3.)* and Lod. Mercatus, who (in his second book *de mulier. affect. cap.* 4.) will have that melancholy of nuns, widows, and more antient maids, to be a peculiar species of melancholy differing from the rest. Some will reduce enthusiasts, extatical and dæmoniacal persons, to this rank, adding [1] *love melancholy* to the first and *lycanthropia.* The most received division is into three kinds. The first proceeds from the sole fault of the *brain,* and is called *head melancholy :* the second sympathetically proceeds from the *whole body,* when the whole temperature is melancholy : the third ariseth from the bowels, liver, spleen, or membrane called *mesenterium,* named *hypochondriacal* or *windy melancholy,* which [2] Laurentius subdivides into three parts, from those three members, *hepatick, splenetick, mesaraick.* *Love melancholy* (which Avicenna calls *illishi)* and *lycanthropia* (which he calls *cucubuthe)* are commonly included in head melancholy : but of this last (which Gerardus de Solo calls, *amoreos,* and most *knight melancholy),* with that of *religious melancholy, virginum, et viduarum* (maintained by Rod. a Castro and Mercatus), and the other kinds of *love melancholy,* I will speak apart by themselves in my third partition. The three precedent species are the subject of my present discourse, which I will anatomize, and treat of, through all their causes, symptomes, cures, together, and apart; that every man, that is in any measure affected with this malady, may know how to examine it in himself, and apply remedies unto it.

   It is a hard matter, I confess, to distinguish these three species one from the other, to express their several causes, symptomes, cures, being that they are so often confounded amongst themselves, having such affinity, that they can scarce be discerned by the most accurate physicians; and so often intermixt with other diseases, that the best experienced have been plunged. Montanus *(consil.* 26.) names a patient that had this disease of melancholy, and *caninus appetitus,* both together ; and *(consil.* 23.) with *vertigo—*[3] Julius Cæsar Claudinus, with stone, gout, jaundice—Trincavellius, with an ague jaundice, *caninus appetitus,* &c. [4] Paulus Regoline, a great doctor in his time, consulted in this case, was so confounded with a confusion of symptomes, that he knew not to what kind of melancholy to

---

[1] Laurentius, cap. 4. de mel.   [2] Cap. 13.   [3] 480. et 116. consult.
consil. 12.   [4] Hildesheim, spicil. 2. fol. 166.

refer it. [1] Trincavellius, Fallopius, and Francanzanus, famous doctors in Italy, all three conferred with about one party at the same time, gave three different opinions: and, in another place, Trincavellius being demanded what he thought of a melancholy young man, to whom he was sent for, ingenuously confessed that he was indeed melancholy, but he knew not to what kind to reduce it. In his seventeenth consultation, there is the like disagreement about a melancholy monk. Those symptomes, which others ascribe to misaffected parts and humours, [2] Herc. de Saxoniâ attributes wholly to distempered spirits, and those immaterial, as I have said. Sometimes they cannot well discern this disease from others. In Reinerus Solinanders Counsels, *sect. consil.* 5. he and Dr. Brande both agreed, that the patients disease was hypochondriacal melancholy. Dr. Matholdus said it was *asthma,* and nothing else. [3] Solinander and Guarionius, lately sent for to the melancholy duke of Cleve, with others, could not define what species it was, or agree amongst themselves; the species are so confounded; as in Cæsar Claudinus his forty fourth consultation for a Polonian count: in his judgement, [4] *he laboured of head melancholy, and that which proceeds from the whole temperature, both at once.* I could give instance of some that have had all three kinds *semel et simul,* and some successively. So that I conclude of our melancholy species, as [5] many politicians do of their pure forms of common-wealths—monarchies, aristocracies, democracies, are most famous in contemplation; but, in practice, they are temperate and usually mixt, (so [6] Polybius enformeth us) as the Lacedæmonian, the Roman of old, German now, and many others. What physicians say of distinct species in their books, it much matters not, since that in their patients bodies they are commonly mixt. In such obscurity therefore, variety and confused mixture of symptomes, causes, how difficult a thing is it to treat of several kinds apart; to make any certainty or distinction among so many casualties, distractions, when seldom two men shall be like affected *per omnia!* 'Tis hard, I confess; yet nevertheless I will adventure through the midst of these perplexities, and, led by the clue or thread of the best writers, extricate my self out of a labyrinth of doubts and errours, and so proceed to the causes.

---

[1] Trincavellius, tom. 1. consil. 15 et 16.   [2] Cap. 13. tract. post. de melan.
[3] Guarion. cons. med. 2.   [4] Laboravit per essentiam, et a toto corpore.
[5] Machiavel, &c. Smithus, de rep. Angl. cap. 8. lib. 1. Buscoldus, discur. polit. discurs. 5. cap. 7. Arist. l. 3. polit. cap. ult. Keckerm. alii, &c.   [6] Lib. 6.

174   *Causes of Melancholy.*   [Part. 1. Sec. 2.

SECT. II.
MEMB. I.
SUBSECT. I.

Causes of Melancholy.   God a cause.

*It is in vain to speak of cures, or think of remedies, until such
time as we have considered of the causes;* so [1]Galen prescribes
(Glauco); and the common experience of others confirms, that
those cures must be unperfect, lame, and to no purpose,
wherein the causes have not first been searched, as [2]Prosper
Calenius well observes in his tract *de atrâ bile* to Cardinal
Cæsius: insomuch that [3]Fernelius *puts a kind of necessity in
the knowledge of the causes, and, without which, it is impossible
to cure or prevent any manner of disease.* Empericks may ease,
and sometimes help, but not thoroughly root out: *sublatâ
caussâ, tollitur effectus,* as the saying is; if the cause be removed, the effect is likewise vanquished. It is a most difficult
thing (I confess) to be able to discern these causes, whence
they are, and, in such [4]variety, to say what the beginning was.
[5]He is happy that can perform it aright. I will adventure to
guess as near as I can, and rip them all up, from the first to
the last, *general,* and *particular* to every *species,* that so they
may the better be descried.

General causes are either *supernatural* or *natural. Supernatural are from God and his angels,* or, *by Gods permission,
from the devil* and his ministers. That God himself is a
cause for the punishment of sin, and satisfaction of his justice,
many examples and testimonies of holy Scriptures make evident unto us: Psal. 107. 17. *Foolish men are plagued for
their offence, and by reason of their wickedness:* Gehazi was
strucken with leprosie (2 *Reg.* 5. 27), Jehoram with dysentery
and flux, and great diseases of the bowels (2 Chron. 21. 15.),
David plagued for numbring his people (1 *Par.* 21,) Sodom
and Gomorrah swallowed up. And this disease is peculiarly
specified, Psal. 127. 12. *He brought down their heart through
heaviness.* Deut. 28. 28. *He stroke them with madness,
blindness, and astonishment of heart.* [6]*An evil spirit was*

---

[1] Primo artis curativæ.   [2] Nostri primum sit propositi affectionum
caussas indagare. Res ipsa hortari videtur; nam alioqui earum curatio manca
et inutilis esset.   [3] Path. lib. 1. cap. 11. Rerum cognoscere caussas, medicis imprimis necessarium; sine quo, nec morbum curare, nec præcavere, licet.
[4] Tanta enim morbi varietas ac differentia, ut non facile dignoscatur, unde initium morbus sumpserit. Melanelius, e Galeno.   [5] Felix, qui potuit rerum
cognoscere caussas !   [6] 1 Sam. 16. 14.

2

Mem. 1. Subs. 1.]   *Causes of Melancholy.*   175

sent by the Lord upon Saul, to vex him. [1] Nebuchadnezzar did eat grass like an oxe; and *his heart was made like the beasts of the field.* Heathen stories are full of such punishments. Lycurgus, because he cut down the vines in the country, was by Bacchus driven into madness; so was Pentheus, and his mother Agave, for neglecting their sacrifice. [2] Censor Fulvius ran mad for untiling Juno's temple, to cover a new one of his own, which he had dedicated to Fortune, [3] *and was confounded to death with grief and sorrow of heart.* When Xerxes would have spoiled [4] Apollos temple at Delphos of those infinite riches it possessed, a terrible thunder came from heaven, and struck 4000 men dead; the rest ran mad. [5] A little after, the like happened to Brennus (lightning, thunder, earthquakes) upon such a sacrilegious occasion. If we may believe our pontificial writers, they will relate unto us many strange and prodigious punishments in this kind, inflicted by their saints;—how [6] Clodovæus, sometime king of France, the son of Dagobert, lost his wits for uncovering the body of S. Denis; and how a [7] sacrilegious Frenchman, that would have stolen away a silver image of S. John, at Birgburge, became frantick on a suddain, raging and tyrannizing over his own flesh;—of a [8] lord of Rhadnor, that, coming from hunting late at night, put his dogs into S. Avans church, (Llan Avan they called it) and, rising betimes next morning, as hunters use to do, found all his dogs mad, himself being suddenly strucken blind;—of Tiridates, an [9] Armenian king, for violating some holy nuns, that was punished in like sort, with loss of his wits. But poets and papists may go together for fabulous tales; let them free their own credits. Howsoever they fain of their Nemesis, and of their saints, or, by the devils means, may be deluded: we find it true, that *ultor a tergo Deus,* [10] *He is God the avenger,* as David stiles him; and that it is our crying sins that pull this and many other maladies on our own heads; that he can, by his angels, which are his ministers, strike and heal (saith [11] Dionysius) whom he will; that he can plague us by his creatures, sun, moon, and stars, which he useth as his instruments, as a husbandman (saith Zanchius) doth an hatchet. Hail, snow, winds, &c.

---

[1] Dan. 5. 21.   [2] Lactant. instit. lib. 2. cap. 8.   [3] Mente captus, et summo animi mœrore consumptus.   [4] Munster. cosmog. lib. 4. cap. 43. De cœlo substernebantur; tamquam insani, de saxis præcipitati, &c.   [5] Livius, lib. 38.   [6] Gaguin. l. 3. c. 4. Quod Dionysii corpus discooperuerat, in insaniam incidit.   [7] Idem, lib. 9. sub Carol. 6. Sacrorum contemptor, templi foribus effractis, dum D. Johannis argenteum simulacrum rapere contendit, simulacrum aversâ facie dorsum ei versat; nec mora, sacrilegus mentis inops, atque in semet insaniens, in proprios artus desævit.   [8] Giraldus Cambrensis, lib. 1. cap. 1. Itiner. Cambriæ.   [9] Delrio, tom. 3. lib. 6. sect. 3. quæst. 3.
[10] Psalm. 44. 1.   [11] Lib. 8. cap. de Hierar.

176   *Causes of Melancholy.*   [Part. 1. Sec. 2.

(¹ Et conjurati veniunt in classica venti ;

as in Joshuas time, as in Pharaohs reign in Ægypt) they are
but as so many executioners of his justice.   He can make the
proudest spirits stoop, and cry out, with Julian the Apostate,
Vicisti, Galilæe ! or, with Apollos priest in ² Chrysostome, *O
cœlum ! o terra! unde hostis hic ?*   What an enemy is this?
and pray with David, acknowledging his power, *I am weakened
and sore broken ; I roar for the grief of mine heart ; mine heart
panteth, &c.* (Psal. 38. 8.)   *O Lord, rebuke me not in thine
anger, neither chastise me in thy wrath* (Psal. 38. 1.)   *Make
me to hear joy and gladness, that the bones which thou hast
broken, may rejoice* (Psal. 51. 8. and verse 12.)   *Restore to
me the joy of thy salvation, and stablish me with thy free
spirit.*   For these causes, belike, ³ Hippocrates would have a
physician take special notice whether the disease come not from
a divine supernatural cause, or whether it follow the course of
nature.   But this is farther discussed by Fran. Valesius *(de
sacr. philos. cap. 8),* ⁴ Fernelius, and ⁵ J. Cæsar Claudinus, to
whom I refer you, how this place of Hippocrates is to be understood.   Paracelsus is of opinion, that such spiritual diseases
(for so he calls them) are spiritually to be cured, and not otherwise.   Ordinary means in such cases will not avail : *non est
reluctandum cum Deo.*   When that monster-taming Hercules
overcame all in the Olympicks, Jupiter at last, in an unknown
shape, wrestled with him; the victory was uncertain, till at
length Jupiter descried himself, and Hercules yielded.   No
striving with supream powers :

Nil juvat immensos Cratero promittere montes :

physicians and physick can do no good; ⁶ *we must submit ourselves under the mighty hand of God,* acknowledge our offences,
call to him for mercy.   If he strike us, *una eademque manus
vulnus opemque feret,* as it is with them that are wounded with
the spear of Achilles ; he alone must help ; otherwise our diseases are incurable, and we not to be relieved.

¹ Claudian.   ² De Babilâ martyre.   ³ Lib. cap. 5. prog.
⁴ Lib. 1. de abditis rerum caussis.   ⁵ Respons. med. 12. resp.   ⁶ 1 Pet.
5. 6.

SUBSECT. II.

A digression of the nature of Spirits, bad Angels, or Devils, and how they cause Melancholy.

How far the power of spirits and devils doth extend, and whether they can cause this or any other disease, is a serious question, and worthy to be considered: for the better understanding of which, I will make a brief digression of the nature of spirits. And, although the question be very obscure, (according to [1] Postellus) *full of controversie and ambiguity*, beyond the reach of humane capacity—*(fateo excedere vires intentionis meæ,)* saith [2] Austin: I confess I am not able to understand it; *finitum de infinito non potest statuere:* we can sooner determine with Tully, *(de nat. deorum,) quid non sint, quam quid sint;* our subtle schoolmen, Cardans, Scaligers, profound Thomists, *Fracastoriana et Ferneliana acies*, are weak, dry, obscure, defective, in these mysteries; and all our quickest wits, as an owles eyes at the suns light, wax dull, and are not sufficient to apprehend them)—yet, as in the rest, I will adventure to say something to this point. In former times, (as we read, Acts 23,) the Sadducees denied that there were any such spirits, devils, or angels. So did Galen the physician, the Peripateticks, even Aristotle himself, as Pomponatius stoutly maintains, and Scaliger in some sort grants; though Dandinus the Jesuite *(com. in lib. 2. de anima)* stifly denies it. *Substantiæ separatæ*, and intelligences, are the same which Christians call angels, and Platonists devils; for they name all the spirits *dæmones*, be they good or bad angels, as Julius Pollux *(Onomasticon, lib. 1. cap. 1.)* observes. Epicures and atheists are of the same mind in general, because they never saw them. Plato, Plotinus, Porphyrius, Jamblicus, Proclus, (insisting in the steps of Trismegistus, Pythagoras, and Socrates) make no doubt of it; nor Stoicks, but that there are such spirits, though much erring from the truth. Concerning the first beginning of them, the [3] Thalmudists say that Adam had a wife called Lilis, before he marryed Eve, and of her he begat nothing but devils. The Turks [4] Alcoran is altogether as absurd and ridiculous in this point; but the scripture informs

---

[1] Lib. 1. c. 7. de orbis concordiâ. In nullâ re major fuit altercatio, major obscuritas, minor opinionum concordia, quam de dæmonibus et substantiis separatis. [2] Lib. 3. de Trinit. cap. 1. [3] Pererius, in Genesin, lib. 4. in cap. 3. v. 23. [4] See Strozzius Cicogna, omnifariæ Mag. lib. 2. c. 15. J. Aubanus, Bredenbachius.

178   *Nature of Devils.*   [Part. 1. Sec. 2.

us Christians, how Lucifer, the chief of them, with his associates, [1] fell from heaven for his pride, and ambition—created
of God, placed in heaven, and sometimes an angel of light, now
cast down into the lower aërial sublunary parts, or into hell,
and *delivered into chains of darkness* (2 Pet. 2. 4.) *to be kept
unto damnation.*

Nature of Devils.]   There is a foolish opinion, which some
hold, that they are the souls of men departed; good and more
noble were deified; the baser groveled on the ground, or in the
lower parts, and were devils; the which, with Tertullian, Porphyrius the philosopher, M. Tyrius, ser. 27. maintains. *These
spirits* he [2] saith, *which we call angels and devils, are nought
but souls of men departed, which, either through love and pity
of their friends yet living, help and assist them, or else persecute their enemies, whom they hated;* as Dido threatned to
persecute Æneas:

> Omnibus umbra locis adero : dabis, improbe, pœnas.

They are (as others suppose) appointed by those higher
powers to keep men from their nativity, and to protect or
punish them, as they see cause; and are called *boni* and *mali
genii* by the Romans—*heroes, lares,* if good, *lemures* or *larvæ,*
if bad—by the Stoicks, governors of countries, men, cities,
saith [3] Apuleius ; *Deos appellant, qui ex hominum numero,
juste ac prudenter vitæ curriculo gubernato, pro numine, postea
ab hominibus præditi fanis et cæremoniis vulgo admittuntur,
ut in Ægypto Osiris, &c.   Præstites* Capella calls them *which
protected particular men as well as princes.*   Socrates had his
dæmonium saturninum et igneum, which, of all spirits, is best,
ad sublimes cogitationes animum erigentem, as the Platonists
supposed; Plotinus, his ; and we Christians, our assisting angel, as Andreas Victorellus, a copious writer of this subject,
Ludovicus de La-Cerda the Jesuite in his voluminous tract *de
Angelo Custode,* Zanchius, and some divines, think.   But this
absurd tenet of Tyrius, Proclus confutes at large in his book
de Animâ et Dæmone.

[4] Psellus, a Christian, and sometimes tutor (saith Cuspinian)
to Michael Parapinatius, emperour of Greece, a great observer
of the nature of devils, holds they are [5] corporeal, and have
aërial bodies; that they are mortal, live and dye (which Martianus Capella likewise maintains, but our Christian philosophers

---

[1] Angelus per superbiam separatus a Deo, qui in veritate non stetit. **Austin.**
[2] Nihil aliud sunt Dæmones, quam nudæ animæ, quæ, corpore deposito, priorem
miserati vitam, cognatis succurrunt, commoti misericordiâ, &c.   [3] De Deo
Socrates.   [4] He lived 500 years since.   [5] Apuleius. Spiritus animalia
sunt animo passibilia, mente rationalia, corpore aëria, tempore sempiterna.

Mem. 1. Subs. 2.]   *Nature of Devils.*   179

explode); that [1] *they are nourished, and have excrements : that they feel pain, if they be hurt* (which Cardan confirms, and Scaliger justly laughs him to scorn for; *si pascantur aëre, cur non pugnant ob puriorem aëra? &c.) or stroken:* and, if their bodies be cut, with admirable celerity they come together again. Austin *(in Gen. lib. 3. lib. arbit.)* approves as much : *mutata casu corpora in deteriorem qualitatem aëris spissioris :* so doth Hierom *(Comment. in epist. ad Ephes. cap.* 3.), Origen, Tertullian, Lactantius, and many ancient fathers of the church, that in their fall, their bodies were changed into a more aërial and gross substance. Bodine *(lib. 4. Theatri Naturæ,)* and David Crusius *(Hermeticæ Philosophiæ lib. 4. cap. 4.)* by several arguments proves angels and spirits to be corporeal: *quidquid continetur in loco, corporeum est : at spiritus continetur in loco,* ergo. *Si spiritus sunt quanti, erunt corporei : at sunt quanti,* ergo. *Sunt finiti, ergo quanti, &c.* [2] Bodine goes further yet, and will have these *animæ separatæ, genii,* spirits, angels, devils, and so likewise souls of men departed, if corporeal (which he most eagerly contends), to be of some shape, and that absolutely round, like sun and moon, because that is the most perfect form, *quæ nihil habet asperitatis, nihil angulis incisum, nihil anfractibus involutum, nihil eminens, sed inter corpora perfecta est perfectissimum :* therefore all spirits are corporeal (he concludes), and in their proper shapes round. That they can assume other aërial bodies, all manner of shapes at their pleasures, appear in what likeness they will themselves: that they are most swift in motion, can pass many miles in an instant, and so likewise [3] transform bodies of others into what shape they please, and with admirable celerity remove them from place to place : (as the angel did Habakkuk to Daniel, and as Philip the deacon was carried away by the spirit, when he had baptized the eunuch ; so did Pythagoras and Appollonius remove themselves and others, with many such feats) that they can represent castles in the aire, pallaces, armies, spectrums, prodigies, and such strange objects to mortal mens eyes, [4] cause smells, savours, &c. deceive all the senses ; most writers of this subject credibly believe ; and that they can foretell future events, and do many strange miracles. Junos image spake to Camillus,

---

[1] Nutriuntur, et excrementa habent; quod pulsata doleant, solido percussa corpore.   [2] Lib. 4. Theol. nat. fol. 535.   [3] Cyprianus, in Epist. Montes etiam et animalia transferri possunt : as the devil did Christ to the top of the pinnacle ; and witches are often translated. See more in Strozzius Cicogna, lib. 3. cap. 4. omnif. mag. Per aëra subducere, et in sublime corpora ferre possunt. Biarmanus.—Percussi dolent, et uruntur in conspicuos cineres. Agrippa, lib. 3. cap. de occul. Philos.   [4] Agrippa, de occult. Philos. lib. 3. cap. 18.

180   *Nature of Devils.*   [Part. 1. Sec. 2.

and Fortunes statue to the Roman matrons, with many such.
Zanchius, Bodine, Spondanus, and others are of opinion that
they cause a true metamorphosis, (as Nebuchadnezzar was really
translated into a beast, Lots wife into a pillar of salt, Ulysses
companions into hogs and dogs by Circes charms) turn themselves and others, as they do witches into cats, dogs, hares,
crows, &c. (Strozzius Cicogna hath many examples, *lib. 3.
omnif. mag. cap. 4. et 5.* which he there confutes, as Austin
likewise doth, *de civ. Dei lib. 18.*)—that they can be seen
when and in what shape, and to whom they will (saith Psellus,
Tametsi nil tale viderim, nec optem videre, though he himself
never saw them nor desired it), and use sometimes carnal copulation (as elsewhere I shall [1] prove more at large) with
women and men. Many will not believe they can be seen;
and if any man shall say, swear, and stifly maintain, (though
he be discreet and wise, judicious and learned) that he hath
seen them, they account him a timourous fool, a melancholy
dizard, a weak fellow, a dreamer, a sick or a mad man; they
contemn him, laugh him to scorn; and yet Marcus, of his
credit, told Psellus that he had often seen them. And Leo
Suavius, a Frenchman, *(c. 8. in Commentar. l. 1. Paracelsi de
vitâ longâ* out of some Platonists) will have the aire to be as
full of them as snow falling in the skies, and that they may be
seen, and withal sets down the means how men may see them;
*Si irreverberatis oculis, sole splendente, versus cœlum con-
tinuaverint obtutus, &c.* and saith moreover he tryed it, *(præ-
missorum feci experimentum)* and it was true, that the Platonists said. Paracelsus confesseth that he saw them divers
times, and conferred with them; and so doth Alexander ab
[2] Alexandro, *that he so found it by experience, when as before
he doubted of it.* Many deny it, saith Lavater, *(de spectris,
part. 1. c. 2. et part. 2. c. 11.) because they never saw themselves:* But, as he reports at large all over his book, especially
c. 19. part. 1, they are often seen and heard, and familiarly
converse with men, as Lod. Vives assureth us, innumerable
records, histories, and testimonies evince in all ages, times,
places, and [3] all travellers besides. In the West Indies, and
our northern climes, *nihil familiarius quam in agris et urbibus
spiritus videre, audire, qui vetent, jubeant, &c.* Hieronymus
(vita Pauli), Basil *(ser.* 40), Nicephorus, Eusebius, Socrates,
Sozomenus, [4] Jacobus Boissardus (in his tract *de spirituum*

---

[1] Part. 3. sect. 2. Mem. 1. Sub. 1. Love Melancholy.   [2] Genial. dierum.
Ita sibi visum et compertum, quum prius, an essent, ambigeret.—Fidem suam
liberet.   [3] Lib. 1. de verit. Fidei. Benzo. &c.   [4] Lib. de Divinatione
et Magiâ.

Mem. 1. Subs. 2.]   *Nature of Devils.*   181

apparitionibus), Petrus Loyerus *(l. de spectris),* Wierus (l. 1.)
have infinite variety of such examples of apparitions of spirits,
for him to read that farther doubts, to his ample satisfaction.
One alone I will briefly insert. A noble man in Germany was
sent embassadour to the King of Sueden (for his name, the
time and such circumstances, I refer you to Boissardus, mine
[1] author). After he had done his business, he sailed for Livonia, on set purpose to see those familiar spirits, which are
there said to be conversant with men, and do their drudgery
works. Amongst other matters, one of them told him where
his wife was, in what room, in what cloaths, what doing, and
brought him a ring from her, which at his return, *non sine
omnium admiratione,* he found to be true ; and so believed
that ever after, which before he doubted of. Cardan *(l.* 19. *de
subtil.)* relates of his father Facius Cardan, that, after the accustomed solemnities, *An.* 1491, 13 August, he conjured up
seven devils in Greek apparel, about 40 years of age, some
ruddy of complexion, and some pale, as he thought : he asked
them many questions; and they made ready answer, that they
were aërial devils, that they lived and died as men did, save
that they were far longer liv'd, (seven or eight hundred
[2] years,) they did as much excel men in dignity, as we do
juments, and were as far excelled again of those that were
above them: our [3] governours and keepers they are moreover, (which [4] Plato in Critias delivered of old,) and subordinate to one another : *ut enim homo homini, sic dæmon dæmoni
dominatur ;* they rule themselves as well as us ; and the spirits
of the meaner sort had commonly such offices, as we make
horse-keepers, neat-herds, and the basest of us, overseers of
our cattle ; and that we can no more apprehend their natures
and functions, than a horse a mans. They knew all things,
but might not reveal them to men ; and ruled and domineered
over us, as we do over our horses ; the best kings amongst us,
and the most generous spirits, were not comparable to the
basest of them. Sometimes they did instruct men and com-
municate their skill, reward and cherish, and sometimes again
terrifie and punish, to keep them in awe, as they thought fit ;
nihil magis cupientes (saith Lysius, *Phys. Stoïcorum) quam
adorationem hominum.* The same authour Cardan in his Hyperchen, out of the doctrine of Stoicks, will have some of these
genii (for so he calls them) to be [5] desirous of mens company,

---

[1] Cap. 8.   Transportavit in Livoniam, cupiditate videndi, &c.   [2] Sic He-
siodus de Nymphis, vivere dicit 10 ætates phœnicum.   [3] Custodes hominum et provinciarum, &c. tanto meliores hominibus, quanto hi brutis animantibus.
[4] Præsides, pastores, gubernatores hominum, ut illi animalium.   [5] Naturâ
familiares ut canes hominibus ; multi aversantur et abhorrent.

182   *Nature of Spirits.*   [Part. 1. Sec. 2.

very affable, and familiar with them, as dogs are: others again
to abhor as serpents, and care not for them. The same, belike,
Trithemius calls *igneos et sublunares, qui nunquam demergunt
ad inferiora, aut vix ullum habent in terris commercium:*
[1] *generally they far excell men in worth, as a man the meanest
worm;* though some of them are *inferiour to those of their own
rank in worth, as the black guard in a princes court, and to
men again, as some degenerate, base rational creatures are excelled of brute beasts.*

That they are mortal, besides these testimonies of Cardan,
Martianus, &c. many other divines and philosophers hold
(post prolixum tempus moriuntur omnes), the [2] Platonists, and
some Rabbines, Porphyrius and Plutarch, as appears by that
relation of Thamus: [3] *The great god Pan is dead:* Apollo Pythius ceased; and so the rest. S. Hierome, in the life of
Paul the eremite, tells a story, how one of them appeared to
S. Antony in the wilderness, and told him as much. [4] Paracelsus, of our late writers, stifly maintains that they are mortal,
live and die, as other creatures do. Zosimus (l. 2.) farther
adds, that religion and policy dies and alters with them. The
[5] Gentiles gods, he saith, were expelled by Constantine; and
together with them, *imperii Romani majestas et fortuna interiit, et profligata est;* the fortune and majesty of the Roman
empire decayed and vanished; as that heathen in [6] Minutius
formerly bragged, when the Jews were overcome by the Romans, the Jews god was likewise captivated by that of Rome;
and Rabsakeh to the Israelites, no god should deliver them out
of the hands of the Assyrians. But these paradoxes of their
power, corporeity, mortality, taking of shapes, transposing
bodies, and carnal copulations, are sufficiently confuted by
Zanch. *(c.* 10. *l.* 4.) Pererius, (in his comment) and Tostatus
(questions on the sixth of Gen.) Th. Aquin. S. Austin, Wierus, Th. Erastus, Delrio, *(tom.* 2. *l.* 2. *quæst.* 29.) Sebastian
Michaelis *(cap.* 2. *de spiritibus),* D. Reinolds *(lect.* 47). They
may deceive the eyes of men, yet not take true bodies, or make
a real metamorphosis: but, as Cicogna proves at large, they
are [7] *illusoriæ et præstigiatrices transformationes (omnif. mag.
lib.* 4. *cap.* 4.), meer illusions and cozenings, like that tale of
Pasetis obulus in Suidas, or that of Autolycus, Mercuries son,

---

[1] Ab homine plus distant, quam homo ab ignobilissimo vernâ; et tamen quidam
ex his ab hominibus superantur, ut homines a feris, &c.   [2] Cibo et potu uti, et
Venere cum hominibus, ac tandem mori. Cicogna, 1. part. lib. 2. c. 3.   [3] Plutarch. de defect. oraculorum.   [4] Lib. de Zilphis et Pygmæis.   [5] Dii gentium a Constantino profligati sunt, &c.   [6] Octavian. dial. Judæorum deum
fuisse Romanorum numinibus unà cum gente captivum.   [7] Omnia spiritibus
plena; et ex eorum concordiâ et discordiâ omnes boni et mali effectus promanant,
omnia humana reguntur. Paradox. veterum, de quo Cicogna, omnif. mag. l. 2.
c. 3.

Mem. 1. Subs. 2.]   *Nature of Spirits.*   183

that dwelt in Parnassus, who got so much treasure by cozenage and stealth.   His father Mercurie, because he could leave
him no wealth, taught him many fine tricks to get means; [1] for
he could drive away mens cattel, and, if any pursued him,
turn them into what shapes he would, and so did mightily
enrich himself; *hoc astu maximam prædam est adsequutus.*
This, no doubt, is as true as the rest; yet thus much in
general, Thomas, Durand, and others grant, that they have
understanding far beyond men, can probably conjecture and
[2] foretell many things; they can cause and cure most diseases,
deceive our senses; they have excellent skill in all arts and
sciences; and that the most illiterate devil is *quovis homine
scientior,* as [3] Cicogna maintains out of others.   They know
the vertues of herbs, plants, stones, minerals, &c. of all creatures, birds, beasts, the four elements, stars, planets; can aptly
apply and make use of them as they see good, perceiving the
causes of all meteors, and the like : *Dant se coloribus,* (as
[4] Austin hath it) *accommodant se figuris, adhærent sonis, sub-
jiciunt se odoribus, infundunt se saporibus, omnes sensus, etiam
ipsam intelligentiam, dæmones fallunt :* they deceive all our
senses, even our understanding itself, at once.   [5] They can
produce miraculous alterations in the aire, and most wonderful effects, conquer armies, give victories; help, further, hurt,
cross, and alter humane attempts and projects, *(Dei permissu)*
as they see good themselves.   [6] When Charles the great intended to make a channel betwixt the Rhine and Danubius,
look, what his workmen did in the day, these spirits flung
down in the night : *ut conatu rex desisteret, pervicere.*   Such
feats can they do.   But that which Bodine (*l. 4. Theat. nat.*)
thinks, (following Tyrius belike and the Platonists) they can
tell the secrets of a mans heart, *aut cogitationes hominum,* is
most false : his reasons are weak, and sufficiently confuted by
Zanch. (*lib. 4. cap. 9.*), Hierom. (*lib. 2. com. in Mat. ad cap.
15.*)   Athanasius (*quæst. 27. ad Antiochum Principem*), and
others.

Orders.] As for those orders of good and bad devils—
which the Platonists hold, is altogether erroneous ; and those

---

[1] Oves, quas abacturus erat, in quascunque formas vertebat.   Pausanias, Hyginus.   [2] Austin. in l. 2. de Gen. ad literam, cap. 17. Partim quia subtilioris
sensûs acumine, partim scientiâ callidiore vigent, et experientiâ propter magnam
longitudinem vitæ, partim ab angelis discunt, &c.   [3] Lib. 3. omnif. mag. cap. 3.
[4] Lib. 18. quæst.   [5] Quum tanta sit et tam profunda spirituum scientia, mirum
non est tot tantasque res visu admirabiles ab ipsis patrari, et quidem rerum natu-
ralium ope, quas multo melius intelligunt, multoque peritius suis locis et temporibus applicare nôrunt quam homo. Cicogna.   [6] Aventinus. Quidquid interdiu
exhauriebatur, noctu explebatur.   Inde pavefacti curatores, &c.

184   *Nature of Spirits.*   [Part 1. Sec. 2.

Ethnicks *boni* and *mali genii* are to be exploded. These
heathen writers agree not in this point among themselves, as
Dandinus notes; *an sint* [1] *mali, non conveniunt;* some will
have all spirits good or bad to us by a mistake : as, if an oxe or
horse could discourse, he would say the butcher was his enemy
because he killed him, the grasier his friend because he fed
him; an hunter preserves and yet kills his game; and is hated
nevertheless of his game ; *nec piscatorem piscis amare potest,*
&c. But Jamblicus, Psellus, Plutarch, and most Platonists,
acknowledge bad, *et ab eorum maleficiis cavendum,* for they are
enemies of man-kind; and this Plato learned in Egypt, that
they quarrelled with Jupiter, [2] and were driven by him down
to hell. That which [3] Apuleius, Xenophon, and Plato contend
of Socrates *dæmonium,* is most absurd; that which Plotinus of
his, that he had likewise *Deum pro dæmonio;* and that which
Porphyry concludes of them all in general, if they be neglected
in their sacrifice, they are angry ; nay, more, as Cardan in his
Hyperchen will, they feed on mens souls : *elementa sunt*
plantis elementum, animalibus plantæ, hominibus animalia,
erunt et homines aliis, non autem diis; nimis enim remota
est eorum natura a nostrâ; quapropter dæmonibus : and so,
belike, that we have so many battels fought in all ages, countries, is to make them a feast, and their sole delight. But to
return to that I said before—if displeased, they fret and chafe,
(for they feed, belike, on the souls of beasts, as we do on
their bodies) and send many plagues amongst us; but, if
pleased, then they do much good; is as vain as the rest, and
confuted by Austin (*l.* 9. *c.* 8 *de Civ. Dei*), Euseb. (*l.* 4.
præpar. Evang. c. 6), and others. Yet thus much I find,
that our school-men and other [4] divines make nine kinds of
bad spirits, as Dionysius hath done of angels. In the first
rank, are those false gods of the Gentiles, which were adored
heretofore in several idols, and gave oracles at Delphos, and
elsewhere; whose prince is Beelzebub. The second rank
is of lyars and æquivocators, as Apollo, Pythius, and the like.
The third are those vessels of anger, inventors of all mischief;
as that Theutus in Plato ; Esay calls them [5] vessels of fury;
their prince is Belial. The fourth are malicious revenging
devils ; and their prince is Asmodæus. The fifth kind are
cozeners, such as belong to magicians and witches; their prince

---

[1] In lib. 2. de animâ, text. 29. Homerus indiscriminatim omnes spiritus dæmones vocat.   [2] A Jove ad inferos pulsi, &c.   [3] De Deo Socratis. Adest
mihi divina sorte dæmonium quoddam, a primâ pueritiâ me sequutum ; sæpe dis-
suadet ; impellit nonnunquam, instar vocis. Plato.   [4] Agrippa, lib. 3. de occul.
ph. c. 18. Zanch. Pictorius, Pererius, Cicogna, l. 3. cap. 1.   [5] Vasa iræ, c. 13.

Mem. 1. Subs. 2.] *Nature of Spirits.* **185**

is Satan. The sixth are those aërial devils, that [1]corrupt the aire, and cause plagues, thunders, fires, &c. spoken of in the Apocalyps, and Paul to the Ephesians names them the princes of the aire; Meresin is their prince. The seventh is a destroyer, captain of the Furies, causing wars, tumults, combustions, uproars, mentioned in the Apocalyps, and called Abaddon. The eighth is that accusing or calumniating devil, whom the Greeks call Διαβολος, that drives men to despair. The ninth are those tempters in several kinds; and their prince is Mammon. Psellus makes six kinds, yet none above the moon. Wierus, in his *Pseudomonarchiá Dæmonis*, out of an old book, makes many more divisions and subordinations, with their several names, numbers, offices, &c. but Gazæus (cited by [2]Lipsius) will have all places full of angels, spirits, and devils, above and beneath the moon, ætherial and aërial, which Austin cites out of *Varro, l. 7. de Civ. Dei, c. 6. The celestial devils above, and aërial beneath,* or as [3]some will, gods above, *semidei* or half gods beneath, *lares, heroes, genii,* which clime higher, if they lived well (as the Stoicks held), but grovel on the ground, as they were baser in their lives, nearer to the earth; and are *manes, lemures, lamiæ,* &c. [4]They will have no place void, but all full of spirits, devils, or some other inhabitants; *Plenum cælum, aër, aqua, terra, et omnia sub terrá,* saith Gazæus; though Anthony Rusca (in his book *de Inferno, lib. 5. cap. 7.*) would confine them to the middle region, yet they will have them every where; [5]not so much as an hair breadth empty in heaven, earth, or waters, above or under the earth. The aire is not so full of flies in summer, as it is at all times of invisible devils: this [6]Paracelsus stifly maintains, and that they have every one their several *chaos;* others will have infinite worlds, and each world his peculiar spirits, gods, angels, and devils, to govern and punish it.

> Singula [7]nonnulli credunt quoque sidera posse
> Dici orbes : terramque appellant sidus opacum,
> Cui minimus divûm præsit.——

[8]Gregorius Tholosanus makes seven kinds of ætherial spirits or angels, according to the number of the seven planets, Saturnine, Jovial, Martial, &c. of which Cardan discourseth, *lib. 20. de subtil.* he calls them *substantias primas; Olympicos dæmones,* Trithemius, *qui præsunt Zodiaco, &c.* and will

---

[1] Quibus datum est nocere terræ et mari, &c. [2] Physiol. Stoïcorum e Senec. lib. 1. c. 28. [3] Usque ad lunam animas esse æthereas, vocarique heroas, lares, genios. [4] Mart. Capella. [5] Nihil vacuum ab his, ubi vel capillum in aëre vel aquam jacias. [6] Lib. de Zilp. [7] Palingenius. [8] Lib. 7. cap. 34. et 5. Syntax. art. mirab.

186   *Nature of Spirits.*   [Part. 1. Sec. 2.

have them to be good angels above, devils beneath the moon ;
their several names and offices he there sets down, and (which
Dionysius of angels) will have several spirits for several countreys, men, offices, &c. which live about them, and as so many
assisting powers, cause their operations ; will have, in a word,
innumerable, and as many of them as there be stars in the
skies. [1] Marcilius Ficinus seems to second this opinion, out
of Plato, or from himself, I know not, (still ruling their inferiours, as they do those under them again, all subordinate ;
and the nearest to the earth rule us ; whom we subdivide into
good and bad angels, call gods or devils, as they help or hurt
us, and so adore, love or hate) but it is most likely from Plato,
for he, relying wholly on Socrates, *quem mori potius quam
mentiri voluisse scribit,* out of Socrates authority alone, made
nine kinds of them : which opinion, belike, Socrates took from
Pythagoras, and he from Trismegistus, he from Zoroaster—
first, God, secondly, ideæ, thirdly, intelligencies, fourthly, arch-
angels, fifthly, angels, sixthly, devils, seventhly, heroes, eightly,
principalities, ninthly, princes ; of which some were absolutely
good, as gods, some bad, some indifferent, *inter deos et homines,*
as heroes and *dæmones,* which ruled men, and were called *genii,*
or (as [2] Proclus and Jamblicus will) the middle betwixt God
and men, principalities and princes, which commanded and
swayed kings and countreys, and had places in the sphears
perhaps; for, as every sphear is higher, so hath it more excellent inhabitants ; which, belike, is that Galilæus a Galilæo
and Kepler aims at in his *Nuncio Siderio,* when he will have
[3] *Saturnine* and *Jovial* inhabitants, and which Tycho Brahe doth
in some sort touch or insinuate in one of his epistles: but these
things [4] Zanchius justly explodes, *cap. 3. lib.* 4, P. Martyr, in
4. Sam. 28.

So that, according to these men, the number of ætherial
spirits must needs be infinite : for, if that be true that some of
our mathematicians say, that if a stone could fall from the
starry heaven, or eighth sphear, and should pass every hour an
hundred miles, it would be sixty-five years, or more, before it
would come to ground, by reason of the great distance of
heaven from earth, which contains (as some say) one hundred
and seventy millions eight hundred and three miles,—besides
those other heavens, (whether they be crystalline or watery,
which Maginus adds) which peradventure holde as much more,

---

[1] Comment. in dial. Plat. de amore, c. 5. Ut sphæra quælibet super nos, ita præ-
stantiores habet habitatores suæ sphæræ consortes, ut habet nostra.   [2] Lib. de
animâ et dæmone. Medii inter deos et homines, divina ad nos, et nostra æqualiter
ad deos ferunt.   [3] Saturninas et Joviales accolas.   [4] In loca detrusi sunt
infra cœlestes orbes, in aërem scilicet et infra, ubi judicio generali reservantur.

Mem. 1. Subs. 2.] *Nature of Devils.* 187

—how many such spirits may it contain? And yet, for all this,
[1] Thomas, Albertus, and most, hold that there be far more
angels than devils.

Sublunary devils, and their kinds.] But, be they more or
less, *quod supra nos, nihil ad nos.* Howsoever, as Martianus
foolishly supposeth, *ætherii dæmones non curant res humanas;*
they care not for us, do not attend our actions, or look for
us; those ætherial spirits have other worlds to reign in, belike,
or business to follow. We are only now to speak in brief of
these sublunary spirits or devils. For the rest our divines determine that the devil hath no power over stars, or heavens.
[2] *Carminibus cœlo possunt deducere lunam, &c.* Those are
poetical fictions; and that they can [3] *sistere aquam fluviis, et
vertere sidera retro, &c.* as Canidia in Horace, 'tis all false.
[4] They are confined, until the day of judgement, to this sublunary world, and can work no further than the four elements,
and as God permits them. Wherefore, of these sublunary
devils, though others divide them otherwise according to their
several places and offices, Psellus makes six kinds, fiery,
aërial, terrestrial, watery, and subterranean devils, besides
those fairies, satyrs, nymphs, &c.

Fiery spirits or devils are such as commonly work by blazing
stars, firedrakes, or *ignes fatui,* which lead men often *in flumina, aut præcipitia,* saith Bodine (*lib. 2. Theat. naturæ,
fol. 221*). *Quos, inquit, arcere si volunt viatores, clarâ voce
Deum appellare, aut pronâ facie terram contingente adorare
oportet: et hoc amuletum majoribus nostris acceptum ferre debemus, &c.* Likewise they counterfeit suns and moons, stars
oftentimes, and sit on ship masts; *in navigiorum summitatibus
visuntur;* and are called *Dioscuri* (as Eusebius, *l. contra Philosophos, c.* 48, informeth us, out of the authority of Zeno-
phanes); or little clouds, *ad motum nescio quem volantes;*
which never appear, saith Cardan, but they signifie some mischief or other to come unto men, though some again will have
them to portend good, and victory to that side they come
towards in sea fights; St. Elmes fires they commonly call them,
and they do likely appear after a sea storm. Radzivilius,
the Polonian duke, calls this apparition *Sancti Germani
sidus;* and saith moreover, that he saw the same after in a
storm, as he was sayling, 1582, from Alexandria to Rhodes.
Our stories are full of such apparitions in all kinds. Some
think they keep their residence in that Hecla, a mountain in

---

[1] Q. 36. art. 9.   [2] Virg. 8. Ec.   [3] Æn. 4.   [4] Austin. Hoc dixi,
ne quis existimet habitare ibi mala dæmonia, ubi solem et lunam et stellas Deus
ordinavit. Et alibi : nemo arbitraretur dæmonem cœlis habitare cum angelis suis,
unde lapsum credimus. Id. Zanch. l. 4. c. 3 de angel. malis. Pererius, in Gen.
cap. 6. lib. 8. in ver. 2.

188   *Digression of Spirits.*   [Part. 1. Sec. 2.

Island, Ætna in Sicily, Lipara, Vesuvius, &c. These devils
were worshipped heretofore by that superstitious πυρομαντεια,
and the like.

Aërial spirits or devils are such as keep quarter, most part,
in the [1] air, cause many tempests, thunder, and lightnings,
tear oaks, fire steeples, houses, strike men and beasts, make it
rain stones (as in Livies time), wooll, frogs, &c. counterfeit
armies in the air, strange noises, swords, &c. as at Vienna before
the coming of the Turks, and many times in Rome, as Scheretzius, *l. de spec. c.* 1, *part.* 1. Lavater, *de spec. part.* 1. *c.* 17,
Julius Obsequens, an old Roman, in his book of prodigies, *ab
urb. cond.* 505, [2] Machiavel hath illustrated by many examples,
and Josephus in his book *de bello Judaico,* before the destruction
of Jerusalem. All which Guil. Postellus (in his first book, *c.* 7.
de orbis concordiâ) useth as an effectual argument (as indeed
it is) to perswade them that will not believe there be spirits or
devils. They cause whirlwinds on a sudden, and tempestuous
storms; which though our meteorologists generally refer to
natural causes, yet I am of Bodines mind (*Theat. nat. l.* 2.)
they are more often caused by those aërial devils, in their several quarters; for *tempestatibus se ingerunt,* saith [3] Rich. Ar-
gentine; as when a desperate man makes away with himself,
which by hanging or drowning they frequently do, (as Kornmannus observes, *de mirac. mort. part.* 7. *c.* 76.) *tripudium
agentes,* dancing and rejoicing at the death of a sinner. These
can corrupt the aire, and cause plagues, sickness, storms, shipwracks, fires, inundations. At Mons Draconis in Italy there is
a most memorable example in [4] Jovianus Pontanus: and nothing
so familiar (if we may believe those relations of Saxo-Gramma-
ticus, Olaus Magnus, Damianus A. Goes) as for witches and
sorcerers, in Lapland, Lithuania, and all over Scandia, to sell
winds to marriners, and cause tempests; which Marcus Paulus
the Venetian relates likewise of the Tartars. These kind of
devils are much [5] delighted in sacrifices, (saith Porphyry)
held all the world in awe, and had several names, idols,
sacrifices in Rome, Greece, Ægypt, and at this day tyrannize over, and deceive those Ethnicks and Indians, being
adored and worshipped for [6] gods: for the Gentiles gods
were devils (as [7] Trismegistus confesseth in his Asclepius;
and he himself could make them come to their images by
magick spells), and are now as much *respected by our*

---

[1] Domus diruunt, muros dejiciunt, immiscent se turbinibus et procellis, et pul-
verem instar columnæ evehunt. Cicogna, l. 5. c. 5.   [2] Quæst. in Liv.
[3] De præstigiis dæmonum, c. 16. Convelli culmina videmus, prosterni sata, &c.
[4] De bello Neapolitano, lib. 5.   [5] Suffitibus gaudent. Idem. Just. Mart. Apol.
pro Christianis.   [6] In Dei imitationem, saith Eusebius.   [7] Dii gentium
dæmonia, &c. ego in eorum statuas pellexi.

Mem. 1. Subs. 2.]   *Digression of Spirits.*   189

papists (saith [1]Pictorius) *under the name of saints.* These
are they which, Cardan thinks, desire so much carnal copulation with witches (*Incubi* and *Succubi*), transform bodies,
and are so very cold, if they be touched; and that serve
magicians. His father had one of them, (as he is not
ashamed to relate[2]) an aërial devil, bound to him for twenty
and eight years. As Agrippas dog had a devil tyed to his col-
ler, some think that Paracelsus (or else Erastus belies him)
had one confined to his sword pummel; others wear them in
rings, &c. Jannes and Jambres did many things of old by
their help, Simon Magus, Cinops, Apollonius Tyaneus, Jamblicus, and Trithemius of late, that shewed Maximilian the
emperour his wife, after she was dead; *et verrucam in collo
ejus* (saith [3]Godolman), so much as the wart in her neck.
Delrio (*lib.* 2.) hath divers examples of their feats; Cicogna,
lib. 3. cap. 3, and Wierus in his book *de præstig. dæmonum,*
Boissardus, *de magis et veneficis.*

Water-devils are those *naiades* or water nymphs which have
been heretofore conversant about waters and rivers. The water
(as Paracelsus thinks) is their chaos, wherein they live. Some
call them *fairies,* and say that Habundia is their queen. These
cause inundations, many times shipwracks, and deceive men
divers wayes, as *Succubæ,* or otherwise, appearing most part
(saith Trithemius) in womens shapes. [4]Paracelsus hath several
stories of them that have lived and been married to mortal
men, and so continued for certain years with them, and
after, upon some dislike, have forsaken them. Such a one
as Egeria, with whom Numa was so familiar, Diana Ceres,
&c. [5]Olaus Magnus hath a long narration of one Hotherus, a
king of Sweden, that, having lost his company as he was hunting one day, met with these water nymphs or fairies, and was
feasted by them; and Hector Boëthius, of Macbeth and Banco,
two Scottish lords, that, as they were wandering in woods, had
their fortunes told them by three strange women. To these
heretofore they did use to sacrifice, by that ὑδρομαντεια, or di-
vination by waters.

Terrestrial devils are those [6]*lares, genii, faunes, satyrs,*
[7]wood-nymphs, foliots, fairies, *Robin Goodfellows, Trulli, &c.*
which as they are most conversant with men, so they do
them most harm. Some think it was they alone that kept the
heathen people in awe of old, and had so many idols and

---

[1] Et nunc sub divorum nomine coluntur a pontificiis.   [2] Lib. 11. de rerum
var.   [3] Lib. 3. cap. 3. de magis et veneficis, &c.   [4] Lib. de Zilphis.
[5] Lib. 3.   [6] Pro salute hominum excubare se simulant; sed in eorum perniciem omnia moliuntur. Aust.   [7] Dryades, Oriades, Hamadryades.

190   *Digression of Spirits.*   [Part. 1. Sec. 2

temples erected to them. Of this range was Dagon amongst
the Philistins, Bel amongst the Babylonians, Astartes amongst
the Sidonians, Baal amongst the Samaritans, Isis and Osiris
amongst the Ægyptians, &c. Some put our [1] fairies into this
rank, which have been in former times adored with much superstition, with sweeping their houses, and setting of a pail
of clean water, good victuals, and the like; and then they should
not be pinched, but find money in their shoes, and be fortunate in their enterprizes. These are they that dance on
heaths and greens, as [2] Lavater thinks with Trithemius, and,
as [3] Olaus Magnus adds, leave that green circle, which we
commonly find in plain fields, which others hold to proceed
from a meteor falling, or some accidental rankness of the
ground; so nature sports herself. They are sometimes seen by
old women and children. Hieron. Pauli, in his description
of the city of Bereino in Spain, relates how they have been
familiarly seen near that town, about fountains and hills: *nonnunquam* (saith Trithemius) *in sua latibula montium simpli-
ciores homines ducunt, stupenda mirantibus ostendentes miracula, molarum sonitus, spectacula, &c.* Giraldus Cambrensis
gives instance in a monk of Wales that was so deluded. [4] Paracelsus reckons up many places in Germany, where they do
usually walk in little coats, some two feet long. A bigger
kind there is of them, called with us *hobgoblins*, and *Robin
Goodfellows*, that would, in those superstitious times, grind
corn for a mess of milk, cut wood, or do any manner of
drudgery work. They would mend old irons in those Æolian
isles of Lipara, in former ages, and have been often seen and
heard. [5] Tholosanus calls them *Trullos* and *Getulos*, and saith
that in his dayes they were common in many places of France.
Dithmarus Bleskenius, in his description of Island, reports for
a certainty, that almost in every family they have yet some such
familiar spirits; and Felix Malleolus, in his book *de crudel.
dæmon.* affirms as much, that these *Trolli* or *Telchines*, are
very common in Norwey, *and* [6] *seen to do drudgery work;*
to draw water, saith Wierus, (*lib. 1. cap. 22.*) dress meat, or
any such thing. Another sort of these there are, which frequent forlorne [7] houses, which the Italians call *foliots*, most
part innoxious, [8] Cardan holds: *They will make strange*

---

[1] Elvas Olaus vocat. lib. 3.   [2] Part 1. cap. 19.   [3] Lib. 3. cap. 11. El-
varum choreas Olaus lib. 3. vocat. Saltum adeo profunde in terras imprimunt, ut
locus insigni deinceps virore orbicularis sit, et gramen non pereat.   [4] Lib. de
Zilph. et Pygmæis, Olaus l. 3.   [5] Lib. 7. cap. 14. Qui et in famulitio viris
et feminis inserviunt, conclavia scopis purgant, patinas mundant, ligna portant,
equos curant, &c.   [6] Ad ministeria utuntur.   [7] Where treasure is hid
(as some think), or some murder, or such like villany committed.   [8] Lib.
16. de rerum varietat.

Mem. 1. Subs. 2.]   *Digression of Spirits.*   191

*noises in the night, howl sometimes pittifully, and then
laugh again, cause great flames and sudden lights, fling stones,
rattle chains, shave men, open doors, and shut them, fling
down platters, stools, chests, sometimes appear in the likenesc
of hares, crows, black dogs, &c.* of which read [1] Pet. Thyræus
the Jesuit (in his Tract *de locis infestis, part.* 1. *et cap.* 4.)
who will have them to be devils, or the souls of damned
men that seek revenge, or else souls out of purgatory that
seek ease. For such examples, peruse [2] Sigismundus Scheretzius, *lib. de spectris, part.* 1. *c.* 1, which he saith he took out
of Luther most part; there be many instances. [3] Plinius Secundus remembers such a house at Athens, which Athenodorus
the philosopher hired, which no man durst inhabit for fear of
devils. Austin *(de Civ. Dei, lib.* 22. *cap.* 8.) relates as much
of Hesperius the tribunes house at Zubeda near their city of
Hippos, vexed with evil spirits to his great hinderance; *cum
afflictione animalium et servorum suorum.* Many such instances are to be read in Niderius *Formicar. lib.* 5. *cap.* 12. 3.
&c. Whether I may call these *Zim* and *Othim,* which Isay
cap. 13. 21. speaks of I make a doubt. See more of these
in the said Scheretz. *lib.* 1. *de spect. cap.* 4: he is full of examples. These kind of devils many times appear to men,
and affright them out of their wits, sometimes walking at
[4] noon-day, sometimes at nights, counterfeiting dead mens
ghosts, as that of Caligula, which (saith Suetonius) was seen
to walk in Lavinias garden, where his body was buried, spirits
haunted, and the house where he dyed : [5] *Nulla nox sine terrore transacta, donec incendio consumpta ;* every night this
hapned ; there was no quietness, till the house was burned.
About Hecla in Island ghosts commonly walk *animas mortuorum simulantes,* saith Jo. Anan. *lib.* 3. *de nat. dæm.*
Olaus, *lib.* 2. *cap.* 2. Natal. Tallopid. *lib. de apparit. spir.*
Kormannus *de mirac. mort. part.* 1. *cap.* 44. Such sights are
frequently seen *circa sepulcra et monasteria,* saith Lavat.
lib. 1. *cap.* 19. in monasteries and about church-yards, *loca
paludinosa, ampla ædificia, solitaria, et cæde hominum no-
tata, &c.* Thyreus adds, *ubi gravius peccatum est commissum, impii, pauperum oppressores, et nequiter insignes habitant.* These spirits often foretell mens deaths, by several
signs, as knocking, groanings, &c. [6] though Rich. Argen-

---

[1] Vel spiritus sunt hujusmodi damnatorum, vel e purgatorio, vel ipsi dæmones,
c. 4.   [2] Quidam lemures domesticis instrumentis noctu ludunt: patinas,
ollas, cantharas, et alia vasa, dejiciunt ; et quidam voces emittunt, ejulant, risum
emittunt, &c. ut canes nigri, feles, variis formis, &c.   [3] Epist. l. 7.   [4] Me-
ridionales dæmones Cicogna calls them, or Alastores, l. 3. cap. 9.   [5] Sueton. c. 69. in Caligulâ.   [6] Strozzius, Cicogna, lib. 3. mag. cap. 5.

2

192   *Digression of Spirits.*   [Part. 1. Sec. 2.

tine, *c.* 18. *de præstigiis dæmonum,* will ascribe these predictions to good angels, out of the authority of Ficinus and
others ; *prodigia in obitu principum sæpius contingunt, &c.* as,
in the Lateran church in [1] Rome, the popes deaths are fore-
told by Silvesters tomb. Near Rupes Nova in Finland, in the
kingdom of Sweden, there is a lake, in which, before the governour of the castle dyes, a *spectrum,* in the habit of Arion
with his harp, appears, and makes excellent musick, like those
blocks in Cheshire, which, (they say) presage death to the
master of the family; or that [2] oak in Lanthadran park in
Cornwall, which foreshews as much. Many families in Europe are so put in mind of their last, by such predictions, and
many men are forewarned (if we may believe Paracelsus) by
familiar spirits, in divers shapes, as cocks, crows, owls, which
often hover about sick mens chambers *vel quia morientium
fœditatem sentiunt,* as [3] Baracellus conjectures, *et ideo super
tectum infirmorum crocitant,* because they smell a corse ; or
for that (as [4] Bernardinus de Bustis thinketh) God permits the
devil to appear in the form of crows, and such like creatures,
to scare such as live wickedly here on earth. A little before
Tullies death, (saith Plutarch) the crows made a mighty noise
about him ; *tumultuose perstrepentes,* they pulled the pillow
from under his head. Rob. Gaguinus, *hist. Franc. lib.* 8.
telleth such another wonderful story at the death of Johannes de Monteforti, a French lord, *anno* 1345. *Tanta
corvorum multitudo ædibus morientis insedit, quantam esse in
Galliâ nemo judicâsset.* Such prodigies are very frequent in
authors. See more of these in the said Lavater, Thyreus, *de
locis infestis, part.* 3. *cap.* 58. Pictorius, Delrio, Cicogna,
lib. 3. *cap.* 9. Necromancers take upon them to raise and lay
them at their pleasures ; and so likewise those which Mizaldus calls *Ambulones,* that walk about midnight on great
heaths and desart places, which (saith [5] Lavater) *draw men out
of the way, and lead them all night a by-way, or quite bar
them of their way.* These have several names in several
places; we commonly call them *Pucks.* In the desarts of
Lop in Asia, such illusions of walking spirits are often perceived, as you may read in M. Paulus the Venetian his travels.
If one lose his company by chance, these devils will call him
by his name, and counterfeit voices of his companions to
seduce him. Hieronym. Pauli, in his book of the hills of

---

[1] Idem, c. 18.   [2] M. Cary. Survey of Cornwall, lib. 2. fol. 140.   [3] Horto
Geniali, fol. 137.   [4] Part. 1. c. 19.   Abducunt eos a rectâ viâ, et viam iter
facientibus intercludunt.   [5] Lib. 1. cap. 44. Dæmonum cernuntur et audiuntur ibi frequentes illusiones ; unde viatoribus cavendum, ne se dissocient,
aut a tergo maneant; voces enim fingunt sociorum, ut a recto itinere abdu-
cant, &c.

Spain, relates of a great [1] mount in Cantabria, where such *spectrums* are to be seen. Lavater and Cicogna have variety of examples of spirits and walking devils in this kind. Sometimes they sit by the high-way side, to give men falls, and make their horses stumble and start as they ride, (if you will believe the relation of that holy man Ketellus, [2] in Nubrigensis,) that had an especial grace to see devils, *gratiam divinitus collatam,* and talk with them, *et impavidus cum spiritibus sermonem miscere,* without offence: and if a man curse and spur his horse for stumbling, they do heartily rejoyce at it; with many such pretty feats.

Subterranean devils are as common as the rest, and do as much harm. Olaus Magnus *(lib.* 6. *cap.* 19.) makes six kinds of them, some bigger, some less. These (saith [3] Munster) are commonly seen about mines of metals, and are, some of them, noxious; some again do no harm. The metal-men in many places account it good luck, a sign of treasure and rich ore, when they see them. Georgius Agricola (in his book *de subterraneis animantibus, cap.* 37.) reckons two more notable kinds of them, which he calls [4] *Gætuli* and *Cobali;* both are *cloathed after the manner of metal-men, and will many times imitate their works.* Their office, as Pictorius and Paracelsus think, is to keep treasure in the earth, that it be not all at once revealed; and, besides, [5] Cicogna averrs, that they are the frequent causes of those horrible earth-quakes, *which often swallow up, not only houses, but whole islands and cities :* in his third book, *cap.* 11, he gives many instances.

The last are conversant about the center of the earth, to torture the souls of damned men to the day of judgement. Their egress and regress some suppose to be about Ætna, Lipara, Mons Hecla in Island, Vesuvius, Terra del Fuego, &c. because many shreeks and fearful cryes are continually heard thereabouts, and familiar apparitions of dead men, ghosts, and goblins.

Their offices, operations, study.] Thus the devil reigns, in a thousand several shapes, *as a roaring lyon, still seeks whom he may devour,* (1 Pet. 5.) by earth, sea, land, air, as yet unconfined, though [6] some will have his proper place the air—all that space betwixt us and the moon, for them that

---

[1] Mons sterilis et nivosus, ubi intempesta nocte umbræ apparent.   [2] Lib. 2. cap. 21. Offendicula faciunt transeuntibus in viâ ; et petulanter rident, cum vel hominem vel jumentum ejus pedes atterere faciant, et maxime si homo maledictis et calcaribus sæviat.   [3] In cosmogr.   [4] Vestiti more metallicorum, gestus et opera eorum imitantur.   [5] Immisso in terræ carceres vento, horribiles terræ motus efficiunt, quibus sæpe non domus modo et turres, sed civitates integræ et insulæ, haustæ sunt.   [6] Hieron. in 3 Ephes. Idem Michaelis c. 4. de spiritibus. Idem Thyreus de locis infestis.

194   *Digression of Spirits.*   [Part. 1. Sec. 2.

transgressed least, and hell for the wickedest of them; *hîc velut in carcere ad finem mundi, tunc in locum funestiorem trudendi,* as Austin holds, *de Civit. Dei, c. 22. lib.* 14. *cap.* 3. *et* 23. But, be where he will, he rageth while he may; to comfort himself (as [1] Lactantius thinks) with other mens falls, he labours all he can to bring them into the same pit of perdition with him : for [2] *mens miseries, calamities, and ruines, are the devils banqueting dishes.* By many temptations and several engines, he seeks to captivate our souls. The lord of lyes saith [3] Austin; *as he was deceived himself, he seeks to deceive others;* the ring-leader to all naughtiness; as he did by Eve and Cain, Sodom and Gomorrha, so would he do by all the world. Sometimes he tempts by covetousness, drunkenness, pleasure, pride, &c. errs, dejects, saves, kills, protects, and rides some men, as they do their horses. He studies our overthrow and generally seeks our destruction ; and, although he pretend many times humane good, and vindicate himself for a god, by curing of several diseases, *ægris sanitatem, et cæcis luminis usum restituendo,* (as Austin declares, *lib.* 10. *de civit. Dei, cap.* 6.) as Apollo, Æsculapius, Isis, of old have done ; divert plagues, assist them in wars, pretend their happiness; yet *nihil his impurius, scelestius, nihil humano generi infestius;* nothing so impure, nothing so pernicious, as may well appear by their tyrannical and bloody sacrifices of men to Saturn and Moloch (which are still in use amongst those barbarous Indians), their several deceits and cozenings to keep men in obedience, their false oracles, sacrifices, their superstitious impositions of fasts, penury, &c. heresies, superstitions, observations of meats, times, &c. by which they [4] crucifie the souls of mortal men, as shall be shewed in our treatise of religious melancholy. *Modico adhuc tempore sinitur malignari,* as [5] Bernard expresseth it : by God's permission he rageth a while, hereafter to be confined to

---

[1] Lactantius, 2. de origine erroris, cap. 15. Hi maligni spiritus per omnem terram vagantur, et solatium perditionis suæ perdendis hominibus operantur. [2] Mortalium calamitates epulæ sunt malorum dæmonum. Synesius.   [3] Dominus mendacii, a seipso deceptus, alios decipere cupit. Adversarius humani generis. Inventor mortis, superbiæ institutor, radix malitiæ, scelerum caput, princeps omnium vitiorum, furit inde in Dei contumeliam, hominum perniciem. De horum conatibus et operationibus, lege Epiphanium, 2 tom. lib. 2. Dionysium, c. 4. Ambros. Epistol. lib. 10. ep. 84. August. de civ. Dei, lib. 5. c. 9. lib. 8. cap. 22. lib. 9. 18. lib. 10. 21. Theophil. in 12 Mat. Pasil. ep. 141. Leonem Ser. Theodoret. in 11 Cor. ep. 22. Chrys. hom. 53. in 12. Gen. Greg. in 1. c. John Barthol. de prop. l. 2. c. 20. Zanch. l. 4. de malis angelis. Perer. in Gen. l. 8. in c. 6. 2. Origen. Sæpe prœliis intersunt; itinera et negotia nostra quæcunque dirigunt, clandestinis subsidiis optatos sæpe præbent successus. Pet. Mar. in Sam. &c. Ruscam de Inferno. [4] Et velut mancipia circumfert. Psellus. [5] Lib. de transmut. Malac. ep.

hell and darkness *which is prepared for him and his angels*, Matt. 25.

How far their power doth extend, it is hard to determine. What the ancients held of their effects, force, and operations, I will briefly shew you. Plato, in Critias, and after him, his followers, gave out that these spirits or devils *were mens governours and keepers, our lords and masters, as we are of our cattle.* [1] *They govern provinces and kingdoms by oracles, auguries,* dreams, rewards, and punishments, prophesies, inspirations, sacrifices, and religious superstitions, varied in as many forms as there be diversity of spirits : they send wars, plagues, peace, sickness, health, dearth, plenty, [2] *adstantes hîc jam nobis, spectantes et arbitrantes, &c.* (as appears by those histories of Thucydides, Livius, Dionysius Halicarnasseus, with many others, that are full of their wonderful stratagems) and were therefore, by those Roman and Greek common-wealths, adored and worshipped for gods, with prayers, and sacrifices, &c. [3] In a word, *nihil magis quærunt, quam metum et admirationem hominum ;* and (as another hath it) *dici non potest, quam impotenti ardore in homines dominium, et divinos cultus, maligni spiritus affectent.* Trithemius, in his book *de septem secundis*, assigns names to such angels as are governours of particular provinces (by what authority I know not), and gives them several jurisdictions. Asclepiades a Grecian, Rabbi Achiba the Jew, Abraham Avenezra, and Rabbi Azareel, Arabians (as I find them cited by [4] Cicogna) farther add, that they are not our governours only, *sed ex eorum concordiâ et discordiâ, boni et mali affectus promanant ;* but as they agree, so do we and our princes, or disagree : stand or fall. Juno was a bitter enemy to Troy, Apollo a good friend, Jupiter indifferent : *Æqua Venus Teucris, Pallas iniqua fuit ;* some are for us still, some against us ; *premente Deo, fert Deus alter opem.* Religion, policy, publick and private quarrels, wars, are procured by them ; and they are [5] delighted perhaps to see men fight, as men are with cocks, bulls, and dogs, bears, &c. Plagues, dearths, depend on them, our *bene* and *male esse*, and almost all our other peculiar actions, (for, as Anthony Rusca contends, *lib.* 5. *cap.* 18, every man hath a good and a bad angel attending of him in particular, all his life long, which Jamblicus calls *dæmonem)* preferments, losses, weddings, deaths, rewards, and punishments, and (as [6] Proclus will) all offices whatsoever : *alii genetricem, alii opificem potes-*

---

[1] Custodes sunt hominum, ut nos animalium : tum et provinciis præpositi regunt auguriis, somniis, oraculis, præmiis, &c. [2] Lipsius, Physiol. Stoïc. lib. 1. cap. 19. [3] Leo Suavis. Idem et Trithemius. [4] Omnif. mag. lib. 2. cap. 23. [5] Ludus deorum sumus. [6] Lib. de animâ et dæmone.

o 2

196   *Digression of Spirits.*   [Part. 1. Sec. 2.

tatem habent, &c. and several names they give them according to their offices, as *Lares, Indigetes, Præstites, &c.*
When the Arcades, in that battel at Chæronea, which was
fought against King Philip for the liberty of Greece, had deceit-
fully carried themselves,—long after, in the very same place,
diis Græciæ ultoribus (saith mine author) they were miserably
slain by Metellus the Roman : so likewise, in smaller matters,
they will have things fall out, as these *boni* and *mali genii*
favour or dislike us. *Saturnini non conveniunt Jovialibus, &c.*
He that is *Saturninus,* shall never likely be preferred. [1] That
base fellows are often advanced, undeserving *Gnathoes,* and
vicious parasites, when as discreet, wise, vertuous, and worthy
men are neglected, and unrewarded, they refer to those domineering spirits, or subordinate *genii:* as they are inclined, or favour
men, so they thrive, are ruled and overcome ; for (as [2] Libanius
supposeth) in our ordinary conflicts and contentions, *genius genio cedit et obtemperat,* one *genius* yields, and is overcome by
another. All particular events almost they refer to these private
spirits : and (as Paracelsus adds) they direct, teach, inspire,
and instruct men.   Never was any man extraordinarily
famous in any art, action, or great commander, that had not
familiarem dæmonem, to inform him, as Numa, Socrates,
and many such, as Cardan illustrates, *cap.* 128. *Arcanis pru-
dentiæ civilis,* [3] *speciali siquidem gratiâ, se a Deo donari as-
serunt magi, a geniis cœlestibus instrui, ab iis doceri.* But
these are most erroneous paradoxes, *ineptæ et fabulosæ nugæ,*
rejected by our divines and Christian Churches. 'Tis true,
they have by God's permission, power over us ; and we find
by experience, that they can [4] hurt, not our fields only, cattel,
goods, but our bodies and minds.   At Hammel in Saxony,
an. 1484. 20 *Junii,* the devil, in the likeness of a pied piper,
carryed away 130 children, that were never after seen. Many
times men are [5] affrighted out of their wits, carried away
quite (as Scheretzius illustrates, *lib.* 1. *c.* 4.) and severally molested by his means. Plotinus the Platonist *(lib.* 14. *advers.
Gnost.)* laughs them to scorn, that hold the devil or spirits can
cause any such diseases.   Many think he can work upon

---

[1] Quoties fit, ut principes novitium aulicum divitiis et dignitatibus pene obruant,
et multorum annorum ministrum, qui non semel pro hero periculum subiit, ne
teruncio donent, &c.   Idem.   Quod philosophi non remunerentur, cum scurra
et ineptus ob insulsum jocum sæpe præmium reportet, inde fit, &c.   [2] Lib.
de cruent. cadaver.   [3] Boissardus, c. 6. magia.   [4] Godelmannus, cap. 3.
lib. 1. de Magis. idem Zanchius, lib. 4. cap. 10 et 11. de malis angelis.   [5] Nocivâ melancholiâ furiosos efficit, et quandoque penitus interficit. G. Picolomineus ; idemque Zanch. cap. 10. lib. 4. Si Deus permittat, corpora nostra movere
possunt, alterare, quovis morborum et malorum genere afficere, imo et in ipsa
penetrare et sævire.

the body, but not upon the mind. But experience pronounceth otherwise, that he can work both upon body and mind. Tertullian is of this opinion (*c. 22.*) [1] *that he can cause both sickness and health,* and that secretly. [2] Taurellus adds *by clancular poysons he can infect the bodies, and hinder the operations of the bowels, though we perceive it not; closely creeping into them,* saith [3] Lipsius, and so crucifie our souls; *et nocivâ melancholiâ furiosos efficit.* For, being a spiritual body, he struggles with our spirits, saith Rogers, and suggests (according to [4] Cardan, *verba sine voce, species sine visu)* envy, lust, anger, &c. as he sees men inclined.

The manner how he performs it, Biarmannus, in his oration against Bodine sufficiently declares. *He* [5] *begins first with the phantasie, and moves that so strongly, that no reason is able to resist.* Now the *phantasie* he moves by mediation of humours; although many physicians are of opinion, that the devil can alter the mind, and produce this disease, of himself. *Quibusdam medicorum visum,* saith [6] Avicenna, *quod melancholia contingat a dæmonio.* Of the same mind is Psellus, and Rhasis, the Arab, *(lib.* 1. *Tract.* 9. *Cont.)* [7] *that this disease proceeds especially from the devil, and from him alone.* Arculanus, *cap.* 6. *in* 9. *Rhasis,* Ælianus Montaltus in his 9 *cap.* Daniel Sennertus, *lib.* 1. *part.* 2. *cap.* 11, confirm as much, that the devil can cause this disease; by reason, many times, that the parties affected prophesie, speak strange language, but *non sine interventu humoris,* not without the humour, as he interprets himself; no more doth Avicenna: *si contingat a dæmonio, sufficit nobis ut convertat complexionem ad choleram nigram, et sit caussa ejus propinqua cholera nigra;* the immediate cause is choler adust; which [8] Pomponatius likewise labours to make good; Galgerandus of Mantua, a famous physician, so cured a dæmoniacal woman in his time, that spake all languages, by purging black choler: and thereupon, belike, this humour of melancholy is called *balneum diaboli,* the devils bath; the devil spying his opportunity of such humours, drives them many times to despair, fury, rage, &c. mingling himself amongst these humours. This is that which Tertullian averrs *corporibus infligunt acerbos casus, animæque repentinos; membra distorquent, occulte repentes, &c.* and, which

[1] Inducere potest morbos et sanitates. [2] Viscerum actiones potest inhibere latenter, et venenis nobis ignotis corpus inficere. [3] Irrepentes corporibus occulto morbos fingunt, mentes terrent, membra distorquent. Lips. Phys. Stoïc. l. 1. c. 19. [4] De rerum. var. l. 16. c. 93. [5] Quum mens immediate decipi nequit, primum movet phantasiam, et ita obfirmat vanis conceptibus, ut nequem facultati æstimativæ, rationive locum relinquat. Spiritus malus invadit animam, turbat sensus, in furorum conjicit. Austin. de vit. beat. [6] Lib. 3. Fen. 1. Tract. 4. c. 18. [7] A dæmone maxime proficisci, et sæpe solo. [8] Lib. de incant.

198 *Digression of Spirits.* [Part. 1. Sec. 2.

Lemnius goes about to prove, *immiscent se mali genii pravis humoribus, atque atræ bili, &c.* and [1] Jason Pratensis, *that the devil, being a slender incomprehensible spirit, can easily insinuate and wind himself into humane bodies, and, cunningly couched in our bowels, vitiate our healths, terrifie our souls with fearful dreams, and shake our mind with furies.* And in another place, *These unclean spirits, settled in our bodies, and now mixt with our melancholy humours, do triumph as it were, and sport themselves as in another heaven.* Thus he argues, and that they go in and out of our bodies, as bees do in a hive, and so provoke and tempt us, as they perceive our temperature inclined of itself, and most apt to be deluded. [2] Agrippa and Lavater are perswaded that this humour invites the devil to it, wheresoever it is in extremity; and, of all other, melancholy persons are most subject to diabolical temptations and illusions, and most apt to entertain them, and the devil best able to work upon them; but, whether by obsession, or possession, or otherwise, I will not determine: 'tis a difficult question, Delrio the Jesuite, *(tom. 3. lib. 6.)* Springer and his colleague, *(mall. malef.)* Pet. Thyreus, the Jesuite, *(lib. de dæmoniacis, de locis infestis, de terrificationibus nocturnis)* Hieronymus Mengus, *(Flagel. dæm.)* and others of that rank of pontificial writers, it seems, by their exorcisms and conjurations, approve of it, having forged many stories to that purpose. A nun did eat a lettice [3] *without grace, or signing it with the sign of the cross,* and was instantly possessed. Durand, *(lib. 6. Rational. c. 86. num. 8)* relates that he saw a wench possessed in Bononia with two devils, by eating an unhallowed pomegranate, as she did afterwards confess, when she was cured by exorcisms. And therefore our papists do sign themselves so often with the sign of the cross, *ne dæmon ingredi ausit,* and exorcise all manner of meats, as being unclean or accursed otherwise, as Bellarmine defends. Many such stories I find amongst pontificial writers, [4] to prove their assertions; let them free their own credits: some few I will recite in this kind out of most approved physicians. Cornelius Gemma *(lib. 2. de nat. mirac. c. 4.)* relates of a young maid, called Katherine Gualter, a coopers daughter, an. 1571, that had such strange passions and convulsions, three men could not sometimes hold her. She purged a live eele, which he saw, a foot and half long, and

---

[1] Cap. de maniâ, lib. de morbis cerebri. Dæmones, quum sint tenues et incomprehensibiles spiritus, se insinuare corporibus humanis possunt, et occulte in visceribus operti, valetudinem vitiare, somniis animas terrere, et mentes furoribus quatere. Insinuant se melancholicorum penetralibus intus, ibique considunt et deliciantur, tamquam in regione clarissimorum siderum, coguntque animum furere.
[2] Lib. 1. cap. 6. occult. philos. part. 1. cap. 1. de spectris. [3] Sine cruce et sanctificatione; sic a dæmone obsessa. dial. [4] Greg. pag. c. 9.

2

Mem. 1. Subs. 3.]   *Causes of Melancholy.*   199

touched himself; but the eele afterward vanished: she vomited some twenty-four pounds of fulsome stuff of all colours, twice a day for fourteen dayes; and, after that, she voided great balls of hair, pieces of wood, pigeons dung, parchment, goose dung, coals; and, after them, two pound of pure blood, and then again coals and stones (of which some had inscriptions) bigger than a walnut, some of them pieces of glass, brass, &c. besides paroxysmes of laughing, weeping, and extasies, &c. *Et hoc (inquit) cum horrore vidi*, this I saw with horrour. They could do no good on her by physick, but left her to the clergy. Marcellus Donatus *(lib. 2. c. 1. de med. mirab.)* hath such another story of a countrey fellow, that had four knives in his belly, *instar serræ dentatos*, indented like a saw, every one a span long, and a wreath of hair like a globe, with much baggage of like sort, wonderful to behold. How it should come into his guts, he concludes, *certe non alio quam dæmonis astutiâ et dolo. Langius (Epist. med. lib. 1. Epist. 38)* hath many relations to this effect, and so hath Christopherus a Vega. Wierus, Skenkius, Scribanius, all agree that they are done by the subtilty and illusion of the devil. If you shall ask a reason of this, 'tis to exercise our patience; for as [1] Tertullian holds, *Virtus non est virtus, nisi comparem habet aliquem in quo superando vim suam ostendat;* 'tis to try us and our faith; 'tis for our offences, and for the punishment of our sins, by Gods permission they do it; *carnifices vindictæ justæ Dei* as [2] Tholosanus stiles them, executioners of his will : or rather as David, *Psal.* 78. ver. 49. *He cast upon them the fierceness of his anger, indignation, wrath, and vexation, by sending out of evil angels.* So did he afflict Job, Saul, the lunaticks and dæmoniacal persons whom Christ cured, Matth. 4. 8. Luke 4. 11. Luke 13. Mark 9. Tobit 8. 3, &c. This, I say, happeneth for a punishment of sin, for their want of faith, incredulity, weakness, distrust, &c.

SUBSECT. III.

Of Witches and Magicians, how they cause Melancholy.

You have heard what the devil can do of himself; now you shall hear what he can perform by his instruments, who are many times worse (if it be possible) than he himself, and to satisfie their revenge and lust, cause more mischief; *multa*

---

[1] Penult. de opific. Dei.   [2] Lib. 28. cap. 26. Tom. 2.

200   *Causes of Melancholy.*   [Part. 1. Sec. 2.

enim mala non egisset dæmon, nisi provocatus a sagis, as
[1] Erastus thinks : much harm had never been done, had he not
been provoked by witches to it.   He had not appeared in Sa-
muels shape, if the witch of Endor had let him alone ; or represented those serpents in Pharaohs presence, had not the magicians urged him unto it : *nec morbos vel hominibus vel brutis
infligeret,* (Erastus maintains) *si sagæ quiescerent ;* men and
cattle might go free, if the witches would let him alone. Many
deny witches at all, or, if there be any, they can do no harm.
Of this opinion is Wierus, *(lib. 3. cap. 53. de præstig. dæm.)*
Austin Lerchemer a Dutch writer, Biarmannus, Ewichius, Eu-
waldus, our countryman Scot : with him in Horace,

> Somnia, terrores magicos, miracula, sagas,
> Nocturnos lemures, portentaque Thessala, risu
> Excipiunt———

they laugh at all such stories : but on the contrary are most
lawyers, divines, physicians, philosophers, Austin, Hemingius,
Danæus, Chytræus, Zanchius, Aretius, &c. Delrio, Springer,
[2] Niderius *(lib. 5 Formicar.)* Cuiatius, Bartolus, *(consil. 6.
tom. 1.)* Bodine, *(dæmoniant. lib. 2. cap. 8)* Godelman, Damhoderius, &c. Paracelsus, Erastus, Scribanius, Camerarius, &c.
The parties by whom the devil deals, may be reduced to these
two—such as command him, in shew at least, as conjurers,
and magicians, (whose detestable and horrid mysteries are
contained in their book called [3] *Arbatell ; dæmones enim ad-
vocati præsto sunt, seque exorcismis et conjurationibus quasi
cogi patiuntur, ut miserum magorum genus in impietate detineant)* or such as are commanded, as witches that deal *ex
parte implicite,* or *explicite,* as the [4] King hath well defined.
Many subdivisions there are, and many several species of sorcerers, witches, inchanters, charmers, &c.   They have been
tolerated heretofore, some of them ; and magick hath been
publickly professed in former times, in [5] Salamanca, [6] Cracovia,
and other places, though after censured by several [7] universities, and now generally contradicted, though practised by
some still, maintained and excused, *tamquam res secreta, quæ
non nisi viris magnis, et peculiari beneficio de cœlo instructis
communicatur* (I use [8] Boissardus his words) ; and so far approved by some princes, *ut nihil ausi aggredi in politicis,*

---

[1] De lamiis.   [2] Et quomodo venefici fiant, enarrat.   [3] De quo plura
legas in Boissardo, lib. 1. de præstig.   [4] Rex Jacobus, Dæmonol. l. 1. c. 3.
[5] An university in Spain, in old Castile.   [6] The chief town in Poland.
[7] Oxford and Paris. See finem P. Lumbardi.   [8] Præfat. de magis et veneficis, lib.

Mem. 1. Subs. 3.]   *Causes of Melancholy.*   201

in sacris, in consiliis, sine eorum arbitrio; they consult still
with them, and dare indeed do nothing without their advice.
Nero and Heliogabalus, Maxentius, and Julianus Apostata,
were never so much addicted to magick of old, as some of
our modern princes and popes themselves are now adayes.
Erricus, king of Sweden, had an [1] inchanted cap, by vertue
of which, and some magical murmur or whispering terms, he
could command spirits, trouble the aire, and make the wind
stand which way he would; insomuch that, when there was
any great wind or storm, the common people were wont to
say, the king now had on his conjuring cap.   But such examples are infinite. That which they can do, is as much almost as
the devil himself, who is still ready to satisfie their desires,
to oblige them the more unto him.   They can cause tempests,
storms; which is familiarly practised by witches in Norway,
Island, as I have proved. They can make friends enemies, and
enemies friends, by philters: *[2] turpes amores conciliare,* enforce love, tell any man where his friends are, about what employed, though in the most remote places: and, if they will,
[3] *bring their sweethearts to them by night, upon a goats back
flying in the aire,* (Sigismund Scheretzius, *part* 1. *cap.* 9. *de
spect.* reports confidently, that he conferred with sundry such,
that had been so carried many miles, and that he heard witches
themselves confess as much) hurt, and infect men and beasts,
vines, corn, cattle, plants, make women abortive, not to conceive, [4] *barren,* men and women unapt and *unable,* married
and unmarried, fifty several wayes, (saith Bodine, *l. 2. c. 2)* flye
in the aire, meet when and where they will, as Cicogna proves,
and (Lavat. *de spec. part.* 2. *c.* 17.) *steal young children out of
their cradles,* ministerio dæmonum, *and put deformed in their
rooms, which we call changelings,* (saith [5] Scheretzius, *part.* 1.
c. 6.) make men victorious, fortunate, eloquent: (and therefore, in those ancient monomachies and combats, they were
searched of old, [6] if they had no magical charms) they can
make [7] stick-frees, such as shall endure a rapiers point, musket
shot, and never be wounded; (of which read more in *Boissardus, cap.* 6. *de Magiá,* the manner of the adjuration, and
by whom 'tis made, where and how to be used *in expeditionibus
bellicis, prœliis, duellis, &c.* with many peculiar instances
and examples) they can walk in fiery furnaces, make men feel

---

[1] Rotatum pileum habebat, quo ventos violentos cieret, aërem turbaret, et in
quam partem, &c.   [2] Erastus.   [3] Ministerio hirci nocturni.
[4] Steriles nuptos et inhabiles.   Vide Petrum de Palude, lib. 4. distinct. 34. Pau-
lum Guiclandum.   [5] Infantes matribus suffurantur; aliis suppositivis in
locum verorum conjectis.   [6] Milles.   [7] D. Luther. in primum
præceptum, et Leon. Varius, lib. 1. de fascino.

202 *Causes of Melancholy.* [Part. 1. Sec. 2.

no pain on the rack, *aut alias torturas sentire;* they can stanch blood, [1]represent dead mens shapes, alter and turn themselves and others into several forms at their pleasures.[2] Agaberta, a famous witch in Lapland, would do as much publickly to all spectatours—*modo pusilla, modo anus, modo procera ut quercus, modo vacca, avis, coluber, &c.* now young, now old, high, low, like a cow, like a bird, a snake, and what not? She could represent to others what forms they most desired to see, shew them friends absent, reveal secrets, *maximâ omnium admiratione, &c.* And yet, for all this subtilty of theirs, (as Lipsius well observes, *Physiolog. Stoïcor. lib. 1. cap.* 17.) neither these magicians, nor devils themselves, can take away gold or letters out of mine or Crassus chest, *et clientelis suis largiri;* for they are base, poor, contemptible fellows, most part: as [3]Bodine notes, they can do nothing *in judicum decreta aut pœnas, in regum consilia vel arcana, nihil in rem nummariam aut thesauros;* they cannot give money to their clients, alter judges decrees, or counsels of kings: these *minuti genii* cannot do it: *altiores genii hoc sibi adservârunt;* the higher powers reserve these things to themselves. Now and then, peradventure, there may be some more famous magicians, (like Simon Magus, [4]Apollonius Tyaneus, Pasetes, Jamblicus, [5]Odo de Stellis) that for a time can build castles in the ayre, represent armies, &c. (as they are [6]said to have done) command wealth and treasure, feed thousands with all variety of meats upon a sudden, protect themselves and their followers, from all princes persecutions, by removing from place to place in an instant, reveal secrets, future events, tell what is done in far countries, make them appear that dyed long since, &c. and do many such miracles, to the worlds terrour, admiration, and opinion of deity to themselves [7]: yet the devil forsakes them at last; they come to wicked ends; and *raro aut nunquam* such impostors are to be found[8]. The vulgar sort of them can work no such feats. But to my purpose—they can, last of all, cure and cause most diseases to such as they love or hate, and this of [9]melancholy amongst the rest. Paracelsus *(tom. 4. de morbis amentium, tract. 1.)* in express words affirms *multi fascinantur in melancholiam;* many are bewitched into melancholy, out of his experience. The same, saith Danæus, *lib. 3. de sortiariis. Vidi, inquit, qui melancholicos morbos*

---

[1] Lavat. Cicog.   [2] Boissardus, de Magis.   [3] Dæmon. lib. 3. c. 3. [4] Vide Philostratum, vitâ ejus; Boissardum de Magis.   [5] Nubrigensis. Lege lib. 1. cap. 19.   [6] Vide Suidam de Paset.   [7] De cruent. cadaver.   [8] Erastus, Adolphus, Scribanius.   [9] Virg. Æneid 4. incantatricem describens; Hæc se carminibus promittit solvere mentes, Quas velit, ast aliis duras immittere curas.

Mem. 1. Subs. 4.] *Causes of Melancholy.* 203

gravissimos induxerunt: I have seen those that have caused melancholy in the most grievous manner, [1] *dryed up womens paps, cured gout, palsie; this and apoplexy, falling-sickness, which no physick could help, solo tactu,* by touch alone. Ruland (*in his* 3. *Cent. Cura* 91.) gives an instance of one David Helde, a young man, who, by eating cakes which a witch gave him, *mox delirare cœpit,* began to dote on a sudden, and was instantly mad. *F. H. D.* in [2] Hildesheim, consulted about a melancholy man, thought his disease was partly magical, and partly natural, because he vomited pieces of iron and lead, and spake such languages as he had never been taught; but such examples are common in Scribanius, Hercules de Saxoniâ, and others. The means by which they work, are usually charms, images, (as that, in Hector Boëthius, of king Duffe) characters stamped of sundry metals, and at such and such constellations, knots, amulets, words, philters, &c. which generally make the parties affected melancholy; as [3] Monavius discourseth at large in an epistle of his to Acolsius, giving instance in a Bohemian baron that was so troubled by a philter taken. Not that there is any power at all in those spells, charms, characters, and barbarous words; but that the devil doth use such means to delude them; *ut fideles inde magos* (saith [4] Libanius) *in officio retineat, tum in consortium malefactorum vocet.*

SUBSECT. IV.

Stars a cause. Signs from Physiognomy, Metoposcopy, Chiromancy.

Natural causes are either *primary* and *universal,* or *secundary* and more *particular.* *Primary* causes are the heavens, planets, stars, &c. by their influence (as our astrologers hold) producing this and such like effects. I will not here stand to discuss, *obiter,* whether stars be causes or signs; or to apologize for judicial astrology. If either Sextus Empiricus, Picus Mirandula, Sextus ab Hemingâ, Pererius, Erastus, Chambers, &c. have so far prevailed with any man, that he will attribute no vertue at all to the heavens, or to sun or moon, more than he doth to their signs at an inn-keepers post, or

---

[1] Godelmannus, cap. 7. lib. 1. Nutricum mammas præsiccant; solo tactu podagram, apoplexiam, paralysin, et alios morbos, quos medicina curare non poterat.
[2] Factus inde maniacus. Spic. 2. fol. 147.   [3] Omnia philtra, etsi inter se differant, hoc habent commune, quod hominem efficiant melancholicum. epist. 231. Scholtzii.   [4] De cruent. cadaver.

204   *Causes of Melancholy.*   [Part. 1. Sec. 2.

tradesmans shop, or generally condemn all such astrological
aphorisms approved by experience—I refer him to Bellan-
tius, Pirovanus, Marascallerus, Goclenius, Sir Christopher
Heydon, &c. If thou shalt ask me what I think, I must answer, (*nam et doctis hisce erroribus versatus sum*) they do incline
but not compell, (no necessity at all: [1] *agunt non cogunt*)
and so gently incline, that a wise man may resist them; *sapiens dominabitur astris;* they rule us; but God rules them.
All this (me thinks) [2] Joh. de Indagine hath comprized in
brief: *quæris a me quantum in nobis operantur astra? &c.
Wilt thou know how far the stars work upon us ? I say they do
but incline, and that so gently, that, if we will be ruled by
reason, they have no power over us ; but if we follow our own
nature, and be led by sense, they do as much in us, as in brute
beasts; and we are no better:* so that, I hope, I may justly conclude with [3] Cajetan, *Cœlum vehiculum divinæ virtutis, &c.* that
the heaven is Gods instrument, by mediation of which he go-
verns and disposeth these elementary bodies—or a great book
whose letters are the stars, (as one calls it) wherein are written many strange things for such as can read—[4] *or an excellent harp, made by an eminent workman, on which he that can
but play, will make most admirable musick.* But to the purpose—

[5] Paracelsus is of opinion, *that a physician, without the
knowledge of stars can neither understand the cause or cure
of any disease—either of this, or gout, not so much as tooth-
ache—except he see the peculiar geniture and scheme of the
party affected.* And for this proper malady, he will have the
principal and primary cause of it proceed from the heaven,
ascribing more to stars than humours, [6] *and that the constel-
lation alone, many times, produceth melancholy, all other
causes set apart.* He gives instance in lunatick persons, that are
deprived of their wits by the moons motion; and, in another
place, refers all to the ascendent, and will have the true and
chief cause of it to be sought from the stars. Neither is it his
opinion only, but of many *Galenists* and philosophers, though

---

[1] Astra regunt homines ; et regit astra Deus.   [2] Chorom. lib. Quæris a me
quantum operantur astra ? dico, in nos nihil astra urgere, sed animos proclives
trahere; qui sic tamen liberi sunt, ut, si ducem sequantur rationem, nihil efficiant; sin vero naturam, id agere quod in brutis fere.   [3] Cœlum vehiculum
divinæ virtutis, cujus mediante motu, lumine, et influentiâ, Deus elementaria corpora ordinat, et disponit. Th. de Veio. Cajetanus in Psa. 104.   [4] Mundus
iste quasi lyra ab excellentissimo quodam artifice concinnata, quam qui nôrit,
mirabiles elIciet harmonias. J. Dee. Aphorismo 11.   [5] Medicus sine cœli
peritiâ nihil est, &c. nisi genesim sciverit, ne tantillum poterit. lib. de podag.
[6] Constellatio in caussâ est: et influentia cœli morbum hunc movet, interdum
omnibus aliis amotis. Et alibi. Origo ejus a cœlo petenda est. Tr. de morbis
amentium.

they not so stifly and peremptorily maintain as much. *This variety of melancholy symptomes proceeds from the stars,* saith [1] Melancthon. The most generous melancholy (as that of Au-
gustus) comes from the conjunction of Saturn and Jupiter in Libra: the bad, (as that of Catiline) from the meeting of Saturn and the moon in Scorpio. Jovianus Pontanus, in his tenth book, and thirteenth chapter *de rebus cœlestibus,* discourseth to this purpose at large. *Ex atrâ bile varii generantur morbi, &c.* [2] *Many diseases proceed from black choler, as it shall be hot or cold; and though it be cold in its own nature, yet it is apt to be heated, as water may be made to boyle, and burn as bad as fire; or made cold as ice; and thence proceed such variety of symptomes; some mad, some solitary; some laugh, some rage, &c.*—the cause of all which intemperance he will have chiefly and primarily proceed from the heavens—[3] *from the position of Mars, Saturn, and Mercury.* His aphorisms be these: [4] Mercury, *in any geniture, if he shall be found in* Virgo *or* Pisces *his opposite sign, and that in the horoscope, irradiated by those quartile aspects of* Saturn *or* Mars, *the child shall be mad or melancholy.* Again, [5] *He that shall have* Saturn *or* Mars, *the one culminating, the other in the fourth house, when he shall be born, shall be melancholy; of which he shall be cured in time, if* Mercury *behold them.* [6] *If the moon be in conjunction or opposition, at the birth-time, with the sun,* Saturn *or* Mars, *or in a quartile aspect with them* (e malo cœli loco, Leoviticus adds) *many diseases are signified; especially the head and brain is like to be mis-affected with pernicious humours, to be melancholy, lunatick, or mad.* Cardan adds, *quartâ lunâ natos,* eclipses, earth-quakes. Garcæus and Leoviticus will have the chief judgement to be taken from the lord of the geniture; or when there is no aspect betwixt the *moon* and *Mercury,* and neither behold the *horoscope,* or *Saturn* and *Mars* shall be lord of the present conjunction or opposition in *Sagittary* or *Pisces,* of the *sun* or *moon,* such persons are commonly epileptick, dote, dæmoniacal, melancholy:

[1] Lib. de animâ, cap. de humorib. Ea varietas in melancholiâ habet cœlestes caussas ☌ ♄ et ♃ in □ ☌ ♂ et ☾ in ♏. [2] Ex atrâ bile varii generantur morbi, perinde ut ipse multum calidi aut frigidi in se habuerit, quum utrique suscipiendo quam aptissima sit, tametsi suâpte naturâ frigida sit. Annon aqua sic afficitur a calore ut ardeat; et a frigore ut in glaciem concrescat? et hæc varietas distinctionum, alii flent, rident, &c. [3] Hanc ad intemperantiam gignendam plurimum confert ♂ et ♄ positus, &c. [4] ☿ Quoties alicujus genitura in ♍ et ♓ adverso signo positus, horoscopum partiliter tenuerit, atque etiam a ♂ vel ♄ □ radio percussus fuerit, natus ab insania vexabitur. [5] Qui ♄ et ♂ habet, alterum in culmine, alterum imo cœlo, cum in lucem venerit, melancholicus erit, a quâ sanabitur, si ☿ illos irradiârit. [6] Hac configuratione natus, aut lunaticus, aut mente captus.

but see more of these aphorisms in the above-named Pontanus, Garcæus, *cap.* 23. de *Jud. genitur.* Schoner. *lib.* 1. *cap.*
8. which he hath gathered out of [1] Ptolemy, Albubater, and
some other Arabians, Junctine, Ranzovius, Lindhout, Origan,
&c. But these men you will reject peradventure, as astrologers, and therefore partial judges; then hear the testimony of
physicians, *Galenists* themselves. [2] Crato confesseth the influence of stars to have a great hand to this peculiar disease ;
so doth Jason Pratensis, Lonicerius *(præfat. de Apoplexiâ)*
Ficinus, Fernelius, &c. [3] P. Cnemander acknowledgeth the
stars an universal cause, the particular from parents, and the
use of the six non-natural things. Baptista Port. *mag. l.* 1.
c, 10, 12, 15, will have them causes to every particular *indi-
viduum.* Instances and examples, to evince the truth of those
aphorisms, are common amongst those astrologian treatises.
Cardan, in his thirty-seventh geniture, gives instance in Math.
Bolognius, Camerar. *hor. natalit. centur.* 7. *genit.* 6. *et* 7. of
Daniel Gare, and others, but see Garcæus, *cap.* 33. Luc.
Gauricus, *Tract.* 6. *de Azemenis, &c.* The time of this melancholy is, when the significators of any geniture are directed
according to art, as the hor. moon, hylech, &c. to the hostile
beams or terms of ♄ and ♂ especially or any fixed star of
their nature, or if ♄, by his revolution or *transitus*, shall offend any of those radical promissors in the geniture.

Other signs there are taken from physiognomy, metopo-
scopy, chiromancy, which because Joh. de Indagine, and Rotman (the landgrave of Hassia his mathematician) not long
since in his Chiromancy, Baptista Porta, in his celestial Physiognomy, have proved to hold great affinity with astrology, to
satisfie the curious, I am the more willing to insert.

The general notions [4] physiognomers give, be these: *black
colour argues natural melancholy; so doth leanness, hirsuteness, broad veins, much hair on the brows,* saith [5] Gratana-
rolus, *cap.* 7. and a little head, out of Aristole; high sanguine
red colour shews head melancholy; they that stutter and are
bald, will be soonest melancholy, as (Avicenna supposeth)
by reason of the driness of their brains. But he that will
know more of the several signs of humours and wits out of
physiognomy, let him consult with old Adamantus and Pole-

---

[1] Ptolemæus, Centiloquio, et quadripartito tribuit omnium melancholicorum
symptomata siderum influentiis.   [2] Arte Medicâ. Accedunt ad has caussas affectiones siderum. Plurimum incitant et provocant influentiæ cœlestes. Velcurio,
lib. 4. cap. 15.   [3] Hildesheim, spicil. 2. de mel.   [4] Joh. de Indag. c. 9.
Montaltus, cap. 22.   [5] Caput parvum qui habent, cerebrum habent et spiritus plerumque angustos.—Facile incidunt in melancholiam rubicundi. Aëtius.
Idem Montaltus, c. 21. e Galeno.

mus, that comment, or rather paraphrase, upon Aristotles Physiognomy, Baptista Portas four pleasant books, Michael Scot *de secretis naturæ,* John de Indagine, Montaltus, Antony Zara, *anat. ingeniorum, sect.* 1. *memb.* 13. *et lib.* 4.

Chiromancy hath these aphorisms to fortell melancholy. Tasnier, *lib.* 5. *cap.* 2. (who hath comprehended the summ of John de Indagine, Tricassus, Corvinus, and others, in his book) thus hath it : [1] *The Saturnine line going from the rascetta through the hand, to Saturns mount, and there intersected by certain little lines, argues melancholy ; so if the vital and natural make an acute angle.* *Aphorism* 100: *The Saturnine, epatick, and natural lines, making a gross triangle in the hand, argue as much ;* which *Goclenius (cap.* 5. *Chiros.)* repeats *verbatim* out of him. In general, they conclude all, that, if *Saturns* mount be full of many small lines and intersections, [2] *such men are most part melancholy, miserable, and full of disquietness, care and trouble, continually vexed with anxious and bitter thoughts, alway sorrowful, fearful, suspicious : they delight in husbandry, buildings, pools, marshes, springs, woods, walks, &c.* Thaddæus Haggesius, in his *Metoposcopia,* hath certain aphorisms derived from *Saturns* lines in the forehead, by which he collects a melancholy disposition ; and [3] Baptista Porta makes observations from those other parts of the body, as, if a spot be over the spleen ; [4] *or in the nails, if it appear black, it signifieth much care, grief, contention, and melancholy.* The reason he refers to the humours, and gives instance in himself, that, for seven years space, he had such black spots in his nails, and all that while was in perpetual law-suites, controversies for his inheritance, fear, loss of honour, banishment, grief, care, &c. and when his miseries ended, the black spots vanished. Cardan, in his book *de libris propriis,* tells such a story of his own person, that, a little before his sons death, he had a black spot, which appeared in one of his nails, and dilated it self as he came nearer to his end. But I am over-tedious in these toyes, which (howsoever, in some mens too severe censures, they may be held absurd and ridiculous) I am the bolder to insert, as not borrowed from circumforanean rogues and Gipsies, but out of the writings of worthy philosophers, and physicians, yet living, some of them,

---

[1] Saturnına, a rascettâ per mediam manum decurrens, usque ad radicem montis Saturni, a parvis lineis intersecta, arguit melancholicos. Aphoris. 78.   [2] Agitantur miseriis, continuis inquietudinibus, neque unquam a solicitudine liberi sunt: anxie affliguntur amarissimis intra cogitationibus, semper tristes, suspiciosi, meticulosi: cogitationes sunt, velle agrum colere, stagna amant et paludes, &c. Jo. de Indagine, lib. 1.   [3] Cœlestis Physiogn. lib. 10.   [4] Cap. 14. lib. 5. Idem. Maculæ in ungulis nigræ, lites, rixas, melancholiam significant, ab humore in corde tali.

208　　　　　*Causes of Melancholy.*　　　[Part. 1. Sec. 2.

and religious professors in famous universities, who are able to patronize that which they have said, and vindicate themselves from all cavillers and ignorant persons.

SUBSECT. V.

Old age a cause.

SECUNDARY peculiar causes efficient (so called in respect of the other precedent (are either *congenitæ, internæ, innatæ,* as they term them, inward, innate, inbred ; or else outward and adventitious, which happen to us after we are born ; congenite or born with us, are either natural, as old age, or *præter naturam* (as [1] Fernelius calls it), that distemperature, which we have from our parents seed, it being an hereditary disease. The first of these, which is natural to all, and which no man living can avoid, is [2] old age, which being cold and dry, and of the same quality as melancholy is, must needs cause it, by diminution of spirits and substance, and increasing of adust humours. Therefore [3] Melancthon avers out of Aristotle, as an undoubted truth *senes plerumque delirásse in senectâ,* that old men familiarly dote, *ob atram bilem,* for black choler, which is then superabundant in them : and Rhasis, that Arabian physician, (in his *Cont. lib.* 1. *cap.* 9.) calls it [4] *a necessary and inseparable accident* to all old and decrepit persons. *After seventy years,* (as the [5] Psalmist saith) *all is trouble and sorrow;* and common experience confirms the truth of it in weak and old persons, especially in such as have lived in action all their lives, had great employments, much business, much command, and many servants to oversee, and leave off *ex abrupto;* as [6] Charles the Fifth did to King Philip, resign up all on a sudden. They are overcome with melancholy in an instant; or, if they do continue in such courses, they dote at last, *(senex bis puer)* and are not able to manage their estates, through common infirmities incident to their age ; full of ache, sorrow, and grief, children again, dizards; they carle many times as they sit, and talk to themselves; they are angry, waspish, displeased with every thing, *suspicious of all, wayward, covetous, hard,* (saith Tully) *self-willed, superstitious, self-conceited, braggers and admirers of themselves,* as [7] Balthasar

---

[1] Lib. 1. Path. c. 11.　　[2] Venit enim, properata malis, inopina senectus : Et dolor ætatem jussit inesse meam. Boëthius, met. 1. de consol. philos.　　[3] Cap. de humoribus, lib. de animâ.　　[4] Necessarium accidens decrepitis, et inseparabile.　　[5] Psal. 90. 10.　　[6] Meteran. Belg. hist. lib. 1.　　[7] Sunt morosi, anxii, et iracundi, et difficiles, senes ; si quærimus, etiam avari. Tull. de senectute.

Mem. 1. Subs. 6.]   *Causes of Melancholy.*   209

Castalio hath truly noted of them.   This natural infirmity is
most eminent in old women, and such as are poor, solitary, live
in most base esteem and beggery, or such as are witches; insomuch that [1] Wierus, Baptista Porta, Ulricus Molitor, Edwicus,
do refer all that witches are said to do, to imagination alone,
and this humour of melancholy.   And, whereas it is controverted,
whether they can bewitch cattle to death, ride in the air upon a
coulstaff out of a chimney-top, transform themselves into cats,
dogs, &c. translate bodies from place to place, meet in companies, and dance, as they do, or have carnal copulation with the
devil, they ascribe all to this redundant melancholy, which domineers in them, to [2] somniferous potions, and natural causes, the
devils policy.   *Non lædunt omnino,* (saith Wierus) *aut quid
mirum faciunt, (de Lamiis, lib. 3. cap. 36.) ut putatur : solam
vitiatam habent phantasiam;* they do no such wonders at all,
only their [3] brains are crazed.   [4] *They think they are witches and
can do hurt, but do not.*   But this opinion Bodine, Erastus,
Danæus, Scribanius, Sebastian Michaelis, Campanella, *(de Sensu
rerum, lib. 4. cap. 9.)* [5] Dandinus the Jesuit, *(lib. 2. de Animâ)*
explode; [6] Cicogna confutes at large.   That witches are melancholy, they deny not, but not out of corrupt phantasie alone, so
to delude themselves and others, or to produce such effects.

SUBSECT. VI.

Parents a cause by propagation.

THAT other inward inbred cause of melancholy is our temperature, in whole or part, which we receive from our parents,
which [7] Fernelius calls *præter naturam,* or unnatural, it being an
hereditary disease; for as he [8] justifies, *quale parentum, maxime
patris, semen obtigerit, tales evadunt similares spermaticæque
partes : quocumque etiam morbo pater, quum generat, tenetur,
cum semine transfert in prolem:* such as the temperature of the
father is, such is the sons; and, look, what disease the father had

[1] Lib. 2. de Aulico. Senes avari, morosi, jactabundi, philauti, deliri, superstitiosi, suspiciosi, &c. Lib. 3. de lamiis, c. 17, et 18.   [2] Solanum, opium, lupi
adeps, lac asini, &c. sanguis infantum, &c.   [3] Corrupta est iis ab humore
melancholico phantasia.   Nymannus.   [4] Putant se lædere, quando non lædunt.   [5] Qui hæc in imaginationis vim referre conati sunt, aut atræ bilis,
inanem prorsus laborem susceperunt.   [6] Lib. 3. cap. 4. omnif. mag.
[7] Lib. 1. c. 11. path.   [8] Ut arthritici, epilep. &c.

VOL. I.   P

210   *Causes of Melancholy.*   [Part. 1. Sec. 2.

when he begot him, his son will have after him, [1] *and is as well
inheritor of his infirmities, as of his lands. And where the complexion and constitution of the father is corrupt, there,* ([2] saith
Roger Bacon) *the complexion and constitution of the son must
needs be corrupt; and so the corruption is derived from the
father to the son.* Now this doth not so much appear in the
composition of the body, according to that of Hippocrates, [3] *in
habit, proportion, scarrs, and other lineaments; but in manners
and conditions of the mind;*

Et patrum in natos abeunt, cum semine, mores.

Seleucus had an anchor on his thigh; so had his posterity, as
Trogus records, *l.* 15. Lepidus (in Pliny, *l.* 7. *c.* 17.) was purblind; so was his son. That famous family of Ænobarbi
were known of old, and so surnamed, from their red beards.
The Austrian lip, and those Indian flat noses, are propagated:
the Bavarian chin, and goggle eyes amongst the Jews, as [4] Bux-
torfius observes. Their voice, pace, gesture, looks are likewise
derived, with all the rest of their conditions and infirmities;
such a mother, such a daughter; their very [5] affections Lemnius contends *to follow their seed, and the malice and bad
conditions of children are many times wholly to be imputed
to their parents.* I need not therefore make any doubt of melancholy, but that it is an hereditary disease. [6] Paracelsus in
express words affirms it, *lib. de morb. amentium, To.* 4.
Tr. 1; so doth [7] Crato in an epistle of his to Monavius: so
doth Bruno Seidelius, in his book *de morbo incurab.* Montaltus
proves *(cap.* 11.) out of Hippocrates and Plutarch, that such
hereditary dispositions are frequent; *et hanc* (inquit) *fieri reor
ob participatam melancholicam intemperantiam* (speaking of
a patient): I think he became so by participation of melancholy. Daniel Sennertus *(lib.* 1. *part.* 2. *cap.* 9.) will have this
melancholy constitution derived not only from the father to the
son, but to the whole family sometimes; *quandoque totis fa-
miliis hæreditativam.* [8] Forestus, in his Medicinal Observations,
illustrates this point with an example of a merchant his pa-

---

[1] Ut filii, non tam possessionum, quam morborum hæredes sint.   [2] Epist.
de secretis artis et naturæ, c. 7.   Nam in hoc quod patres corrupti sunt, generant
filios corruptæ complexionis, et compositionis; et filii eorum, eâdem de caussâ,
se corrumpunt; et sic derivata corruptio a patribus ad filios.   [3] Non tam (inquit Hippocrates) gibbos et cicatrices oris et corporis habitum agnoscis ex iis, sed
verum incessum, gestus, mores, morbos, &c.   [4] Synagog. Jud.   [5] Affectus parentum in fœtus transeunt, et puerorum malitia parentibus imputanda, l. 4.
cap. 3. de occult. nat. mirac.   [6] Ex pituitosis pituitosi, ex biliosis biliosi, ex
lienosis et melancholicis melancholici.   [7] Ep. 174. in Scoltz. Nascitur nobiscum illa, aliturque, et una cum parentibus habemus malum hunc. Jo. Pelesius,
lib. 2. de curâ humanorum affectuum.   [8] Lib. 10. observ. 15.

tient, that had this infirmity by inheritance; so doth Rodericus a Fonseca, (*Tom.* 1. *consul.* 69.) by an instance of a young man that was so affected *ex matre melancholicâ*, had a melancholy mother, *et victu melancholico*, and bad diet together. Ludovicus Mercatus, a Spanish physician, (in that excellent tract, which he hath lately written of hereditary diseases, *Tom.2. oper. lib.* 5.) reckons up leprosie, as those [1] Galbots in Gascony, hereditary lepers, pox, stone, gout, epilepsie, &c. Amongst the rest, this and madness after a set time comes to many, which he calls a miraculous thing in nature, and sticks for ever to them as an incurable habit. And, that which is more to be wondered at, it skips in some families the father, and goes to the son, [2] *or takes every other, and sometimes every third, in a lineal descent, and doth not alwayes produce the same, but some like, and a symbolizing disease.* These secundary causes hence derived, are commonly so powerful, that (as [3] Wolphius holds) *sæpe mutant decreta siderum;* they do often alter the primary causes, and decrees of the heavens. For these reasons, belike, the church and common-wealth, humane and divine laws, have conspired to avoid hereditary diseases, forbidding such marriages as are any whit allyed ; and, as Mercatus adviseth all families, to take such, *si fieri possit, quæ maxime distant naturâ,* and to make choice of those who are most differing in complexion from them; if they love their own, and respect the common good. And sure, I think, it hath been ordered by Gods especial providence, that in all ages, there should be, (as usually there is) once in [4] six hundred years, a transmigration of nations to amend and purify their blood, as we alter seed upon our land, and that there should be as it were an inundation of those northern Goths and Vandales, and many such like people which came out of that continent of Scandia, and Sarmatia (as some suppose), and over-ran, as a deluge, most part of Europe and Africk, to alter (for our good) our complexions, which were much defaced with hereditary infirmities, which by our lust and intemperance we had contracted. A sound generation of strong and able men were sent amongst us, as those northern men usually are, innocuous, free from riot, and free from diseases: to qualifie and make us as those poor naked Indians are generally at this day, and those about Brasile, (as a late [5] writer observes) in the isle of Maragnan, free from

---

[1] Maginus, Geog. [2] Sæpe non eundem, sed similem producit effectum, et illæso parente transit in nepotem. [3] Dial. præfix. genituris Leovitici. [4] Bodin. de rep. cap. de periodis reip. [5] Claudius Abaville, Capuchion, in his voyage to Maragnan. 1614. c. 45. Nemo fere ægrotus, sano omnes et robusto corpore, vivunt annos 120, 140, sine medicinâ. Idem. Hector Boëthius de insulis Orchad. et Damianus a Goes de Scandiâ.

212   *Causes of Melancholy.*   [Part. 1. Sec. 2.

all hereditary diseases, or other contagion, whereas, without
help of physick, they live commonly an hundred and twenty
years or more; as in the Orchades and many other places. Such
are the common effects of temperance, and intemperance: but
I will descend to particulars, and shew by what means, and by
whom especially, this infirmity is derived unto us.

Filii ex senibus nati raro sunt firmi temperamenti : old
mens children are seldom of a good temperament, (as Scoltzius
supposeth, *consult.* 177) and therefore most apt to this disease :
and, as [1] Levinus Lemnius farther adds, old men beget, most
part, wayward, peevish, sad, melancholy sons, and seldom
merry. He that begets a child on a full stomach, will either
have a sick child, or a crazed son (as [2] Cardan thinks, *contradict. med. lib.* 1. *contradict.* 18); or, if the parents be sick
or have any great pain of the head, or megrim, head-ache
([3] Hieronymus Wolfius doth instance in a child of Sebastian
Castalio's), or if a drunken man get a child, it will never likely
have a good brain, as Gellius argues, *lib.* 12. *cap.* 1. *Ebrii
gignunt ebrios ;* one drunkard begets another, saith [4] Plutarch,
(sym. lib. 1. *quæst.* 5.) whose sentence [5] Lemnius approves,
l. 1. *c.* 4. Alsarius Crutius *Gen. de qui sit med. cent.* 3.
fol. 182. Macrobius *lib.* 1. Avicenna *lib.* 3. *Fen.* 21.
Tract. 1. *cap.* 8. and Aristotle himself *sect.* 2. *prob.* 4.
Foolish, drunken, or hair-brain women, most part bring forth
children like unto themselves *morosos et languidos ;* and so
likewise he that lyes with a menstruous woman. *Intemperantia
Veneris, quam in nautis præsertim insectatur* [6] *Lemnius, qui
uxores ineunt, nullâ menstrui decursus ratione habitâ, nec ob-
servato interlunio, præcipua caussa est, noxia, perniciosa ;
(concubitum hunc exitialem ideo, et pestiferum, vocat Rodericus a Castro, Lusitanus ; detestantur ad unum omnes medici)
tum et quartâ lunâ concepti, infelices plerumque et amentes,
delirit, stolidi, morbosi, impuri, invalidi, tetrâ lue sordidi,
minime vitales, omnibus bonis corporis atque animi destituti ;
ad laborem nati, si seniores (inquit* [7] *Eustathius) ut Hercules,
et alii.* [8] *Judæi maxime insectantur fœdum hunc et immundum apud Christianos concubitum, ut illicitum abhorrent, et
apud suos prohibent ; et quod Christiani toties leprosi,
amentes, tot morbilli, impetigines, alphi, psoræ, cutis et*

---

[1] Lib. 4. c. 3. de occult. nat. mir. Tetricos plerumque filios senes progenerant
et tristes, rarius exhilaratos.   [2] Coitus super repletionem pessimus, et filii
qui tum gignuntur, aut morbosi sunt, aut stolidi.   [3] Dial. præfix. Leovitico.
[4] L. de ed. liberis.   [5] De occul. nat. mor. Temulentæ et stolidæ mulieres
liberos plerunque producunt sibi similes.   [6] Lib. 2. c. 8. de occult. nat. mir.
Good master schoolmaster, do not English this.   [7] De nat. mul. lib. 3. cap. 4.
[8] Buxdorphius, c. 13. Synag. Jud. Ezek. 18.

*faciei decolorationes, tam multi morbi epidemici, acerbi, et
venenosi sint, in hunc immundum concubitum rejiciunt ; et cru-
deles in pignora vocant, qui, quartâ lunâ profluente hac mensium illuvie, concubitum hunc non perhorrescunt.* Damnavit
olim divina lex, et morte mulctavit hujusmodi homines (Lev. 18.
20) ; *et inde nati si qui deformes aut mutili, pater dilapidatus,
quod non contineret ab* [1]*immundâ muliere. Gregorius Magnus,
petenti Augustino numquid apud* [2] *Britannos hujusmodi concubitum toleraret, severe prohibuit viris suis tum misceri fœminas
in consuetis suis menstruis, &c.* I spare to English this which
I have said. Another cause some give—inordinate diet, as if a
man eat garlick, onions, fast over-much, study too hard, be
over-sorrowful, dull, heavy, dejected in mind, perplexed in his
thoughts, fearful, &c. *their children* (saith [3] Cardan *subtil.
lib.* 18) *will be much subject to madness and melancholy ; for,
if the spirits of the brain be fusled or mis-affected by such
means at such a time, their children will be fusled in the brain ;
they will be dull, heavy, timorous, discontented all their lives.*
Some are of opinion, and maintain that paradox or problem,
that wise men beget commonly fools. Suidas gives instance in
Aristarchus the grammarian ; *duos reliquit filios, Aristarchum
et Aristachorum, ambos stultos ;* and (which [4] Erasmus urgeth
in his Moria) fools beget wise men. *Card. subtil. l.* 12. gives
this cause: *quoniam spiritus sapientium ob studium resolvuntur,
et in cerebrum feruntur a corde :* because their natural spirits
are resolved by study, and turned into animal; drawn from the
heart, and those other parts, to the brain. Lemnius subscribes
to that of Cardan, and assigns this reason, *quod persolvant debitum languide, et oscitanter ; unde fœtus a parentum generositate
desciscit :* they pay their debt (as Paul calls it) to their wives
remisly; by which means their children are weaklings, and
many times idiots and fools.

Some other causes are given, which properly pertain to, and
proceed from, the mother. If she be over-dull, heavy, angry,
peevish, discontented, and melancholy not only at the time of
conception, but even all the while she carries the child in her
womb, (saith Fernelius, *path. l.* 1. 11) her son will be so likewise affected ; and worse, (as [5] Lemnius adds, *l.* 4. *c.* 7) if she
grieve over-much, be disquieted, or by any casualty be affrighted
and terrified by some fearful object, heard or seen, she endan-

---

[1] Drusius, obs. lib. 3. cap. 20.   [2] Bed. Eccl. hist. lib. 1. c. 27. respon. 10.
[3] Nam spiritus cerebri si tum male afficiantur, tales procreant ; et quales fuerint
affectus, tales filiorum : ex tristibus tristes, ex jucundis jucundi nascuntur, &c.
[4] Fol. 229. mer. Socrates children were fools. Sab.   [5] De occult. nat. mer.
Pica, morbus mulierum.

214   *Causes of Melancholy.*   [Part. 1. Sec. 2.

gers her child, and spoils the temperature of it; for the strange
imagination of a woman works effectually upon her infant,
that (as Baptista Porta proves, *Physiog. cœlestis, l. 5. c. 2*) she
leaves a mark upon it; which is most especially seen in such as
prodigiously long for such and such meats: the child will love
those meats, saith Fernelius, and be addicted to like humours.
[1] *If a great-bellied woman see a hare, her child will often have
an hare-lip*, as we call it. Garcœus, *de Judiciis geniturarum,
c. 33.* hath a memorable example of one Thomas Nickell, born
in the city of Brandeburge, 1551, [2] *that went reeling and stag-
gering all the dayes of his life, as if he would fall to the
ground, because his mother, being great with child, saw a
drunken man reel in the street.* Such an other I find in Martin
Wenrichius, *com. de ortu monstrorum, c.* 17. [3] I saw, (saith he)
at Wittenberge in Germany, a citizen that looked like a carkass.
*I asked him the cause; he replied, his mother when she bore
him in her womb, saw a carkass by chance, and was so sore
affrighted with it, that* ex eo fœtus ei assimilatus; *from a
ghastly impression, the child was like it.*

So many several wayes are we plagued and punished for our
fathers defaults; in so much that (as Fernelius truly saith)
[4] *it is the greatest part of our felicity to be well-born; and it
were happy for humane kind, if only such parents, as are sound
of body and mind, should be suffered to marry.* An husbandman will sow none but the best and choicest seed upon his
land; he will not rear a bull or an horse, except he be right
shapen in all parts, or permit him to cover a mare, except he
be well assured of his breed; we make choice of the best rams
for our sheep, rear the neatest kine, and keep the best dogs;
quanto id diligentius in procreandis liberis observandum! and
how careful then should we be in begetting of our children! In
former time, some [5] countreys have been so chary in this behalf,
so stern, that, if a child were crooked or deformed in body or
mind, they made him away; so did the Indians of old (by the
relation of Curtius), and many other well-governed common-
wealths, according to the discipline of those times. Here-

---

[1] Baptista Porta, loco præd. Ex leporum intuitu pleræque infantes edunt bifido superiore labello.   [2] Quasi mox in terram collapsurus, per omnem vitam
incedebat, cum mater gravida ebrium hominem sic incedentem viderat.   [3] Ci-
vem facie cadaverosâ, qui dixit, &c.   [4] Optimum bene nasci; maxima pars
felicitatis nostræ bene nasci; quamobrem præclare humano generi consultum videretur, si soli parentes bene habiti et sani liberis operam darent.   [5] Infantes infirmi præcipitio necati. Bohemus, lib. 3. c. 3. Apud Lacones olim.
Lipsius, epist. 85. cent. ad Belgas, Dionysio Villerio, Siquos aliquâ membrorum
parte inutiles notaverint, necari jubent.

Mem. 2. Subs. 1.]　　*Causes of Melancholy.*　　215

tofore, in Scotland, (saith [1] Hect. Boëthius) *if any were visited with the falling sickness, madness, gout, leprosie, or any such dangerous disease, which was likely to be propagated from the father to the son, he was instantly gelded; a woman kept from all company of men: and if by chance, having some such disease, she were found to be with child, she with her brood were buried alive:* and this was done for the common good, lest the whole nation should be injured or corrupted. A severe doom, you will say, and not to be used amongst Christians, yet more to be looked into than it is. For now, by our too much facility in this kind, in giving way for all to marry that will, too much liberty and indulgence in tolerating all sorts, there is a vast confusion of hereditary diseases, no family secure, no man almost free from some grievous infirmity or other. When no choice is had, but still the eldest must marry, as so many stallions of the race; or, if rich, be they fools or dizzards, lame or maimed, unable, intemperate, dissolute, exhaust through riot, (as he said) [2]*jure hæreditario sapere jubentur;* they must be wise and able by inheritance; it comes to pass that our generation is corrupt; we have many weak persons, both in body and mind, many feral diseases raging amongst us, crazed families, *parentes peremptores;* our fathers bad; and we are like to be worse.

MEMB. II.

SUBSECT. I.

Bad diet a cause. Substance. Quality of meats.

ACCORDING to my proposed method, having opened hitherto these secundary causes, which are inbred with us, I must now proceed to the outward and adventitious, which happen unto us after we are born. And those are either evident, remote; or inward, antecedent, and the nearest: continent causes some call them. These outward, remote, precedent causes are subdivided again into *necessary* and *not necessary*. *Necessary* (because we cannot avoid them, but they will alter us, as they are used, or abused) are those six non-natural things, so much spoken of amongst physicians, which are principal causes of this disease: for, almost in every consultation, whereas they

---

[1] Lib. 1. de veterum Scotorum moribus. Morbo comitiali, dementiâ, maniâ, leprâ, &c. aut simili labe, quæ facile in prolem transmittitur, laborantes inter eos, ingenti factâ indagine, inventos, ne gens fœdâ contagione læderetur, ex iis natâ, castraverunt; mulieres hujusmodi procul a virorum consortio ablegârunt; quod si harum aliqua concepisse inveniebatur, simul cum fetu nondum edito, defodiebatur viva.　　[2] Euphormio Satyr.

216   *Causes of Melancholy.*   [Part. 1. Sec. 2.

shall come to speak of the causes, the fault is found, and this
most part objected to the patient ; *peccavit circa res sex non
naturales :* he hath still offended in one of those six.   Montanus, (*consil. 22.*) consulted about a melancholy Jew, gives that
sentence ; so did Frisemelica in the same place ; and, in his two
hundred forty fourth counsel, censuring a melancholy souldier,
assigns that reason of his malady : [1]*He offended in all those six
non-natural things, which were the outward causes, from which
came those inward obstructions ;* and so in the rest.

These six non-natural things are diet, retention and evacuation, which are more material than the other, because they
make new matter, or else are conversant in keeping or expelling it.   The other four are, air, exercise, sleeping, waking,
and perturbations of the mind, which only alter the matter.
The first of these is diet, which consists in meat and drink,
and causeth melancholy, as it offends in substance or accidents,
that is, quantity, quality, or the like.   And well it may be
called a material cause, since that, as [2] Fernelius holds, *it hath
such a power in begetting of diseases, and yields the matter
and sustenance of them ; for neither air, nor perturbations,
nor any of those other evident causes, take place or work this
effect, except the constitution of body and preparation of
humours do concur ; that a man may say, this diet is the
mother of diseases, let the father be what he will ; and from
this alone, melancholy and frequent other maladies arise.*
Many physicians, I confess, have written copious volumes of
this one subject, of the nature and qualities of all manner of
meats ; as, namely, Galen, Isaac the Jew ; Halyabbas, Avicenna, Mesue, also four Arabians ; Gordonius, Villanovanus,
Wecker, Johannes Bruerinus, *sitologia de Esculentis et Poculen-
tis*, Michael Savanarola, *Tract. 2. cap.* 8.   Anthony Fumanellus,
lib. de regimine senum, Curio in his comment on *Schola
Salerna,* Godefridus Stekius *arte med.* Marsilius Cognatus, Ficinus, Ranzovius, Fonseca, Lessius, Magninus, *regim. sanitatis,*
Frietagius, Hugo Fridevallius, &c. besides many other in
[3] English ; and almost every peculiar physician discourseth at
large of all peculiar meats in his chapter of Melancholy.   Yet,
because these books are not at hand to every man, I will briefly
touch what kind of meats ingender this humour, through their
several species, and which are to be avoided.   How they alter

---

[1] Fecit omnia delicta, quæ fieri possunt, circa res sex non naturales ; et eæ
fuerunt caussæ extrinsecæ, ex quibus postea ortæ sunt obstructiones.   [2] Path.
l. 1. c. 2.   Maximam in gignendis morbis vim obtinet, pabulum, materiamque
morbi suggerens : nam nec ab aëre, nec a perturbationibus, vel aliis evidentibus
caussis morbi sunt, nisi consentiat corporis præparatio, et humorum constitutio.
Ut semel dicam, una gula est omnium morborum mater, etiamsi alius est genitor.
Ab hâc morbi sponte sæpe emanant, nullâ aliâ cogente caussâ.   [3] Cogan,
Eliot, Vauhan, Vener.

2

[Mem. 2. Subs. 1.] *Causes of Melancholy.* 217

and change the matter, spirits first, and after humours, by
which we are preserved, and the constitution of our body,
Fernelius and others will shew you. I hasten to the thing
it self: and, first, of such diet as offends in substance.

Beef.] Beef, a strong and hearty meat (cold in the first
degree, dry in the second, saith Gal. *l. 3. c. 1. de alim. fac.*) is
condemned by him, and all succeeding authors, to breed gross
melancholy blood ; good for such as are sound, and of a strong
constitution, for labouring men, if ordered aright, corned,
young, of an ox, for all gelded meats in every species are held
best ; or, if old, [1]such as have been tired out with labour, are
preferred. Aubanus and Sabellicus commend Portugal beef
to be the most savoury, best, and easiest of digestion ; we
commend ours : but all is rejected and unfit for such as lead a
resty life, any ways inclined to melancholy, or dry of complexion. *Tales* (Galen thinks) *de facili melancholicis ægritu-
dinibus capiuntur.*

Pork.] Pork, of all meats, is most nutritive in his own nature, but altogether unfit for such as live at ease, or are any
ways unsound of body or mind; too moist, full of humours,
and therefore *noxia delicatis,* saith Savanarola, *ex earum usu
ut dubitetur, an febris quartana generetur :* naught for queasie
stomachs, in so much, that frequent use of it may breed a
quartan ague.

Goat.] Savanarola discommends goats flesh, and so doth
[2]Bruerinus, *l. 13. c.* 19, calling it a filthy beast, and rammish ;
and therefore supposeth it will breed rank and filthy substance :
yet kid, such as are young and tender, Isaac excepts, Bruerinus, and Galen, *l. 1. c. 1. de alimentorum facultatibus.*

Hart.] *Hart, and red deer,* [3] *hath an evil name; it yields
gross nutriment ;* a strong and great grained meat, next unto
a horse, which although some countries eat, as Tartars and
they of China, yet [4]Galen condemns. Young foals are as
commonly eaten in Spain, as red deer, and, to furnish their
navies, about Malaga especially, often used. But such meats
ask long baking or seething, to qualifie them ; and yet all will
not serve.

Venison, Fallow Deer.] All venison is melancholy, and
begets bad blood : a pleasant meat in great esteem with us
(for we have more parks in England than there are in all
Europe besides) in our solemn feasts. 'Tis somewhat better,

---

[1] Frietagius.   [2] Non laudatur, quia melancholicum præbet alimentum.
[3] Male alit cervina (inquit Frietagius) : crassissimum et atribilarium suppeditat
alimentum.   [4] Lib. de subtiliss. diætâ. Equina caro et asinina equinis
danda est hominibus et asininis.

218   *Causes of Melancholy.*   [Part. 1. Sec. 2.

hunted, than otherwise, and well prepared by cookery; but
generally bad, and seldom to be used.

Hare.] Hare, a black meat, melancholy, and hard of digestion: it breeds *incubus*, often eaten, and causeth fearful dreams;
so doth all venison, and is condemned by a jury of physicians.
Mizaldus and some others say that hare is a merry meat, and
that it will make one fair, as Martials epigram testifies to
Gellia; but this is *per accidens*, because of the good sport it
makes, merry company, and good discourse that is commonly
at the eating of it, and not otherwise to be understood.

Conies.] [1] Conies are of the nature of hares. Magninus
compares them to beef, pig, and goat, *Reg. sanit. part. 3. c.* 17:
yet young rabbets, by all men, are approved to be good.

Generally, all such meats as are hard of digestion, breed melancholy. Aretæus, *lib.* 7. *cap.* 5, reckons up heads and feet,
[2] bowels, brains, entrals, marrow, fat, blood, skins, and those
inward parts, as heart, lungs, liver, spleen, &c. They are rejected by Isaac, *lib.* 2. *part.* 3. Magninus, *part.* 3. *cap.* 17.
Bruerinus, *lib.* 12. Savanarola, *Rub.* 32. *Tract.* 2.

Milk.] Milk, and all that comes of milk, as butter and
cheese, curds, &c. increase melancholy (whey only excepted,
which is most wholesome). [3] Some except asses milk. The
rest, to such as are sound, is nutritive and good, especially for
young children; but, because soon turned to corruption, [4]not
good for those that have unclean stomacks, are subject to head-
ach, or have green wounds, stone, &c. Of all cheeses, I take
that kind which we call Banbury cheese to be the best. *Ex
vetustis pessimus*, the older, stronger, and harder, the worst, as
Langius discourseth in his Epistle to Melancthon, cited by Mizaldus, Isaac, *p.* 5. *Gal.* 3. *de cibis boni succi, &c.*

Fowl.] Amongst fowl, [5]peacocks and pigeons, all fenny fowl,
are forbidden, as ducks, geese, swans, herns, cranes, coots,
didappers, waterherns, with all those teals, curs, sheldrakes,
and peckled fowls, that come hither in winter out of Scandia,
Muscovy, Greenland, Friezland, which half the year are covered all over with snow, and frozen up. Though these be fair
in feathers, pleasant in taste, and have a good outside (like hypocrites), white in plumes, and soft, their flesh is hard, black, unwholesome, dangerous, melancholy meat. *Gravant et putre-
faciunt stomachum*, saith Isaac, *part.* 5. *de vol.* their young ones
are more tolerable; but young pigeons he quite disproves.

---

[1] Parum absunt a naturâ leporum. Bruerinus, l. 13. cap. 25. pullorum tenera
et optima.   [2] Illaudabilis succi nauseam provocant.   [3] Piso. Altomar.
[4] Curio. Frietagius, Magninus. part. 3. cap. 17.—Mercurialis, de affect. lib. 1.
c. 10, excepts all milk meats in hypochondriacal melancholy.   [5] Wecker,
Syntax. theor. p. 2. Isaac, Bruer. lib. 15. cap. 30, et 31.

Mem. 2. Subs. 1.]   *Causes of Melancholy.*   219

Fishes.] Rhasis and [1] Magninus discommend all fish, and say, they breed *viscosities*, slimy nutriment, little and humorous nourishment; Savanarola adds cold, moist; and phlegmatick, Isaac; and therefore unwholesome for all cold and melancholy complexions. Others make a difference, rejecting only, among fresh-water fish, eel, tench, lamprey, craw-fish (which Bright approves, *cap.* 6), and such as are bred in muddy and standing waters, and have a taste of mud, as Franciscus Bonsuetus poetically defines. (*Lib. de aquatilibus*)

> Nam pisces omnes, qui stagna lacusque frequentant,
>   Semper plus succi deterioris habent.

> All fish, that standing pools and lakes frequent,
> Do ever yield bad juyce and nourishment.

Lampreys, Paulus Jovius (*c.* 34. *de piscibus fluvial.*) highly magnifies, and saith, none speak against them, but *inepti* and *scrupulosi;* some scrupulous persons; but [2] eels (*c.* 33.) he ab-horreth: *in all places, at all times, all physicians detest them, especially about the solstice.* Gomesius (*lib.* 1. *c.* 22. de sale) doth immoderately extol sea-fish, which others as much vilifie, and, above the rest, dryed, sowced, indurate fish, as ling, fumados, red-herrings, sprats, stock-fish, haberdine, poor-john, all shell-fish. [3] Tim. Bright excepts lobster and crab. Mes-sarius commends salmon, which Bruerinus contradicts, *lib.* 22. *c.* 17. Magninus rejects congre, sturgeon, turbot, mackerel, skate.

Carp is a fish, of which I know not what to determine. Fran-ciscus Bonsuetus accounts it a muddy fish. Hippolytus Sal-vianus, in his book *de Piscium naturâ et præparatione*, which was printed at Rome in folio, 1554, (with most elegant pic-tures) esteems carp no better than a slimy watery meat. Pau-lus Jovius, on the other side, disallowing tench, approves of it; so doth Dubravius in his books of fish-ponds. Frietagius [4] extols it for an excellent wholesome meat, and puts it amongst the fishes of the best rank; and so do most of our countrey gentlemen, that store their ponds almost with no other fish. But this controversie is easily decided, in my judgment, by Bruerinus, *l.* 22. *c.* 13. The difference riseth from the site and nature of pools, [5] sometimes muddy, sometimes sweet: they are in taste as the place is, from whence they be taken. In

---

[1] Cap. 18. part. 3.   [2] Omni loco et omni tempore medici detestantur an-guillas, præsertim circa solstitium. Damnantur tum sanis tum ægris.   [3] Cap. 6. in his Tract of Melancholy.   [4] Optime nutrit, omnium judicio, inter primæ notæ pisces gustu præstanti.   [5] Non est dubium, quin, pro vivariorum situ ac naturâ, magnas alimentorum sortiantur differentias, alibi suaviores, alibi lutulentiores.

220 Causes of Melancholy. [Part. 1. Sec. 2.

like manner almost, we may conclude of other fresh-fish. But see more in Rondeletius, Bellonius, Oribasius, *lib.* 7. *cap.* 22. Isaac, *l.* 1. especially Hippolytus Salvianus, who is *instar omnium, solus, &c.* Howsoever they may be wholesome and approved, much use of them is not good. P. Forestus, in his Medicinal Observations, [1] relates, that Carthusian fryers, whose living is most part fish, are more subject to melancholy that any other order ; and that he found by experience, being sometimes their physician ordinary at Delph in Holland. He exemplifies it with an instance of one Buscodnese, a Carthusian of a ruddy colour, and well liking, that, by solitary living and fish-eating, became so misaffected.

Herbs.] Amongst herbs to be eaten, I find gourds, cowcumbers, coleworts, melons, disallowed, but especially cabbage. It causeth troublesome dreams, and sends up black vapours to the brain. Galen, (*loc. affect. l.* 3. *c.* 6) of all herbs, condemns cabbage ; and Isaac, *lib.* 2. *c.* 1. *animæ gravitatem facit,* it brings heaviness to the soul. Some are of opinion, that all raw herbs and sallets breed melancholy blood, except bugloss and lettice. Crato (*consil.* 21. *lib.* 2) speaks against all herbs and worts, except borrage, bugloss, fennel, parsly, dill, bawm, succory. Magninus, (*regim. sanitatis,* 3. *part. cap.* 31.) *omnes herbæ simpliciter malæ, viâ cibi :* all herbs are simply evil to feed on (as he thinks). So did that scoffing cook in [2] Plautus hold.

————Non ego cœnam condio, ut alii coqui solent,
Qui mihi condita prata in patinis proferunt,
Boves qui convivas faciunt, herbasque aggerunt.

Like other cooks, I do not supper dress,
    That put whole meadows into a platter,
And make no better of the guests than beeves,
    With herbs and grass to feed them fatter.

Our Italians and Spaniards do make a whole dinner of herbs and sallets (which our said Plautus calls *cœnas terrestres,* Horace, *cœnas sine sanguine) ;* by which means, as he follows it,

[3] Hic homines tam brevem vitam colunt——
Qui herbas hujusmodi in alvum suum congerunt :
Formidolosum dictu, non esu modo,
Quas herbas pecudes non edunt, homines edunt,

Their lives, that eat such herbs, must needs be short ;
And 'tis a fearful thing for to report,

[1] Observat. 16. lib. 10.   [2] Pseudolus, act. 3. scen. 2.   [3] Plautus, ibid.

That men should feed on such a kind of meat,
Which very juments would refuse to eat.

[1] They are windy, and not fit therefore to be eaten of all men raw, though qualified with oyl, but in broths, or otherwise. See more of these in every [2] husbandman and herbalist.

Roots.] Roots (*etsi quarundam gentium opes sint*, saith Bruerinus—the wealth of some countries, and sole food) are windy and bad, or troublesome to the head; as onyons, garlick, scallions, turneps, carrets, radishes, parsnips. Crato (*lib. 2. consil.* 11) disallows all roots; though [3] some approve of parsnips and potatoes. [4] Magninus is of Cratos opinion—[5]*they trouble the mind, sending gross fumes to the brain, make men mad*, especially garlick, onyons, if a man liberally feed on them a year together. Guianerius (*tract.* 15. *cap.* 2) complains of all manner of roots, and so doth Bruerinus, even parsnips themselves, which are the best; *Lib.* 9. *cap.* 14. *pastinacarum usus succos gignit improbos.*

Fruits.] Crato (*consil.* 21. *lib.* 1) utterly forbids all manner of fruits, as pears, apples, plums, cherries, strawberries, nuts, medlers, serves, &c. *Sanguinem inficiunt*, saith Villanovanus; they infect the blood; and putrifie it, Magninus holds, and must not therefore be taken, *viâ cibi, aut quantitate magnâ*, not to make a meal of, or in any great quantity. [6] Cardan makes that a cause of their continual sickness at Fessa in Africk, *because they live so much on fruits, eating them thrice a day.* Laurentius approves of many fruits, in his *Tract of Melancholy*, which others disallow, and, amongst the rest, apples, (which some likewise commend) sweetings, pairmains, pippins, as good against melancholy; but to him that is any way inclined to or touched with this malady, [7] Nicholas Piso, in his *Practicks*, forbids all fruits, as windy, or to be sparingly eaten at least, and not raw. Amongst other fruits, [8] Bruerinus (out of Galen) excepts grapes and figs; but I find them likewise rejected.

Pulse.] All pulse are naught, beans, pease, fitches, &c. they fill the brain (saith Isaac) with gross fumes, breed black, thick blood, and cause troublesome dreams. And therefore, that which Pythagoras said to his scholars of old, may be for ever applyed to melancholy men, *A fabis abstinete;* eat no

---

[1] Quare rectius valetudini suæ quisque consulet, qui, lapsûs priorum parentum memor, eas plane vel omiserit vel parce degustârit. Kersleius, cap. 4. de vero usu med. [2] In Mizaldo de Horto, P. Crescent. Herbastein, &c. [3] Cap. 13. part. 3. Bright, in his Tract of Mel. [4] Intellectum turbant, producunt insaniam. [5] Audivi, (inquit Magnin.) quod, si quis ex iis per annum continue comedat, in insaniam caderet. c. 13. Improbi succi sunt. cap. 12. [6] De rerum varietat. In Fessâ plerumque morbosi, quod fructus comedant ter in die. [7] Cap. de mel. [8] Lib. 11. c. 3.

222   *Causes of Melancholy.*   [Part. 1. Sec. 2.

pease nor beans. Yet, to such as will needs eat them, I
would give this counsel; to prepare them according to those
rules that Arnoldus Villanovanus and Frietagius prescribe, for
eating and dressing fruits, herbs, roots, pulse, &c.

Spices.] Spices cause hot and head melancholy, and are,
for that cause, forbidden by our physicians, to such men as
are inclined to this malady, as pepper, ginger, cinnamon,
cloves, mace, dates, &c. hony and sugar. [1] Some except
hony : to those that are cold, it may be tolerable ; but [2]*dulcia
se in bilem vertunt;* they are obstructive. Crato therefore forbids all spice (in a consultation of his for a melancholy schoolmaster), *omnia aromatica, et quidquid sanguinem adurit:* so
doth Fernelius, *consil.* 45 ; Guianerius, *tract.* 15. *c.* 2 : Mercurialis, *cons.* 189. To these I may add all sharp and sowre
things, luscious, and over-sweet, or fat, as oyl, vinegar, verjuice, mustard, salt; as sweet things are obstructive, so these
are corrosive. Gomesius (in his books *de sale, l.* 1. *c.* 21.)
highly commends salt ; so do Codronchus in his tract, *de sale
absinthii,* Lemn. *l.* 3. *c.* 9. *de occult. nat. mir.* Yet common
experience finds salt, and salt-meats, to be great procurers of
this disease : and for that cause, belike, those Egyptian priests
abstained from salt, even so much as in their bread, *ut sine
perturbatione anima esset,* saith mine authour—that their
souls might be free from perturbations.

Bread.] Bread that is made of baser grain, as pease, beans,
oats, rye, or [3]over-hard baked, crusty, and black, is often
spoken against as causing melancholy juyce and wind. John
Mayor, in the first book of his History of Scotland, contends
much for the wholesomeness of oaten bread. It was objected
to him, then living at Paris in France, that his countrymen
fed on oats and base grain, as a disgrace; but he doth ingenuously confess, Scotland, Wales, and a third part of England,
did most part use that kind of bread; that it was as wholsome
as any grain, and yielded as good nourishment. And yet
Wecker (out of Galen), calls it horse meat, and fitter for
juments than men, to feed on. But read Galen himself, (*Lib.*
1. *De cibis boni et mali succi*) more largely discoursing of corn
and bread.

Wine.] All black wines, over-hot, compound, strong thick
drinks, as Muscadine, Malmsie, Allegant, Rumny, Brown-
bastard, Metheglen, and the like, of which they have thirty
several kinds in Muscovy—all such made drinks are hurtful in
this case, to such as are hot, or of a sanguine cholerick com-

---

[1] Bright (c. 6.) excepts hony.   [2] Hor. apud Scoltzium, consil. 186.   [3] Ne
comedas crustam, choleram quia gignit adustam.   Schol. Sal.

Mem. 2. Subs. 1.]   *Causes of Melancholy.*   223

plexion, young, or inclined to head-melancholy: for many times
the drinking of wine alone causeth it.   Arculanus (*c.* 16. *in* 9.
Rhasis) puts in [1]wine for a great cause, especially if it be immoderately used. Guianerius (*Tract.* 15. *c.* 2) tells a story of
two Dutchmen, to whom he gave entertainment in his house,
that, [2]*in one months space, were both melancholy by drinking of
wine:* one did nought but sing, the other sigh.   Galen (*l. de
caussis morb. c.* 3), Matthiolus (on Dioscorides) and, above all
other, Andreas Bachius, (*l.* 3. 18, 19, 20) have reckoned upon
those inconveniences that come by wine.   Yet, notwithstanding
all this, to such as are cold, or sluggish melancholy, a cup of
wine is good physick; and so doth Mercurialis grant, *consil.* 25.
In that case, if the temperature be cold, as to most melancholy
men it is, wine is much commended, if it be moderately used.
    Cider, Perry.]   Cider and Perry are both cold and windy
drinks, and, for that cause, to be neglected; and so are all
those hot spiced strong drinks.
    Beer.]   Beer, if it be over new or over stale, over strong, or
not sod, smell of the cask, sharp, or sowr, is most unwholesome, frets, and gauls, &c.   Henricus Ayrerus, in [3]a consultation of his, for one that laboured of *hypochondriacal* melancholy, discommends beer; so doth [4]Crato (in that excellent
counsel of his, *lib.* 2. *consil.* 21) as too windy, because of the
hop.   But he means, belike, that thick black Bohemian beer
used in some other parts of [5]Germany.

———————————————nil spissius illâ,
Dum bibitur; nil clarius est, dum mingitur; unde
Constat, quod multas fæces in corpore linquat—

Nothing comes in so thick;
Nothing goes out so thin;
It must needs follow, then,
The dregs are left within—

as that old [6]poet scoffed, calling it *Stygiæ monstrum conforme
paludi,* a monstrous drink, like the river *Styx.*   But let them
say as they list, to such as are accustomed unto it, *'tis a most
wholesome* ([7]so Polydor Virgil calleth it) *and a pleasant drink;*
it is more subtil and better for the hôp, that rarifies it, and
hath an especial vertue against melancholy, as our herbalists
confess, Fuchsius approves, *lib.* 2. *sect.* 2. *instit. cap.* 11. and
many others.

---

[1] Vinum turbidum.   [2] Ex vini potentis bibitione, duo Alemanni in uno mense
melancholici facti sunt.   [3] Hildesheim, spicil. fol. 373.   [4] Crassum generat
sanguinem.   [5] About Dantzick, Inspruck, Hamburg, Lypsick.   [6] Henricus
Abrincensis.   [7] Potus tum salubris tum jucundus, l. 1.

224   *Causes of Melancholy.*   [Part. 1. Sec. 2.

Waters.] Standing waters, thick and ill coloured, such
as come forth of pools and motes, where hemp hath been
steeped, or slimy fishes live, are most unwholesome, putrified,
and full of mites, creepers, slimy, ·muddy, unclean, corrupt,
impure, by reason of the suns heat, and still standing. They
cause foul distemperatures in the body and mind of man, are
unfit to make drink of, to dress meat with, or to be [1] used
about men inwardly or outwardly. They are good for many
domestical uses, to wash horses, water cattle, &c. or in time
of necessity, but not otherwise. Some are of opinion, that
such fat standing waters make the best beer, and that seething
doth defecate it, as [2] Cardan holds (*lib. 13. subtil.*) *it mends
the substance and savour of it;* but it is a paradox. Such
beer may be stronger, but not so wholesome as the other, as
[3] Jobertus truly justifieth, out of Galen, (*Paradox. dec. 1.
Paradox. 5*) that the seething of such impure waters doth
not purge or purifie them. Pliny (*lib. 31. c. 3.*) is of the
same tenent; and P. Crescentius, *agricult. lib. 1. et lib. 4. c.*
11. *et c.* 45. Pamphilius Herilachus, *l. 4. de nat. aquarum,*
such waters are naught, not to be used, and (by the testimony of [4] Galen) breed *agues, dropsies, pleurisies, splenetick
and melancholy passions, hurt the eyes, cause a bad temperature, and ill disposition of the whole body, with bad colour.*
This Jobertus stifly maintains, (*Paradox. lib. 1, part. 5*) that
it causeth bleer eyes, bad colour, and many loathsome diseases
to such as use it. This, which they say, stands with good
reason; for, as geographers relate, the water of Astracan
breeds worms in such as drink it. [5] Axius, or (as now called)
Verduri, the fairest river in Macedonia, makes all cattle
black that taste of it. Aliacmon, now Peleca, another stream
in Thessaly, turns cattle most part white, *si potui ducas.*
I. Aubanus Bohemus referrs that [6] *struma,* or poke of the
Bavarians and Styrians, to the nature of their waters, as
[7] Munster doth that of the Valesians, in the Alps: and [8] Bodine
supposeth the stuttering of some families in Aquitania, about
Labden, to proceed from the same cause, *and that the filth
is derived from the water to their bodies.* So that they
that use filthy, standing, ill-coloured, thick, muddy water,
must needs have muddy, ill-coloured, impure, and infirm
bodies: and, because the body works upon the mind, they

---

[1] Galen. l. 1. de san. tuend. Cavendæ sunt aquæ quæ ex stagnis hauriuntur,
et quæ turbidæ et male olentes, &c.   [2] Innoxium reddit et bene olentem.
[3] Contendit hæc vitia coctione non emendari.   [4] Lib. de bonitate aquæ. Hy-
dropem auget, febres putridas, splenem, tusses: nocet oculis; malum habitum
corporis et colorem.   [5] Mag. Nigritatem inducit, si pecora biberint.
[6] Aquæ ex nivibus coactæ strumosos faciunt.   [7] Cosmog. l. 3. cap. 36.
[8] Method. hist. cap. 5. Balbutiunt Labdoni in Aquitaniâ ob aquas; atque hi
morbi ab aquis in corpora derivantur.

Mem. 2. Subs. 2.] *Dyet a Cause.* 225

shall have grosser understandings, dull, foggy, melancholy spirits, and be really subject to all manner of infirmities.

To these noxious simples, we may reduce an infinite number of compound, artificial, made dishes, of which our cooks afford us a great variety, as taylors do fashions in our apparel. Such are [1] puddings stuffed with blood, or otherwise composed, baked meats, sowced, indurate meats, fryed, and broiled, buttered meats, condite, powdred, and over-dryed, [2] all cakes, simnels, buns, cracknels, made with butter, spice, &c. fritters, pancakes, pies, salsages, and those several sawces, sharp, or over sweet, of which *scientia popinæ*, (as Seneca calls it) hath served those [3] Apician tricks, and perfumed dishes, which Adrian the Sixth, pope, so much admired in the accounts of his predecessour *Leo decimus ;* and which prodigious riot and prodigality have invented in this age. These do generally ingender gross humours, fill the stomach with crudities, and all those inward parts with obstructions. Montanus (*consil.* 22) gives instance in a melancholy Jew, that, by eating such tart sawces, made dishes, and salt meats, with which he was over-much delighted, became melancholy, and was evil affected. Such examples are familiar and common.

SUBSECT. II.

Quantity of Dyet a cause.

THERE is not so much harm proceeding from the substance it self of meat, and quality of it, in ill-dressing and preparing, as there is from the quantity, disorder of time and place, unseasonable use of it, [4] intemperance, over-much or over-little taking of it. A true saying it is, *Plures crapula quam gladius ;* this gluttony kills more than the sword ; this *omnivorantia, et homicida gula,* this all devouring, and murdering gut. And that of [5] Pliny is truer; *simple diet is the best : heaping up of several meats, is pernicious, and sawces worse ; many dishes bring many diseases.* [6] Avicen cryes out, that *nothing is worse*

---

[1] Edulia ex sanguine et suffocato parta. Hildesheim. [2] Cupedia vero, placentæ, bellaria, commentaque alia curiosa pistorum et coquorum gustui servientium conciliant morbos tum corpori tum animo insanabiles. Philo Judæus, lib. de victimis, P. Jov. vitâ ejus. [3] As lettice steeped in wine, birds fed with fennel and sugar, as a popes concubine used in Avignion. Stephan. [4] Animæ negotium illa facessit, et de templo Dei immundum stabulum facit. Peletius, 10. c. [5] Lib. 11. c. 52. Homini cibus utilissimus simplex ; acervatio ciborum pestifera, et condimenta perniciosa ; multos morbos multa fercula ferunt. [6] 31 Dec. 2. c. Nihil deterius quam si tempus justo longius comedendo protrahatur, et varia ciborum genera conjungantur ; inde morborum scaturigo, quæ ex repugnantiâ humorum oritur.

VOL. I.   Q

226   *Dyet a Cause.*   [Part. 1. Sec. 2.

*than to feed on many dishes, or to protract the time of meals
longer than ordinary ; from thence proceed our infirmities; and
'tis the fountain of all diseases, which arise out of the repugnancy of gross humours.* Thence, saith [1] Fernelius, come crudities, wind, oppilations, *cacochymia, plethora, cachexia, bradypepsia : [2] hinc subitæ mortes, atque intestata senectus ;* suddain
death, &c. and what not ?

As a lamp is choaked with a multitude of oyl, or a little
fire with overmuch wood quite extinguished; so is the natural
heat, with immoderate eating, strangled in the body. *Perniciosa sentina est abdomen insaturabile,* one saith—an insatiable paunch is a pernicious sink, and the fountain of all diseases, both of body and mind. [3] Mercurialis will have it a
peculiar cause of this private disease. Solenander (*consil. 5.
sect. 3*) illustrates this of Mercurialis, with an example of one
so melancholy, *ab intempestivis comissationibus,* unseasonable feasting. [4] Crato confirms as much, in that often cited
counsel, *21. lib. 2,* putting superfluous eating for a main cause.
But what need I seek farther for proofs ? Hear [5] Hippocrates
himself, *lib. 2, aphoris. 10. Impure bodies, the more they
are nourished, the more they are hurt ; for the nourishment is
putrified with vicious humours.*

And yet, for all this harm, which apparently follows surfet-
ting and drunkenness, see how we luxuriate and rage in this
kind. Read what Johannes Stuckius hath written lately of
this subject, in his great volume *De Antiquorum Conviviis,* and
of our present age : *quam [6] portentosæ cœnæ,* prodigious sup-
pers : [7] *qui, dum invitant ad cœnam, efferunt ad sepulcrum,*
what Fagos, Epicures, Apicios, Heliogables our times afford ?
Lucullus ghost walks still ; and every man desires to sup in
Apollo ; Æsops costly dish is ordinarily served up.

———— [8] Magis illa juvant, quæ pluris emuntur :

the dearest cates are best; and 'tis an ordinary thing to bestow twenty or thirty pound on a dish, some thousand crowns
upon a dinner. [9] Muley-Hamet, king of Fez and Morocco,
spent three pound on the sawce of a capon : it is nothing in
our times: we scorn all that is cheap. *We loath the very
[10] light,* (some of us, as Seneca notes) *because it comes free ; and*

---

[1] Path. l. 1. c. 14.   [2] Juv. Sat. 5.   [3] Nimia repletio ciborum facit
melancholicum.   [4] Comestio superflua cibi, et potûs quantitas nimia.   [5] Im-
pura corpora quanto magis nutris, tanto magis lædis : putrefacit enim alimentum
vitiosus humor.   [6] Vid. Goclen. de portentosis cœuis, &c. Puteani Com.
[7] Amb. lib. de Jeju. cap. 14.   [8] Juvenal.   [9] Guicciardin.   [10] Na. quæst. 4.
ca. ult. fastidio est lumen gratuitum ; dolet quod solem, quod spiritum, emere non
possimus, quod hic aër, non emptus, ex facili, &c. adeo nihil placet, nisi quod ca-
rum est.

we are *offended with the suns heat, and those cool blasts, be-cause we buy them not.* This air we breath is so common, *we care not for it;* nothing pleaseth but what is dear. And, if we be [1] witty in any thing, it is *ad gulam :* if we study at all, it is *erudito luxu,* to please the palat, and to satisfie the gut. *A cook of old was a base knave* (as [2] Livy complains), *but now a great man in request; cookery is become an art, a noble science: cooks are gentlemen : venter deus.* They wear *their brains in their bellies, and their guts in their heads,* (as [3] Agrippa taxed some parasites of his time) rushing on their own destruction, as if a man should run upon the point of a sword ; *usque dum rumpantur, comedunt :* [4] all day, all night, let the physician say what he will—imminent danger and feral diseases are now ready to seize upon them—they will eat till they vomit, (*edunt ut vomant ; vomunt ut edant,* saith Seneca ; which Dion re-lates of Vitellius, *Solo transitu ciborum nutriri judicatus :* his meat did pass through, and away) or till they burst again. [5] *Strage animantium ventrem onerant ;* and rake over all the world, as so many [6] slaves, belly-gods, and land-serpents ; *et totus orbis ventri nimis angustus ;* the whole world cannot satisfie their appetite. [7] *Sea, land, rivers, lakes, &c. may not give content to their raging guts.* To make up the mess, what immoderate drinking in every place ! *Senem potum pota trahe-bat anus ;* how they flock to the tavern ! as if they were *fruges consumere nati,* born to no other end, but to eat and drink, (like Offellius Bibulus, that famous Roman parasite, *qui, dum vixit, aut bibit aut minxit*) as so many casks to hold wine ; yea, worse than a cask, that marrs wine, and it self is not marred by it. Yet these are brave men ; Silenus ebrius was no braver : *et quæ fuerunt vitia, mores sunt :* 'tis now the fashion of our times, an honour : *nunc vero res ista eo rediit* (as Chrysost. serm. 30. in 5. Ephes. comments) *ut effeminatæ ridendæque ignaviæ loco habeatur, nolle inebriari ;* 'tis now come to that pass, that he is no gentleman, a very milk-sop, a clown, of no bring-ing up, that will not drink, fit for no company : he is your only gallant that plays it off finest, no disparagement now to stagger in the streets, reel, rave, &c. but much to his fame and renown ; as, in like case, Epidicus told Thesprio his fellow servant, in the [8] poet. *Ædepol ! facinus improbum,* one urged : the other replied, *At jam alii fecere idem ; erit illi illa res hònori :* 'tis

---

[1] Ingeniosi ad gulam.   [2] Olim vile mancipium, nunc in omni æstimati-one ; nunc ars haberi cœpta, &c.   [3] Epist. 28. l. 7. quorum in ventre inge-nium, in patinis, &c.   [4] In lucem cœnat Sertorius.   [5] Seneca.   [6] Man-cipia, gulæ, dapes non sapore sed sumptu æstimantes. Seneca, consol. ad Hel-viam.   [7] Sævientia guttura satiare non possunt fluvii et maria. Æneas Sylvius, de miser. curial.   [8] Plautus.

Q 2

228   *Dyet a Cause.*   [Part. 1. Sec. 2.

now no fault, there be so many brave examples to bear one
out ; 'tis a credit to have a strong brain, and carry his liquor
well: the sole contention, who can drink most, and fox his
fellow soonest. 'Tis the *summum bonum* of our *tradesmen,*
their felicity, life and soul, (*tantâ dulcedine affectant,* saith
Pliny, *lib.* 14. *cap.* 12, *ut magna pars non aliud vitæ præmium
intelligat*) their chief comfort, to be merry together in an ale-
house or tavern, as our modern Muscovites do in their mede-
inns, and Turks in their coffee-houses, which much resemble
our taverns: they will labour hard all day long, to be drunk at
night, and spend *totius anni labores* (as St. Ambrose adds) in a
tipling feast; convert day into night, as Seneca taxeth some
in his times, *pervertunt officia noctis et lucis;* when we rise,
they commonly go to bed, like our Antipodes,

> Nosque ubi primus equis Oriens afflavit anhelis,
> Illis sera rubens accendit lumina Vesper.

So did Petronius in Tacitus, Heliogabalus in Lampridius,

> ———— [1] Noctes vigilabat ad ipsum
> Mane ; diem totum stertebat.————

Smyndiris the Sybarite never saw the sun rise or set, so much
as once in twenty years. Verres, against whom Tully so much
inveighs, in winter he never was *extra tectum, vix extra lectum,* never almost out of bed, [2] still wenching, and drinking;
so did he spend his time, and so do myriads in our dayes.
They have *gymnasia bibonum,* schools and rendezvous ; these
Centaures and Lapithæ toss pots and bowls, as so many balls,
invent new tricks, as salsages, anchoves, tobacco, caveare,
pickled oysters, herrings, fumadoes, &c. innumerable salt-
meats to increase their appetite, and study how to hurt themselves by taking antidotes, [3] *to carry their drink the better :*
[4] *and, when naught else serves, they will go forth, or be conveyed out, to empty their gorge, that they may return to drink
afresh.* They make laws, *insanas leges, contra bibendi fal-
lacias,* and [5] brag of it when they have done, crowning that
man that is soonest gone, as their drunken predecessours
have done, (*[6] quid ego video? Ps. Cum coronâ Pseudo-
lum ebrium tuum*) and, when they are dead, will have a

---

[1] Hor.   [2] Diei brevitas conviviis, noctis longitudo stupris, conterebatur.
[3] Et, quo plus capiant, irritamenta excogitantur.   [4] Foras portantur, ut ad
convivium reportentur ; repleri ut exhauriant, et exhaurire ut bibant. Ambros.
[5] Ingentia vasa, velut ad ostentationem, &c.   [6] Plautus.

Mem. 2. Subs. 2.] *Dyet a Cause.* 229

can of wine, with [1] Marons old woman, to be engraven on their tombs. So they triumph in villany, and justifie their wickedness, with Rabelais, that French Lucian, "drunkenness is better for the body than physick, because there be more old drunkards, than old physicians." Many such frothy arguments they have, [2] inviting and encouraging others to do as they do, and love them dearly for it (no glew like to that of good fellowship). So did Alcibiades in Greece, Nero, Bonosus, Heliogabalus in Rome (or Alegabalus rather, as he was stiled of old, as [3] Ignatius proves out of some old coyns) ; so do many great men still, as [4] Heresbachius observes. When a prince drinks till his eyes stare, like Bitias in the poet,

——————— ([5] ille impiger hausit
Spumantem pateram)———

and comes off clearly, sound trumpets, fife and drums, the spectators will applaud him ; *the* [6] *bishop himself,* (if he belye them not) *with his chaplain, will stand by, and do as much ; O dignum principe haustum !* 'twas done like a prince. *Our Dutchmen invite all comers with a pail and a dish : velut infundibula, integras obbas exhauriunt, et in monstrosis poculis ipsi monstrosi monstrosius epotant, making barrels of their bellies. Incredibile dictu,* (as [7] one of their own countrey-men complains) [8] *quantum liquoris immodestissima gens capiat, &c. How they love a man that will be drunk, crown him and honour him for it,* hate him that will not pledge him, stab him, kill him : a most intolerable offence, and not to be forgiven. [9] *He is a mortal enemy that will not drink with him,* as Munster relates of the Saxons. So, in Poland, he is the best servitor, and the honestest fellow, (saith Alexander Gaguinus) [10] *that drinketh most healths to the honour of his master :* he shall be rewarded as a good servant, and held the bravest fellow, that carries his liquor best ; when as a brewers horse will bare much more than any sturdy drinker ; yet, for his noble exploits in this kind, he shall be accounted a most valiant man ; for [11] *tam inter epulas fortis vir esse potest ac in bello,* as much valour is to be found in feasting, as in fighting ; and some of our city captains,

---

[1] Lib. 3. Anthol. c. 20.   [2] Gratiam conciliant potando.   [3] Notis ad Cæsares.   [4] Lib. de educandis principum liberis.   [5] Virg.   [6] Idem. strenui potoris episcopi sacellanus, cum ingentem pateram exhaurit princeps. [7] Bohemus, in Saxoniâ. Adeo immoderate et immodeste ab ipsis bibitur, ut, in compotationibus suis, non cyathis solum et cantharis sat infundere possint, sed impletum mulctrale apponant, et scutellâ injectâ hortantur quemlibet ad libitum potare.   [8] Dictu incredibile, quantum hujusce liquoris immodesta gens capiat : plus potantem amicissimum habent, et serto coronant, inimicissimum e contra qui non vult, et cæde et fustibus expiant.   [9] Qui potare recusat, hostis habetur, et cæde nonnumquam res expiatur.   [10] Qui melius bibit pro salute domini, melior habetur minister.   [11] Græc. poëta apud Stobæum, ser. 18.

230   *Dyet a Cause.*   [Part. 1. Sec. 2.

and carpet knights, will make this good, and prove it. Thus
they many times wilfully pervert the good temperature of their
bodies, stifle their wits, strangle nature, and degenerate into
beasts.

Some again are in the other extream, and draw this mischief
on their heads by too ceremonious and strict diet, being over-
precise, cockney-like, and curious in their observation of meats,
times, as that *Medicina statica* prescribes—just so many ounces
at a dinner (which Lessius enjoins), so much at supper; not a
little more, nor a little less, of such meat, and at such hours;
a dyet drink in the morning, cock-broth, China-broth, at dinner,
plumb-broth, a chicken, a rabbit, rib of a rack of mutton, wing
of a capon, the merry thought of a hen, &c.—to sounder bodies,
this is too nice and most absurd. Others offend in over-much
fasting; pining a dayes, (saith [1] Guianerius) and waking a
nights, as many Moors and Turks in these our times do. *Anchorites, monks, and the rest of that superstitious rank,* (as the
same Guianerius witnesseth, *that he hath often seen to have
hapned in his time*) *through immoderate fasting, have been frequently mad.* Of such men, belike, Hippocrates speaks, (1
Aphor. 5.) when as he saith, [2] *they more offend in too sparing
diet, and are worse damnified, than they that feed liberally,
and are ready to surfeit.*

SUBSECT. III.

*Custom of Dyet, Delight, Appetite, Necessity, how they cause
or hinder.*

No rule is so general, which admits not some exception; to
this therefore which hath been hitherto said, (for I shall otherwise put most men out of commons) and those inconveniences
which proceed from the substance of meats, an intemperate or
unseasonable use of them, custom somewhat detracts, and quali-
fies, according to that of Hippocrates, 2 *Aphoris.* 50. [3] *Such
things as we have been long accustomed to, though they be evil
in their own nature, yet they are less offensive.* Otherwise it

---

[1] Qui de die jejunant, et nocte vigilant, facile cadunt in melancholiam; et qui
naturæ modum excedunt, c. 5. tract. 15. c. 2. Longâ famis tolerantiâ, ut iis sæpe
accidit qui tanto cum fervore Deo servire cupiunt per jejunium, quod maniaci
efficiantur, ipse vidi sæpe.   [2] In tenui victu ægri delinquunt; ex quo fit ut
majori afficiantur detrimento, majorque fit error tenui quam pleniore victu.
[3] Quæ longo tempore consueta sunt, etiamsi deteriora, minus assuetis molestare
solent.

Mem. 2. Subs. 3.]   *Causes of Melancholy.*   231

might well be objected, that it were a meer [1]tyranny to live
after those strict rules of physick; for custom [2]doth alter nature
it self; and, to such as are used to them, it makes bad meats
wholesome, and unseasonable times to cause no disorder. Cider
and perry are windy drinks; (so are all fruits windy in themselves, cold most part) yet, in some shires of [3]England, Normandy in France, Guipuscova in Spain, 'tis their common
drink; and they are no whit offended with it.   In Spain, Italy,
and Africk, they live most on roots, raw herbs, camels [4]milk,
and it agrees well with them; which to a stranger will cause
much grievance.   In Wales, *lacticiniis vescuntur,* (as Hum-
frey Lluyd confesseth, a Cambro-Brittain himself, in his elegant epistle to Abraham Ortelius) they live most on white
meats; in Holland, on fish, roots, [5]butter; and so at this day
in Greece, as [6]Bellonius observes, they had much rather feed
on fish than flesh.   With us, *maxima pars victûs in carne consistit;* we feed on flesh most part, (saith [7]Polydor Virgil) as
all northern countreys do; and it would be very offensive to us
to live after their dyet, or they to live after ours: we drink
beer, they wine: they use oyl, we butter: we in the north are
[8]great eaters, they most sparing in those hotter countreys: and
yet they and we, following our own customs, are well pleased.
An Æthiopian of old, seeing an European eat bread, wondred,
quomodo stercoribus vescentes viveremus, how we could eat
such kind of meats: so much differed his countrey-men from
ours in dyet, that (as mine [9]author infers), *si quis illorum victum apud nos æmulari vellet;* if any man should so feed with
us, it would be all one to nourish, as *cicuta, aconitum,* or *hellebor* it self.   At this day, in China, the common people live,
in a manner, altogether on roots and herbs; and, to the
wealthiest, horse, ass, mule, dogs, cat-flesh is as delightsome as
the rest: so [10]Mat. Riccius the Jesuit relates, who lived many
years amongst them.   The Tartars eat raw meat, and most
commonly [11]horse-flesh, drink milk and blood, as the Nomades
of old—

[1] Qui medice vivit, misere vivit.   [2] Consuetudo altera natura.   [3] Here-
fordshire, Gloucestershire, Worcestershire.   [4] Leo Afer. l. 1. solo camelorum
lacte contenti, nil præterea deliciarum ambiunt.   [5] Flandri vinum butyro dilu-
tum bibunt (nauseo referens): ubique butyrum, inter omnia fercula et bellaria, locum obtinet. Steph. præfat. Herod.   [6] Delectantur Græci piscibus magis quam
carnibus.   [7] Lib. 1. hist. Ang.   [8] P. Jovius descrip. Britonum. They sit,
eat and drink all day at dinner in Island, Muscovy, and those northern parts.
[9] Suidas, vit. Herod. nihilo cum eo melius quam siquis cicutam, aconitum, &c.
[10] Expedit. in Sinas, lib. 1. c. 3. hortensium herbarum et olerum apud Sinas quam
apud nos longe frequentior usus; complures quippe de vulgo reperias nullâ aliâ re,
vel tenuitatis vel religionis caussâ, vescentes. Equos, mulos, asellos, &c. æque
fere vescuntur, ac pabula omnia, Mat. Riccius, lib. 5. c. 13.   [11] Tartari mulis,
equis vescuntur, et crudis carnibus, et fruges contemnunt, dicentes, hoc jumentorum pabulum et boum, non hominum.

232   *Causes of Melancholy.*   [Part. 1. Sec. 2.

(Et lac concretum cum sanguine potat equino).

They scoff at our Europæans for eating bread, which they call
tops of weeds, and horse-meat, not fit for men ; and yet Scaliger
accounts them a sound and witty nation, living an hundred
years ; even in the civilest countrey of them, they do thus,
as Benedict the Jesuit observed in his travels, from the great
Mogors court by land to Paquin, which Riccius contends to
be the same with Cambulu in Cataia. In Scandia, their bread
is usually dryed fish, and so likewise in the Shetland Isles ; and
their other fare, as in Island, (saith [1] Dithmarus Bleskenius)
butter, cheese, and fish ; their drink, water, their lodging on
the ground. In America, in many places, their bread is roots,
their meat palmitos, pinas, potatos, &c. and such fruits. There
be of them, too, that familiarly drink [2] salt sea water, all their
lives, eat [3] raw meat, grass, and that with delight : with some,
fish, serpents, spiders ; and in divers places they [4] eat mans
flesh raw, and rosted, even the emperour [5] Metazuma himself.
In some coasts again, [6] one tree yields them coquernuts, meat
and drink, fire-fuel, apparel (with his leaves), oyl, vinegar,
cover for houses, &c. and yet these men, going naked, feeding
coarse, live commonly a hundred years, are seldom or never
sick ; all which dyet our physicians forbid. In Westphaling,
they feed most part on fat meats and wourts, knuckle-deep,
and call it [7] *cerebrum Jovis :* in the Low Countreys, with
roots ; in Italy, frogs and snails are used. The Turks, saith
Busbequius, delight most in fryed meats. In Muscovy, garlick
and onions are ordinary meat and sauce, which would be pernicious to such as are unaccustomed to them, delightsome to
others ; and all is [8] because they have been brought up unto it.
Husbandmen, and such as labour, can eat fat bacon, salt gross
meat, hard cheese, &c. *(O dura messorum ilia !)* coarse bread
at all times, go to bed and labour upon a full stomach ; which,
to some idle persons, would be present death, and is against the
rules of physick ; so that custom is all in all. Our travellers
[9] find this by common experience : when they come in far countreys, and use their dyet, they are suddenly offended ; as our
Hollanders and Englishmen, when they touch upon the coasts
of Africk, those Indian capes and islands, are commonly mo-

---

[1] Islandiæ descriptione. Victus eorum butyro, lacte, caseo consistit : pisces
loco panis habent ; potus aqua, aut serum ; sic vivunt sine medicinâ multi ad
annos 200.   [2] Laet. occident. Ind. descrip. l. 11. c. 10. Aquam marinam
bibere sueti absque noxâ.   [3] Davies second voyage.   [4] Patagones.
[5] Benzo et Fer. Cortesius, lib. novus orbis inscrip.   [6] Linscoften, c. 56. palmæ
instar, totius orbis arboribus longe præstantior.   [7] Lips. ep.   [8] Teneris
assuescere multum.   [9] Repentinæ mutationes noxam pariunt. Hippocrat.
aphorism. 21. ep. 6. sect. 3.

Mem. 2. Subs. 3.]   *Causes of Melancholy.*   233

lested with calentures, fluxes, and much distempered by reason of their fruits. [1] *Peregrina, essi suavia, solent vescentibus
perturbationes insignes adferre;* strange meats, though pleasant, cause notable alterations and distempers.   On the other
side, use or custom mitigates or makes all good again.   Mithridates, by often use, (which Pliny wonders at) was able to
drink poyson; and a maid, (as Curtius records) sent to Alexander from king Porus, was brought up with poyson from
her infancy. The Turks (saith Bellonius, *lib. 3. cap.* 15.)
eat opium familiarly, a dram at once, which we dare not take
in grains.   [2] Garcius ab Horto writes of one whom he saw at
Goa in the East Indies, that took ten drams of opium in three
dayes; and yet *consulto loquebatur,* spake understandingly; so
much can custom do.   [3] Theophrastus speaks of a shepherd
that could eat hellebor in substance.   And therefore Cardan
concludes (out of Galen) *consuetudinem utcunque ferendam,
nisi valde malam;* custom is however to be kept, except it be
extreme bad.   He adviseth all men to keep their old customs,
and that by the authority of [4] Hippocrates himself: *dandum
aliquid tempori, ætati, regioni, consuetudini,* and therefore to
[5] continue as they began, be it diet, bath, exercise, &c. or
whatsoever else.

   Another exception is delight, or appetite to such and such
meats.   Though they be hard of digestion, melancholy ; yet as
(Fuchsius excepts, *cap.* 6. *lib.* 2. *Instit. sect.* 2) [6] *the stomach doth
readily digest, and willingly entertain such meats we love most
and are pleasing to us, abhors on the other side such as we
distaste;* which Hippocrates confirms, *Aphoris.* 2. 38.   Some
cannot endure cheese, out of a secret antipathy, or to see a
roasted duck, which to others is a [7] delightsome meat.

   The last exception is necessity, poverty, want, hunger, which
drives men many times to do that which otherwise they are
loath, cannot endure, and thankfully to accept of it; as beverage
in ships, and, in sieges of great cities, to feed on dogs, cats, rats,
and men themselves.   Three out-laws, in [8] Hector Boëthius,
being driven to their shifts, did eat raw flesh, and flesh of such
fowl as they could catch, in one of the Hebrides, for some few
moneths. These things do mitigate or disannul that which
hath been said of melancholy meats, and make it more tolerable ; but, to such as are wealthy, live plenteously, at ease,
may take their choice, and refrain if they will, these viands are

[1] Bruerinus, l. 1. c. 23.   [2] Simpl. med. c. 4. l. 1.   [3] Heurnius, l. 3.
c. 19. prax. med.   [4] Aphoris. 17.   [5] In dubiis consuetudinem sequatur adolescens, et in cœptis perseveret.   [6] Qui cum voluptate assumuntur
cibi, ventriculus avidius complectitur, expeditiusque concoquit: et, quæ displi-
cent, aversatur.   [7] Nothing against a good stomach, as the saying is.
[8] Lib. 7. Hist. Scot.

234   *Retention and Evacuation, Causes.*   [Part. 1. Sec. 2.

to be forborn, if they be inclined to or suspect melancholy, as they tender their healths: otherwise, if they be intemperate, or disordered in their dyet, at their peril be it. *Qui monet, amat. Ave, et cave.*

SUBSECT. IV.

Retention and Evacuation a cause, and how.

Of retention and evacuation there be divers kinds, which are either concomitant, assisting, or sole causes many times of melancholy. [1] Galen reduceth defect and abundance to this head; others, [2] *all that is separated or remains.*

Costiveness.]   In the first rank of these, I may well reckon up costiveness, and keeping in of our ordinary excrements, which, as it often causeth other diseases, so this of melancholy in particular. [3] Celsus (*lib.* 1. *cap.* 3) *saith it produceth inflammation of the head, dulness, cloudiness, head-ach, &c.* Prosper Calenus (*lib. de atrâ bile*) will have it distemper not the organ only, [4] *but the mind it self by troubling of it:* and sometimes it is a sole cause of madness, as you may read in the first book of [5] Skenkius his Medicinal Observations. A young merchant, going to Nordeling fair in Germany, for ten dayes space never went to stool: at his return, he was grievously melancholy, [6] thinking that he was robbed, and would not be perswaded, but that all his money was gone. His friends thought he had some *philtrum* given him; but Cnelinus, a physician, being sent for, found his [7] costiveness alone to be the cause, and thereupon gave him a clister, by which he was speedily recovered. Trincavellius (*consult. 35. lib.* 1) saith as much of a melancholy lawyer, to whom he administered physick; and Rodericus a Fonseca (*consult. 85. tom.* 2) [8] of a patient of his, that for eight dayes was bound, and therefore melancholy affected. Other retentions and evacuations there are, not simply necessary, but at some times; as Fernelius accounts them, (*Path. lib.* 1, *cap.* 15) as suppression of emrods, monethly issues in women, bleeding at nose, immoderate, or no use at all of Venus; or any other ordinary issues.

[9] Detention of emrods, or monethly issues, Villanovanus (*Breviar. lib.* 1. *cap.* 18) Arculanus, (*cap.* 16. *in.* 9. *Rhasis*) Vittorius Faventinus, (*pract. mag. Tract.* 2. *cap.* 15) Bruel, &c.

---

[1] 30. artis.   [2] Quæ excernuntur aut subsistunt. inflammationes, capitis dolores, caligines, crescunt. mentis agitationem parere solent.   [5] Cap. de mel. hominem agnosceret.   [7] Alvus astrictus caussa. siccum habet, et nihil reddit.   [9] Sive per nares, sive hæmorrhoïdes.   [3] Ex ventre suppresso,   [4] Excrementa retenta   [6] Tam delirus, ut vix se   [8] Per octo dies alvum

Mem. 2. Subs. 4.]   *Retention and Evacuation, Causes.*   235

put for ordinary causes. Fuchsius (*l. 2. sect. 5. c.* 30) goes farther, and saith, [1] *that many men, unseasonably cured of the emrods, have been corrupted with melancholy ; seeking to avoid Scylla, they fall into Charybdis.* Galen (*l. de hum. commen. 3. ad text.* 26) illustrates this by an example of Lucius Martius, whom he cured of madness, contracted by this means : and [2] Skenkius hath other two instances of two melancholy and mad women, so caused from the suppression of their moneths. The same may be said of bleeding at the nose, if it be suddenly stopt, and have been formerly used, as [3] Villanovanus urgeth ; and [4] Fuchsius (*lib. 2. sect. 5. cap.* 33) stifly maintains, *that without great danger, such an issue may not be stayed.*

Venus omitted produceth like effects. Matthiolus (*epist. 5. l. penult.*) [5] *avoucheth of his knowledge, that some through bashfulness abstained from venery, and thereupon became very heavy and dull; and some others, that were very timorous, melancholy, and beyond all measure sad.* Oribasius (*Med. Collect. l.* 6. *c.* 37) speaks of some, [6] *That, if they do not use carnal copulation, are continually troubled with heaviness and head-ach; and some in the same case by intermission of it.* Not-use of it hurts many ; Arculanus (*c.* 6. *in* 9. *Rhasis*) and Magninus (*part. 3. cap.* 5) think, because [7] *it sends up poisoned vapours to the brain and heart.* And so doth Galen himself hold, that, if this *natural seed be over-long kept (in some parties) it turns to poison.* Hieronymus Mercurialis, in his chapter of Melancholy, cites it for an especial cause of this malady, [8] *priapismus, satyriasis, &c.* Haliabbas (5 *Theor. c.* 36) reckons up this and many other diseases. Villanovanus (*Breviar. l.* 1. *c.* 18) saith, he *knew* [9] *many monks and widows, grievously troubled with melancholy, and that from this sole cause.* [10] Ludovicus Mercatus (*l.* 2. *de mulierum affect. cap.* 4) and Rodericus a Castro (*de morbis mulier. l.* 2. *c.* 3) treat largely of this subject, and will have it produce a peculiar kind of melancholy, in stale maids, nuns, and widows *ob suppressionem mensium et Venerem omissam, timidæ, mœstæ,*

---

[1] Multi, intempestive ab hæmorrhoidibus curati, melancholiâ correpti sunt. Incidit in Scyllam, &c.   [2] Lib. 1. de Maniâ.   [3] Breviar. l. 7. c. 18. [4] Non sine magno incommodo ejus, cui sanguis a naribus promanat, noxii sanguinis vacuatio impediri potest.   [5] Novi quosdam, præ pudore a coitu abstinentes, torpidos pigrosque factos ; nonnullos etiam melancholicos præter modum, mœstos, timidosque.   [6] Nonnulli, nisi coëant, assidue capitis gravitate infestantur. Dicit se novisse quosdam tristes, et ita factos ex intermissione Veneris. [7] Vapores venenatos mittit sperma ad cor et cerebrum. Sperma, plus diu retentum, transit in venenum.   [8] Graves producit corporis et animi ægritudines.   [9] Ex spermate supra modum retento, monachos et viduas melancholicos sæpe fieri vidi.   [10] Melancholia orta a vasis seminariis in utero.

236   *Retention and Evacuation, Causes.* [Part. 1. Sec. 2.

anxiæ, verecundæ, suspiciosæ, languentes, consilii inopes, cum summâ vitæ et rerum meliorum desperatione, &c. they are melancholy in the highest degree, and all for want of husbands. Ælianus Montaltus (*cap.* 37. *de melanchol.*) confirms as much out of Galen; so doth Wierus. Christopherus a Vega (*de art. med. lib.* 3. *cap.* 14) relates many such examples of men and women, that he had seen so melancholy. Felix Plater, in the first book of his Observations, [1] *tells a story of an antient gentleman in Alsatia, that married a young wife, and was not able to pay his debts in that kind for a long time together, by reason of his several infirmities. But she, because of this inhibition of Venus, fell into a horrible fury, and desired every one that came to see her, by words, looks, and gestures to have to do with her, &c.* [2] Bernardus Paternus, a physician, saith, he knew *a good honest godly priest, that, because he would neither willingly marry, nor make use of the stews, fell into grievous melancholy fits.* Hildesheim (*spicil.* 2.) hath such another example of an Italian melancholy priest, in a consultation had anno 1580. John Pratensis gives instance in a married man, that, from his wifes death abstaining, [3] *after marriage, became exceeding melancholy;* Rodericus a Fonseca, in a young man so mis-affected, *tom.* 2. *consult.* 85. To these you may add, if you please, that conceited tale of a Jew, so visited in like sort, and so cured, out of Poggius Florentinus.

Intemperate Venus is, all out, as bad in the other extream. Galen (*l.* 6. *de morbis popular. sect.* 5. *text.* 26) reckons up melancholy amongst those diseases which are [4] *exasperated by venery:* so doth Avicenna, (2. 3. *c.* 11) Oribasius, (*loc. citat.*) Ficinus, (*lib.* 2. *de sanitate tuendâ*) Marsilius Cognatus, Montaltus, (*cap.* 27) Guianerius, (*Tract.* 3. *cap.* 2) Magninus, (*cap.* 5. *part.* 3) [5] gives the reason, because [6] *it infrigidates and dryes up the body, consumes the spirits; and would therefore have all such as are cold and dry, to take heed of and to avoid it, as a mortal enemy.* Jacchinus (*in* 9 *Rhasis, cap.* 15) ascribes the same cause, and instanceth in a patient of his, that married a young wife in a hot summer, [7] *and so*

---

[1] Nobilis senex Alsatus juvenem uxorem duxit: at ille, colico dolore et multis morbis correptus, non potuit præstare officium mariti, vix inito matrimonio ægrotus. Illa in horrendum furorem incidit, ob Venerem cohibitam, ut omnium eam invisentium congressum, voce, vultu, gestu, expeteret: et, quum non consentirent, molossos Anglicanos magno expetiit clamore. [2] Vidi sacerdotem optimum et pium, qui, quod nollet uti Venere, in melancholica symptomata incidit. [3] Ob abstinentiam a concubitu incidit in melancholiam. [4] Quæ a coitu exacerbantur. [5] Superfluum coitum caussam ponunt. [6] Exsiccat corpus, spiritus consumit, &c. caveant ab hoc sicci, velut inimico mortali. [7] Ita exsiccatus, ut e melancholico statim fuerit insanus ; ab humectantibus curatus.

Mem. 2. Subs. 4.] *Retention and Evacuation, Causes.* 237

dryed himself with chamber-work, that he became, in short space, from melancholy, mad: he cured him by moistning remedies. The like example I find in Lælius a Fonte Eugubinus (*consult.* 129) of a gentlemen of Venice, that, upon the same occasion, was first melancholy, afterwards mad. Read in him the story at large.

Any other evacuation stopped will cause it, as well as these above named, be it bile, [1] ulcer, issue, &c. Hercules de Saxoniâ, (*lib.* 1. *cap.* 16) and Gordonius verefie this out of their experience. They saw one wounded in the head, who, as long as the sore was open, *lucida habuit mentis intervalla,* was well; but, when it was stopped, *rediit melancholia,* his melancholy fit seized on him again.

Artificial evacuations are much like in effect, as hot-houses, baths, blood-letting, purging, unseasonably and immoderately used. [2] Baths dry too much, if used in excess, be they natural or artificial, and offend, extream hot, or cold; [3] one dries, the other refrigerates, over-much. Montanus (*consil.* 137) saith they over-heat the liver. Joh. Struthius (*Stigmat. artis, l.* 4. *c.* 9) contends, [4] *that if one stay longer than ordinary at the bath, go in too oft, or at unseasonable times, he putrifies the humours in his body.* To this purpose writes Magninus *l.* 3. *c.* 5). Guianerius (*Tract.* 15. *c.* 21) utterly disallows all hot baths in melancholy adust. [5] *I saw* (saith he) *a man that laboured of the gout, who, to be freed of his malady, came to the bath, and was instantly cured of his disease, but got another worse, and that was madness.* But this judgment varies, as the humour doth, in hot or cold. Baths may be good for one melancholy man, bad for another; that which will cure it in this party, may cause it in a second.

Phlebotomy.] Phlebotomy, many times neglected, may do much harm to the body, when there is a manifest redundance of bad humours and melancholy blood; and when these humours heat and boyl, if this be not used in time, the parties affected so inflamed, are in great danger to be mad; but if it be unadvisedly, importunely, immoderately, used, it doth as much harm by refrigerating the body, dulling the spirits, and consuming them. As Joh. [6] Curio, in his tenth chapter, well reprehends, such kind of letting blood doth more hurt than good: [7] *the humours rage much more than they did before; and is so far from avoiding melancholy, that it increaseth it, and*

---

[1] Ex cauterio et ulcere exsiccato. [2] Gord. c. 10. lib. 1. discommends cold baths, as noxious. [3] Siccum reddunt corpus. [4] Si quis longius moretur in iis, aut nimis frequenter aut importune utatur, humores putrefacit. [5] Ego anno superiore quemdam guttosum vidi adustum, qui, ut liberaretur de guttâ, ad balnea accessit, et, de guttâ liberatus, maniacus factus est. [6] On Schola Salernitana. [7] Calefactio et ebullitio per venæ incisionem magis sæpe incitatur et augetur; majore impetu humores per corpus discurrunt.

238   *Bad Air, a Cause.*   [Part. 1. Sec. 2.

weakeneth the sight. [1] Prosper Calenus observes as much of all
phlebotomy, except they keep a very good diet after it : yea,
and, as [2] Leonartus Jacchinus speaks out of his own experience,
[3] *the blood is much blacker to many men after their letting
of blood, than it was at first.* For this cause, belike, Salust.
Salvinianus (*l. 2. c.* 1) will admit or hear of no blood-letting
at all in this disease, except it be manifest it proceeds from
blood. He was (it appears, by his own words in that place)
master of an hospital of mad men, [4] *and found, by long experience, that this kind of evacuation, either in head, arm, or any
other part, did more harm than good.* To this opinion of his
[5] Felix Plater is quite opposite : *though some wink at, disallow,
and quite contradict, all phlebotomy in melancholy, yet by long
experience I have found innumerable so saved, after they had
been twenty, nay, sixty times let blood, and to live happily after
it. It was an ordinary thing of old, in Galens time, to take at
once from such men six pound of blood, which we now dare
scarce take in ounces : sed viderint medici :* great books are
written of this subject.

Purging upward and downward, in abundance of bad humours
omitted may be for the worst ; so likewise, as in the precedent,
if over-much, too frequent or violent, it [6] weakeneth their
strength, saith Fuchsius (*l. 2. sect. 2. c.* 17) : or, if they be
strong or able to endure physick, yet it brings them to an ill
habit ; they make their bodies no better than apothecaries shops ;
this, and such like infirmities, must needs follow.

SUBSECT. V.

Bad Air a Cause of Melancholy.

AIR is a cause of great moment, in producing this or any
other disease, being that it is still taken into our bodies by
respiration, and our more inner parts. [7] *If it be impure and
foggy, it dejects the spirits, and causeth diseases by infection
of the heart,* as Paulus hath it (*lib.* 1. *c.* 49), Avicenna,
(*l.* 1) Gal. (*de san. tuendâ*), Mercurialis, Montaltus, &c.
[8] Fernelius saith, *a thick air thickneth the blood and hu-*

---

[1] Lib. de flatulentâ Melancholiâ. Frequens sanguinis missio, corpus extenuat.
[2] In 9 Rhasis. Atram bilem parit, et visum debilitat.   [3] Multo nigrior spectatur sanguis post dies quosdam, quam fuit ab initio.   [4] Non laudo eos qui
in desipientiâ docent secandam esse venam frontis, quia spiritus debilitantur
inde, et ego longâ experientiâ observavi in proprio xenodochio, quod desipientes
ex phlebotomiâ magis læduntur, et magis desipiunt ; et melancholici sæpe fiunt
inde pejores.   [5] De mentis alienat. cap. 3. etsi multos hoc improbâsse
sciam, innumeros hac ratione sanatos longâ observatione cognovi, qui vigesies,
sexagies venas tundendo, &c.   [6] Vires debilitat.   [7] Impurus aër
spiritus dejicit ; infecto corde gignit morbos.   [8] Sanguinem densat, et humores, P. l. c. 13.

Mem. 2. Subs. 5.]   *Causes of Melancholy.*   239

mours. [1] Lemnius reckons up two main things, most profitable and most pernicious to our bodies—air and diet: and this peculiar disease nothing sooner causeth ([2] Jubertus holds) *than the air wherein we breath and live.* [3] Such as is the air, such be our spirits: and, as our spirits, such are our humours. It offends, commonly, if it be too [4] hot and dry, thick, fuliginous, cloudy, blustering, or a tempestuous air. Bodine (in his fifth book *de repub. cap.* 1. *et cap.* 5. of his Method of History) proves that hot countreys are most troubled with melancholy, and that there are therefore in Spain, Africk, and Asia Minor, great numbers of mad men, insomuch that they are compelled, in all cities of note, to build peculiar hospitals for them. Leo [5] Afer *(lib. 3. de Fessâ urbe)*, Ortelius, and Zuinger, confirm as much. They are ordinarily so cholerick in their speeches, that scarce two words pass without railing or chiding in common talk, and often quarrelling in their streets. [6] Gordonius will have every man take notice of it: *Note this,* (saith he) *that in hot countreys, it is far more familiar than in cold:* although this we have now said be not continually so; for, as [7] Acosta truly saith, under the æquator it self, is a most temperate habitation, wholsome air, a paradise of pleasure: the leaves ever green, cooling showres. But it holds in such as are intemperately hot, as [8] Johannes a Meggen found in Cyprus, others in Malta, Apulia, and the [9] Holy Land, where, at some seasons of the year, is nothing but dust, their rivers dryed up, the air scorching hot, and earth inflamed ; insomuch that many pilgrims going barefoot, for devotion sake, from Joppa to Jerusalem upon the hot sands, often run mad, or else quite overwhelmed with sand, *profundis arenis,* as in many parts of Africk, Arabia Deserta, Bactriana, now Charassan, when the west wind blows, [10] *involuti arenis transeuntes necantur.* [11] Hercules de Saxoniâ, a professor in Venice, gives this cause, why so many Venetian women are melancholy, *quod diu sub sole degant,* they tarry too long in the sun, Montanus *(consil. 21),* amongst other causes, assigns this, why that Jew his patient was mad *quod tam multum exposuit se calori et frigori ;* he exposed himself so much to heat and cold. And, for that reason,

---

[1] Lib 3. cap. 3.   [2] Lib. de quartanâ. Ex aëre ambiente contrahitur humor melancholicus.   [3] Qualis aër, talis spiritus ; et cujusmodi spiritus, humores.   [4] Ælianus Montaltus, c. 11. calidus et siccus, frigidus et siccus, paludinosus, crassus.   [5] Multa hic in xenodochiis fanaticorum millia, quæ strictissime catenata servantur.   [6] Lib. med. part. 2. c. 19. Intellige, quod in calidis regionibus frequenter accidit mania, in frigidis autem tarde.   [7] Lib. 2.   [8] Hodopericon, c. 7.   [9] Apulia æstivo calore maxime fervet, ita ut ante finem Maii pene exusta sit.   [10] Maginus, Pers.   [11] Pantheo, seu Pract. med. l. 1. c. 16.   Venetæ mulieres, quæ diu sub sole vivunt, aliquando melancholicæ evadunt.

240   *Causes of Melancholy.*   [Part. 1. Sec. 2.

in Venice, there is little stirring in those brick-paved streets in
summer about noon; they are most part then asleep; as they
are likewise in the great Mogors countreys, and all over the
East Indies. At Aden, in Arabia, as [1] Lodovicus Vertomannus
relates in his travels, they keep their markets in the night,
to avoid extremity of heat; and in Ormus, like cattle in a pasture, people of all sorts lye up to the chin in water all day long.
At Braga in Portugal, Burgos in Castile, Messina, in Sicily,
all over Spain and Italy, their streets are most part narrow, to
avoid the sun-beams. The Turks wear great turbans, *ad fu-*
gandos solis radios, to refract the sun-beams; and much inconvenience that hot air of Bantam in Java yields to our
men, that sojourn there for traffick; where it is so hot, [2] *that*
they that are sick of the pox, lye commonly bleaching in the
sun, to dry up their sores. Such a complaint I read of those
Isles of Cape Verde, fourteen degrees from the equator: they
do *male audire :* [3] one calls them the unhealthiest clime of
the world, for fluxes, fevers, frenzies, calentures, which commonly seize on sea-faring men that touch at them, and all by
reason of a hot distemperature of the air. The hardiest men
are offended with this heat; and stiffest clowns cannot resist
it, as Constantine affirms, *Agricul. l. 2. c.* 45. They that are
naturally born in such air may not [4] endure it, as Niger records
of some part of Mesopotamia, now called Diarbecha; *qui-*
busdam in locis sævienti æstu adeo subjecta est, ut pleraque
animalia fervore solis et cæli extinguantur ; 'tis so hot there in
some places, that men of the countrey and cattle are killed
with it; and [5] Adricomius, of Arabia Felix, by reason of myrrhe,
frankincense, and hot spices there growing, the air is so obnoxious to their brains that the very inhabitants at some
times cannot abide it, much less weaklings and strangers.
[6] Anatus Lusitanus (*cent.* 1. *curat.* 45) reports of a young maid,
that was one Vincent a curriers daughter, some thirty years of
age, that would wash her hair in the heat of the day (in July)
and so let it dry in the sun, [7] *to make it yellow; but by that*
means, tarrying too long in the heat, she inflamed her head,
and made her self mad.

Cold air in the other extream, is almost as bad as hot; and so
doth Montaltus esteem of it, (*c.* 11) if it be dry withal. In those
northern countreys, the people are therefore generally dull,

---

[1] Navig. l. 2. c. 4. commercia nocte, horâ secundâ, ob nimios, qui sæviunt interdiu, æstus, exercent.   [2] Morbo Gallico laborantes exponunt ad solem, ut
morbos exsiccent.   [3] Sir. Rich. Haukins, in his Observations, sect. 13.
[4] Hippocrates. 3. Aphorismorum, idem ait.   [5] Idem Maginus in Persiâ.
[6] Descrip. Ter. sanct.   [7] Quum ad solis radios in leone longam moram
traheret, ut capillos flavos redderet, in maniam incidit.

2

Mem. 2. Subs. 5.]   *Bad Air, a Cause.*

heavy, and many witches; which (as I have before quoted)
Saxo Grammaticus, Olaus, Baptista Porta, ascribe to melancholy. But these cold climes are more subject to natural melancholy (not this artificial) which is cold and dry : for which
cause [1] Mercurius Britannicus, belike, puts melancholy men
to inhabit just under the pole. The worst of the three is a
[2] thick, cloudy, misty, foggy air, or such as comes from fens,
moorish grounds, lakes, muckhils, draughts, sinks, where any
carkasses, or carrion lyes, or from whence any stinking fulsom
smell comes. Galen, Avicenna, Mercurialis, new and old physicians, hold that such air is unwholsom, and ingenders melancholy, plagues, and what not ? [3] Alexandretta, an haven town
in the Mediterranean sea, Saint John de Ullua, an haven in
Nova-Hispania, are much condemned for a bad air, so as
Durazzo in Albania, Lithuania, Ditmarsh, Pomptinæ paludes
in Italy, the territories about Pisa, Ferrara, &c. Rumney
marsh with us, the hundreds in Essex, the fens in Lincolnshire. Cardan (*de rerum varietate, l.* 17. *c.* 96) finds fault with
the site of those rich and most populous cities in the Low
Countreys, as Bruges, Gant, Amsterdam, Leyden, Utrecht,
&c. the air is bad, and so at Stockholm in Sweden, Regium
in Italy, Salisbury with us, Hull and Lin. They may be
commodious for navigation, this new kind of fortification, and
many other good necessary uses : but are they so wholsom ?
Old Rome hath descended from the hills to the valley ; 'tis the
site of most of our new cities, and held best to build in
plains, to take the opportunity of rivers. Leander Albertus
pleads hard for the air and site of Venice, though the black
moorish lands appear at every low water. The sea, fire, and
smoke, (as he thinks) qualifie the air : and [4] some suppose that
a thick foggy air helps the memory, as in them of Pisa in
Italy ; and our Cambden (out of Plato) commends the site of
Cambridge, because it is so near the fens   But, let the site of
such places be as it may, how can they be excused that have a
delicious seat, a pleasant air, and all that nature can afford,
and yet, through their own nastiness and sluttishness, immund
and sordid manner of life, suffer their air to putrifie, and
themselves to be choked up? Many cities in Turkey do
male audire in this kind: Constantinople it self, where commonly carryon lyes in the street. Some find the same fault in
Spain, even in Madrit, the kings seat, a most excellent air, a
pleasant site ; but the inhabitants are slovens, and the streets
uncleanly kept.

---

[1] Mundus alter et idem, seu Terra Australis incognita.   [2] Crassus et turbidus
aër tristem efficit animam.   [3] Commonly called Scandarone, in Asia Minor.
[4] Atlas Geographicus. Memoriâ valent Pisani, quod crassiore fruantur aëre.

VOL. I.   R

242   *Causes of Melancholy.*   [Part. 1. Sec. 2.

A troublesom tempestuous air is as bad as impure ; rough, and foul weather, impetuous winds, cloudy dark dayes, as it is commonly with us : *cœlum visu fœdum,* [1] Polydore calls it—a filthy sky, *et in quo facile generantur nubes ;* as Tullies brother Quintus wrote to him in Rome, being then quæ stor in Britain. *In a thick and cloudy air,* (saith Lemnius) *men are tetrick, sad, and pievish: and if the western winds blow, and that there be a calm, or a fair sunshine day, there is a kind of alacrity in mens minds; it cheers up men and beasts: but if it be a turbulent, rough, cloudy, stormy weather, men are sad, lumpish, and much dejected, angry, waspish, dull, and melancholy.* This was [2] Virgils experiment of old,

> Verum, ubi tempestas, et cœli mobilis humor,
> Mutavere vices, et Jupiter humidus Austris. . . . .
> Vertuntur species animorum, et pectora motus
> Concipiunt alios————

> But, when the face of heaven changed is
> To tempests, rain, from seasons fair,
> Our minds are altered, and in our breasts
> Forthwith some new conceits appear.

And who is not weather-wise against such and such conjunctions of planets, moved in foul weather, dull and heavy in such tempestuous seasons? [3] *Gelidum contristat Aquarius annum;* the time requires, and the autumn breeds it; winter is like unto it, ugly, foul, squalid ; the air works on all men, more or less, but especially on such as are melancholy, or inclined to it, as Lemnius holds : [4] *they are most moved with it; and those which are already mad, rave downright, either in or against a tempest. Besides, the devil many time takes his opportunity of such storms ; and, when the humours by the air be stirred, he goes on with them, exagitates our spirits, and vexeth our souls; as the sea-waves, so are the spirits and humours in our bodies tossed with tempestuous winds and storms.* To such as are melancholy therefore, Montanus (*consil.* 24) will have tempestuous and rough air to be avoided, and (*consil.* 27) all night air, and would not have them to walk abroad, but in a pleasant day. Lemnius (*lib. 3. cap. 3.*) discommends the south and eastern winds, commends the north. Montanus

---

[1] Lib. 1. hist. lib. 1. cap. 41. Aurâ densâ ac caliginosâ tetrici homines existunt, et subtristes. Et cap. 3. Flante subsolano et Zephyro, maxima in mentibus hominum alacritas existit, mentisque erectio, ubi cœlum solis splendore nitescit. Maxima dejectio mœrorque, siquando aura caliginosa est.   [2] Geor.   [3] Hor.
[4] Mens quibus vacillat, ab aëre cito offenduntur ; et multi insani apud Belgas ante tempestates sæviunt, aliter quieti. Spiritus quoque aëris, et mali genii, aliquando se tempestatibus ingerunt, et menti humanæ se latenter insinuant, eamque vexant, exagitant ; et, ut fluctus marini, humanum corpus ventis agitatur.
2

Mem. 2. Subs. 6.] *Immoderate Exercise a Cause.* 243

(*consil.* 31) [1] *will not any windows to be opened in the night:*
(*consil.* 29. *et consil.* 230) he discommends especially the south
wind, and nocturnal air: so doth [2] Plutarch : the night and
darkness makes men sad ; the like do all subterranean vaults,
dark houses in caves and rocks ; desert places cause melancholy
in an instant, especially such as have not been used to it, or
otherwise accustomed. Read more of air in Hippocrates,
Aëtius, *lib.* 3. *a c.* 171. *ad* 175. Oribasius, *à c.* 1. *ad* 22.
Avicen. *l.* 1. *can. Fen.* 2. *doc.* 2. *Fen.* 1. *c.* 123. *to the* 12, &c.

SUBSECT. VI.

Immoderate Exercise a Cause, and how. Solitariness, Idleness.

NOTHING so good, but it may be abused. Nothing better
than exercise (if opportunely used) for the preservation of the
body: nothing so bad, if it be unseasonable, violent, or over-
much. Fernelius (out of Galen, *Path. lib.* 1. *cap.* 16) saith,
[3] *that much exercise and weariness consumes the spirits and substance, refrigerates the body ; and such humours which nature
would have otherwise concocted and expelled, it stirs up and
makes them rage ; which being so enraged, diversely affect, and
trouble the body and mind.* So doth it, if it be unseasonably
used, upon a full stomach, or when the body is full of crudities,
which Fuchsius so much inveighs against, (*Lib.* 2. *instit. sect.* 2.
cap. 4) giving that for a cause, why school-boys in Germany
are so often scabbed, because they use exercise presently after
meats. [4] Bayerus puts in a caveat against such exercise, because
it [5] *corrupts the meat in the stomach, and carries the same juice
raw, and as yet undigested, into the veins* (saith Lemnius), *which
there putrifies, and confounds the animal spirits.* Crato (*consil.*
21. *l.* 2) [6] protests against all such exercise after meat, as being
the greatest enemy to concoction that may be, and cause of
corruption of humours, which produce this and many other
diseases. Not without good reason then, doth Sallust, Salvianus (*l.* 2. *c.* 1), and Leonartus Jacchinus (*in* 9 *Rhasis*) Mercurialis, Arculanus, and many other, set down [7] immoderate exercise as a most forcible cause of melancholy.

---

[1] Aër noctu densatur, et cogit mœstitiam. [2] Lib. de Iside et Osiride.
[3] Multa defatigatio spiritus viriumque substantiam exhaurit, et corpus refrigerat.
Humores corruptos, qui aliter a naturâ concoqui et domari possint, et demum
blande excludi, irritat, et quasi in furorem agit, qui postea (mota Camarina) tetro
vapore corpus varie lacessunt, animumque. [4] In Veni mecum, Libro sic in-
scripto. [5] Instit. ad vit. Christ. cap. 44. Cibos crudos in venas rapit, qui pu-
trescentes illic spiritus animales inficiunt. [6] Crudi hæc humoris copia per
venas aggeritur ; unde morbi multiplices. [7] Immodicum exercitium.

R 2

244 *Causes of Melancholy.* [Part. 1. Sec. 2

Opposite to exercise is idleness (the badge of gentry), or want of exercise, the bane of body and mind, the nurse of naughtiness, step-mother of discipline, the chief author of all mischief, one of the seven deadly sins, and a sole cause of this and many other maladies, the devils cushion, (as [1] Gualter calls it) his pillow and chief reposal: *for the mind can never rest, but still meditates on one thing or other: except it be occupied about some honest business, of his own accord it rusheth into melancholy.* [2] *As too much and violent exercise offends on the one side, so doth an idle life on the other* (saith Crato): *it fills the body full of flegm, gross humours, and all manner of obstructions, rheums, catarrhs, &c.* Rhasis (*cont. lib.* 1. *tract.* 9) accounts of it as the greatest cause of melancholy. [3] *I have often seen,* (saith he) *that idleness begets this humour more than any thing else.* Montaltus (*c.* 1.) seconds him out of his experience: [4] *they that are idle are far more subject to melancholy, than such as are conversant or employed about any office or business.* [5] Plutarch reckons up idleness for a sole cause of the sickness of the soul; *there are those* (saith he) *troubled in mind, that have no other cause but this.* Homer (*Iliad* 1) brings in Achilles eating of his own heart in his idleness, because he might not fight. Mercurialis, *consil.* 86, for a melancholy young man, urgeth [6] it as a chief cause: why was he melancholy? because idle. Nothing begets it sooner, encreaseth and continueth it oftener, than idleness;— a disease familiar to all idle persons, an inseparable companion to such as live at ease, (*pingui otio desidiose agentes*) a life out of action, and have no calling or ordinary employment to busie themselves about; that have small occasions; and, though they have, such is their laziness, dulness, they will not compose themselves to do ought; they cannot abide work, though it be necessary, easie, as to dress themselves, write a letter, or the like. Yet, as he that is benummed with cold, sits still shaking, that might relieve himself with a little exercise or stirring, do they complain, but will not use the facile and ready means to do themselves good; and so are still tormented with melancholy. Especially if they had been formerly brought up to

---

[1] Hom. 31. in 1. Cor. 6. Nam, quum mens hominis quiescere non possit, sed continuo circa varias cogitationes discurrat, nisi honesto aliquo negotio occupetur, ad melancholiam sponte delabitur.   [2] Crato, consil. 21. Ut immodica corporis exercitatio nocet corporibus, ita vita deses et otiosa : otium animal pituitosum reddit, viscerum obstructiones, et crebras fluxiones, et morbos concitat. [3] Et vidi quod una de rebus quæ magis generat melancholiam, est otiositas. [4] Reponitur otium ab aliis caussa ; et hoc a nobis observatum, eos huic malo magis obnoxios qui plane otiosi sunt, quam eos qui aliquo munere versantur exsequendo. [5] De Tranquil. animæ. Sunt quos ipsum otium in animi conjicit ægritudinem. [6] Nihil est quod æque melancholiam alat ac augeat, ac otium et abstinentia a corporis et animi exercitationibus.

Mem. 2. Subs. 6.] *Idleness a Cause.* 245

business, or to keep much company, and upon a sudden come
to lead a sedentary life, [1] it crucifies their souls, and seizeth on
them in an instant; for, whilest they are any ways imployed,
in action, discourse, about any business, sport or recreation, or
in company to their liking, they are very well; but, if alone or
idle, tormented instantly again: one days solitariness, one
hours sometimes, doth them more harm, than a weeks physick, labour and company can do good. Melancholy seizeth
on them forthwith, being alone, and is such a torture, that, as
wise Seneca well saith, *malo mihi male quam molliter esse*, I
had rather be sick than idle. This idleness is either of body
or mind. That of body is nothing but a kind of benumming
laziness, intermitting exercise, which (if we may believe [2] Fernelius) *causeth crudities, obstructions, excremental humours,
quencheth the natural heat, dulls the spirits, and makes them
unapt to do any thing whatsoever.*

[3] Neglectis urenda filix innascitur agris.

As fern grows in untild grounds, and all manner of weeds, so
do gross humours in an idle body: *ignavum corrumpunt otia
corpus.* A horse in a stable, that never travels, a hawk in a
mew, that seldom flies, are both subject to diseases; which, left
unto themselves, are most free from any such incumbrances.
An idle dog will be mangy; and how shall an idle person think
to escape? Idleness of the mind is much worse than this of
the body: wit without employment, is a disease, [4] *ærugo
animi, rubigo ingenii:* the rust of the soul, [5] a plague, a hell
it self; *maximum animi nocumentum,* Galen calls it. [6] *As
in a standing pool, worms and filthy creepers increase, (et vitium capiunt, ni moveantur, aquæ;* the water itself putrifies,
and air likewise, if it be not continually stirred by the wind) *so
do evil and corrupt thoughts in an idle person;* the soul is con-
taminated. In a common-wealth, where is no public enemy,
there is, likely, civil wars, and they rage upon themselves;
this body of ours, when it is idle, and knows not how to bestow it self, macerates and vexeth it self with cares, griefs,
false fears, discontents, and suspicions; it tortures and preys
upon his own bowels, and is never at rest. Thus much I dare
boldly say, he or she that is idle, be they of what condition
they will, never so rich, so well allied, fortunate, happy—let

---

[1] Nihil magis excæcat intellectum, quam otium. Gordonius, de observat. vit.
hum. lib. 1.   [2] Path. lib. 1. cap. 17. exercitationis intermissio, inertem calorem,
languidos spiritus, et ignavos, et ad omnes actiones segniores, reddit; cruditates,
obstructiones, et excrementorum proventus facit.   [3] Hor. Ser. 1. Sat. 3.
[4] Seneca.   [5] Mœrorem animi, et maciem, Plutarch calls it.   [6] Sicut in
stagno generantur vermes, sic in otioso malæ cogitationes. Sen.

246   *Causes of Melancholy.*   [Part. 1. Sec. 2.

them have all things in abundance, and felicity, that heart can wish and desire, all contentment—so long as he, or she, or they, are idle, they shall never be pleased, never well in body and mind, but weary still, sickly still, vexed still, loathing still, weeping, sighing, grieving, suspecting, offended with the world, with every object, wishing themselves gone or dead, or else carried away with some foolish phantasie or other. And this is the true cause that so many great men, ladies, and gentlewomen, labour of this disease in countrey and city; for idleness is an appendix to nobility; they count it a disgrace to work, and spend all their days in sports, recreations, and pastimes, and will therefore take no pains, be of no vocation; they feed liberally, fare well, want exercise, action, employment, (for to work, I say, they may not abide) and company to their desires; and thence their bodies become full of gross humours, wind, crudities, their minds disquieted, dull, heavy, &c. Care, jealousie, fear of some diseases, sullen fits, weeping fits, seize too [1] familiarly on them : for, what will not fear and phantasie work in an idle body? what distempers will they not cause? When the children of Israel murmured [2] against Pharaoh in Ægypt, he commanded his officers to double their task, and let them get straw themselves, and yet make their full number of brick: for the sole cause why they mutiny, and are evil at ease, is, *they are idle.* When you shall hear and see so many discontented persons in all places where you come, so many several grievances, unnecessary complaints, fears, suspicions [3], the best means to redress it, is to set them awork, so to busie their minds; for the truth is, they are idle. Well they may build castles in the air for a time, and sooth up themselves with phantastical and pleasant humours ; but in the end they will prove as bitter as gall; they shall be still, I say, discontent, suspicious, [4]fearful, jealous, sad, fretting and vexing of themselves ; so long as they be idle, it is impossible to please them. *Otio qui nescit uti, plus habet negotii, quam qui negotium in negotio,* as that [5] Agellius could observe: he that knows not how to spend his time, hath more business, care, grief, anguish of mind, than he that is most busie in the midst of all his business. *Otiosus animus nescit quid volet :* an idle person (as he follows it) knows not when he is well, what he would have, or whither he would go ; *quum illuc ventum est, illinc lubet;* he is tired out with every thing, displeased with all, weary of his life : *nec bene domi, nec militiæ,* neither at

---

[1] Now this leg, now that arm, now their head, heart, &c.   [2] Exod. 5.
[3] (For they cannot well tell what aileth them, or what they would have themselves) my heart, my head, my husband, my son, &c.   [4] Pro. 18. Pigrum dejiciet timor—Heautontimorumenon.   [5] Lib. 19. c. 10.

Mem. 2. Subs. 6.]   *Idleness a Cause.*   247

home or abroad; *errat, et præter vitam vivit;* he wanders, and lives besides himself. In a word, what the mischievous effects of laziness and idleness are, I do not find any where more accurately expressed, than in these verses of Philolaches in the [1] Comical Poet, which, for their elegancy, I will in part insert.

> Novarum ædium esse arbitror similem ego hominem,
> Quando hic natus est.   Ei rei argumenta dicam.
> Ædes quando sunt ad amussim expolitæ,
> Quisque laudat fabrum, atque exemplum expetit, &c.
> At ubi illo migrat nequam homo indiligensque, &c.
> Tempestas venit, confringit tegulas, imbricesque, &c.
> Putrefacit aër operam fabri, &c.
> *Dicam* ut homines similes esse ædium arbitremini.
> Fabri parentes fundamentum substruunt liberorum ;
> Expoliunt, docent literas, nec parcunt sumptui.
> Ego autem sub fabrorum potestate frugi fui ;
> Postquam autem migravi in ingenium meum,
> Perdidi operam fabrorum illico, oppido
> Venit ignavia ; ea mihi tempestas fuit,
> Adventuque suo grandinem et imbrem attulit.
> Illa mihi virtutem deturbavit, &c.

A young man is like a fair new house : the carpenter leaves it well built, in good repair, of solid stuff; but a bad tenant lets it rain in, and, for want of reparation, fall to decay, &c. Our parents, tutors, friends, spare no cost to bring us up in our youth, in all manner of vertuous education ; but when we are left to our selves, idleness, as a tempest, dries all vertuous motions out of our minds; *et nihili sumus;* on a sudden, by sloth and such bad wayes, we come to nought.

Cozen german to idleness, and a concomitant cause, which goes hand in hand with it, is [2] *nimia solitudo,* too much solitariness—by the testimony of all physicians, cause and symptome both : but as it is here put for a cause, it is either coact, enforced, or else voluntary. Enforced solitariness is commonly seen in students, monks, friers, anchorites, that by their order and course of life, must abandon all company, society of other men, and betake themselves to a private cell; *otio superstitioso seclusi* (as Bale and Hospinian well term it), such as are the Carthusians of our time, that eat no flesh (by their order), keep perpetual silence, never go abroad; such as live in prison, or some desert place, and cannot have company, as many of our countrey gentlemen do in solitary houses ; they must either be alone without companions, or live beyond their means, and

---

[1] Plautus, Mostel.   [2] Piso, Montaltus, Mercurialis, &c.

248   *Causes of Melancholy.*   [Part. 1. Sec. 2.

entertain all comers as so many hosts, or else converse with
their servants and hinds, such as are unequal, inferior to
them, and of a contrary disposition: or else, as some do, to
avoid solitariness, spend their time with leud fellows in taverns,
and in ale-houses, and thence addict themselves to some unlawful disports, or dissolute courses. Divers again are cast
upon this rock of solitariness for want of means, or out of a
strong apprehension of some infirmity, disgrace: or, through
bashfulness, rudeness, simplicity, they cannot apply themselves
to others company. *Nullum solum infelici gratius solitudine, ubi nullus sit qui miseriam exprobret.* This enforced
solitariness takes place, and produceth his effect soonest, in
such as have spent their time jovially, peradventure in all
honest recreations, in good company, in some great family or
populous city, and are upon a sudden confined to a desart
country cottage far off, restrained of their liberty, and barred
from their ordinary associates. Solitariness is very irksom
to such, most tedious, and a sudden cause of great inconvenience.

Voluntary solitariness is that which is familiar with melancholy, and gently brings on, like a Siren, a shooing-horn, or
some Sphinx, to this irrevocable gulf: [1] a primary cause Piso
calls it: most pleasant it is at first, to such as are melancholy
given, to lie in bed whole dayes, and keep their chambers, to
walk alone in some solitary grove, betwixt wood and water, by
a brook side, to meditate upon some delightsome and pleasant
subject, which shall affect them most; *amabilis insania,* and
mentis gratissimus error. A most incomparable delight it is
so to melancholize, and build castles in the air, to go smiling
to themselves, acting an infinite variety of parts, which they
suppose, and strongly imagine they represent, or that they see
acted or done. *Blanda quidem ab initio,* saith Lemnius, to
conceive and meditate of such pleasant things sometimes,
[2] *present, past, or to come,* as Rhasis speaks. So delightsome
these toyes are at first, they could spend whole days and
nights without sleep, even whole years alone in such contemplations, and phantastical meditations, which are like
unto dreams; and they will hardly be drawn from them,
or willingly interrupt. So pleasant their vain conceits are,
that they hinder their ordinary tasks and necessary business; they cannot address themselves to them, or almost to
any study or imployment: these phantastical and bewitching
thoughts so covertly, so feelingly, so urgently, so continually,
set upon, creep in, insinuate, possess, overcome, distract, and

---

[1] A quibus malum, velut a primariâ caussâ, occasionem nactum est.   [2] Jucunda rerum præsentium, præteritarum, et futurarum meditatio.

Mem. 2. Subs. 6.] *Idleness a Cause.* 249

detain them, they cannot, I say, go about their more necessary business, stave off, or extricate themselves, but are ever musing, melancholizing, and carried along, as he (they say) that is led round about an heath with a *Puck* in the night. They run earnestly on in this labyrinth of anxious and solicitous melancholy meditations, and cannot well or willingly refrain, or easily leave off, winding and unwinding themselves, as so many clocks, and still pleasing their humours, until at last the scene is turned upon a sudden, by some bad object: and they, being now habituated to such vain meditations and solitary places, can endure no company, can ruminate of nothing but harsh and distasteful subjects. Fear, sorrow, suspicion, *subrusticus pudor,* discontent, cares and weariness of life, surprize them in a moment; and they can think of nothing else: continually suspecting, no sooner are their eyes open, but this infernal plague of melancholy seizeth on them, and terrifies their souls, representing some dismal object to their minds, which now, by no means, no labour, no perswasions, they can avoid; *hæret lateri lethalis arundo;* they may not be rid of it; [1] they cannot resist. I may not deny but that there is some profitable meditation, contemplation, and kind of solitariness, to be embraced, which the fathers so highly commended—[2] Hierom, Chrysostom, Cyprian, Austin, in whole tracts, which Petrarch, Erasmus, Stella, and others, so much magnifie in their books—a paradise, an heaven on earth, if it be used aright, good for the body, and better for the soul; as many of those old monks used it, to divine contemplations; as Simulus, a courtier in Adrians time, Dioclesian the emperour, retired themselves, &c. in that sense, *Vatia solus scit vivere;* Vatia lives alone; which the Romans were wont to say, when they commended a countrey life; or to the bettering of their knowledge, as Democritus, Cleanthes, and those excellent philosophers, have ever done, to sequester themselves from the tumultuous world; or, as in Plinies villa Laurentana, Tullies Tusculan, Jovius study, that they might better *vacare studiis et Deo,* serve God and follow their studies. Methinks, therefore, our too zealous innovators were not so well advised in that general subversion of abbies and religious houses, promiscuously to fling down all. They might have taken away those gross abuses crept in amongst them, rectified such inconveniences, and not so far to have raved and raged against those fair buildings, and everlasting monuments of our forefathers devotion, consecrated to pious

---

[1] Facilis descensus Averni; Sed revocare gradum, superasque evadere ad auras, Hic labor, hoc opus est. Virg.   [2] Hieronymus, ep. 72. dixit oppida et urbes videri sibi tetros carceres, solitudinem Paradisum; solum scorpionibus infestum, sacco amictus, humi cubans, aquâ et herbis victitans, Romanis prætulit deliciis.

250 *Causes of Melancholy.* [Part. 1. Sec. 2.

uses. Some monasteries and collegiate cells might have been well spared, and their revenues otherwise imployed; here and there one, in good towns or cities at least, for men and women of all sorts and conditions to live in, to sequester themselves from the cares and tumults of the world, that were not desirous or fit to marry, or otherwise willing to be troubled with common affairs, and know not well where to bestow themselves, to live apart in, for more conveniency, good education, better company sake; to follow their studies (I say) to the perfection of arts and sciences, common good, and, as some truly devoted monks of old had done, freely and truly to serve God: for these men are neither solitary, nor idle, as the poet made answer to the husbandman in Æsop, that objected idleness to him, he was never so idle as in his company; or that Scipio Africanus in [1] Tully, *numquam minus solus, quam quum solus; numquam minus otiosus, quam quum esset otiosus;* never less solitary than when he was alone, never more busie, than when he seemed to be most idle. It is reported by Plato, in his dialogue *de Amore,* in that prodigious commendation of Socrates, how, a deep meditation coming into Socrates mind by chance, he stood still musing, *eodem vestigio cogitabundus,* from morning to noon; and, when as then he had not yet finished his meditation, *perstabat cogitans;* he so continued till the evening: the souldiers (for he then followed the camp) observed him with admiration, and on set purpose watched all night; but he persevered immovable *ad exortum solis,* till the sun rose in the morning, and then, saluting the sun, went his wayes. In what humour constant Socrates did thus, I know not, or how he may be affected: but this would be pernicious to another man; what intricate business might so really possess him, I cannot easily guess. But this is *otiosum otium;* it is far otherwise with these men, according to Seneca: *omnia nobis mala solitudo persuadet;* this solitude undoeth us: *pugnat cum vitâ sociali;* 'tis a destructive solitariness. These men are devils, alone, as the saying is; *homo solus aut deus, aut dæmon;* a man, alone, is either a saint or a devil; *mens ejus aut languescit, aut tumescit;* and [2] *væ soli!* in this sense; woe be to him that is so alone! These wretches do frequently degenerate from men, and, of sociable creatures, become beasts, monsters, inhumane, ugly to behold, *misanthropi;* they do even loath themselves, and hate the company of men, as so many Timons, Nebuchadnezzars, by too much indulging to these pleasing humours, and through their own default. So that which Mercurialis (*consil.* 11) sometimes expostulated with his melancholy patient, may be justly applied to every

[1] Offic. 3.   [2] Eccl. 4.

Mem. 2. Subs. 7.]   *Sleeping and waking, Causes.*   251

solitary and idle person in particular : [1] *natura de te videtur conqueri posse, &c. nature may justly complain of thee, that, whereas she gave thee a good wholesome temperature, a sound body, and God hath given thee so divine and excellent a soul, so many good parts and profitable gifts, thou hast not only contemned and rejected, but hast corrupted them, polluted them, overthrown their temperature, and perverted those gifts with riot, idleness, solitariness, and many other wayes : thou art a traitour to God and Nature, an enemy to thy self and to the world. Perditio tua ex te ;* thou hast lost thy self wilfully, cast away thy self; *thou thy self art the efficient cause of thine own misery, by not resisting such vain cogitations, but giving way unto them.*

SUBSECT. VII.

Sleeping and waking, Causes.

WHAT I have formerly said of exercise, I may now repeat of sleep. Nothing better than moderate sleep; nothing worse than it, if it be in extreams, or unseasonably used. It is a received opinion, that a melancholy man cannot sleep overmuch : *somnus supra modum prodest,* as an only antidote ; and nothing offends them more, or causeth this malady sooner, than waking. Yet in some cases, sleep may do more harm than good, in that flegmatick, swinish, cold, and sluggish melancholy, which Melancthon speaks of, that thinks of waters, sighing most part, &c. [2] It duls the spirits (if overmuch) and senses, fills the head full of gross humours, causeth distillations, rheumes, great stores of excrements in the brain, and all the other parts, as [3] Fuchsius speaks of them, that sleep like so many dormice. Or, if it be used in the day time, upon a full stomach, the body ill composed to rest, or after hard meats, it increaseth fearful dreams, *incubus,* night walking, crying out, and much unquietness. Such sleep prepares the body, as [4] one observes, to *many perilous diseases.* But, as I have said, waking overmuch is both a symptome and an ordinary cause. *It causeth driness of the brain, frensie, dotage, and makes the*

---

[1] Natura de te videtur conqueri posse, quod, cum ab eâ temperatissimum corpus adeptus sis; tam præclarum a Deo ac utile donum, non contempsisti modo, verum corrupisti, fœdâsti, prodidisti, optimam temperaturam otio, crapulâ, et aliis vitæ erroribus, &c.   [2] Path. lib. cap. 17.   Fern. corpus infrigidat ; omnes sensus, mentisque vires, torpore debilitat.   [3] Lib. 2. sect. 2. cap. 4. Magnam excrementorum vim cerebro et aliis partibus coacervat.   [4] Jo. Retzius, lib. de rebus 6 non naturalibus.   Præparat corpus talis somnus ad multas periculosas ægritudines.

252   *Causes of Melancholy.*   [Part. 1. Sec. 2.

body dry, lean, hard, and ugly to behold, as [1] Lemnius hath it.
*The temperature of the brain is corrupted by it, the humours
adust, the eyes made to sink into the head, choler increased,
and the whole body inflamed;* and (as may be added out of Galen, 3. *de sanitate tuendá, Avicenna* 3. 1) [2] *it overthrows the
natural heat; it causeth crudities, hurts concoction* ; and what
not? Not without good cause, therefore, Crato, (*consil.* 21.
lib. 2), Hildesheim (*spicil.* 2. *de delir. et Maniá*), Jacchinus, Arculanus (on *Rhasis*), Guianerius, and Mercurialis, reckon up
this overmuch waking, as a principal cause.

MEMB. III. SUBSECT. I.

*Passions and Perturbations of the Mind, how they cause
Melancholy.*

As that Gymnosophist, in [3] Plutarch, made answer to Alexander (demanding which spake best), every one of his fellows,
did speak better than the other; so may I say of these causes,
to him that shall require which is the greatest, every one is
more grievous than other, and this of passion the greatest of
all; a most frequent and ordinary cause of melancholy, [4] *fulmen
perturbationum* (Piccolomineus calls it), this thunder and lightning of perturbation, which causeth such violent and speedy
alterations in this our microcosm, and many times subverts the
good estate and temperature of it: for, as the body works upon
the mind, by his bad humours, troubling the spirits and sending gross fumes into the brain, and so *per consequens*, disturb-
ing the soul, and all the faculties of it.

———————————————[5] Corpus onustum :
Hesternis vitiis, animum quoque prægravat unà,

with fear, sorrow, &c. which are ordinary symptomes of this
disease : so, on the other side, the mind most effectually
works upon the body, producing by his passions and perturbations, miraculous alterations, as melancholy, despair, cruel
diseases, and sometimes death it self; insomuch that it is most
true which Plato saith in his Charmides; *omnia corporis
mala ab animá procedere:* all the [6] mischiefs of the body

---

[1] Instit. ad vitam optimam, c. 26. cerebro siccitatem adfert, phrenesin et delirium: corpus aridum facit, squalidum, strigosum ; humores adurit; temperamen-
tum cerebri corrumpit; maciem inducit: exsiccat corpus, bilem accendit, pro-
fundos reddit oculos, calorem auget.   [2] Naturalem calorem dissipat;
læsâ concoctione, cruditates facit. Attenuant juvenum vigilatæ corpora noctes.
[3] Vita Alexand.   [4] Grad. 1. c. 14.   [5] Hor.   [6] Perturbationes clavi
sunt, quibus corpori animus ceu patibulo affigitur. Jamb. de myst.

[Mem. 3. Subs. 1.] *Perturbations of the Mind.* 253

proceed from the soul: and Democritus in [1] Plutarch urgeth, *Damnatum iri animam a corpore;* if the body should, in this behalf, bring an action against the soul, surely the soul would be cast and convicted, that by her supine negligence, had caused such inconveniences, having authority over the body, and using it for an instrument, as a smith doth his hammer, saith [2] Cyprian, imputing all those vices and maladies to the mind. Even so doth [3] Philostratus, *non coinquinatur corpus, nisi consensu animæ;* the body is not corrupted, but by the soul. [4] Lodovicus Vives will have such turbulent commotions proceed from ignorance, and indiscretion. All philosophers impute the miseries of the body to the soul, that should have governed it better by command of reason, and hath not done it. The Stoicks are altogether of opinion (as [5] Lipsius and [6] Piccolomineus record) that a wise man should be απαθης. without all manner of passions and perturbations whatsoever, as [7] Seneca reports of Cato, the [8] Greeks of Socrates, and [9] Jo. Aubanus of a nation in Africk, so free from passion, or rather so stupid, that, if they be wounded with a sword, they will only look back. [10] Lactantius (*2 instit.*) will exclude *fear from a wise man;* others except all, some the greatest passions. But, let them dispute how they will, set down in *thesi,* give precepts to the contrary; we find that of [11] Lemnius true by common experience; *no mortal man is free from these perturbations:* or if he be so, sure he is either a god, or a block. They are born and bred with us, we have them from our parents by inheritance: *a parentibus habemus malum hunc assem,* saith [12] Pelezius; *nascitur unà nobiscum, aliturque;* 'tis propagated from Adam; Cain was melancholy, [13] as Austin hath it; and who is not? Good discipline, education, philosophy, divinity, (I cannot deny) may mitigate and restrain these passions in some few men at some times; but, most part, they domineer, and are so violent, [14] that as a torrent, (*torrens velut aggere rupto*) bears down all before, and overflows his banks, *sternit agros, sternit sata*—they overwhelm reason, judgement, and pervert the temperature of the body. *Fertur* [15] *equis auriga, neque audit currus habenas.* Now such a man (saith [16] Austin) *that is so led, in a wise mans eye, is no better*

---

[1] Lib. de sanitat. tuend.   [2] Proleg. de virtute Christi. Quæ utitur corpore, ut faber malleo.   [3] Vita Apollonii, lib. 1.   [4] Lib. de anim. ab inconsiderantiâ, et ignorantiâ omnes animi motus.   [5] De Physiol. Stoic.   [6] Grad. 1. c. 32.   [7] Epist. 104.   [8] Ælianus.   [9] Lib. 1. cap. 6. si quis ense percusserit eos, tantum respiciunt.   [10] Terror in sapiente esse non debet. [11] De occult. nat. mir. l. 1. c. 16. Nemo mortalium, qui affectibus non ducatur: qui non movetur, aut saxum aut Deus est.   [12] Instit. l. 2. de humanorum affect. mórborumque curat.   [13] Epist. 105.   [14] Granatensis.   [15] Virg. [16] De civit. Dei, l. 14. c. 9. qualis in oculis hominum, qui inversis pedibus ambulat, talis in oculis sapientum, cui passiones dominantur.

254   *Causes of Melancholy.*   [Part. 1. Sec. 2.

than he that stands upon his head. It is doubted by some, *gravioresne morbi a perturbationibus, an ab humoribus,* whether humours or perturbations cause the more grievous maladies. But we find that of our Saviour (*Mat.* 26, 41) most true: *the spirit is willing; the flesh is weak;* we cannot resist; and this of [1] Philo Judæus: *perturbations often offend the body, and are most frequent causes of melancholy, turning it out of the hinges of his health.* Vives compares them to [2] *winds upon the sea; some only move, as those great gales; but others turbulent, quite overturn the ship.* Those which are light, easie, and more seldom, to our thinking, do us little harm, and are therefore contemned of us: yet if they be reiterated, [3] *as the rain* (saith Austin) *doth a stone, so do these perturbations penetrate the mind,* [4] and (as one observes) *produce an habit of melancholy at the last,* which having gotten the mastery in our souls, may well be called diseases.

How these passions produce this effect, [5] Agrippa hath handled at large, *Occult. Philos. l.* 11. *c.* 63; Cardan, *l.* 14. *subtil.* Lemnius, *l.* 1. *c.* 12. *de occult. nat. mir. et lib.* 1. *cap.* 16; Suarez, *Met. disput.* 18. *sect.* 1. *art.* 25; T. Bright, *cap.* 12. of his Melancholy Treatise; Wright the Jesuit, in his book of the Passions of the Mind, &c.—thus in brief—To our imagination cometh, by the outward sense or memory, some object to be known (residing in the foremost part of the brain), which he misconceiving or amplifying, presently communicates to the heart, the seat of all affections. The pure spirits forthwith flock from the brain to the heart, by certain secret channels, and signifie what good or bad object was presented; [6] which immediately bends it self to prosecute or avoid it, and, withal, draweth with it other humours to help it. So, in pleasure, concur great store of purer spirits; in sadness, much melancholy blood; in ire, choler. If the imagination be very apprehensive, intent, and violent, it sends great store of spirits to or from the heart, and makes a deeper impression, and greater tumult: as the humours in the body be likewise prepared, and the temperature it self ill or well disposed, the passions are longer and stronger: so that the first step and fountain of all our grievances in this

---

[1] Lib. de Decal. passiones maxime corpus offendunt et animam, et frequentissimæ caussæ melancholiæ, dimoventes ab ingenio et sanitate pristinâ, l. 3. de animâ.   [2] Fræna et stimuli animi; velut in mari quædam auræ leves, quædam placidæ, quædam turbulentæ; sic in corpore quædam affectiones excitant tantum, quædam ita movent, ut de statu judicii depellant.   [3] Ut gutta lapidem, sic paullatim hæ penetrant animum.   [4] Usu valentes, recte morbi animi vocantur.   [5] Imaginatio movet corpus, ad cujus motum excitantur humores, et spiritus vitales, quibus alteratur.   [6] Eccles. 13. 26. The heart alters the countenance to good or evil: and distraction of the mind causeth distemperature of the body.

Mem. 3. Subs. 2.]   *Of the Force of Imagination.*   255

kind is ¹*læsa imaginatio,* which, mis-informing the heart, causeth all these distemperatures, alteration and confusion of spirits and humours; by means of which, so disturbed, concoction is hindered, and the principal parts are much debilitated; as ² Dr. Navarra well declared, being consulted by Montanus about a melancholy Jew.   The spirits so confounded, the nourishment must needs be abated, bad humours increased, crudities and thick spirits ingendred, with melancholy blood.   The other parts cannot perform their functions, having the spirits drawn from them by vehement passion, but fail in sense and motion: so we look upon a thing, and see it not; hear and observe not; which otherwise would much affect us, had we been free.   I may therefore conclude with ³ Arnoldus, *maxima vis est phantasiæ: et huic uni fere, non autem corporis intemperiei, omnis melancholiæ caussa est ascribenda :* great is the force of imagination; and much more ought the cause of melancholy to be ascribed to this alone, than to the distemperature of the body.   Of which imagination, because it hath so great a stroke in producing this malady, and is so powerful of it self, it will not be improper to my discourse, to make a brief digression, and speak of the force of it, and how it causeth this alteration. Which manner of digression howsoever some dislike, as frivolous and impertinent, yet I am of ⁴ Beroaldus his opinion, *such digressions do mightily delight and refresh a weary reader ; they are like sawce to a bad stomach ; and I do therefore most willingly use them.*

SUBSECT. II.

Of the Force of Imagination.

WHAT Imagination is, I have sufficiently declared in my digression of the anatomy of the soul.   I will only now point at the wonderful effects and power of it; which, as it is eminent in all, so most especially it rageth in melancholy persons, in keeping the species of objects so long, mistaking, amplifying them by continual and ⁵ strong meditation, until at length it produceth in some parties real effects, causeth this, and many

---

¹ Spiritus et sanguis a læsâ imaginatione contaminantur; humores enim mutati actiones animi immutant. Piso.   ² Montani consil. 22. Hæ vero quomodo causent melancholiam, clarum : et quod concoctionem impediant, et membra principalia debilitent.   ³ Breviar. l. 1. cap. 18.   ⁴ Solent hujusmodi egressiones favorabiliter oblectare, et lectorem lassum jucunde refovere, stomachumque nauseantem, quodam quasi condimento, reficere: et ego libenter excurro.   ⁵ Ab imaginatione oriuntur affectiones, quibus anima componitur, aut turbatur. Jo. Sarisbur. Matolog. lib. 4. c. 10.

256   *Causes of Melancholy.*   [Part. 1. Sec. 2.

other maladies. And, although this phantasie of ours be a
subordinate faculty to reason, and should be ruled by it, yet in
many men, through inward or outward distemperatures, defect
of organs, which are unapt or hindered, or otherwise contami-
nated, it is likewise unapt, hindred, and hurt. This we see
verified in sleepers, which, by reason of humours and concourse
of vapours troubling the phantasie, imagine many times absurd
and prodigious things, and in such as are troubled with *incubus,*
or witch-ridden (as we call it) : if they lie on their backs, they
suppose an old woman rides and sits so hard upon them, that
they are almost stifled for want of breath : when there is nothing offends, but a concourse of bad humours, which trouble
the phantasie. This is likewise evident in such as walk in the
night in their sleep, and do strange feats : [1] these vapours move
the phantasie, the phantasie the appetite, which, moving the
animal spirits, causeth the body to walk up and down, as if they
were awake.   Fracast. (*l. 3. de intellect.*) refers all extasies to
this force of imagination ; such as lye whole dayes together in a
trance, as that priest whom [2] Celsus speaks of, that could separate himself from his senses when he list, and lie like a dead
man void of life and sense.   Cardan brags of himself, that he
could do as much, and that when he list.   Many times such
men, when they come to themselves, tell strange things of heaven and hell, what visions they have seen ; as that S[r]. Owen in
Matthew Paris, that went into St. Patricks Purgatory, and the
monk of Evesham in the same author. Those common apparitions in Bede and Gregory, Saint Bridgets revelations, Wier, *l. 3.*
de lamiis c. 11, Cæsar Vanninus in his Dialogues, &c. reduceth,
(as I have formerly said) with all those tales of witches progresses, dancing, riding, transformations, operations, &c. to the
force of [3] imagination, and the [4] devils allusions. The like effects
almost are to be seen in such as are awake; how many chimæras,
anticks, golden mountains, and castles in the air, do they build
unto themselves ! I appeal to painters, mechanicians, mathematicians.   Some ascribe all vices to a false and corrupt imagination, anger, revenge, lust, ambition, covetousness, which
prefers falshood, before that which is right and good, deluding
the soul with false shews and suppositions. [5] Bernardus Penottus
will have heresie and superstition to proceed from this fountain ;
as he falsely imagineth, so he believeth; and as he conceiveth of
it, so it must be, and it shall be ; *contra gentes* he will have it

[1] Scalig. exercit.   [2] Qui, quoties volebat, mortuo similis jacebat, auferens
se a sensibus ; et, quum pungeretur, dolorem non sensit.   [3] Idem Nymannus,
orat. de Imaginat.   [4] Verbis et unctionibus se consecrant dæmoni pessimæ
mulieres, qui iis ad opus suum utitur, et earum phantasiam regit, ducitque ad
loca ab ipsis desiderata : corpora vero earum sine sensu permanent, quæ umbrâ
cooperit diabolus, ut nulli sint conspicua ; et post, umbrâ sublatâ, propriis corporibus eas restituit, l. 3. c. 11. Wier.   [5] Denario medico.

Mem. 3. Subs. 2.] *Of the Force of Imagination.* 257

so. But most especially in passions and affections, it shews strange and evident effects : what will not a fearful man conceive in the dark? what strange forms of bugbears, devils, witches, goblins? Lavater imputes the greatest cause of spectrums, and the like apparitions, to fear, which, above all other passions, begets the strongest imagination (saith [1] Wierus) ; and so likewise love, sorrow, joy, &c. Some die suddenly, as she that saw her son come from the battel at Cannæ, &c. Jacob the patriarch, by force of imagination, made peckled lambs, laying peckled rods before his sheep. Persina, that Æthiopian queen in Heliodorus, by seeing the picture of Perseus and Andromeda, in stead of a blackmoor, was brought to bed of a fair white child ; in imitation of whom, belike, an hard favoured fellow in Greece, because he and his wife were both deformed, to get a good brood of children, *elegantissimas imagines in thalamo collocavit,* &c. hung the fairest pictures he could buy for money in his chamber, *that his wife, by frequent sight of them, might conceive and bear such children.* And, if we may believe Bale, one of Pope Nicholas the thirds concubines, by seeing of [2] a bear, was brought to bed of a monster. *If a woman* (saith [3] Lemnius) *at the time of her conception, think of another man present or absent, the child will be like him.* Great-bellied women, when they long, yield us prodigious examples in this kind, as moles, warts, scars, harelips, monsters, especially caused in their children by force of a depraved phantasie in them. *Ipsam speciem, quam animo effigiat, fetui inducit :* she imprints that stamp upon her child, which she [4] conceives unto her self. And therefore Lodovicus Vives (*lib. 2.* de *Christ. fem.*) gives a special caution to greatbellied women, [5] *that they do not admit such absurd conceits and cogitations, but by all means avoid those horrible objects, heard or seen, or filthy spectacles.* Some will laugh, weep, sigh, groan, blush, tremble, sweat, at such things as are suggested unto them by their imagination. Avicenna speaks of one that could cast himself into a palsie when he list ; and some can imitate the tunes of birds and beasts, that they can hardly be discerned. Dagobertus and Saint Francis scars and wounds, like to those of Christ (if at the least any such were),

---

[1] Solet timor, præ omnibus affectibus, fortes imaginationes gignere ; post, amor &c. l. 3. c. 8.　　[2] Ex viso urso, talem peperit.　　[3] Lib. 1. cap. 4. de occult. nat. mir. Si, inter amplexus et suavia, cogitet de uno aut alio absente, ejus effigies solet in fetu elucere.　　[4] Quid non fetui, adhuc matri unito, subitâ spirituum vibratione, per nervos, quibus matrix cerebro conjuncta est, imprimit imprægnatæ imaginatio? ut, si imaginetur malum granatum, illius notas secum proferet fetus ; si leporem, infans editur supremo labello bifido, et dissecto. Vehemens cogitatio movet rerum species. Wier. l. 3. cap. 8.　　[5] Ne, dum uterum gestent, admittant absurdas cogitationes · sed et visu, audituque fœda et horrenda devitent.

VOL. I.　　　　　　　　　S

258   *Causes of Melancholy.*   [Part. 1. Sec. 2.

[1] Agrippa supposeth to have hapned by force of imagination.
That some are turned to wolves, from men to women, and
women again to men, (which is constantly believed) to the same
imagination; or from men to asses, dogs, or any other shapes—
[2] Wierus ascribes all those famous transformations to imagination. That, in *hydrophobia*, they seem to see the picture
of a dog still in their water; [3] that melancholy men, and sick
men, conceive so many phantastical visions, apparitions to
themselves, and have such absurd suppositions, as that they are
kings, lords, cocks, bears, apes, owls; that they are heavy, light,
transparent, great and little, senseless and dead, (as shall be
shewn more at large, in our [4] Sections of Symptomes) can be
imputed to nought else, but to a corrupt, false, and violent imagination. It works not in sick and melancholy men only, but
even most forcibly sometimes in such as are sound: it makes
them suddenly sick, and [5] alters their temperature in an instant. And sometimes a strong conceit or apprehension, as
[6] Valesius proves, will take away diseases: in both kinds, it
will produce real effects. Men, if they see but another man
tremble, giddy or sick of some fearful disease, their apprehension and fear is so strong in this kind, that they will have the
same disease. Or if, by some sooth-sayer, wise-man, fortune-
teller, or physician, they be told they shall have such a disease,
they will so seriously apprehend it, that they will instantly
labour of it—a thing familiar in China (saith Riccius the
Jesuit:) [7] *if it be told them that they shall be sick on such a day,*
when that day comes, they will surely be sick, and will be so
terribly afflicted, that sometimes they dye upon it. Dr. Cotta
(in his Discovery of ignorant Practitioners of Physick, *cap.* 8.)
hath two strange stories to this purpose, what phansie is able
to do; the one of a parsons wife in Northamptonshire, *anno*
1607, that, coming to a physician, and told by him that she was
troubled with the *sciatica,* as he conjectured, (a disease she was
free from) the same night after her return, upon his words fell
into a grievous fit of a *sciatica :* and such another example he
hath of another good wife, that was so troubled with the cramp;
after the same manner she came by it, because her physician
did but name it. Sometimes death itself is caused by force of
phantasie. I have heard of one, that, coming by chance in

---

[1] Occult. Philos. l. 1. c. 64.   [2] Lib. 3. de Lamiis, cap. 10.   [3] Agrippa,
lib. 1. cap. 64.   [4] Sect. 3. memb. 1. subsect. 3.   [5] Malleus malefic. fol.
77. Corpus mutari potest in diversas ægritudines, ex forti apprehensione.   [6] Fr.
Vales. l. 5. cont. 6. Nonnumquam etiam morbi diuturni consequuntur, quandoque curantur.   [7] Expedit. in Sinas, l. 1. c. 9. Tantum porro multi præ-
dictoribus hisce tribuunt, ut ipse metus fidem faciat : nam, si prædictum iis fuerit
tali die eos morbo corripiendos, ii, ubi dies advenerit, in morbum incidunt : et, vi
metûs afflicti, cum ægritudine, aliquando etiam cum morte, colluctantur.

Mem. 3. Subs. 2.]   *Of the Force of Imagination.*   259

company of him that was thought to be sick of the plague (which was not so,) fell down suddenly dead. Another was sick of the plague with conceit. One, seeing his fellow let blood, falls down in a swoun. Another (saith [1] Cardan, out of Aristotle) fell down dead, (which is familiar to women at any ghastly sight) seeing but a man hanged. A Jew in France (saith [2] Lodovicus Vives) came by chance over a dangerous passage or plank, that lay over a brook, in the dark, without harm; the next day, perceiving what danger he was in, fell down dead. Many will not believe such stories to be true, but laugh commonly, and deride when they hear of them: but let these men consider with themselves, (as [3] Peter Byarus illustrates it) if they were set to walk upon a plank on high, they would be giddy, upon which they dare securely walk upon the ground. Many, (saith Agrippa) [4] *strong hearted men otherwise, tremble at such sights: dazel, and are sick, if they look but down from an high place; and what moves them but conceit?* As some are so molested by phantasie; so some again, by fancy alone and a good conceit, are as easily recovered. We see commonly the tooth-ach, gout, falling-sickness, biting of a mad dog, and many such maladies, cured by spells, words, characters, and charms; and many green wounds, by that now so much used *unguentum armarium,* magnetically cured; which Crollius and Goclenius in a book of late have defended, Libavius in a just tract as stifly contradicts, and most men controvert. All the world knows there is no vertue in such charms, or cures, but a strong conceit and opinion alone, (as [5] Pomponatius holds) *which forceth a motion of the humours, spirits, and blood; which takes away the cause of the malady from the parts affected.* The like we may say of our magical effects, superstitious cures, and such as are done by mountebanks and wizards. *As, by wicked incredulity, many men are hurt* (so saith [6] Wierus of charms, spells, &c.) *we find, in our experience, by the same means many are relieved.* An empirick oftentimes, and a silly chirurgion, doth more strange cures, than a rational physician. Nymannus gives a reason—because the patient puts his confidence in him; [7] which Avicenna *prefers before art, precepts, and all remedies whatsoever.* 'Tis opinion alone, (saith [8] Cardan) that makes or marrs physicians; and he doth the best

---

[1] Subtil. 18.   [2] Lib. 3. de animâ, cap. de mel.   [3] Lib. de Peste.
[4] Lib. 1. cap. 63. Ex alto despicientes, aliqui præ timore contremiscunt, caligant, infirmantur; sic singultus, febres, morbi comitiales, quandoque sequuntur, quandoque recedunt.   [5] Lib. de Incantatione. Imaginatio subitum humorum et spirituum motum infert; unde vario affectu rapitur sanguis, ac unâ morbificas caussas partibus affectis eripit.   [6] L. 3. cap. 18. de præstig. Ut impiâ credulitate quis læditur, sic et levari eundem credibile est, usuque observatum.
[7] Ægri persuasio et fiducia omni arti et consilio et medicinæ præferenda. Avicen.
[8] Plures sanat, in quem plures confidunt. lib. de sapientiâ.

s 2

260 *Causes of Melancholy.* [Part. 1. Sec. 2.

cures, according to Hippocrates, in whom most trust. So diversly doth this phantasie of ours affect, turn, and wind, so imperiously command our bodies, which, as another [1] *Proteus, or a cameleon, can take all shapes, and is of such force* (as Ficinus adds) *that it can work upon others, as well as ourselves.* How can otherwise blear-eyes in one man cause the like affection in another? Why doth one man's yawning [2] make another yawn? one mans pissing, provoke a second many times to do the like? Why doth scraping of trenchers offend a third, or hacking of files? Why doth a carkass bleed, when the murtherer is brought before it, some weeks after the murther hath been done? Why do witches and old women fascinate and bewitch children? but (as Wierus, Paracelsus, Cardan, Mizaldus, Valleriola, Cæsar Vanninus, Campanella, and many philosophers think) the forcible imagination of the one party moves and alters the spirits of the other. Nay more, they can cause and cure not only diseases, maladies, and several infirmities, by this means, (as Avicenna, *de anim. l. 4. sect. 4.* supposeth) in parties remote, but move bodies from their places, cause thunder, lightning, tempests; which opinion Alkindus, Paracelsus, and some others, approve of; so that I may certainly conclude, this strong conceit or imagination is *astrum hominis,* and the rudder of this our ship, which reason should steer, but, over-born by phantasie, cannot manage, and so suffers it self and this whole vessel of ours to be over-ruled, and often overturned. Read more of this in Wierus, *l. 3. de Lamiis, c.* 8, 9, 10. Franciscus Valesius *med. controv. l.* 5. *cont.* 6. Marcellus Donatus, *l. 2. c.* 1. *de hist. med. mirabil.* Levinus Lemnius, *de occult. nat. mir. l.* 1. *c.* 12. Cardan, *l.* 18. *de rerum var.* Corn. Agrippa, *de occult. Philos. cap.* 64, 65. Camerarius, 1. *Cent. cap.* 54. *horarum subcis.* Nymannus, *in orat. de Imag.* Laurentius, and him that is *instar omnium,* Fienus, a famous physician of Antwerp, that wrote three books *de viribus imaginationis.* I have thus far digressed, because this imagination is the *medium deferens* of passions, by whose means they work and produce many times prodigious effects; and as the phantasie is more or less intended or remitted, and their humours disposed, so do perturbations move more or less, and make deeper impression.

---

[1] Marcilius Ficinus, l. 13. c. 18. de theolog. Platonicâ. Imaginatio est tanquam Proteus vel chamæleon, corpus proprium et alienum nonnumquam afficiens.
[2] Cur oscitantes oscitent. Wierus.

SUBSECT. III.

Division of Perturbations.

PERTURBATIONS and passions, which trouble the phantasie, though they dwell between the confines of sense and reason, yet they rather follow sense than reason, because they are drowned in corporeal organs of sense. They are commonly [1] reduced into two inclinations, *irascible* and *concupiscible*. The Thomists subdivide them into eleven, six in the *coveting*, and five in the *invading*. Aristotle reduceth all to pleasure and pain; Plato, to love and hatred; [2] Vives, to good and bad. If good, it is present, and then we absolutely joy and love: or to come, and then we desire or hope for it: if evil, we absolutely hate it: if present, it is sorrow; if to come, fear. These four passions [3] Bernard compares *to the wheels of a chariot, by which we are carried in this world.* All other passions are subordinate under these four, or six, as some will—love, joy, desire, hatred, sorrow, fear. The rest, as anger, envy, emulation, pride, jealousie, anxiety, mercy, shame, discontent, despair, ambition, avarice, &c. are reducible unto the first: and, if they be immoderate, they [4] consume the spirits; and melancholy is especially caused by them. Some few discreet men there are, that can govern themselves, and curb in these inordinate affections, by religion, philosophy, and such divine precepts of meekness, patience, and the like; but most part, for want of government, out of indiscretion, ignorance, they suffer themselves wholly to be led by sense, and are so far from repressing rebellious inclinations, that they give all encouragement unto them, leaving the reins, and using all provocations to further them. Bad by nature, worse by art, discipline, [5] custom, education, and a perverse will of their own, they follow on, wheresoever their unbridled affections will transport them, and do do more out of custom, self will, than out of reason. *Contumax voluntas* (as Melancthon calls it) *malum facit:* this stubborn will of ours perverts judgement, which sees and knows what should and ought to be done, and yet will not do it. *Mancipia gulæ*, slaves to their several lusts and appetite, they precipitate and plunge [6] themselves into a labyrinth of cares:

---

[1] T. W. Jesuit.   [2] 3. de Animâ.   [3] Ser. 35. Hæ quatuor passiones sunt tamquam rotæ in curru, quibus vehimur hoc mundo.   [4] Harum quippe immoderatione, spiritus marcescunt. Fernel. l. 1. Path. c. 18.   [5] Malâ consuetudine depravatur ingenium, ne bene faciat. Prosper Calenus. l. de atrâ bile. Plura faciunt homines e consuetudine, quam e ratione.—A teneris assuescere multum est.—Video meliora proboque; Deteriora sequor. Ovid.   [6] Nemo læditur, nisi a seipso.

262   *Causes of Melancholy.*   [Part. 1. Sec. 2.

blinded with lust, blinded with ambition, [1] *they seek that at Gods hands, which they may give unto themselves, if they could but refrain from those cares and perturbations, wherewith they continually macerate their mindes.* But giving way to these violent passions of fear, grief, shame, revenge, hatred, malice, &c. they are torn in pieces, as Actæon was with his dogs, and [2] crucifie their own souls.

SUBSECT. IV.

Sorrow, a Cause of Melancholy.

Sorrow. Insanus dolor.] In this catalogue of passions, which so much torment the soul of man, and cause this malady, (for I will briefly speak of them all, and in their order) the first place in this irascible appetite may justly be challenged by *sorrow—* an inseparable companion, [3] *the mother and daughter of melancholy, her epitome, symptome, and chief cause.* As Hippocrates hath it, they beget one another and tread in a ring; for sorrow is both cause and symptome of this disease. How it is a symptome, shall be shewed in his place. That it is a cause, all the world acknowledgeth. *Dolor nonnullis insaniæ caussa fuit, et aliorum morborum insanabilium,* saith Plutarch to Apollonius; a cause of madness, a cause of many other diseases; a sole cause of this mischief, [4] Lemnius calls it. So doth Rhasis, *cont. l.* 1. *tract.* 9. Guianerius, *tract.* 15. c. 5. And, if it take root once, it ends in despair, as [5] Felix Plater observes, and (as in [6] Cebes table) may well be coupled with it. [7] Chrysostom, in his seventeenth epistle to Olympia, describes it to be *a cruel torture of the soul, a most inexplicable grief, poisoned worm, consuming body and soul, and gnawing the very heart, a perpetual executioner, continual night, pro-*

---

[1] Multi se in inquietudinem præcipitant: ambitione et cupiditatibus excæcati, non intelligunt se illud a diis petere, quod sibi ipsis, si velint, præstare possint, si curis et perturbationibus, quibus assidue se macerant, imperare vellent.   [2] Tanto studio miseriarum caussas, et alimenta dolorum, quærimus; vitamque, secus felicissimam, tristem et miserabilem efficimus. Petrarch. præfat. de Remediis, &c. [3] Timor et mœstitia, si diu perseverent, caussa et soboles atri humoris sunt, et in circulum se procreant. Hipp. Aphoris. 23. l. 6. Idem Montaltus, cap. 19. Victorius Faventinus, pract. imag.   [4] Multi ex mœrore et metu huc delapsi sunt. Lemn. lib. i. cap. 16.   [5] Multa cura et tristitia faciunt accedere melancholiam: (cap. 3. de mentis alien.) si altas radices agat, in veram fixamque degenerant melancholiam, et in desperationem desinit. [6] Ille, luctus; ejus vero soror desperatio simul ponitur.   [7] Animarum crudele tormentum, dolor inexplicabilis, tinea, non solum ossa, sed corda, pertingens, perpetuus carnifex, vires animæ consumens, jugis nox et tenebræ profundæ, tempestas, et turbo, et febris non apparens, omni igne validius incendens, longior, et pugna finem non habens —Crucem circumfert dolor, faciemque omni tyranno crudeliorem præ se fert.

found darkness, a whirlwind, a tempest, an ague not appearing, heating worse than any fire, and a battle that hath no end. It crucifies worse than any tyrant: no torture, no strappado, no bodily punishment, is like unto it. 'Tis the eagle, without question, which the poets fained to gnaw [1] Prometheus heart; *and no heaviness is like unto the heaviness of the heart* (Ecclus. 25. 15, 16). [2] *Every perturbation is a misery; but grief a cruel torment*, a domineering passion. As in old Rome, when the Dictator was created, all inferiour magistracies ceased —when grief appears, all other passions vanish. *It dries up the bones* (saith Solomon, *c.* 17. Prov.); makes them hollow-ey'd, pale, and lean, furrow-faced, to have dead looks, wrinkled brows, riveled cheeks, dry bodies, and quite perverts their temperature, that are misaffected with it; as Elenora, that exil'd mournful duchess, (in our [3] English Ovid) laments to her noble husband, Humphrey duke of Gloucester—

> Sawest thou those eyes, in whose sweet cheerful look,
> Duke Humphrey once such joy and pleasure took,
> Sorrow hath so despoil'd me of all grace,
> Thou couldst not say this was my Elnors face.
> Like a foul Gorgon, &c.

[4] *It hinders concoction, refrigerates the heart, takes away stomach, colour, and sleep; thickens the blood* ([5] Fernelius, *l.* 1. *c.* 18. *de morb. caussis*), *contaminates the spirits,* ([6] Piso) overthrows the natural heat, perverts the good estate of body and mind, and makes them weary of their lives, cry out, howl, and roar, for very anguish of their souls. David confessed as much: (Psal. 38. 8.) *I have roared for the very disquietness of my heart:* and (Psal. 119. 4. part. 4. v.) *my soul melteth away for very heaviness:* (vers. 38) *I am like a bottle in the smoak.* Antiochus complained that he could not sleep, and that his heart fainted for grief. [7] Christ himself, *vir dolorum*, out of an apprehension of grief, did sweat blood, (Mark 14): his soul was heavy to the death, and no sorrow was like unto his. Crato (*consil.* 21. *l.* 2) gives instance in one that was so melancholy by reason of [8] grief; and Montanus (*consil.* 30) in a noble

---

[1] Nat. Comes, Mythol. l. 4. c. 6.   [2] Tully, 3. Tusc. omnis perturbatio miseria; et carnificina est dolor.   [3] M. Drayton, in his Her. ep.   [4] Crato consil. 21. lib. 2. mœstitia universum infrigidat corpus, calorem innatum extinguit, appetitum destruit.   [5] Cor refrigerat tristitia, spiritus exsiccat, innatumque calorem obruit, vigilias inducit, concoctionem labefactat, sanguinem incrassat, exaggeratque melancholicum succum.   [6] Spiritus et sanguis hoc contaminatur. Piso.   [7] Marc. 6. 16. 11.   [8] Mœrore maceror, marcesco, et consenesco, miser: ossa atque pellis sum miserâ macritudine. Plaut.

264   *Causes of Melancholy.*   [Part. 1. Sec. 2.

matron, *¹ that had no other cause of this mischief.* J. S. D.
(in Hildesheim) fully cured a patient of his, that was much
troubled with melancholy, and for many years; *² but afterwards
by a little occasion of sorrow, he fell into his former fits, and was
tormented as before.* Examples are common, how it causeth
melancholy, *³ desperation,* and sometimes death it self; for
(Ecclus. 38. 15) *of heaviness comes death. Worldly sorrow
causeth death.* (2 Cor. 7. 10. Psal. 31. 10.) *My life is wasted
with heaviness, and my years with mourning.* Why was Hecuba
said to be turned to a dog? Niobe, into a stone? but that for
grief she was senseless and stupid. Severus the emperour
*⁴ dyed for grief; and how *⁵ many myriads besides!

> Tanta illi est feritas, tanta est insania luctûs.

Melancthon gives a reason of it—*⁶ the gathering of much melancholy blood about the heart; which collection extinguisheth
the good spirits, or at least dulleth them; sorrow strikes the
heart, makes it tremble and pine away, with great pain : and
the black blood, drawn from the spleen, and diffused under the
ribs on the left side, makes those perilous hypochondriacal convulsions, which happen to them that are troubled with sorrow.*

SUBSECT. V.

Fear, a Cause.

Cosen german to *sorrow,* is *fear,* or rather a sister,—*fidus
Achates,* and continual companion—an assistant and a principal agent in procuring of this mischief; a cause and symptome
as the other. In a word, as *⁷ Virgil of the Harpies, I may
justly say of them both,

> Tristius haud illis monstrum ; nec sævior ulla
> Pestis, et ira Deûm, Stygiis sese extulit undis.

> A sadder monster, or more cruel plague so fell,
> Or vengeance of the Gods, ne'er came from Styx or Hell.

---

¹ Malum inceptum et actum a tristitiâ solâ.   ² Hildesheim, spicil. 2. de
melancholiâ. Mœrore animi postea accedente, in priora symptomata incidit.
³ Vives, 3. de animâ, c. de mœrore, Sabin. in Ovid.   ⁴ Herodian. l. 3. Mœrore
magis quam morbo consumptus est.   ⁵ Bothwellius atribilarius obiit, Brizarrus
Genuensis hist. &c.   ⁶ Mœstitiâ cor quasi percussum constringitur, tremit, et
languescit, cum acri sensu doloris. In tristitiâ, cor fugiens attrahit ex splene
lentum humorem melancholicum, qui, effusus sub costis in sinistro latere, hypo-
chondriacos flatus facit; quod sæpe accidit iis qui diuturnâ curâ et mœstitiâ con-
flictantur. Melancthon.   ⁷ Lib. 3. Æn. 4.

Mem. 3. Subs. 5.]   *Fear, a Cause.*   265

This foul fiend of fear was worshipped heretofore as a God by the Lacedæmonians, and most of those other torturing [1] affections, and so was sorrow, amongst the rest, under the name of Angerona Dea; they stood in such awe of them, as Austin (*de Civitat. Dei, lib.* 4. *cap.* 8) noteth out of Varro. Fear was commonly [2] adored and painted in their temples with a lions head; and (as Macrobius records, l. 10. Saturnalium) [3] *In the calends of January, Angerona had her holy day, to whom, in the temple of Volupia, or goddess of pleasure, their augures and bishops did yearly sacrifice; that, being propitious to them, she might expel all cares, anguish, and vexation of the mind, for that year following.* Many lamentable effects this fear causeth in men, as to be red, pale, tremble, sweat; [4] it makes sudden cold and heat to come over all the body, palpitation of the heart, syncope, &c. It amazeth many men that are to speak, or shew themselves in publick assemblies, or before some great personages, as Tully confessed of himself, that he trembled still at the beginning of his speech; and Demosthenes that great orator of Greece, before Philippus. It confounds voice and memory, as Lucian wittily brings in Jupiter Tragœdus so much afraid of his auditory, when he was to make a speech to the rest of the gods, that he could not utter a ready word, but was compelled to use Mercuries help in prompting. Many men are so amazed and astonished with fear, they know not where they are, what they say, [5] what they do; and (that which is worst) it tortures them, many dayes before, with continual affrights and suspicion. It hinders most honourable attempts, and makes their hearts ake, sad and heavy. They that live in fear, are never free, [6] resolute, secure, never merry, but in continual pain; that, as Vives truly said, *nulla est miseria major quam metus;* no greater misery, no rack, no torture, like unto it; ever suspicious, anxious, solicitous, they are childishly drooping without reason, without judgement, [7] *especially if some terrible object be offered,* as Plutarch hath it. It causeth oftentimes sudden madness, and almost all manner of diseases, as I have sufficiently illustrated in my [8] digression of the Force of Imagination, and shall do more at large in my

---

[1] Et metum ideo deam sacrârunt, ut bonam mentem concederet. Varro, Lactantius, Aug.   [2] Lilius Girald. Syntag. 1. de diis miscellaneis.   [3] Calendis Jan. feriæ sunt divæ Angeronæ, cui pontifices in sacello Volupiæ sacra faciunt, quod angores et animi solicitudines propitiata propellat.   [4] Timor inducit frigus, cordis palpitationem, vocis defectum, atque pallorem. Agrippa, l. l. c. 63. Timidi semper spiritus habent frigidos. Mont.   [5] Effusas cernens fugientes agmine turmas, Quis mea nunc inflat cornua? Faunus ait. Aliciat.   [6] Metus non solum memoriam consternat, sed et institutum animi omne et laudabilem conatum impedit. Thucydides.   [7] Lib. de fortitudine et virtute Alexandri. Ubi prope res adfuit terribilis.   [8] Sect. 2. Mem. 3. Subs. 2.

266　　　　　　*Causes of Melancholy.*　　[Part. 1. Sec. 2.

section of [1]Terrours. Fear makes our imagination conceive what it list, invites the devil to come to us, (as [2]Agrippa and Cardan avouch), and tyrannizeth over our phantasie more than all other affections, especially in the dark. We see this verified in most men; as [3]Lavater saith, *quæ metuunt, fingunt;* what they fear they conceive, and faign unto themselves; they think they see goblins, haggs, devils, and many times become melancholy thereby. Cardan (*subtil. lib.* 18) hath an example of such an one, so caused to be melancholy (by sight of a bug-bear) all his life after. Augustus Cæsar durst not sit in the dark; *nisi aliquo assidente*, saith [4]Suetonius, *numquam tene-bris evigilavit.* And 'tis strange what women and children will conceive unto themselves, if they go over a church-yard in the night, lye or be alone in a dark room; how they sweat and tremble on a sudden. Many men are troubled with future events, foreknowledge of their fortunes, destinies, as Severus the emperour, Adrian, and Domitian: *quod sciret ultimum vitæ diem*, saith Suetonius, *valde solicitus:* much tortured in mind because he foreknew his end; with many such, of which I shall speak more opportunely in [5]another place. Anxiety, mercy, pitty, indignation, &c. and such fearful branches derived from these two stems of fear and sorrow, I voluntarily omit. Read more of them in [6]Carolus Pascalius, [7]Dandinus, &c.

SUBSECT. VI.

Shame and Disgrace, Causes.

SHAME and disgrace cause most violent passions, and bitter pangs. *Ob pudorem et dedecus publicum, ob errorem commissum, sæpe moventur generosi animi* (Felix Plater, *lib. 3. de alienat. mentis):* Generous minds are often moved with shame, to despair, for some publick disgrace. And *he* (saith Philo, *lib. 2. de provid. Dei*) [8]*that subjects himself to fear, grief, ambition, shame, is not happy, but altogether miserable, tortured with continual labour, care, and misery.* It is as forcible a batterer as any of the rest. [9]*Many men neglect the tumults of the world, and care not for glory, and yet they are*

---

[1]Sect. 2. Mem. 4. Subs. 3.　　　[2] Subtil. 18. lib. Timor attrahit ad se dæmonas. Timor et error multum in hominibus possunt.　　[3] Lib. de Spectris, ca. 3. Fortes raro spectra vident, quia minus timent.　　[4] Vitâ ejus.　　[5] Sect. 2. Memb. 4. Subs. 7.　　[6] De virt. et vitiis.　　[7] Com. in Arist. de Animâ.　　[8] Qui mentem subjecit timoris dominationi, cupiditatis, doloris, ambitionis, pudoris, felix non est, sed omnino miser: assiduis laboribus torquetur et miseriâ. [9] Multi contemnunt mundi strepitum, reputant pro nihilo gloriam, sed timent infamiam, offensionem, repulsam. Voluptatem severissime contemnunt; in dolore sunt molliores: gloriam negligunt; franguntur infamiâ.

Mem. 3. Subs. 6.]   *Shame and Disgrace, Causes.*   267

afraid of infamy, repulse, disgrace : (*Tul. offic. l.* 1.) *they can severely contemn pleasure, bear grief indifferently; but they are quite* [1] *battered and broken with reproach and obloquy* (*siquidem vita et fama pari passu ambulant*), and are so dejected many times for some public injury, disgrace, as a box on the ear by their inferiour, to be overcome of their adversary, foiled in the field, to be out in a speech, some foul fact committed or disclosed, &c. that they dare not come abroad all their lives after, but melancholize in corners, and keep in holes. The most generous spirits are most subject to it. *Spiritus altos frangit et generosos :* Hieronym. Aristotle, because he could not understand the motion of Euripus, for grief and shame drowned himself : Cælius Rodoginus (*antiquar. lec. lib.* 29. *cap.* 8.) *Homerus pudore consumptus,* was swallowed up with this passion of shame, [2] *because he could not unfold the fisherman's riddle.* Sophocles killed himself, [3] *for that a tragedy of his was hissed off the stage.* (Valer. Max. *lib.* 9. *cap.* 12.) Lucretia stabbed her self; and so did [4] *Cleopatra, when she saw that she was reserved for a triumph, to avoid the infamy.* Antonius the Roman, [5] *after he was overcome of his enemy, for three days space sat solitary in the fore-part of the ship, abstaining from all company, even of Cleopatra her self, and afterwards, for very shame, butchered himself.* (Plutarch. vitâ ejus.) Apollonius Rhodius [6] *wilfully banished himself, forsaking his countrey, and all his dear friends, because he was out in reciting his poems* (Plinius, *lib.* 7. *cap.* 23). Ajax ran mad, because his arms were adjudged to Ulysses. In China, 'tis an ordinary thing for such as are excluded in those famous tryals of theirs, or should take degrees, for shame and grief to lose their wits [7] (Mat. Riccius, *expedit. ad Sinas, l.* 3. *c.* 9). Hostratus the fryer took that book which Reuclin had writ against him, under the name of *Epist. obscurorum virorum,* so to heart, that, for shame and grief, he made away himself [8] (*Jovius, in elogiis*). A grave and learned minister, and an ordinary preacher at Alcmar in Holland, was (one day, as he walked in the fields for his recreation) suddenly taken with a lask or looseness, and thereupon compelled to retire to the next

---

[1] Gravius contumeliam ferimus quam detrimentum, ni abjecto nimis animo simus. Plut. in Timol.   [2] Quod piscatoris ænigma solvere non posset.   [3] Ob tragœdiam explosam, mortem sibi gladio conscivit.   [4] Cum vidit in triumphum se servari, caussâ ejus ignominiæ vitandæ mortem sibi conscivit. Plut.   [5] Bello victus, per tres dies sedit in prorâ navis, abstinens ab omni consortio, etiam Cleopatræ ; postea se interfecit.   [6] Cum male recitâsset Argonautica, ob pudorem exulavit.   [7] Quidam, præ verecundiâ simul et dolore, in insaniam incidunt, eo quod a literatorum gradu in examine excluduntur.   [8] Hostratus cucullatus adeo graviter ob Reuclini librum, qui inscribitur, Epistolæ obscurorum virorum, dolore simul et pudore sauciatus, ut seipsum interfecerit.

268   *Causes of Melancholy.*   [Part. 1. Sec. 2.

ditch; but, being [1] surprized at unawares by some gentle-women of his parish wandering that way, was so abashed, that he did never after shew his head in publick, or come into the pulpit, but pined away with melancholy: (Pet. Forestus, *med. observat. lib.* 10. *observat.* 12.) So shame amongst other passions can play his prize.

I know there be many base, impudent, brazen-faced rogues, that will [2] *nullá pallescere culpá*, be moved with nothing, take no infamy or disgrace to heart, laugh at all; let them be proved perjured, stigmatized, convict rogues, thieves, traitours, lose their ears, be whipped, branded, carted, pointed at, hissed, re-viled, and derided, (with [3] Ballio the baud in Plautus) they rejoyce at it; *cantores probos! babæ!* and *bombax!* what care they? We have too many such in our times.

> —— Exclamat Melicerta perîsse
> Frontem de rebus.

Yet a modest man, one that hath grace, a generous spirit, ten-der of his reputation, will be deeply wounded, and so grievously affected with it, that he had rather give myriads of crowns, lose his life, than suffer the least defamation of honour, or blot in his good name. And, if so be that he cannot avoid it,—as a nightingale, *quæ, cantando victa, moritur* (saith [4] Mizaldus) dies for shame, if another bird sing better—he languisheth and pineth away in the anguish of his spirit.

SUBSECT. VII.

Envy, Malice, Hatred, Causes.

Envy and malice are two links of this chain; and both (as Guianerius, *Tract.* 15. *cap.* 2. proves out of Galen, 3 *Apho-rism. com.* 22.) [5] *cause this malady by themselves, especially if their bodies be otherwise disposed to melancholy.* 'Tis Valescus de Taranta and Felix Platerus observation: [6] *envy so gnawes many men's hearts, that they become altogether melancholy.* And therefore, belike, Solomon (*Prov.* 14. 13.) calls it, *the rotting of the bones;* Cyprian, *vulnus occultum.*

---

[1] Propter ruborem confusus, statim cœpit delirare, &c. ob suspicionem, quod vili illum crimine accusarent.   [2] Horat.   [3] Ps. Impudice. B. Ita est. Ps. sceleste. B. dicis vera. Ps. verbero. B. quippini? Ps. furcifer. B. factum optime. Ps. sociofraude. B. sunt mea istæc. Ps. parricida. B. perge tu. P. sacrilege. B. fa-teor. Ps. perjure. B. vera dicis. Ps. pernicies adolescentum. B. acerrime. Ps. fur. B. babæ! Ps. fugitive. B. bombax! Ps. fraus populi. B. planissime. Ps. impure leno, cœnum. B. cantores probos! Pseudolus, act. 1. scen. 3.   [4] Cent. 7. e Plinio.   [5] Multos videmus, propter invidiam et odium, in melancholiam incidisse; et illos potissimum quorum corpora ad hanc apta sunt.   [6] Invidia affligit homines adeo et corrodit, ut hi melancholici penitus fiant.

Mem. 3. Subs. 7.] *Envy, Malice, Hatred, Causes.*

—————[1] Siculi non invenêre tyranni
Majus tormentum :

the Sicilian tyrants never invented the like torment. It crucifies their souls, withers their bodies, makes them hollow-ey'd, [2] pale, lean, and ghastly to behold (Cyprian, *ser. 2. de zelo et livore*). [3] *As a moth gnaws a garment,* so (saith Chrysostome) *doth envy consume a man;* to be a living anatomy, a *skeleton; to be a lean and* [4] *pale carcass, quickned with a* [5] *fiend* (Hall, *in Charact.*); for, so often as an envious wretch sees another man prosper, to be enriched, to thrive, and be fortunate in the world, to get honours, offices, or the like, he repines, and grieves:

—————[6] intabescitque videndo
Successus hominum. . . . .
Suppliciumque suum est :

he tortures himself, if his equal, friend, neighbour be preferred, commended, do well : if he understand of it, it gauls him afresh ; and no greater pain can come to him, than to hear of another mans well-doing; 'tis a dagger at his heart, every such object. He looks at him (as they that fell down in Lucians rock of honour) with an envious eye, and will damage himself to do the other a mischief, (*Atque cadet subito, dum super hoste cadat*) as he did, in Æsop, lose one eye willingly, that his fellow might lose both, or that rich man, in [7] Quintilian, that poysoned the flowers in his garden, because his neighbours bees should get no more honey from them. His whole life is sorrow; and every word he speaks, a *satyre;* nothing fats him but other mens ruines; for to speak in a word, envy is nought else but *tristitia de bonis alienis,* sorrow for other mens good, be it present, past or to come; *et gaudium de adversis,* and [8] joy at their harms, opposite to mercy, [9] which grieves at other mens mischances, and misaffects the body in another kind; so Damascen defines it, *lib. 2. de orthod. fid.* Thomas, 2. 2. *quæst.* 36. *art.* 1. Aristotle, *l. 2. Rhet. c. 4. et* 10. Plato, *Philebo.* Tulley, 3. *Tusc.* Greg. Nic. *l. de virt.*

[1] Hor.   [2] His vultus minax, torvus aspectus, pallor in facie, in labiis tremor, stridor in dentibus, &c.   [3] Ut tinea corrodit vestimentum, sic invidia eum, qui zelatur, consumit.   [4] Pallor in ore sedet, macies in corpore toto. Nusquam recta acies; livent rubigine dentes.   [5] Diaboli expressa imago, toxicum charitatis, venenum amicitiæ, abyssus mentis ; non est eo monstrosius monstrum, damnosius damnum : urit, torret, discruciat, macie et squalore conficit. Austin. Domin. prim. Advent.   [6] Ovid.   [7] Declam. 13, linivit flores maleficis succis, in venenum mella convertens.   [8] Statuis cereis Basilius eos comparat, qui liquefiunt ad præsentiam solis, quâ alii gaudent et ornantur ; muscis alii, quæ ulceribus gaudent, amœna prætereunt, sistunt in fœtidis.   [9] Misericordia etiam, quæ tristitia quædam est, sæpe miserantis corpus male afficit. Agrippa, l. 1. cap. 63.

270   *Causes of Melancholy.*   [Part. 1. Sec. 2.

animæ. c. 12. Basil, *de Invidiâ.* Pindarus, *Od.* 1. *ser.* 5; and
we find it true. 'Tis a common disease, and almost natural to
us, (as [1] Tacitus holds) to envy another mans prosperity: and
'tis in most men an incurable disease. [2] *I have read,* saith
Marcus Aurelius, *Greek, Hebrew, Chaldee authors; I have
consulted with many wise men, for a remedy for envy: I could
find none, but to renounce all happiness, and to be a wretch,
and miserable for ever.* 'Tis the beginning of hell in this life,
and a passion not to be excused. [3] *Every other sin hath some
pleasure annexed to it, or will admit of an excuse; envy alone
wants both. Other sins last but for a while: the gut may be
satisfied; anger remits; hatred hath an end; envy never
ceaseth.* (Cardan, *lib.* 2. *de sap.*) Divine and humane examples
are very familiar: you may run and read them, as that of Saul
and David, Cain and Abel; *angebat illum non proprium peccatum, sed fratris prosperitas,* saith Theodoret; it was his
brothers good fortune gauled him. Rachel envied her sister,
being barren, (Gen. 30) Josephs brethren, him (Gen. 37).
David had a touch of this vice, as he confesseth ([4] Psal. 37), [5] Jeremy and [6] Habbakuk: they repined at others good; but in the
end they corrected themselves. Psal. 75. *Fret not thyself, &c.*
Domitian spited Agricola for his worth, [7] *that a private man
should be so much glorified.* [8] Cæcinna was envyed of his fellow-citizens, because he was more richly adorned. But of all
others, [9] women are most weak: *ob pulchritudinem, invidæ
sunt feminæ* (Musæus): *aut amat, aut odit; nihil est tertium*
(Granatensis): they love, or hate: no medium amongst them.
Implacabiles plerumque læsæ mulieres. Agrippina like, [10] *a
woman, if she see her neighbour more neat or elegant, richer in
tires, jewels, or apparel, is enraged, and like a lioness sets upon
her husband, rails at her, scoffs at her, and cannot abide her;*
so the Roman ladies, in Tacitus, did at Solonina, Cæcinna's wife,
[11] *because she had a better horse, and better furniture; as if she
had hurt them with it, they were much offended.* In like sort
our gentlewomen do at their usual meetings; one repines or

---

[1] Insitum mortalibus a naturâ recentem aliorum felicitatem ægris oculis intueri.
Hist. l. 2. Tacit.   [2] Legi Chaldæos, Græcos, Hebræos; consului sapientes,
pro remedio invidiæ; hoc enim inveni, renunciare felicitati, et perpetuo miser
esse.   [3] Omne peccatum aut excusationem secum habet, aut voluptatem;
sola invidia utrâque caret. Reliqua vitia finem habent; ira defervescit; gula sa-
tiatur; odium finem habet, invidia numquam quiescit.   [4] Urebat me æmulatio propter stultos.   [5] Hier. 12. 1.   [6] Hab. 1.   [7] Invidit privati
nomen supra principis attolli.   [8] Tacit. Hist. lib. 2. part. 6.   [9] Perituræ
dolore et invidiâ, si quam viderint ornatiorem se in publicum prodiisse. Platina,
dial. amorum.   [10] Ant. Guianerius, lib. 2. cap. 8. vit. M. Aurelii. Femina, vici-
nam elegantius se vestitam videns, leænæ instar in virum insurgit, &c.   [11] Quod
insignis equo et ostro veheretur, quamquam nullius cum injuriâ, ornatum illum,
tamquam læsæ, gravabantur.

scoffs at anothers bravery and happiness. Myrsine, an Attick wench, was murthered of her fellows, [1] *because she did excel the rest in beauty* (Constantine, *Agricult. l.* 11. *c.* 7). Every village will yield such examples.

SUBSECT. VIII.

Æmulation, Hatred, Faction, Desire of Revenge, Causes.

Out of this root of envy, [2] spring those feral branches of faction, hatred, livor, emulation, which cause the like grievances, and are *serræ animæ*, the sawes of the soul, [3] *consternationis pleni affectus*, affections full of desperate amazement: or, as Cyprian descibes emulation, it is, [4] *a moth of the soul, a consumption, to make another mans happiness his misery, to torture, crucifie and execute himself, to eat his own heart. Meat and drink can do such men no good; they do always grieve, sigh, and groan, day and night without intermission; their breast is torn asunder:* and a little after, [5] *whosoever he is, whom thou dost emulate and envy, he may avoid thee; but thou canst neither avoid him, nor thyself. Wheresoever thou art, he is with thee; thine enemy is ever in thy breast; thy destruction is within thee; thou art a captive, bound hand and foot, as long as thou art malicious and envious, and canst not be comforted. It was the devils overthrow;* and, whensoever thou art thoroughly affected with this passion, it will be thine. Yet no perturbation so frequent, no passion so common.

> [6] Καὶ κεραμεὺς κεραμεῖ κοτέει, καὶ τέκτονι τέκτων·
> Καὶ πτωχὸς πτωχῷ φθονέει, καὶ αοιδὸς αοιδῷ.

> A potter emulates a potter;
> One smith envies another;
> A beggar emulates a beggar;
> A singing man his brother.

---

[1] Quod pulchritudine omnes excelleret, puellæ indignatæ occiderunt.   [2] Late patet invidiæ fecunda pernicies; et livor radix omnium malorum, fons cladium: inde odium surgit, æmulatio. Cyprian. ser. 2. de Livore.   [3] Valerius, l. 3. cap. 9.   [4] Qualis est animi tinea, quæ tabes pectoris, zelare in altero, vel aliorum felicitatem suam facere miseriam, et velut quosdam pectori suo admovere carnifices, cogitationibus et sensibus suis adhibere tortores, qui se intestinis cruciatibus lacerent? Non cibus talibus lætus, non potus potest esse jucundus; suspiratur semper et gemitur, et doletur dies et noctes; pectus sine intermissione laceratur.   [5] Quisquis est ille, quem æmularis, cui invides, is te subterfugere potest; at tu non te: ubicunque fugeris, adversarius tuus tecum est; hostis tuus semper in pectore tuo est, pernicies intus inclusa: ligatus es, vinctus, zelo dominante captivus: nec solatia tibi ulla subveniunt: hinc diabolus inter initia statim mundi, et periit primus, et perdidit. Cyprian. ser 2. de zelo et livore.   [6] Hesiod. op. et dies.

272   *Causes of Melancholy.*   [Part. 1. Sec. 2.

Every society, corporation, and private family, is full of it;
it takes hold almost of all sorts of men, from the prince to the
ploughman; even amongst gossips it is to be seen: scarce three
in a company, but there is siding, faction, emulation, between
two of them, some *simultas,* jarr, private grudge, heart-burning
in the midst of them. Scarce two gentlemen dwell together
in the country, (if they be not near kin or linked in marriage)
but there is emulation betwixt them and their servants, some
quarrel or some grudge betwixt their wives or children, friends
and followers, some contention about wealth, gentry, precedency, &c. by means of which, (like the frog in [1] Æsop,
*that would swell till she was as big as an ox, but burst her
self at last*) they will stretch beyond their fortunes, callings, and strive so long, that they consume their substance in
law-suits, or otherwise in hospitality, feasting, fine clothes,
to get a few bumbast titles; for *ambitiosâ paupertate labora-
mus omnes;* to out-brave one another, they will tire their bodies,
macerate their souls, and through contentions or mutual invitations, beggar themselves. Scarce two great scholars in an
age, but with bitter invectives they fall foul one on the other,
and their adherents—Scotists, Thomists, Reals, Nominals,
Plato, and Aristole, Galenists and Paracelsians, &c. it holds
in all professions.

Honest [2] emulation in studies, in all callings, is not to be dis-
liked: 'tis *ingeniorum cos,* as one calls it—the whetstone of wit,
the nurse of wit and valour; and those noble Romans, out of
this spirit, did brave exploits. There is a modest ambition, as
Themistocles was roused up with the glory of Miltiades;
Achilles trophies moved Alexander.

> [3] Ambire semper stulta confidentia est;
> Ambire numquam deses arrogantia est.

'tis a sluggish humour not to emulate or to sue at all, to with-
draw himself, neglect, refrain from such places, honours, offices,
through sloth, niggardliness, fear, bashfulness, or otherwise,
to which, by his birth, place, fortunes, education, he is called,
apt, fit, and well able to undergo: but, when it is immoderate,
it is a plague and a miserable pain. What a deal of money did
Henry the eighth, and Francis the first, king of France, spend
at that [4] famous interview! and how many vain courtiers, seeking each to outbrave other, spent themselves, their lively-hood
and fortunes, and dyed beggars! [5] Adrian the emperour was so
galled with it, that he killed all his equals; so did Nero. This

---

[1] Rana, cupida æquandi bovem, se distendebat, &c.   [2] Æmulatio alit ingenia. Paterculus, poster. Vol.   [3] Grotius, Epig. lib. 1.   [4] Anno
1519, betwixt Ardes and Quinc.   [5] Spartian.

passion made [1] Dionysius the tyrant banish Plato and Philoxenus the poet, because they did excell and eclipse his glory, as
he thought; the Romans exile Coriolanus, confine Camillus,
murder Scipio; the Greeks, by ostracism, to expel Aristides,
Nicias, Alcibiades, imprison Theseus, make away Phocion, &c.
When Richard the first, and Philip of France, were fellow souldiers together at the siege of Acon, in the Holy land, and
Richard had approved himself to be the more valiant man, in so
much that all mens eyes were upon him, it so gauled Philip,
(Francum urebat regis victoria, saith mine [2] author; *tam ægre
ferebat Richardi gloriam, ut carpere dicta, calumniari facta)*
that he cavilled at all his proceedings, and fell at length to open
defiance. He could contain no longer, but, hasting home, in-
vaded his territories, and professed open war. *Hatred stirs up
contention (Prov.* 10. 12); and they break out at last into immortal enmity, into virulency, and more than Vatinian hate and
rage; [3] they persecute each other, their friends, followers, and
all their posterity, with bitter taunts, hostile wars, scurril invectives, libels, calumnies, fire, sword, and the like, and will not
be reconciled. Witness that Guelf and Gibelline faction in
Italy; that of the Adurni and Fregosi in Genoa; that of Cneius
Papirius and Quintus Fabius in Rome; Cæsar and Pompey;
Orleans and Burgundy in France; York and Lancaster in
England. Yea, this passion so rageth [4] many times, that it subverts, not men only, and families, but even populous cities.
[5] Carthage and Corinth can witness as much; nay, flourishing
kingdoms are brought into a wilderness by it. This hatred,
malice, faction, and desire of revenge, invented first all those
racks, and wheels, strappadoes, brazen bulls, feral engines,
prisons, inquisitions, severe laws, to macerate and torment one
another. How happy might we be, and end our time with
blessed days, and sweet content, if we could contain our selves,
and, as we ought to do, put up injuries, learn humility, meekness, patience, forget and forgive, (as in [6] Gods word we are
enjoyned), compose such small controversies amongst our
selves, moderate our passions in this kind, *and think better of
others* (as [7] Paul would have us) *than of our selves; be of like
affection one towards another, and not avenge our selves, but
have peace with all men.* But being that we are so peevish and
perverse, insolent and proud, so factious and seditious, so mali-

---

[1] Plutarch.   [2] Johannes Heraldus, l. 2. c. 12. de bello sac.   [3] Nulla
dies tantum poterit lenire furorem.—Æterna bella pace sublatâ gerunt.—Jurat
odium, nec ante invisum esse desinit, quam esse desiit. Paterculus, vol. 1.   [4] Ita
sævit hæc Stygia ministra, ut urbes subvertat aliquando, deleat populos, provin-
cias alioqui florentes redigat in solitudines, mortales vero miseros in profundâ miseriarum valle miserabiliter immergat.   [5] Carthago, æmula Romani imperii,
funditus interiit. Sallust. Catil.   [6] Paul. 3. Col.   [7] Rom. 12.

VOL. I.   T

274   *Causes of Melancholy.*   [Part. 1. Sec. 2.

cious and envious, we do *invicem angariare*, maul and vex one another, torture, disquiet, and precipitate our selves into that gulf of woes and cares, aggravate our misery, and melancholy, heap upon us hell and eternal damnation.

SUBSECT. IX.

Anger, a Cause.

ANGER, a perturbation, which carries the spirits outwards, preparing the body to melancholy, and madness it self— *ira furor brevis est;* and (as [1] Piccolomineus accounts it) one of the three most violent passions. [2] Aretæus sets it down for an especial cause (so doth Seneca, ep. 18. l. 1) of this malady. [3] Magninus gives the reason; *ex frequenti irâ supra modum calefiunt;* it over-heats their bodies; and, if it be too frequent, it breaks out into manifest madness, saith S. Ambrose. 'Tis a known saying; *furor fit læsa sæpius patientia;* the most patient spirit that is, if he be often provoked, will be incensed to madness; it will make a devil of a saint: and therefore Basil (belike) in his Homily *de Irâ,* calls it *tenebras rationis, morbum animæ, et dæmonem pessimum;* the darkning of our understanding, and a bad angel. [4] Lucian (*in Abdicato, Tom.* 1.) will have this passion to work this effect, especially in old men and women. *Anger and calumny* (saith he) *trouble them at first, and, after a while, break out into open madness: many things cause fury in women, especially if they love or hate overmuch, or envy, be much grieved or angry; these things, by little and little, lead them on to this malady.* From a disposition, they proceed to a habit; for there is no difference betwixt a mad man, and an angry man, in the time of his fit. Anger, as Lactantius describes it, (*L. de Irâ Dei, ad Donatum, c.* 5) is [5] *sæva animi tempestas, &c.* a cruel tempest of the mind, *making his eyes sparkle fire, and stare, teeth gnash in his head, his tongue stutter, his face pale or red; and what more filthy imitation can be of a mad man.*

---

[1] Grad. l. c. 54.   [2] Ira, et mœror, et ingens animi consternatio, melancholicos facit. Aretæus. Ira immodica gignit insaniam.   [3] Reg. sanit. parte 2. c. 8. In apertam insaniam mox ducitur iratus.   [4] Gilberto Cognato interprete. Multis, et præsertim senibus, ira impotens insaniam facit, et importuna calumnia: hæc initio perturbat animum; paullatim vergit ad insaniam. Porro mulierum corpora multa infestant, et in hunc morbum adducunt præcipue si quæ oderint aut invideant, &c. hæc paullatim in insaniam tandem evadunt. [5] Sæva animi tempestas, tantos excitans fluctus, ut statim ardescant oculi, os tremat, lingua titubet, dentes concrepent, &c.

Mem. 3. Subs. 9.] *Anger, a Cause.* 275

[1] Ora tument irâ; fervescunt sanguine venæ;
Lumina Gorgoneo sævius angue micant.

They are void of reason, inexorable, blind, like beasts and monsters for the time, say and do they know not what, curse, swear, rail, fight, and what not? How can a mad man do more? as he said in the comedy, [2] *iracundiâ non sum apud me;* I am not mine own man. If these fits be immoderate, continue long, or be frequent, without doubt they provoke madness. Montanus (*consil.* 21) had a melancholy Jew to his patient; he ascribes this for a principal cause: *irascebatur levibus de caussis;* he was easily moved to anger. Ajax had no other beginning of his madness; and Charles the Sixth, that lunatick French king, fell into this misery, out of the extremity of his passion, desire of revenge, and malice; [3] incensed against the duke of Britain, he could neither eat, drink, nor sleep for some days together; and in the end, about the calends of July, 1392, he became mad upon his horse-back, drawing his sword, striking such as came near him promiscuously, and so continued all the days of his life. (*Æmil. lib.* 10. *Gal. hist.*) Hegesippus (*de excid. urbis Hieros. l.* 1. *c.* 37) hath such a story of Herod, that, out of an angry fit, became mad, and [4] leaping out of his bed, he killed Josippus, and played many such Bedlam pranks. The whole court could not rule him for a long time after. Sometimes he was sorry and repented, much grieved for that he had done, *postquam deferbuit ira;* by and by outrageous again. In hot cholerick bodies, nothing so soon causeth madness, as this passion of anger, besides many other diseases, as Pelesius observes, (*Cap.* 21. *l.* 1. *de hum. affect. caussis*) *Sanguinem imminuit, fel auget:* and, as [5] Valesius controverts, (*Med. controv. lib.* 5. *contro.* 8.) many times kills them quite out. If this were the worst of this passion it were more tolerable: [6] *but it ruines and subverts whole towns,* [7] *cities, families, and kingdoms. Nulla pestis humano generi pluris stetit,* saith Seneca, (*de Irâ, lib.* 1.) no plague hath done mankind so much harm. Look into our histories; and you shall almost meet with no other subject, but what a company [8] of hare-brains have done in their rage. We may do well, therefore, to put this in our precession amongst the rest; *From all blindness of heart, from pride, vain-glory, and hypocrisie, from envy, hatred, and malice, anger, and all such pestiferous perturbations, good Lord, deliver us!*

---

[1] Ovid.　　[2] Terence.　　[3] Infensus Britanniæ duci, et in ultionem versus, nec cibum cepit, nec quietem; ad Calendas Julias, 1392, comites occidit. [4] Indignatione nimiâ furens, animique impotens, exsiliit de lecto: furentem non capiebat aula, &c.　　[5] An ira possit hominem interimere.　　[6] Abernethy. [7] As Troy, sævæ memorem Junonis ob iram.　　[8] Stultorum regum et populorum continet æstus.

T 2

276   *Causes of Melancholy.*   [Part. 1. Sec. 2.

SUBSECT. X.

Discontents, Cares, Miseries, &c. Causes.

DISCONTENTS, cares, crosses, miseries, or whatsoever it is that shall cause any molestation of spirits, grief, anguish, and perplexity, may well be reduced to this head. Preposterously placed here, in some mens judgements, they may seem : yet, in that Aristotle in his [1] Rhetorick defines these cares, as he doth envy, emulation, &c. still by grief, I think I may well rank them in this irascible row; being that they are, as the rest, both causes and symptomes of this disease, producing the like inconveniences, and are, most part, accompanied with anguish and pain (the common etymology will evince it—*cura, quasi corura); dementes curæ, insomnes curæ, damnosæ curæ, tristes, mordaces, carnifices, &c.* biting, eating, gnawing, cruel, bitter, sick, sad, unquiet, pale, tetrick, miserable, intolerable cares (as the poets [2] call them) ; worldly cares, and are as many in number as the sea sands. [3] Galen, Fernelius, Felix Plater, Valescus de Taranta, &c. reckon afflictions, miseries, even all these contentions and vexations of the mind, as principal causes, in that they take away sleep, hinder concoction, dry up the body, and consume the substance of it. They are not so many in number, but their causes be as divers, and not one of a thousand free from them, or that can vindicate himself, whom that *Ate dea*—

[4] Per hominum capita molliter ambulans,
   Plantas pedum teneras habens—

   Over mens heads walking aloft,
   With tender feet treading so soft—

Homers goddess Ate, hath not involved into this discontented [5] rank, or plagued with some misery or other. Hyginus (*fab. 220*) to this purpose hath a pleasant tale. Dame Cura by chance went over a brook, and, taking up some of the dirty slime, made an image of it. Jupiter, eftsoons coming by, put life to it; but Cura and Jupiter could not agree what name to give him, or who should own him. The matter was referred to

---

[1] Lib. 2. Invidia est dolor, et ambitio est dolor, &c.   [2] Insomnes, Claudianus. tristes, Virg. mordaces, Luc. edaces, Hor. mœstæ, amaræ, Ovid. damnosæ, inquietæ, Mart. urentes, rodentes, Mant. &c.   [3] Galen. l. 3. c. 7, de locis affectis. Homines sunt maxime melancholici, quando vigiliis multis, et solicitudinibus, et laboribus, et curis, fuerint circumventi.   [4] Lucian Podag.
[5] Omnia imperfecta, confusa, et perturbatione plena. Cardan.

Mem. 3. Subs. 10.] *Discontents, Cares, &c.* 277

Saturn as judge : he gave this arbitrement: his name shall be *Homo ab humo: Cura eum possideat quamdiu vivat:* Care shall have him whil'st he lives: Jupiter his soul, and Tellus his body, when he dies. But, to leave tales—A general cause, a continuate cause, an inseparable accident to all men, is discontent, care, misery. Were there no other particular affliction (which who is free from ?) to molest a man in this life, the very cogitation of that common misery were enough to macerate, and make him weary of his life ; to think that he can never be secure, but still in danger, sorrow, grief, and persecution. For, to begin at the hour of his birth, as [1] Pliny doth elegantly describe it, *he is born naked, and falls* [2] *a whining at the very first ; he is swadled and bound up, like a prisoner ; cannot help himself ; and so he continues to his lives end ; cujusque feræ pabulum,* saith [3] Seneca, impatient of heat and cold, impatient of labour, impatient of idleness, exposed to Fortunes contumelies. To a naked mariner Lucretius compares him, cast on shore by shipwrack, cold and comfortless in an unknown land: [4] No estate, age, sex, can secure himself from this common misery. *A man, that is born of a woman, is of short continuance, and full of trouble* (Job 14. 1. 22) ; *and, while his flesh is upon him, he shall be sorrowful : and, while his soul is in him, it shall mourn. All his days are sorrow and his travels grief: his heart also taketh not rest in the night ;* (Ecclus. 2. 23. and 2. 11.) *all that is in it, is sorrow and vexation of spirit ;* [5] *ingress, progress, regress, egress, much alike. Blindness seizeth on us in the beginning, labour in the middle, grief in the end, errour in all. What day ariseth to us, without some grief, care or anguish ? or what so secure and pleasing a morning have we seen, that hath not been overcast before the evening ?* One is miserable, another ridiculous, a third odious. One complains of this grievance, another of that. *Aliquando nervi, aliquando pedes, vexant,* (Seneca) *nunc destillatio, nunc hepatis morbus ; nunc deest, nunc superest, sanguis :* now the head akes, then the feet, now the lungs, then the liver, &c. *Huic census exuberat ; sed est pudori degener sanguis, &c.* He is rich, but base born ; he is noble, but poor : a third hath means ; but he wants health, peradventure, or wit to manage his estate. Children vex one, wife a second, &c. *Nemo facile cum conditione suâ concordat,* no man is

---

[1] Lib. 7. nat. hist. cap. 1. Hominem nudum et ad vagitum edit natura. Flens ab initio, devinctus jacet, &c.
[2] Δακρυχεων γενομην, και δακρυσας αποθνησκω·
Τῳ γενος ανθρωπων πολυδακρυτον, ασθενες, οικτρον.
Lacrymans natus sum, et lacrymans morior, &c. [3] Ad Marinum. [4] Boëthius. [5] Initium cæcitas, progressum labor, exitum dolor, error omnia : quem tranquillum, quæso, quem non laboriosum aut anxium diem egimus? Petrarch.

278   *Causes of Melancholy.*   [Part. 1. Sec. 2.

pleased with his fortune; a pound of sorrow is familiarly mixt
with a dram of content: little or no joy, little comfort, but
[1] every where danger, contention, anxiety in all places.   Go
where thou wilt; and thou shalt find discontents, cares, woes,
complaints, sickness, diseases, incumbrances, exclamations. *If
thou look into the market, there* (saith [2] Chrysostom) *is brawling
and contention ; if to the court, there knavery and flattery, &c.
if to a private mans house, there's cark and care, heaviness,
&c.*   As he said of old,

[3] Nil homine in terrâ spirat miserum magis almâ :

No creature so miserable as man, so generally molested, [4] *in
miseries of body, in miseries of mind, miseries of heart, in
miseries asleep, in miseries awake, in miseries, wheresoever he
turns,* as Bernard found.   *Numquid tentatio est vita humana
super terram ?*   A meer temptation is our life ; (Austin. *confess. lib.* 10. *cap.* 28) *catena perpetuorum malorum : et quis
potest molestias et difficultates pati ?*   Who can endure the
miseries of it ?   [5] *In prosperity we are insolent and intolerable,
dejected in adversity, in all fortunes foolish and miserable.* [6] *In
adversity, I wish for prosperity; and, in prosperity, I am afraid
of adversity.   What mediocrity may be found? where is no
temptation? what condition of life is free?* [7] *Wisdom hath
labour annexed to it, glory envy ; riches and cares, children and
incumbrances, pleasure and diseases, rest and beggery, go together ; as if a man were therefore born* (as the Platonists hold)
to be punished in this life, for some precedent sins; or that, as
[8] Pliny complains, *Nature may be rather accounted a step-
mother, than a mother unto us, all things considered : no creatures life so brittle, so full of fear, so mad, so furious ; only man
is plagued with envy, discontent, griefs, covetousness, ambition,
superstition.*   Our whole life is an Irish sea, wherein there is
nought to be expected, but tempestuous storms, and troublesome waves, and those infinite ;

[1] Ubique periculum, ubique dolor, ubique naufragium, in hoc ambitu, quocunque
me vertam. Lipsius.   [2] Hom. 10. Si in forum iveris, ibi rixæ, et pugnæ; si in
curiam, ibi fraus, adulatio; si in domum privatam, &c.   [3] Homer.   [4] Multis repletur homo miseriis, corporis miseriis, animi miseriis, dum dormit, dum
vigilat, quocunque se vertit. Lususque rerum temporumque nascimur.   [5] In
blandiente fortunâ intolerandi, in calamitatibus lugubres, semper stulti et miseri.
Cardan.   [6] Prospera in adversis desidero, et adversa prosperis timeo ; quis
inter hæc medius locus, ubi non sit humanæ vitæ tentatio ?   [7] Cardan. consol. Sapientiæ labor annexus, gloriæ invidia, divitiis curæ, soboli solicitudo, volup-
tati morbi, quieti paupertas, ut quasi luendorum scelerum caussâ nasci hominem
possis cum Platonistis agnoscere.   [8] Lib. 7. cap. 1.   Non satis æstimare, an
melior parens natura homini, an tristior noverca, fuerit. Nulli fragilior vita,
pavor, confusio, rabies major ; uni animantium ambitio data, luctus, avaritia; uni
superstitio.

Mem. 3. Subs. 10.] *Discontents, Cares, &c.* 279

(¹ Tantum malorum pelagus aspicio,
Ut non sit inde enatandi copia)

no Halcyonian times, wherein a man can hold himself secure,
or agree with his present estate: but, as Boëthius inferrs, ² *there
is something in every one of us, which before tryal, we seek,
and, having tryed, abhor;* ³ *we earnestly wish, and eagerly
covet, and are eftsoons weary of it.* Thus, betwixt hope and
fear, suspicions, angers,

⁴ Inter spemque metumque, timores inter et iras,

betwixt falling in, falling out, &c. we bangle away our best
dayes, befool out our times, we lead a contentious, discontent,
tumultuous, melancholy, miserable life; insomuch that, if we
could foretel what was to come, and it put to our choice, we
should rather refuse, than accept of, this painful life. In a
word, the world itself is a maze, a labyrinth of errours, a desart,
a wilderness, a den of thieves, cheaters, &c. full of filthy puddles,
horrid rocks, precipitiums, an ocean of adversity, an heavy
yoke, wherein infirmities and calamities overtake and follow
one another, as the sea-waves; and, if we scape Scylla, we fall
foul on Charybdis; and so, in perpetual fear, labour, anguish,
we run from one plague, one mischief, one burden, to another,
duram servientes servitutem; and you may as soon separate
weight from lead, heat from fire, moystness from water, bright-
ness from the sun, as misery, discontent, care, calamity, danger,
from a man. Our towns and cities are but so many dwellings
of human misery, *in which, grief and sorrow,* (⁵ as he right well
observes out of Solon) *innumerable troubles, labours of mortal
men, and all manner of vices, are included, as in so many pens.*
Our villages are like mole-hills, and men as so many emmets,
busie, busie still, going to and fro, in and out, and crossing
one anothers projects, as the lines of several *sea-cards* cut each
other in a globe or map; *now light and merry,* but (⁶ as
one follows it) *by-and-by sorrowful and heavy; now hoping,
then distrusting; now patient, to morrow crying out; now
pale, then red; running, sitting, sweating, trembling, halting,
&c.* Some few amongst the rest, or perhaps one of a thousand, may be *pullus Jovis,* in the worlds esteem, *gallinæ*

---

¹ Euripides.　² De consol. l. 2. Nemo facile cum conditione suâ concordat. Inest singulis quod imperiti petant, experti horreant.　³ Esse in honore
juvat, mox displicet.　⁴ Hor.　⁵ Borrhæus in 6. Joh. Urbes et oppida
nihil aliud sunt quam humanarum ærumnarum domicilia, quibus luctus et mœror,
et mortalium varii infinitique labores, et omnis generis vitia, quasi septis includuntur.　⁶ Nat. Chytreus, de lit. Europæ. Lætus nunc, mox tristis; nunc
sperans, paullo post diffidens; patiens hodie, cras ejulans; nunc pallens, rubens,
currens, sedens, claudicans, tremens, &c.

280 *Causes of Melancholy.* [Part. 1. Sec. 2.

filius albæ, an happy and fortunate man, *ad invidiam felix,* because rich, fair, well allied, in honour and office; yet peradventure ask himself, and he will say, that, of all others, [1] he is most miserable and unhappy. A fair shooe *hic soccus novus, elegans,* as he [2] said; *sed nescis ubi urat;* but thou knowest not where it pincheth. It is not another mans opinion can make me happy : but (as [3] Seneca well hath it) *he is a miserable wretch, that doth not account himself happy : though he be soveraign lord of the world, he is not happy, if he think himself not to be so ; for what availeth it what thine estate is, or seem to others, if thou thy self dislike it?* A common humour it is of all men to think well of other mens fortunes, and dislike their own :

> [4] Cui placet alterius, sua nimirum est odio, sors :

but [5] *quî fit, Mæcenas, &c.* how comes it to pass? what's the cause of it? Many men are of such a perverse nature, they are well pleased with nothing, (saith [6] Theodoret) *neither with riches, nor poverty : they complain when they are well, and, when they are sick, grumble at all fortunes, prosperity and adversity ; they are troubled in a cheap year, in a barren : plenty, or not plenty, nothing pleaseth them, war nor peace, with children, nor without.* This, for the most part, is the humour of us all, to be discontent, miserable and most unhappy, as we think at least; and shew me him that is not so, or that ever was otherwise. Quintus Metellus his felicity is infinitely admired amongst the Romans, insomuch, that (as [7] Paterculus mentioneth of him) you can scarce find, of any nation, order, age, sex, one for happiness to be compared unto him : he had, in a word, *bona animi, corporis, et fortunæ,* goods of mind, body, and fortune; so had P. Mutianus [8] Crassus. Lampsaca, that Lacedæmonian lady, was such another in [9] Plinies conceit, *a kings wife, a kings mother, a kings daughter;* and all the world esteemed as much of Polycrates of Samos. The Greeks brag of their Socrates, Phocion, Aristides ; the Psophidians in particular of their Aglaüs, *omni vitâ felix, ab omni periculo immunis* (which, by the way, Pausanias held impossible ;) the Romans of their [10] Cato,

---

[1] Sua cuique calamitas præcipua. [2] Cn. Græcinus. [3] Epist. 9. l. 7. Miser est qui se beatissimum non judicat; licet imperet mundo, non est beatus, qui se non putat: quid enim refert, qualis status tuus sit, si tibi videtur malus? [4] Hor. ep. l. 1. 4. [5] Hor. ser. 1. sat. 1. [6] Lib. de curat. Græc. affec. cap. 6. de provident. Multis nihil placet; atque adeo et divitias damnant, et paupertatem; de morbis expostulant; bene valentes, graviter ferunt; atque, ut semel dicam, nihil eos delectat, &c. [7] Vix ullius gentis, ætatis, ordinis, hominem invenies, cujus felicitatem fortunæ Metelli compares. Vol. 1. [8] P. Crassus Mutianus quinque habuisse dicitur rerum bonarum maxima, quod esset ditissimus, quod esset nobilissimus, eloquentissimus, jurisconsultissimus, pontifex maximus. [9] Lib. 7. Regis filia, regis uxor, regis mater. [10] Qui nihil unquam mali aut dixit, aut fecit, quod aliter facere non potuit.

Mem. 3. Subs. 10.]   *Discontents, Cares, &c.*   281

Curius, Fabricius, for their composed fortunes, and retired estates, government of passions, and contempt of the world: yet none of all these was happy or free from discontent—neither Metellus, Crassus, nor Polycrates; for he died a violent death, and so did Cato: and how much evil doth Lactantius and Theodoret speak of Socrates!—a weak man—and so of the rest.   There is no content in this life; but (as [1] he said) *all is vanity and vexation of spirit;* lame and imperfect.   Hadst thou Sampsons hair, Milos strength, Scanderbegs arm, Solomons wisdom, Absaloms beauty, Crœsus his wealth, *Pasetis obulum,* Cæsars valour, Alexanders spirit, Tullys or Demosthenes eloquence, Gyges ring, Perseus Pegasus, and Gorgons head, Nestors years to come, all this would not make thee absolute, give thee content and true happiness in this life, or so continue it.   Even in the midst of all our mirth, jollity, and laughter, is sorrow and grief; or, if there be true happiness amongst us, 'tis but for a time :

[2] Desinit in piscem mulier formosa superne :

a fair morning turns to a lowring afternoon.   Brutus and Cassius, once renowned, both eminently happy—yet you shall scarce find two (saith Paterculus) *quos fortuna maturius destituerit,* whom fortune sooner forsook.   Hannibal, a conqueror all his life, met with his match, and was subdued at last :

Occurrit forti, qui mage fortis erat.

One is brought in triumph, as Cæsar into Rome, Alcibiades into Athens, *coronis aureis donatus,* crowned, honoured, admired; by-and-by his statues demolished, he hissed out, massacred, &c.   [3] Magnus Gonsalva, that famous Spaniard, was of the prince and people at first honoured, approved; forthwith confined and banished.   *Admirandas actiones graves plerumque sequuntur invidiæ, et acres calumniæ* ('tis Polybius his observation;) grievous enmities, and bitter calumnies, commonly follow renowned actions.   One is born rich, dies a beggar; sound to day, sick to morrow; now in most flourishing estate, fortunate and happy, by-and-by deprived of his goods by foreign enemies, robbed by thieves, spoiled, captivated, impoverished, as they of [4] Rabbah, *put under iron saws, and under iron harrows, and under axes of iron, and cast into the tile-kiln.*

[5] Quid me felicem toties jactâstis, amici ?
Qui cecidit stabili non erat ille gradu.

---

[1] Solomon, Eccles. 1. 14.   [2] Hor. Art. Poët.   [3] Jovius, vitâ ejus.
[4] 2 Sam. 12. 31.   [5] Boëthius, lib. 1. met. 1.

282 *Causes of Melancholy.* [Part. 1. Sec. 2.

He that erst marched like Xerxes with innumerable armies, as rich as Crœsus, now shifts for himself in a poor cock-boat, is bound in iron chains, with Bajazet the Turk, and a foot-stool with Aurelian, for a tyrannizing conqueror to trample on. So many casualties there are, that, as Seneca said of a city consumed with fire, *una dies interest inter maximam civitatem et nullam,* one day betwixt a great city, and none; so many grievances from outward accidents, and from our selves, our own indiscretion, inordinate appetite; one day betwixt a man and no man. And (which is worse) as if discontents and miseries would not come fast enough upon us, *homo homini dæmon;* we maul, persecute, and study how to sting, gaul, and vex one another with mutual hatred, abuses, injuries; preying upon, and devouring, as so many [1] ravenous birds; and, as juglers, panders, bawds, cosening one another; or raging as [2] wolves, tygers, and devils, we take a delight to torment one another; men are evil, wicked, malicious, treacherous, and [3] naught, not loving one another, or loving themselves, not hospitable, charitable, nor sociable as they ought to be, but counterfeit, dissemblers, ambodexters, all for their own ends, hard-hearted, merciless, pittiless; and, to benefit themselves, they care not what mischief they procure to others. [4] Praxinoë and Gorgo, in the poet, when they had got in to see those costly sights, they then cryed *bene est,* and would thrust out all the rest; when they are rich themselves, in honour, preferred, full, and have even that they would, they debar others of those pleasures which youth requires, and they formerly have enjoyed. He sits at table in a soft chair at ease; but he doth not remember in the mean time, that a tired waiter stands behind him, *an hungry fellow ministers to him full: he is a thirst that gives him drink,* (saith [5] Epictetus) *and is silent whiles he speaks his pleasure; pensive, sad, when he laughs. Pleno se proluit auro;* he feasts, revels, and profusely spends, hath variety of robes, sweet musick, ease, and all the pleasure the world can afford, whilst many an hunger-starved poor creature pines in the street, wants clothes to cover him, labours hard all day long, runs, rides for a trifle, fights peradventure from sun to sun, sick and ill, weary, full of pain and grief, is in great distress and sorrow of heart. He

---

[1] Omnes hic aut captantur, aut captant; aut cadavera quæ lacerantur, aut corvi qui lacerant. Petron.　　[2] Homo omne monstrum est; ille nam superat feras; luposque et ursos pectore obscuro tegit. Heins.　　[3] Quod Paterculus de populo Romano, durante bello Punico, per annos 115, aut bellum inter eos, aut belli præparatio, aut infida pax, idem ego de mundi accolis.　　[4] Theocritus, Idyll. 15.　　[5] Qui sedet in mensâ, non meminit sibi otioso ministrare negotiosos, edenti esurientes, bibenti sitientes, &c.

Mem. 3. Subs. 10.] *Discontents, Cares, &c.* **283**

lothes and scorns his inferiour, hates or emulates his equal, envies his superiour, insults over all such as are under him, as if he were of another species, a demi-god, not subject to any fall, or humane infirmities. Generally they love not, are not beloved again : they tire out others bodies with continual labour, they themselves living at ease, caring for none else, *sibi nati ;* and are so far many times from putting to their helping hand, that they seek all means to depress, even most worthy and well deserving, better than themselves, those whom they are, by the laws of nature, bound to relieve and help, as much as in them lyes ; they will let them cater-waul, starve, beg and hang, before they will any wayes (though it be in their power) assist or ease : [1] so unnatural are they for the most part, so unregardful, so hard-hearted, so churlish, proud, insolent, so dogged, of so bad a disposition. And, being so brutish, so devilishly bent one towards another, how is it possible, but that we should be discontent of all sides, full of cares, woes, and miseries ?

If this be not a sufficient proof of their discontent and misery, examine every condition and calling apart. Kings, princes, monarchs, and magistrates, seem to be most happy ; but look into their estate, you shall [2] find them to be most encombred with cares, in perpetual fear, agony, suspicion, jealousie ; that, as [3] he said of a crown, if they knew but the discontents that accompany it, they would not stoop to take it up. *Quem mihi regem dabis,* (saith Chrysostom) *non curis plenum ?* what king canst thou shew me, not full of cares? [4] *Look not on his crown, but consider his afflictions ; attend not his number of servants, but multitude of crosses. Nihil aliud potestas culminis, quam tempestas mentis,* as Gregory seconds him : soveraignty is a tempest of the soul : Sylla like, they have brave titles, but terrible fits—*splendorem titulo, cruciatum animo ;* which made [5] Demosthenes vow, *si vel ad tribunal, vel ad interitum duceretur,* if to be a judge, or to be condemned, were put to his choice, he would be condemned. Rich men are in the same predicament : what their pains are, *stulti nesciunt, ipsi sentiunt*—they feel, fools perceive not, as I shall prove elsewhere ; and their wealth is brittle, like childrens rattles : they come and go ; there is no certainty in them ; those whom they elevate, they do as suddenly depress, and leave in a vale of misery. The

---

[1] Quando in adolescentiâ suâ ipsi vixerint lautius, et liberius voluptates suas expleverint, illi gnatis imponunt duriores continentiæ leges. [2] Lugubris Ate luctuque fero regum tumidas obsidet arces.—Res est inquieta felicitas. [3] Plus aloës quam mellis habet.—Non humi jacentem tolleres. Valer. l. 7. c. 3. [4] Non diadema aspicias, sed vitam afflictione refertam, non catervas satellitum, sed curarum multitudinem. [5] As Plutarch relateth.

2

284   *Causes of Melancholy.*   [Part. 1. Sec. 2.

middle sort of men are so many asses to bear burdens; or, if
they be free, and live at ease, they spend themselves, and consume their bodies and fortunes with luxury and riot, contention, emulation, &c. The poor I reserve for another [1] place,
and their discontents.

For particular professions, I hold, as of the rest, there's no
content or security in any. On what course will you pitch?
how resolve? To be a divine? 'tis contemptible in the worlds
esteem: to be a lawyer? 'tis to be a wrangler: to be a physician? [2] *pudet lotii;* 'tis loathed: a philosopher? a mad man:
an alchymist? a beggar: a poet? *esurit,* an hungry jack: a
musician? a player: a school-master? a drudge: an husbandman? an emmet: a merchant? his gains are uncertain: a me-
chanician? base: a chirurgion? fulsome: a tradesman? a [3] lyar:
a taylor? a thief: a serving-man? a slave: a souldier? a
butcher: a smith, or a metal-man? the pot's never from's nose:
a courtier? a parasite. As he could find no tree in the wood
to hang himself, I can shew no state of life to give content.
The like you may say of all ages; children live in a perpetual
slavery, still under that tyrannical government of masters: young
men, and of riper years, subject to labour, and a thousand cares
of the world, to treachery, falsehood, and cozenage:

> [4]————Incedit per ignes,
> Suppositos cineri doloso:

[5] old are full of aches in their bones, cramps and convulsions,
silicernia, dull of hearing, weak-sighted, hoary, wrinckled,
harsh, so much altered as that they cannot know their own
face in a glass, a burden to themselves and others: after
seventy years, *all is sorrow* (as David hath it); they do not
live, but linger. If they be sound, they fear diseases; if sick,
weary of their lives: *non est vivere, sed valere, vita.* One
complains of want, a second of servitude, [6] another of a secret
or incurable disease, of some deformity of body, of some loss,
danger, death of friends, shipwrack, persecution, imprisonment, disgrace, repulse, [7] contumely, calumny, abuse, injury,
contempt, ingratitude, unkindness, scoffs, flouts, unfortunate
marriage, single life, too many children, no children, false
servants, unhappy children, barrenness, banishment, oppression,
frustrate hopes, and ill success, &c.

---

[1] Sect. 2. mem. 4. subsect. 6.   [2] Stercus et urina, medicorum fercula
prima.   [3] Nihil lucrantur, nisi admodum mentiendo. Tull. Offic.   [4] Hor.
l. 2. od. 1.   [5] Rarus felix idemque senex. Seneca, in Herc. Œtæo.   [6] Omitto
ægros, exsules, mendicos, quos nemo audet felices dicere. Card. lib. 8. c. 46. de
rer. var.   [7] Spretæque injuria formæ.

Cætera de genere hoc (adeo sunt multa) loquacem
Delassare valent Fabium———

talking Fabius will be tyred before he can tell half of them ;
they are the subject of whole volumes, and shall (some of them)
be more opportunely dilated elsewhere.   In the mean time,
thus much I may say of them, that generally they crucifie the
soul of man, [1] attenuate our bodies, dry them, wither them,
rivel them up like old apples, and make them as so many ana-
tomies ([2] *ossa atque pellis est totus, ita curis macet);* they
cause *tempus fœdum et squalidum,* cumbersome dayes, *ingrataque tempora,* slow, dull, and heavy times; make us howl, roar,
and tear our hairs (as Sorrow did in [3] Cebes table), and groan
for the very anguish of our souls. Our hearts fail us, as Davids
did, (Psal. 40. 12) *for innumerable troubles that compassed him;*
and we are ready to confess with Hezekiah, (Isa. 58. 17) *behold! for felicity, I had bitter grief:* to weep with Heraclitus,
to curse the day of our birth, with Jeremy (20. 14) and our
stars with Job; to hold that axiom of Silenus, [4] *better never to
have been born, and the best next of all, to dye quickly;* or, if
we must live, to abandon the world, as Timon did, creep into
caves and holes, as our anchorites; cast all into the sea, as
Crates Thebanus; or, as Cleombrotus Ambraciotes four hundred auditors, precipitate our selves to be rid of these miseries.

SUBSECT. XI.

Concupiscible Appetite, as Desires, Ambition, Causes.

THESE concupiscible and irascible appetites are as the two
twists of a rope, mutually mixt one with the other, and both
twining about the heart; both good, (as Austin holds, *l.* 14. *c.*
9. *de civ. Dei.*) [5] *if they be moderate; both pernitious if they
be exorbitant.* This concupiscible appetite, howsoever it may
seem to carry with it a shew of pleasure and delight, and our
concupiscences most part affect us with content and a pleasing
object, yet if they be in extreams, they rack and wring us on
the other side.   A true saying it is, *desire hath no rest,* is infinite in it self, endless, and (as [6] one calls it) a perpetual rack,

---

[1] Attenuant vigiles corpus miserabile curæ.   [2] Plautus.   [3] Hæc, quæ
crines revellit, Ærumna.   [4] Optimum non nasci, aut cito mori.   [5] Bonæ,
si rectam rationem sequuntur; malæ, si exorbitant.   [6] Tho. Bouvie. Prob. 18.

286   *Causes of Melancholy.*   [Part. 1. Sec. 2.

[1] or horse-mill (according to Austin), still going round as in a ring. They are not so continual, as divers: *facilius atomos dinumerare possem,* (saith [2] Bernard) *quam motus cordis; nunc hæc, nunc illa cogito:* you may as well reckon up the motes in the sun, as them. [3] *It extends it self to every thing* (as Guianerius will have it) *that is superfluously sought after,* or to any [4]*fervent desire* (as Fernelius interprets it: be it in what kind soever, it tortures, if immoderate, and is (according to [5] Plater and others) an especial cause of melancholy. *Multuosis concupiscentiis dilaniantur cogitationes meæ,* [6] Austin confessed— that he was torn a-pieces with his manifold desires; and so doth [7] Bernard complain, *that he could not rest for them a minute of an hour: this I would have, and that, and then I desire to be such and such.* 'Tis a hard matter therefore to confine them, being they are so various and many, and unpossible to apprehend all. I will only insist upon some few of the chief, and most noxious in their kind, as that exorbitant appetite and desire of honour, which we commonly call *ambition;* love of money, which is *covetousness,* and that greedy desire of gain; *self-love,* pride, and inordinate desire of *vain-glory* or applause; *love of study* in excess; *love of women* (which will require a just volume of it self). Of the other I will briefly speak, and in their order.

Ambition, a proud covetousness or a dry thirst of honour, a great torture of the mind, composed of envy, pride, and covetousness, a gallant madness, one [8] defines it, a pleasant poyson, Ambrose, *a canker of the soul; an hidden plague;* [9] Bernard, *a secret poyson, the father of livor, and mother of hypocrisie, the moth of holiness, and cause of madness, crucifying and disquieting all that it takes hold of.* [10] Seneca calls it, *rem solicitam, timidam, vanam, ventosam,* a windy thing, a vain, solicitous, and fearful thing; for, commonly, they that, like Sisyphus, roll this restless stone of ambition, are in a perpetual agony, still [11] perplexed, *semper taciti, tristesque recedunt,* (Lucretius) doubtful, timorous, suspicious, loth to offend in word or deed, still cogging, and colloguing, embracing, capping, cringing, applauding, flattering, fleering, visiting, waiting at mens doors, with all affability, counterfeit honesty,

---

[1] Molam asinariam.   [2] Tract. de Inter. c. 92.   [3] Circa quamlibet rem mundi hæc passio fieri potest, quæ superflue diligatur.   [4] Ferventius desiderium.   [5] Imprimis vero appetitus, &c. 3. de alien. ment.   [6] Conf. l. c. 29.   [7] Per diversa loca vagor; nullo temporis momento quiesco; talis et talis esse cupio; illud atque illud habere desidero.   [8] Ambros. l. 3. super Lucam. ærugo animæ.   [9] Nihil animum cruciat, nihil molestius inquietat; secretum virus, pestis occulta, &c. epist. 126.   [10] Ep. 88.   [11] Nihil infelicius his; quantus iis timor, quanta dubitatio, quantus conatus, quanta solicitudo! nulla illis a molestiis vacua hora.

Mem. 3. Subs. 11.] *Ambition, a Cause.* 287

and humility [1]. If that will not serve, if once this humour (as [2] Cyprian describes it) possess his thirsty soul, *ambitionis salsugo ubi bibulam animam possidet,* by hook and by crook he will obtain it; *and from his hole he will climbe to all honours and offices, if it be possible for him to get up; flattering one, bribing another, he will leave no means unessay'd to win all.* [3] It is a wonder to see how slavishly these kind of men subject themselves, when they are about a sute, to every inferiour person; what pains they will take, run, ride, cast, plot, countermine, protest and swear, vow, promise, what labours undergo, early up, down late; how obsequious and affable they are, how popular and courteous, how they grin and fleer upon every man they meet; with what feasting and inviting, how they spend themselves and their fortunes, in seeking that, many times, which they had much better be without (as [4] Cineas the orator told Pyrrhus); with what waking nights, painful hours, anxious thoughts, and bitterness of mind, *inter spemque metumque,* distracted and tired, they consume the interim of their time. There can be no greater plague for the present. If they do obtain their sute, which with such cost and solicitude they have sought, they are not so freed, their anxiety is anew to begin; for they are never satisfied; *nihil aliud nisi imperium spirant;* their thoughts, actions, endeavours are all for soveraignty and honour; like [5] Lues Sforsia (that huffing duke of Milan, *a man of singular wisdom, but profound ambition, born to his own, and to the destruction of Italy*) though it be to their own ruine, and friends undoing, they will contend; they may not cease; but as a dog in a wheel, a bird in a cage, or a squirrel in a chain, (so [6] Budæus compares them) [7] they climbe and climbe still with much labour, but never make an end, never at the top. A knight would be a baronet, and then a lord, and then a vicount, and then an earl, &c. a doctor a dean, and then a bishop: from tribune to prætor: from bailiff to mayor: first this office, and then that: as Pyrrhus, (in [8] Plutarch) they will first have Greece, then Africk, and then Asia, and swell with Æsops frog so long, till in the end they burst or come down, with Sejanus, *ad Gemonias scalas,* and

---

[1] Semper attonitus, semper pavidus quid dicat, faciatve: ne displiceat, humilitatem simulat, honestatem mentitur.   [2] Cypr. Prolog. ad ser. to. 2. Cunctos honorat, universis inclinat, subsequitur, obsequitur; frequentat curias, visitat optimates, amplexatur, applaudit, adulatur; per fas et nefas e latebris, in omnem gradum ubi aditus patet, se ingerit, discurrit.   [3] Turbæ cogit ambitio regem inservire, ut Homerus Agamemnonem querentem inducit.   [4] Plutarchus. Quin convivemur, et in otio nos oblectemus, quoniam in promptu id nobis sit, &c.   [5] Jovius, hist. l. 1. Vir singulari prudentiâ, sed profundâ ambitione; ad exitium Italiæ natus.   [6] Ut hedera arbori adhæret, sic ambitio, &c. [7] Lib. 3. de contemptu rerum fortuitarum. Magno conatu et impetu moventur; super eodem centro rotati, non proficiunt, nec ad finem perveniunt.   [8] Vita Pyrrhi.

288   *Causes of Melancholy.*   [Part. 1. Sec. 2.

break their own necks; or as Evangelus the piper, (in Lucian)
that blew his pipe so long, till he fell down dead. If he chance
to miss, and have a canvas, he is in a hell on the other side;
so dejected, that he is ready to hang himself, turn heretick,
Turk, or traytor, in an instant. Enraged against his enemies,
he [1] rails, swears, fights, slanders, detracts, envies, murders;
and, for his own part, *si appetitum explere non potest, furore
corripitur;* if he cannot satisfie his desire, (as [2] Bodine writes)
he runs mad: so that, both wayes, hit or miss, he is distracted
so long as his ambition lasts; he can look for no other but
anxiety and care, discontent and grief, in the mean time—[3]madness itself, or violent death, in the end. The event of this is
common to be seen in populous cities, or in princes courts; for
a courtiers life (as Budæus describes it) *is a [4] gallimaufry of
ambition, lust, fraud, imposture, dissimulation, detraction,
envy, pride; the court, a common conventicle of flatterers,
time-servers; politicians, &c.* or (as [5] Anthony Perez will)
the suburbs of hell it self. If you will see such discontented
persons, there you shall likely find them: [6] and (which he observed of the markets of old Rome)

Qui perjurum convenire vult hominem, mitto in Comitium;
Qui mendacem et gloriosum, apud Cloacinæ sacrum ;
Dites, damnosos maritos, sub Basilicâ quærito, &c.

Perjur'd knaves, knights of the post, lyers, crackers, bad husbands, &c. keep their several stations, they do still, and alwayes did, in every common-wealth.

SUBSECT. XII.

Φιλαργυρια, *Covetousness, a Cause.*

PLUTARCH (in his [7] book whether the diseases of the
body be more grievous than those of the soul) is of opinion, *if you will examine all the causes of our miseries in
this life, you shall find them, most part, to have had their*

---

[1] Ambitio in insaniam facile delabitur, si excedat. Patritius, l. 4. tit. 20. de
regis instit.   [2] Lib. 5. de rep. cap. 1.   [3] Imprimis vero appetitus, seu
concupiscentia nimia rei alicujus honestæ vel inhonestæ, phantasiam lædunt;
unde multi ambitiosi, philauti, irati, avari, insani, &c. Felix Plater, l. 3. de
mentis alien.   [4] Aulica vita colluvies ambitionis, cupiditatis, simulationis,
imposturæ, fraudis, invidiæ, superbiæ Titanicæ: diversorium aula, et commune
conventiculum, assentandi artificum, &c. Budæus de asse. lib. 5.   [5] In his
Aphor.   [6] Plautus, Curcul. act. 4. sce. 1.   [7] Tom. 2. Si examines,
omnes miseriæ caussas vel a furioso contendendi studio, vel ab injustâ cupiditate,
originem traxisse scies.—Idem fere Chrysostomus, Com. in c. 6. ad Romam
ser. 11.

Mem. 3. Subs. 12.] *Covetousness, a Cause.* 289

*beginning from stubborn anger, that furious desire of conten-
tion, or some unjust or immoderate affection, as covetousness,
&c.* From whence *are wars and contentions amongst you?*
[1]St. James asks: I will add usury, fraud, rapine, simony, oppression, lying, swearing, bearing false witness, &c. are they
not from this fountain of covetousness, that greediness in getting, tenacity in keeping, sordidity in spending? that they are
so wicked, [2]*unjust against God, their neighbour, themselves,*
all comes hence. *The desire of money is the root of all evil,
and they that lust after it, pierce themselves through with many
sorrows,* 1 Tim. 6. 10. Hippocrates therefore, in his epistle
to Crateva an herbalist, gives him this good counsel, that, if
it were possible, [3]*amongst other hearbs, he should cut up that
weed of covetousness by the roots, that there be no remainder
left ; and then know this for a certainty, that, together with
their bodies, thou maist quickly cure all the diseases of their
minds:* for it is indeed the pattern, image, epitome, of all
melancholy, the fountain of many miseries, much discontent,
care and woe—this *inordinate or immoderate desire of gain,
to get or keep money,* as [4]Bonaventure defines it ; or, as Austin
describes it, a madness of the soul; Gregory, a torture; Chrysostom, an unsatiable drunkenness ; Cyprian, blindness, *spe-
ciosum supplicium,* a plague subverting kingdoms, families,
an [5]incurable disease ; Budæus, an ill habit, [6]*yielding to no
remedies* ; (neither Æsculapius nor Plutus can cure them)
a continual plague, saith Solomon, and vexation of spirit,
another hell. I know there be some of opinion, that covetous
men are happy, and worldly-wise, that there is more pleasure
in getting wealth than in spending, and no delight in the
world like unto it. 'Twas Bias problem of old, *With what
art thou not weary? with getting money.* [7]*What is most
delectable? to gain.* What is it, trow you, that makes a poor
man labour all his life time, carry such great burdens, fare
so hardly, macerate himself, and endure so much misery, undergo such base offices with so great patience, to rise up early,
and lye down late, if there were not an extraordinary delight
in getting and keeping of money? What makes a merchant,
that hath no need, *satis superque domi,* to range over all

---

[1] Cap. 4. 1.   [2] Ut sit iniquus in Deum, in proximum, in seipsum.   [3] Si
vero, Crateva, inter cæteras herbarum radices, avaritiæ radicem secare posses
amaram, ut nullæ reliquiæ essent, probe scito, &c.   [4] Cap. 6. Diætæ salutis. Avaritia est amor immoderatus pecuniæ vel acquirendæ vel retinendæ.
[5] Malus est morbus, maleque afficit avaritia, siquidem censeo, &c. Avaritia
difficilius curatur quam insania ; quoniam hac omnes fere medici laborant. Hip.
ep. Abderit.   [6] Ferum profecto dirumque ulcus animi, remediis non cedens,
medendo exasperatur.   [7] Quâ re non es lassus? lucrum faciendo. Quid
maxime delectabile? lucrari.

VOL. I.   U

290 *Causes of Melancholy.* [Part. 1. Sec. 2.

the world, through all those intemperate [1] zones of heat and cold, voluntarily to venture his life, and be content with such miserable famine, nasty usage, in a stinking ship, if there were not a pleasure and hope to get money, which doth season the rest, and mitigate his indefatigable pains? What makes them go into the bowels of the earth, an hundred fathom deep, endangering their dearest lives, enduring damps and filthy smells, (when they have enough already, if they could be content, and no such cause to labour) but an extraordinary delight they take in riches? This may seem plausible at first shew, a popular and strong argument; but let him that so thinks, consider better of it; and he shall soon perceive that it is far otherwise than he supposeth; it may be haply pleasing at the first, as, most part, all melancholy is; for such men likely have some *lucida intervalla,* pleasant symptomes intermixt: but you must note that of [2] Chrysostome, *'tis one thing to be rich, another to be covetous :* generally they are all fools, dizards, mad-men, [3] miserable wretches, living besides themselves, *sine arte fruendi,* in perpetual slavery, fear, suspicion, sorrow, and discontent; *plus aloës quam mellis habent;* and are, indeed, *rather possessed by their money, than possessors;* as [4] Cyprian hath it, *mancipati pecuniis,* bound prentise to their goods, as [5] Pliny; or as Chrysostom, *servi divitiarum,* slaves and drudges to their substance; and we may conclude of them all, as [6] Valerius doth of Ptolemæus king of Cyprus, *he was in title a king of that island, but in his mind, a miserable drudge of money :*

—————————[7] Potiore metallis
Libertate carens——

wanting his liberty, which is better than gold. Damasippus the Stoick (in Horace) proves that all mortal men dote by fits, some one way, some another, but that covetous men [8] are madder than the rest: and he that shall truly look into their estates, and examine their symptomes, shall find no better of them, but that they are all [9] fools, as Nabal was, *re et nomine* (1 *Reg.* 15): for, what greater folly can there be, or [10] madness, than to macerate himself when he need not? and when

[1] Extremos currit mercator ad Indos. Hor.   [2] Hom. 2. Aliud avarus, aliud dives.   [3] Divitiæ, ut spinæ, animum hominis timoribus, solicitudinibus, angoribus, mirifice pungunt, vexant, cruciant. Greg. in Hom.   [4] Epist. ad Donat. cap. 2.   [5] Lib. 9. ep. 30.   [6] Lib. 9. cap. 4. Insulæ rex titulo, sed animo pecuniæ miserabile mancipium.   [7] Hor. 10. lib. 1. [8] Danda est hellebori multo pars maxima avaris.   [9] Luke 12. 20. Stulte, hac nocte eripiam animam tuam.   [10] Opes quidem mortalibus sunt dementia. Theog.

Mem. 3. Subs. 12.]   *Covetousness, a Cause.*   291

(as Cyprian notes) [1] *he may be freed from his burden, and cased of his pains, will go on still, his wealth increasing, when he hath enough, to get more, to live besides himself,* to starve his *genius,* keep back from his wife [2] and children, neither letting them nor other friends use or enjoy that which is theirs by right, and which they much need perhaps : like a - hog, or dog in the manger, he doth only keep it, because it shall do nobody else good, hurting himself and others ; and, for a little momentary pelf, damn his own soul. They are commonly sad and tetrick by nature, as Achabs spirit was because he could not get Naboths vineyard (1 *Reg.* 22) ; and, if he lay out his money at any time, though it be to necessary uses, to his own childrens good, he brawls and scolds ; his heart is heavy ; much disquieted he is, and loth to part from it : *miser abstinet, et timet uti* (Hor). He is of a wearish, dry, pale constitution, and cannot sleep for cares and worldly business ; his riches (saith Solomon) will not let him sleep, and unnecessary business which he heapeth on himself : or if he do sleep, 'tis a very unquiet, interrupt, unpleasing sleep, with his bags in his arms,

>   —— congestis undique saccis
>   Indormit inhians ;

and though he be at a banquet, or at some merry feast, *he sighs for grief of heart* (as [3] Cyprian hath it), *and cannot sleep, though he be upon a down bed ; his wearish body takes no rest,* [4] *troubled in his abundance, and sorrowful in plenty, unhappy for the present, and more unhappy in the life to come* (Basil). He is a perpetual drudge, [5] *restless in his thoughts, and never satisfied,* a slave, a wretch, a dust-worm ; *semper quod idolo suo immolet, sedulus observat ;* (Cypr. *prolog. ad sermon.*) still seeking what sacrifice he may offer to his golden god, *per fas et nefas,* he cares not how ; his trouble is endless : [6] *crescunt divitiæ ; tamen curtæ nescio quid semper abest rei :* his wealth increaseth, and the more he hath, the more [7] he wants, like Pharoahs lean kine, which devoured the fat, and were not satisfied. [8] Austin therefore defines covetousness, *quarumlibet*

---

[1] Ed. 2. lib. 2. Exonerare cum se posset et relevare ponderibus, pergit magis fortunis augentibus pertinaciter incubare   [2] Non amicis, non liberis, non ipsi sibi quidquam impertit ; possidet ad hoc tantum, ne possidere alteri liceat, &c. Hieron. ad Paulin.   Tam deest quod habet, quam quod non habet.   [3] Epist. 2. lib. 2.   Suspirat in convivio, bibat licet gemmis, et toro molliore marcidum corpus condiderit, vigilat in plumâ.   [4] Angustatur ex abundantiâ, contristatur ex opulentiâ, infelix præsentibus bonis, infelicior in futuris.   [5] Illorum cogitatio nunquam cessat, qui pecunias supplere diligunt. Guianer. tract. 15. c. 17.   [6] Hor. 3. Od. 24.   Quo plus sunt potæ, plus sitiuntur aquæ. [7] Hor. l. 2. Sat. 6. O si angulus ille proximus accedat, qui nunc denormat agellum !   [8] Lib.3. de lib. arbit. Immoritur studiis, et amore senescit habendi.

u 2

292   *Causes of Melancholy.*   [Part. 1. Sec. 2.

rerum inhonestam et insatiabilem cupiditatem, an unhonest
and unsatiable desire of gain; and, in one of his epistles, compares it to hell, [1] *which devours all, and yet never hath enough,
a bottomless pit,* an endless misery: *in quem scopulum avaritiæ
cadaverosi senes ut plurimum impingunt;* and, that which is
their greatest corrosive, they are in continual suspicion, fear, and
distrust. He thinks his own wife and children are so many
thieves, and go about to cozen him, his servants are all false:

Et divûm atque hominum clamat continuo fidem,
Rem suam periisse, seque eradicarier,
De suo tigillo fumus si quâ exit foras,

If his doors creek, then out he cryes anon,
His goods are gone, and he is quite undone.

Timidus Plutus, an old proverb—as fearful as Plutus: so doth
Aristophanes, and Lucian, bring him in fearful still, pale,
anxious, supicious, and trusting no man. [2] *They are afraid of
tempests for their corn, they are afraid of their friends, least
they should ask something of them, beg or borrow; they are
afraid of their enemies, lest they hurt them; thieves, lest they
rob them; they are afraid of war, and afraid of peace, afraid
of rich, and afraid of poor; afraid of all.* Last of all, they are
afraid of want, that they shall dye beggers; which makes them
lay up still, and dare not use that they have: (what if a dear
year come, or dearth, or some loss?) and were it not that they
are loth to [3] lay out money on a rope, they would be hanged
forthwith, and sometimes dye to save charges, and make away
themselves, if their corn and cattle miscarry, though they have
abundance left, as [4] Agellius notes. [5] Valerius makes mention
of one, that in a famine sold a mouse for two hundred pence,
and famished himself. Such are their cares, [6] griefs and perpetual
fears. These symptomes are elegantly expressed by Theophrastus in his character of a covetous man: [7] *lying in bed,
he askes his wife whether she shut the trunks and chests fast,
the capcase be sealed, and whether the hall door be bolted;
and though she say all is well, he riseth out of his bed in his*

---

[1] Avarus vir inferno est similis, &c. modum non habet, hoc egentior, quo plura
habet.   [2] Erasm. Adag. chil. 3. cent. 7. pro. 72. Nulli fidentes, omnium
formidant opes: ideo pavidum malum vocat Euripides: metuunt tempestates ob
frumentum, amicos ne rogent, inimicos ne lædant, fures ne rapiant; bellum timent, pacem timent, summos, medios, infimos.   [3] Hall Char.   [4] Agellius, lib. 3. c. 1. Interdum eo sceleris perveniunt, ob lucrum ut vitam propriam
commutent.   [5] Lib. 7. cap. 6.   [6] Omnes perpetuo morbo agitantur; sus-
picatur omnes timidus, sibique ob aurum insidiari putat, nunquam quiescens.
Plin. Prœm. lib. 14.   [7] Cap. 18. In lecto jacens, interrogat uxorem an
arcam probe clausit, an capsula, &c. E lecto surgens nudus, et absque calceis,
accensâ lucernâ omnia obiens et lustrans, et vix somno indulgens.

shirt, bare foot, and bare legged, to see whether it be so, with a dark lanthorn searching every corner, scarce sleeping a wink all night. Lucian, in that pleasant and witty dialogue called Gallus, brings in Micyllus the cobler disputing with his cock, sometimes Pythagoras; where, after much speech *pro* and *con*, to prove the happiness of a mean estate, and discontents of a rich man, Pythagoras his cock in the end, to illustrate by examples that which he had said, brings him to Gniphon the usurers house at mid-night, and after that to Eucrates; whom they found both awake, casting up their accounts, and telling of their money, [1] lean, dry, pale, and anxious, still suspecting lest some body should make a hole through the wall, and so get in; or, if a rat or mouse did but stir, starting upon a sudden, and running to the door, to see whether all were fast. Plautus, in his Aulularia, makes old Euclio [2] commanding Staphyla his wife to shut the doors fast, and the fire to be put out, lest any body should make that an errant to come to his house: when he washed his hands, [3] he was loth to fling away the foul water; complaining that he was undone, because the smoak got out of his roof. And, as he went from home, seeing a crow scrat upon the muck-hill, returned in all haste, taking it for *malum omen*, an ill sign, his money was digged up; with many such. He that will but observe their actions, shall find these and many such passages, not feigned for sport, but really performed, verified indeed by such covetous and miserable wretches; and that it is,

—————————[4] manifesta phrenesis,
Ut locuples moriaris, egenti vivere fato—

a meer madness, to live like a wretch, and dye rich.

SUBSECT. XIII.

Love of Gaming, &c. and Pleasures immoderate; Causes.

It is a wonder to see, how many poor distressed miserable wretches, one shall meet almost in every path and street, begging for an alms, that have been well descended, and sometimes in flourishing estate, now ragged, tattered, and ready to

---

[1] Curis extenuatus, vigilans, et secum supputans. [2] Cave, quemquam alienum in ædes intromiseris. Ignem extingui volo, ne caussæ quidquam sit, quod te quisquam quæritet. Si bona Fortuna veniat, ne intromiseris. Occlude sis fores ambobus pessulis. Discrucior animi, quia domo abeundum est mihi. Nimis hercule invitus abeo; nec, quid agam, scio. [3] Plorat aquam profundere, &c. periit dum fumus de tigillo exit foras. [4] Juv. Sat. 14.

294   *Causes of Melancholy.*   [Part. 1. Sec. 2.

be starved, lingring out a painful life, in discontent and grief
of body and mind, and all through immoderate lust, gaming,
pleasure, and riot. 'Tis the common end of all sensual Epicures and brutish prodigals, that are stupified and carried away
headlong with their several pleasures and lusts. Cebes, in his
table, S. Ambrose, in his second book of Abel and Cain, and,
amongst the rest, Lucian, in his tract *de Mercede conductis*,
hath excellent well deciphered such mens proceedings in his
picture of *Opulentia*, whom he feigns to dwell on the top of a
high mount, much sought after by many suitors. At their first
coming, they are generally entertained by *Pleasure* and *Dalli-
ance*, and have all the content that possibly may be given, so
long as their money lasts; but, when their means fail, they
are contemptibly thrust out at a back door, headlong, and
there left to *Shame, Reproach, Despair.* And he, at first that
had so many attendants, parasites, and followers, young and
lusty, richly array'd, and all the dainty fare that might be had,
with all kind of welcome and good respect, is now upon a
sudden stript of all, [1] pale, naked, old, diseased, and forsaken,
cursing his stars, and ready to strangle himself; having no
other company but *Repentance, Sorrow, Grief, Derision,
Beggery*, and *Contempt*, which are his daily attendants to his
lives end. As the [2] prodigal son had exquisite musick, merry
company, dainty fare at first, but a sorrowful reckoning in
the end; so have all such vain delights and their followers.
[3] *Tristes voluptatum exitus, ut quisquis voluptatum suarum
reminisci volet, intelliget:* as bitter as gall and wormwood
is their last; grief of mind, madness it self. The ordinary
rocks upon which such men do impinge and precipitate themselves, are cards, dice, hawks, and hounds, (*insanum venandi
studium*, one calls it—*insanæ substructiones*) their mad structures, disports, playes, &c. when they are unseasonably used,
imprudently handled, and beyond their fortunes.—Some men
are consumed by mad phantastical buildings, by making galleries, cloisters, taraces, walks, orchards, gardens, pools, rillets,
bowers, and such like places of pleasure, (*inutiles domos*,
[4] Xenophon calls them) which howsoever they be delightsome
things in themselves, and acceptable to all beholders, an ornament, and befitting some great men, yet unprofitable to others
and the sole overthrow of their estates. Forestus, in his observations, hath an example of such a one that became melancholy
upon the like occasion, having consumed his substance in an

---

[1] Ventricosus, nudus, pallidus, lævâ pudorem occultans, dextrâ seipsum stran-
gulans. Occurrit autem exeunti Pœnitentia, his miserum conficiens, &c.
[2] Luke 15.   [3] Boëthius.   [4] In Œconom. Quid si nunc ostendam
eos qui magnâ vi argenti domus inutiles ædificant? inquit Socrates.

Mem. 3. Subs. 13.] *Love of Gaming, &c.* 295

unprofitable building, which would afterward yield him no advantage. Others, I say, are [1] overthrown by those mad sports of hawking and hunting—honest recreations, and fit for some great men, but not for every base inferiour person. Whilst they will maintain their faulkoners, dogs, and hunting nags, their wealth (saith [2] Salmutze) *runs away with hounds, and their fortunes flye away with hawks:* they persecute beasts so long, till, in the end, they themselves degenerate into beasts (as [3] Agrippa taxeth them), [4] Actæon like; for, as he was eaten to death by his own dogs, so do they devour themselves and their patrimonies, in such idle and unnecessary disports, neglecting in the mean time their more necessary business, and to follow their vocations. Over-mad too sometimes are our great men in delighting and doting too much on it; [5] *when they drive poor husbandmen from their tillage* (as [6] Sarisburiensis objects, *Polycrat. l. 1. c.* 4), *fling down countrey farms, and whole towns, to make parks and forests, starving men to feed beasts, and* [7] *punishing in the mean time such a man that shall molest their game, more severely than him that is otherwise a common hacker, or a notorious thief.* But great men are some wayes to be excused: the meaner sort have no evasion why they should not be counted mad. Poggius, the Florentine, tells a merry story to this purpose, condemning the folly and impertinent business of such kind of persons. A physician of Milan, (saith he) that cured mad men, had a pit of water in his house, in which he kept his patients, some up to the knees, some to the girdle, some to the chin, *pro modo insaniæ*, as they were more or less affected. One of them by chance, that was well recovered, stood in the door, and, seeing a gallant ride by with a hawk on his fist, well mounted, with his spaniels after him, would needs know to what use all this preparation served. He made answer, to kill certain fowl. The patient demanded again, what his fowl might be worth, which he killed in a year. He replyed, five or ten crowns; and when he urged him farther what his dogs, horse, and hawks, stood him in, he told him

---

[1] Sarisburiensis, Polycrat. l. 1. c. 4. Venatores omnes adhuc institutionem redolent Centaurorem. Raro invenitur quisquam eorum modestus et gravis, raro continens, et, ut credo, sobrius unquam. [2] Pancirol. Tit. 23. Avolant opes cum accipitre. [3] Insignis venatorum stultitia, et supervacanea cura eorum, qui, dum nimium venationi insistunt, ipsi, abjectâ omni humanitate, in feras degenerant, ut Actæon, &c. [4] Sabin. in Ovid. Met. [5] Agrippa, de vanit. scient. Insanum venandi studium, dum a novalibus arcentur agricolæ, subtrahunt prædia rusticis, agri colonis præcluduntur, sylvæ et prata pastoribus, ut augeantur pascua feris.—Majestatis reus agricola, si gustârit. [6] A novalibus suis agricolæ, dum feræ habeant vagandi libertatem: istis ut pascua augeantur prædia subtrahuntur, &c. Sarisburiensis. [7] Feris quam hominibus æquiores. Cambd. de Guil. Conq. qui 36 ecclesias matrices depopulatus est ad Forestam Novam. Mat. Paris.

296   *Causes of Melancholy.*   [Part. 1. Sec. 2.

four hundred crowns. With that the patient bade him be gone
as he loved his life and welfare ; " for, if our master come and
find thee here, he will put thee in the pit amongst mad men,
up to the chin ;" taxing the madness and folly of such vain
men, that spend themselves in those idle sports, neglecting
their business and necessary affairs. Leo Decimus, that hunting pope, is much discommended by [1] Jovius in his life, for his
immoderate desire of hawking and hunting, in so much, that
(as he saith) he would sometimes live about Ostia weeks and
moneths together, leave suitors [2] unrespected, bulls and pardons
unsigned, to his own prejudice, and many private mens loss :
[3] *and if he had been by chance crossed in his sport, or his game
not so good, he was so impatient, that he would revile and miscall
many times men of great worth with most bitter taunts, look so
sowr, be so angry and waspish, so grieved and molested, that it
is incredible to relate it.* But, if he had good sport, and been
well pleased on the other side, *incredibili munificentiâ*, with
unspeakable bounty and munificence, he would reward all his
fellow hunters and deny nothing to any suiter, when he was in
that mood. To say truth, 'tis the common humour of all gamesters, as Galatæus observes : if they win, no men living are so
jovial and merry ; but, [4] if they lose, though it be but a trifle,
two or three games at tables, or dealings at cards for two pence
a game, they are so cholerick and testy, that no man may
speak with them, and break many times into violent passions,
oaths, imprecations, and unbeseeming speeches, little differing
from mad men for the time. Generally of all gamesters and
gaming, if it be excessive, thus much we may conclude, that
whether they win or lose for the present, their winnings are not
munera fortunæ, sed insidiæ, as that wise Seneca determines—
not fortunes gifts, but baits; the common catastrophe is
[5] beggery : [6] *ut pestis vitam, sic adimit alea pecuniam;* as the
plague takes away life, so doth gaming goods; for [7] *omnes nudi,
inopes et egeni ;*

    [8] Alea Scylla vorax, species certissima furti,
      Non contenta bonis, animum quoque perfida mergit,
      Fœda, furax, infamis, iners, furiosa, ruina.

---

[1] Tom. 2. de vitis illustrium, l. 4. de vit. Leon. 10.   [2] Venationibus adeo
perdite studebat et aucupiis.   [3] Aut infeliciter venatus, tam impatiens inde,
ut summos sæpe viros acerbissimis contumeliis oneraret ; et incredibile est, quali
vultus animique habitu dolorem iracundiamque præferret, &c.   [4] Unicuique
autem hoc a naturâ insitum est, ut doleat, sicubi erraverit aut deceptus sit.
[5] Juven. Sat. 8. Nec enim loculis comitantibus itur ad casum tabulæ; positâ sed
luditur arcâ.—Lemnius, instit. c. 44. Mendaciorum quidem, et perjuriorum, et
paupertatis, mater est alea ; nullam habens patrimonii reverentiam, quum illud
effuderit, sensim in furta delabitur et rapinas. Saris. Polycrat. l. 1. c. 5.
[6] Damhoderus.   [7] Dan. Souter.   [8] Petrar. dial. 27.

Mem. 3. Subs. 13.]   *Love of Gaming, &c.*   297

For a little pleasure they take, and some small gains and get-
tings now and then, their wives and children are wringed in the
mean time; and they themselves, with the loss of body and soul,
rue it in the end. I will say nothing of those prodigious prodigals, [1]*perdendæ pecuniæ genitos*, (as he taxed Anthony) *qui
patrimonium sine ullâ fori calumniâ amittunt*, (saith [2] Cyprian),
and [3] mad Sybaritical spendthrifts, *quique unâ comedunt patrimonia mensâ;* that eat up all at a breakfast, at a supper, or
amongst bauds, parasites, and players; consume themselves
in an instant, (as if they had flung it into [4] Tyber) with great
wagers, vain and idle expences, &c. not themselves only, but
even all their friends; as a man desperately swimming drowns
him that comes to help him, by suretiship and borrowing they
will willingly undo all their associates and allies; [5] *irati pecuniis*, as he saith—angry with their money. [6] *What with a
wanton eye, a liquorish tongue, and a gamesome hand,* when
they have undiscreetly impoverished themselves, mortgaged
their wits together with their lands, and entombed their ances-
tors fair possessions in their bowels, they may lead the rest of
their dayes in prison, as many times they do, and there repent
at leisure: and, when all is gone, begin to be thrifty: but *sera
est in fundo parsimonia :* 'tis then too late to look about; their
[7] end is misery, sorrow, shame, and discontent. And well they
deserve to be infamous and discontent, [8] *catamidiari in amphitheatro*, (as by Adrian the emperours edict they were of old;
decoctores bonorum suorum ; so he calls them—prodigal fools)
to be publickly shamed, and hissed out of all societies, rather
than to be pittied or relieved. [9] The Tuscans and Bœotians
brought their bankrupts into the market place in a bier, with
an empty purse carried before them, all the boys following,
where they sat all day, *circumstante plebe*, to be infamous and
ridiculous. At [10] Padua in Italy, they have a stone called the
stone of turpitude, near the senate house, where spendthrifts,
and such as disclaim nonpayments of debts, do sit with their
hinder parts bare, that, by that note of disgrace, others may be
terrified from all such vain expence, or borrowing more than
they can tell how to pay. The [11] civilians of old set guardians
over such brain-sick prodigals, as they did over mad-men, to
moderate their expences, that they should not so loosely consume their fortunes, to the utter undoing of their families.

---

[1] Sallust.   [2] Tom. 3. Ser. de aleâ.   [3] Plutus, in Aristoph. calls
all such gamesters mad men; Si in insanum hominem contigero. Spontaneum ad
se trahunt furorem : et os, et nares, et oculos, rivos faciunt furoris et diversoria.
Chrys. hom. 71.   [4] Paschasius Justus. l. 1. de aleâ.   [5] Seneca.
[6] Hall.   [7] In Sat. 11. Sed deficiente crumenâ, et crescente gulâ, quis te
manet exitus—rebus in ventrem mersis ?   [8] Spartian. Adriano.   [9] Alex.
ab Alex. l. 6. c. 10. Idem Gerbelius, l. 5. Græ. disc.   [10] Fines Moris.   [11] Jus-
tinian. in Digestis.

298 Causes of Melancholy. [Part. 1. Sec. 2.

I may not here omit those two main plagues, and common dotages of humane kind, wine and women, which have infatuated and besotted myriads of people. They go commonly together.

[1] Qui vino indulget, quemque alea decoquit, ille
In Venerem putris.

To whom is sorrow, saith Solomon, (Prov. 23. 39) to whom is wo, but to such a one as loves drink? It causeth torture, (*vino tortus et irâ*) and bitterness of mind (*Sirac.* 31. 21). *Vinum furoris*, Jeremy calls it (*chap.* 15), wine of madness, as well he may; for *insanire facit sanos*, it makes sound men sick and sad, and wise men [2] mad, to say and do they know not what. *Accidit hodie terribilis casus* (saith [3] St. Austin): hear a miserable accident: Cyrillus son this day, in his drink, *matrem prægnantem nequiter oppressit, sororem violare voluit, patrem occidit fere, et duas alias sorores ad mortem vulneravit*—would have violated his sister, killed his father, &c. A true saying it was of him, *vino dari lætitiam et dolorem;* drink causeth mirth and drink causeth sorrow; drink causeth *poverty and want,* (Prov. 21.) *shame and disgrace. Multi ignobiles evasere ob vini potum, &c.* (Austin) *amissis honoribus, profugi aberrârunt:* many men have made shipwrack of their fortunes, and go like rogues and beggers, having turned all their substance into *aurum potabile,* that otherwise might have lived in good worship and happy estate; and for a few hours pleasure (for their *Hilary* term's but short), or [4]*free madness* (as Seneca calls it), purchase unto themselves eternal tediousness and trouble.

That other madness is on women. *Apostatare facit cor,* (saith the wise man) [5]*atque homini cerebrum minuit.* Pleasant at first she is (like Dioscorides Rhododaphne, that fair plant to the eye, but poyson to the taste); the rest as bitter as wormwood in the end, (Prov. 5. 4.) and sharpe as a two-edged sword (7. 21.) *Her house is the way to hell, and goes down to the chambers of death.* What more sorrowful can be said? They are miserable in this life, mad, beasts, led like [6] *oxen to the slaughter:* and (that which is worse) whoremasters and drunkards shall be judged; *amittunt gratiam,* (saith Austin) *perdunt gloriam, incurrunt damnationem æternam.* They lose grace and glory:

———————[7] brevis illa voluptas
Abrogat æternum cœli decus.——

they gain hell and eternal damnation.

[1] Persius, Sat. 5.   [2] Poculum quasi sinus, in quo sæpe naufragium faciunt, jacturâ tum pecuniæ tum mentis. Erasm. in Prov. Calicum remiges. chil. 4. cent. 7. Pro. 41.   [3] Ser. 33. ad frat. in Eremo.   [4] Liberæ unius horæ insaniam æterno temporis tædio pensant.   [5] Menander.   [6] Prov. 5.   [7] Merlin. Cocc.

SUBSECT. XIV.

Philautia, or Self-love, Vain-glory, Praise, Honour, Immoderate Applause, Pride, over-much Joy, &c. Causes.

SELF-LOVE, pride, and vain-glory, [1] *cæcus amor sui*, (which Chrysostome calls one of the devils three great nets ; [2] Bernard, *an arrow which pierceth the soul through, and slayes it ; a slye insensible enemy, not perceived*) are main causes. Where neither anger, lust, covetousness, fear, sorrow, &c. nor any other perturbation, can lay hold, this will slily and insensibly pervert us. *Quem non gula vicit, philautia superavit* (saith Cyprian): whom surfeiting could not overtake, self-love hath overcome. [3] *He that hath scorned all money, bribes, gifts, upright otherwise and sincere, hath inserted himself to no fond imagination, and sustained all those tyrannical concupiscences of the body, hath lost all his honour, captivated by vain-glory.* (Chrysostom. *sup. Jo.*) *Tu sola animum mentemque peruris, gloria:* a great assault and cause of our present malady— although we do most part neglect, take no notice of it, yet this is a violent batterer of our souls, causeth melancholy and dotage. This pleasing humour, this soft and whispering popular air, *amabilis insania*, this delectable frensie, most irrefragable passion, *mentis gratissimus error*, this acceptable disease, which so sweetly sets upon us, ravisheth our senses, lulls our souls asleep, puffs up our hearts as so many bladders, and that without all feeling, [4] in so much as *those that are misaffected with it, never so much as once perceive it, or think of any cure.* We commonly love him best in this [5] malady, that doth us most harm, and are very willing to be hurt: *adulationibus nostris libenter favemus* (saith [6] Jerome): we love him, we love him for it: [7] *O Bonciari, suave, suave fuit a te tali hæc tribui;* 'twas sweet to hear it: and, as [8] Pliny doth ingenuously confess to his dear friend Augurinus, *all thy writings are most acceptable, but those especially that speak of us :* again, a little after to Maximus, [9] *I cannot express how pleasing it is to me to hear my*

---

[1] Hor. [2] Sagitta, quæ animam penetrat, leviter penetrat, sed non leve infligit vulnus. sup. cant. [3] Qui omnem pecuniarum contemtum habent, et nulli imaginationi totius mundi se immiscuerint, et tyrannicas corporis concupiscentias sustinuerint, hi multoties, capti a vanâ gloriâ, omnia perdiderunt. [4] Hac correpti non cogitant de medelâ. [5] Di, talem a terris avertite pestem. [6] Ep. ad Eustochium, de custod. virgin. [7] Lips. Ep. ad Bonciarium. [8] Ep. lib. 9. Omnia tua scripta pulcherrima existimo, maxime tamen illa quæ de nobis. [9] Exprimere non possum, quam sit jucundum, &c.

300   *Causes of Melancholy.*   [Part. 1. Sec. 2.

self commended. Though we smile to ourselves, at least ironi-
cally, when parasites bedawb us with false *encomions,* as many
princes cannot chuse but do, *quum tale quid nihil intra se
repererint,* when they know they come as far short, as a mouse
to an elephant, of any such vertues; yet it doth us good.
Though we seem many times to be angry, [1] *and blush at our
own praises, yet our souls inwardly rejoice: it puffs us up;
'tis fallax suavitas, blandus dæmon, makes us swell beyond our
bounds, and forget our selves.* Her two daughters are lightness
of mind, immoderate joy and pride, not excluding those other
concomitant vices, which [2] Jodocus Lorichius reckons up—
bragging, hypocrisie, pievishness, and curiosity.

N ow the common cause of this mischief ariseth from our
selves or others: [3] we are active and passive. It proceeds inwardly from our selves, as we are active causes, from an overweening conceit we have of our good parts, own worth, (which
indeed is no worth) our bounty, favour, grace, valour, strength,
wealth, patience, meekness, hospitality, beauty, temperance,
gentry, knowledge, wit, science, art, learning, our [4] excellent
gifts and fortunes, for which (Narcissus like) we admire, flatter, and applaud our selves, and think all the world esteems
so of us; and, as deformed women easily believe those that
tell them they be fair, we are too credulous of our own good
parts and praises, too well perswaded of our selves. We brag
and vendicate our [5] own works, (and scorn all others in respect
of us; *inflati scientiâ,* saith Paul) our wisdom, [6] our learning:
all our geese are swans; and we as basely esteem and vilifie
other mens, as we do over-highly prize and value our own.
We will not suffer them to be in *secundis,* no not in *tertiis;*
what! *mecum confertur Ulysses?* they are *mures, muscæ,
culices, præ se,* nitts and flies compared to his inexorable and
supercilious, eminent and arrogant worship; though indeed
they be far before him. Only wise, only rich, only fortunate, valorous, and fair, puffed up with this tympany of self-
conceit, as the proud [7] Pharisee, they are not (as they suppose) *like other men,* of a purer and more precious metal [8];
Soli rei gerendæ sunt efficaces (which that wise Periander held
of such): [9] *meditantur omne qui prius negotium, &c. Novi
quemdam* (saith [10] Erasmus) I knew one so arrogant that he

---

[1] Hieron. Et, licet nos indignos dicimus, et calidus rubor ora perfundat, attamen
ad laudem suam intrinsecus animæ lætantur.   [2] Thesaur. Theo.   [3] Nec
enim mihi cornea fibra est. Per.   [4] E manibus illis Nascentur violæ. Pers. 1.
Sat.   [5] Omnia enim nostra supra modum placent.   [6] Fab. l. 10. c. 3. Ri-
dentur, mala qui componunt carmina; verum Gaudent scribentes, et se venerantur,
et ultro, Si taceas, laudant quidquid scripsere, beati. Hor. ep. 2. l. 2.   [7] Luke
18. 10.   [8] De meliore luto finxit præcordia Titan.   [9] Auson. sap.   [10] Chil.
3. cent. 10. pro. 97.   Qui se crederet neminem ullâ in re præstantiorem.

Mem. 3. Subs. 14.] *Philautia, or Self-love, &c.* 301

thought himself inferiour to no man living, like [1] Callisthenes the philosopher, that neither held Alexanders acts, or any other subject, worthy of his pen, such was his insolency; or Seleucus, king of Syria, who thought none fit to contend with him but the Romans; *[2] eos solos dignos ratus quibuscum de imperio certaret.* That which Tully writ to Atticus long since, is still in force—*[3] there was never yet true poet or orator, that thought any other better than himself.* And such for the most part, are your princes, potentates, great philosophers, historiographers, authors of sects or heresies, and all our great scholars, as [4] Hierom defines: *a natural philosopher is glories creature, and a very slave of rumour, fame, and popular opinion:* and, though they write *de contemptu gloriæ,* yet (as he observes) they will put their names to their books. *Vobis et famæ me semper dedi* saith Trebellius Pollio, I have wholly consecrated my self to you and fame. *'Tis all my desire, night and day, 'tis all my study to raise my name.* Proud [5] Pliny seconds him; *Quamquam O! &c.* and that vainglorious [6] orator is not ashamed to confess in an Epistle of his to Marcus Lecceius, *ardeo incredibili cupiditate, &c. I burn with an incredible desire to have my [7] name registered in thy book.* Out of this fountain proceed all those cracks and brags, —[8] *speramus carmina fingi posse linenda cedro, et lævi servanda cupresso*—[9] *Non usitatâ nec tenui ferar pennâ* —*nec in terrâ morabor longius. Nil parvum aut humili modo, nil mortale, loquor. Dicar, quâ violens obstrepit Aufidus*—*Exegi monumentum ære perennius.—Jamque opus exegi, quod nec Jovis ira, nec ignis, &c. cum venit illa dies, &c. parte tamen meliore mei super alta perennis astra ferar, nomenque erit indelebile nostrum*—(This of Ovid I have paraphrased in English—

<blockquote>
And when I am dead and gone,
My corps laid under a stone,
My fame shall yet survive,
And I shall be alive;
In these my works for ever,
My glory shall persever, &c.)
</blockquote>

---

[1] Tanto fastu scripsit, ut Alexandri gesta inferiora scriptis suis existimaret. Jo. Vossius, lib. 1. cap. 9. de hist. [2] Plutarch, vit. Catonis. [3] Nemo unquam poëta aut orator, qui quemquam se meliorem arbitraretur. [4] Consol. ad Pammachium. Mundi philosophus, gloriæ animal, et popularis auræ et rumorum venale mancipium. [5] Epist. 5. Capitoni suo. Diebus ac noctibus, hoc solum cogito, si quâ me possum levare humo. Id voto meo sufficit, &c. [6] Tullius. [7] Ut nomen meum scriptis tuis illustretur.—Inquies animus studio æternitatis noctes et dies angebatur. Heinsius, orat. funeb. de Scal. [8] Hor. art. Poët. [9] Od. ult. l. 3. Jamque opus exegi—Vade, liber felix! Palingen. lib. 18.

302   *Causes of Melancholy*.   [Part. 1. Sec. 2.

and that of Ennius,

> Nemo me lacrymis decoret, neque funera fletu
> Faxit : cur ? volito vivu' per ora virum.—

with many such proud strains, and foolish flashes, too common
with writers. Not so much as Democharis on the [1] Topicks,
but he will be immortal. Typotius, *de famâ*, shall be famous;
and well he deserves, because he writ of fame ; and every trivial poet must be renowned,

> ———plausuque petit clarescere vulgi.

This puffing humour it is, that hath produced so many great
tomes, built such famous monuments, strong castles, and
Mausolean tombs, to have their acts eternized,

> Digito monstrari, et dicier, " Hic est!"

to see their names inscribed, as Phryne on the walls of Thebes,
Phryne fecit. This causeth so many bloody battles,

> ———et noctes cogit vigilare serenas ;

long journeys,

> Magnum iter intendo ; sed dat mihi gloria vires———

gaining honour, a little applause, pride, self-love, vain-glory—
that is it which makes them take such pains, and break out
into those ridiculous strains, this high conceit of themselves, to
[2] scorn all others, *ridiculo fastu et intolerando contemtu,* (as
[3] Palæmon the grammarian contemned Varro, *secum et natas
et morituras literas jactans*) and brings them to that height of
insolency, that they cannot endure to be contradicted, [4] *or hear
of any thing but their own commendation*, which Hierom
notes of such kind of men: and (as [5] Austin well seconds him)
*'tis their sole study, day and night, to be commended and ap-
plauded ;* when as indeed, in all wise mens judgements, *quibus
cor sapit*, they are [6] mad, empty vessels, funges, beside themselves, derided, *et ut camelus in proverbio, quærens cornua,
etiam quas habebat aures amisit ;* their works are toyes, as an
almanack out of date, [7] *auctoris pereunt garrulitate sui :* they
seek fame and immortality, but reap dishonour and infamy ;
they are a common obloquy, *insensati*, and come far short of
that which they suppose or expect. ([8] *O puer, ut sis vitalis,*

---

[1] In lib. 8.   [2] De ponte dejicere.   [3] Sueton. lib. de gram.   [4] Nihil
libenter audiunt, nisi laudes suas.   [5] Epis. 56. Nihil aliud dies noctesque
cogitant, nisi ut in studiis suis laudentur ab hominibus.   [6] Quæ major dementia aut dici aut excogitari potest, quam sic ob gloriam cruciari? Insaniam
istam, Domine, longe fac a me. Austin. conf. lib. 10. cap. 37.   [7] Mart.
l. 5. 51.   [8] Hor. Sat. l. 1. 2.

metuo.) Of so many myriads of poets, rhetoricians, philosophers, sophisters, (as [1] Eusebius well observes) which have written in former ages, scarce one of a thousands works remains; *nomina et libri simul cum corporibus interierunt:* their books and bodies are perished together. It is not, as they vainly think, they shall surely be admired and immortal: as one told Philip of Macedon insulting after a victory, that his shadow was no longer than before, we may say to them,

> Nos demiramur, sed non cum deside vulgo,
> Sed velut Harpyias, Gorgonas, et Furias:

> We marvail too, not as the vulgar we,
> But as we Gorgons, Harpy, or Furies see:

or, if we do applaud, honour, and admire—*quota pars*, how small a part, in respect of the whole world, never so much as hears our names! how few take notice of us! how slender a tract, as scant as Alcibiades his land in a map! And yet every man must and will be immortal, as he hopes, and extend his fame to our Antipodes, when as half, no not a quarter of his own province or city, neither knows nor hears of him: but, say they did, what's a city to a kingdom, a kingdom to Europe, Europe to the world, the world it self that must have an end, if compared to the least visible star in the firmament, eighteen times bigger than it? and then, if those stars be infinite, and every star there be a sun, as some will, and as this sun of ours hath his planets about him, all inhabited; what proportion bear we to them? and where's our glory? *Orbem terrarum victor Romanus habebat*, as he cracked in Petronius; all the world was under Augustus; and so, in Constantines time, Eusebius brags he governed all the world: *universum mundum præclare admodum administravit——et omnes orbis gentes imperatori subjectæ:* so of Alexander it is given out, the four monarchies, &c. when as neither Greeks nor Romans ever had the fifteenth part of the now known world, nor the half of that which was then described. What braggadocians are they and we then! *quam brevis hic de nobis sermo!* as [2] he said: [3]*pudebit aucti nominis:* how short a time, how little a while, doth this fame of ours continue! Every private province, every small territory and city, when we have all done, will yield as generous spirits, as brave examples in all respects, as famous as ourselves—Cadwallader in Wales, Rollo in Normandy—Robbin-hood and Little John are as much renowned in Sherwood, as Cæsar in Rome, Alexander in Greece, or his Hephæstion,

---

[1] Lib. cont. Philos. cap. 1. [2] Tull. Som. Scip. [3] Boëthius.

304   *Causes of Melancholy.*   [Part. 1. Sec. 2.

[1] *Omnis ætas omnisque populus in exemplum et admirationem venit :* every town, city, book, is full of brave souldiers, senators, scholars; and though [2] Brasidas was a worthy captain, a good man, and, as they thought, not to be matched in Lacedæmon, yet, as his mother truly said, *plures habet Sparta Brasidâ meliores ;* Sparta had many better men than ever he was; and, howsoever thou admirest thyself, thy friend, many an obscure fellow the world never took notice of, had he been in place or action, would have done much better than he, or he, or thyself.

Another kind of mad men there is, opposite to these, that are insensibly mad, and know not of it—such as contemn all praise and glory, think themselves most free, when as indeed they are most mad: *calcant, sed alio fastu :* a company of cynicks, such as are monks, hermites, anachorites, that contemn the world, contemn themselves, contemn all titles, honours, offices, and yet, in that contempt, are more proud than any man living whatsoever. They are proud in humility; proud in that they are not proud; *sæpe homo de vanæ gloriæ contemtu vanius gloriatur,* as Austin hath it (*confess. lib.* 10. *cap.* 38): like Diogenes *intus gloriantur,* they brag inwardly, and feed themselves fat with self-conceit of sanctity, which is no better than hypocrisie. They go in sheeps russet, many great men that might maintain themselves in cloth of gold, and seem to be dejected, humble, by their outward carriage, when as inwardly they are swollen full of pride, arrogancy, and self-conceit. And therefore Seneca adviseth his friend Lucilius, [3] *in his attire and gesture, outward actions, especially to avoid all such things as are more notable in themselves ; as a rugged attire, hirsute head, horrid beard, contempt of money, coarse lodging, and whatsoever leads to fame that opposite way.*

All this madness yet proceeds from ourselves; the main engin which batters us, is from others; we are meerly passive in this business; from a company of parasites and flatterers, that, with immoderate praise, and bumbast epithetes, glozing titles, false elogiums, so bedawb and applaud, gild over many a silly and undeserving man, that they clap him quite out of his wits. *Res imprimis violenta est laudum placenta,* as Hierom notes: this common applause is a most violent thing, (a drum, a fife, a trumpet, cannot so animate) that fattens men, erects and dejects them in an instant.

---

[1] Putean. Cisalp. hist. lib. 1.   [2] Plutarch. Lycurgo.   [3] Epist. 5. Illud te admoneo, ne eorum more, qui non proficere, sed conspici cupiunt, facias aliqua, quæ in habitu tuo, aut genere vitæ, notabilia sint. Asperum cultum, et intonsum caput, negligentiorem barbam, indictum argento odium, cubile humi positum, et quidquid aliud laudem perversâ viâ sequitur, devita.

[1] Palma negata macrum, donata reducit opimum.

It makes them fat and lean, as frost doth conies. [2] *And who is that mortal man that can so contain himself, that if he be immoderately commended and applauded, will not be moved?* Let him be what he will, those parasites will overturn him: if he be a king, he is one of the nine worthies, more than a man, a God forthwith [3] (*edictum Domini Deique nostri*); and they will sacrifice unto him;

———————[4] divinos, si tu patiaris, honores
Ultro ipsi dabimus, meritasque sacrabimus aras.

If he be a souldier, then Themistocles, Epaminondas, Hector, Achilles, *duo fulmina belli, triumviri terrarum, &c.* and the valour of both Scipios is too little for him; he is *invictissimus, serenissimus, multis tropæis ornatissimus, naturæ dominus,* although he be *lepus galeatus,* indeed a very coward, a milk sop, [5] and (as he said of Xerxes) *postremus in pugnâ, primus in fugâ,* and such a one as never durst look his enemy in the face. If he be a big man, then is he a Sampson, another Hercules: if he pronounce a speech, another Tully or Demosthenes (as of Herod in the Acts, *the voyce of God, and not of man*): if he can make a verse, Homer, Virgil, &c. And then my silly weak patient takes all these elogiums to himself: if he be a scholar so commended for his much reading, excellent style, method, &c. he will eviscerate himself like a spider, study to death:

Laudatas ostentat avis Junonia pennas:

peacock-like, he will display all his feathers. If he be a souldier, and so applauded, his valour extoll'd, though it be *impar congressus,* as that of Troilus and Achilles—*infelix puer*—he will combat with a giant, run first upon a breach: as another [6] Philippus, he will ride into the thickest of his enemies. Commend his house-keeping, and he will beggar himself: commend his temperance, he will starve himself.

———————laudataque virtus
Crescit; et immensum gloria calcar habet.

he is mad, mad, mad! no whoe with him;

Impatiens consortis erit;

---

[1] Hor.   [2] Quis vero tam bene modulo suo metiri se novit, ut eum assiduæ et immodicæ laudationes non moveant? Hen. Steph.   [3] Mart.   [4] Stroza.   [5] Justin.   [6] Livius. Gloriâ tantum elatus, non irâ, in medios hostes irruere, quod, completis muris, conspici se pugnantem, a muro spectantibus, egregium ducebat.

VOL. I.   X

306   *Causes of Melancholy.*   [Part. 1. Sec. 2.

he will over the [1] Alpes, to be talked of, or to maintain his
credit.   Commend an ambitious man, some proud prince or
potentate : *si plus æquo laudetur* (saith [2] Erasmus) *cristas eri-
git, exuit hominem, Deum se putat :* he sets up his crest, and
will be no longer a man, but a God.

> ———————[3] nihil est, quod credere de se
> Non audet, quum laudatur, Dîs æqua potestas.

How did this work with Alexander, that would needs be Jupiters son, and go, like Hercules, in a lions skin ?   Domitian, a
God, ([4]*Dominus Deus noster sic fieri jubet*) like the [5] Persian
kings, whose image was adored by all that came into the city
of Babylon.   Commodus the emperour was so gulled by his
flattering parasites, that he must be called Hercules.   [6] Antonius the Roman would be crowned with ivy, carried in a
chariot, and adored for Bacchus.   Cotys, king of Thrace, was
married to [7] Minerva, and sent three several messengers, one
after another, to see if she were come to his bed-chamber.
Such a one was [8] Jupiter Menecrates, Maximinus Jovianus,
Dioclesianus Herculeus, Sapor the Persian king, brother of
the sun and moon, and our modern Turks, that will be Gods
on earth, kings of kings, Gods shadow, commanders of all that
may be commanded, our kings of China and Tartaria in
this present age.   Such a one was Xerxes, that would whip
the sea, fetter Neptune, *stultâ jactantiâ*, and send a challenge
to Mount Athos ; and such are many sottish princes, brought
into a fools paradise by their parasites. 'Tis a common humour,
incident to all men, when they are in great places, or come
to the solstice of honour, have done, or deserved well, to
applaud and flatter themselves.   *Stultitiam suam produnt, &c.*
(saith [9] Platerus) your very tradesmen, if they be excellent,
will crack and brag, and shew their folly in excess.   [10] They
have good parts; and they know it : you need not tell them of
it ; out of a conceit of their worth, they go smiling to themselves, and perpetual meditation of their trophies and plaudites :
they run at the last quite mad, and lose their wits.   Petrarch,
(*lib.* 1. *de contemtu mundi*) confessed as much of himself;

[1] I, demens, et sævas curre per Alpes : Aude aliquid, &c.   Ut pueris placeas,
et declamatio fias. Juv. Sat. 10.   [2] In Mor. Encom.   [3] Juvenal. Sat. 4.
[4] Sueton. c. 12. in Domitiano.   [5] Brisonius.   [6] Antonius, ab assentatori-
bus evectus, Liberum se Patrem appellari jussit, et pro deo se venditavit.   Redi-
mitus hederâ, et coronâ velatus aureâ, et thyrsum tenens, cothurnisque succinc-
tus, curru, velut Liber Pater, vectus est Alexandriæ. Pater. vol. post.   [7] Minervæ nuptias ambiit, tanto furore percitus, ut satellites mitteret ad videndum
num dea in thalamum venisset, &c.   [8] Ælian. lib 12.   [9] De mentis alienat.
cap. 3.   [10] Sequiturque superbia formam. Livius, lib. 11.   Oraculum est,
vivida sæpe ingenia luxuriare hac, et evanescere ; multosque sensum penitus
amisisse.   Homines intuentur, ac si ipsi non essent homines.

Mem. 3. Subs. 15.]   *Study, a Cause.*   307

and Cardan (in his fifth book of wisdom) gives an instance in a
smith of Milan, a fellow citizen of his, [1] one Galeus de Rubeis, that being commended for refinding of an instrument of
Archimedes, for joy ran mad.   Plutarch (in the life of Arta-
xerxes) hath such a like story of one Chamus a souldier, that
wounded king Cyrus in battel, and *grew thereupon so* [2] *arrogant, that, in a short space after, he lost his wits.* So, many
men, if any new honour, office, preferment, booty, treasure,
possession, or patrimony, *ex insperato*, fall unto them, for immoderate joy, and continual meditation of it, cannot sleep, [3] or
tell what they say or do : they are so ravished on a sudden,
and with vain concits transported, there is no rule with them.
Epaminondas therefore, the next day after his Leuctrian victory, [4] *came abroad all squalid and submiss,* and gave no other
reason to his friends of so doing, than that he perceived himself
the day before, by reason of his good fortune, to be too insolent,
overmuch joyed.   That wise and vertuous lady [5] queen Ka-
tharin, dowager of England, in private talk, upon like occasion,
said, *that* [6] *she would not willingly endure the extremity of
either fortune; but if it were so that of necessity she must undergo the one, she would be in adversity, because comfort was
never wanting in it ; but still counsel and government were defective in the other ;* they could not moderate themselves.

SUBSECT. XV.

*Love of Learning, or overmuch Study. With a digression
of the Misery of Scholars, and why the Muses are melancholy.*

LEONARTUS Fuchsius (*Instit. lib. 3. sect. 1. cap. 1*), Felix
Plater (*lib. 3. de mentis alienat.*), Herc. de Saxoniâ (*Tract.
post. de melanch. cap. 3*), speak of a [7] peculiar fury, which
comes by overmuch study.   Fernelius (*lib. 1. cap. 18*) [8] puts
study, contemplation, and continual meditation, as an especial
cause of madness ; and in his 86 *consul.* cites the same words.

---

[1] Galeus de Rubeis, civis noster, faber ferrarius, ob inventionem instrumenti,
cochleæ olim Archimedis dicti, præ lætitiâ insanivit.   [2] Insaniâ postmodum
correptus, ob nimiam inde arrogantiam.   [3] Bene ferre magnam disce fortunam.
Hor.—Fortunam reverenter habe, quicunque repente Dives ab exili progrediere
loco. Ausonius.   [4] Processit squalidus et submissus, ut hesterni diei gaudium intemperans hodie castigaret.   [5] Uxor Hen. VIII.   [6] Neutrius se
fortunæ extremum libenter experturam dixit : sed, si necessitas alterius subinde
imponeretur, optare se difficilem et adversam ; quod in hac nulli unquam defuit
solatium, in alterâ multis consilium, &c. Lod. Vives.   [7] Peculiaris furor qui
ex literis fit.   [8] Nihil magis auget, ac assidua studia, et profundæ cogitationes.

x 2

308   *Causes of Melancholy.*   [Part. 1. Sec. 2.

Jo. Arculanus (*in lib. Rhasis ad Almansorem, cap.* 16) amongst
other causes, reckons up *studium vehemens :* so doth Levinus
Lemnius (*lib. de occul. nat. mirac. lib.* 1. *cap.* 16). [1] *Many
men* (saith he) *come to this malady by continual* [2] *study, and
night-waking ; and of all other men, scholars are most subject
to it :* and such (Rhasis adds) [3] *that have commonly the finest
wits* (*Cont. lib.* 1. *tract.* 9). Marcilius Ficinus (*de sanit. tuendâ,
lib.* 1. *cap.* 7) puts melancholy amongst one of those five principal plagues of students: 'tis a common maul unto them all,
and almost in some measure an inseparable companion.
Varro (belike for that cause) calls *tristes philosophos et severos.*
Severe, sad, dry, tetrick, are common epithetes to scholars :
and [4] Patritius, therefore, in the Institution of Princes,
would not have them to be great students: for (as Machiavel
holds) study weakens their bodies, dulls their spirits, abates
their strength and courage ; and good scholars are never
good souldiers ; which a certain Goth well perceived; for,
when his countrey-men came into Greece, and would have
burned all their books, he cryed out against it, by all means
they should not do it: [5] *leave them that plague which in
time will consume all their vigour, and martial spirits.*
The [6] Turks abdicated Cornutus, the next heir, from the empire, because he was so much given to his book ; and 'tis the
common tenent of the world, that learning dulls and dimi-
nisheth the spirits, and so, *per consequens,* produceth melancholy.

Two main reasons may be given of it, why students should
be more subject to this malady than others. The one is, they
live a sedentary, solitary life, *sibi et Musis,* free from bodily
exercise, and those ordinary disports which other men use;
and many times, if discontent and idleness concur with it
(which is too frequent), they are precipitated into this gulf on a
sudden : but the common cause is overmuch study ; too much
learning (as [7] Festus told Paul) hath made thee mad : 'tis that
other extreme which effects it. So did Trincavellius (*lib.* 1.
consil. 12. *et* 13.) find by his experience, in two of his patients, a young baron, and another, that contracted this malady
by too vehement study ; so Forestus (*observat. l.* 10. *observ.*

---

[1] Non desunt, qui ex jugi studio, et intempestivâ lucubratione, huc devene-
runt: hi, præ cæteris, enim plerumque melancholiâ solent infestari.   [2] Study
is a continual and earnest meditation, applyed to some thing with great desire.
Tully.   [3] Et illi qui sunt subtilis ingenii et multæ præmeditationis, de facili
incidunt in melancholiam.   [4] Ob studiorum solicitudinem, lib. 5. tit. 5.
[5] Gaspar Ens. Thesaur. Polit. Apoteles. 31. Græcis hanc pestem relinquite, quæ
dubium non est quin brevi omnem iis vigorem ereptura Martiosque spiritus ex-
haustura sit, ut ad arma tractanda plane inhabiles futuri sint.   [6] Knolles,
Turk. Hist.   [7] Act. 26. 24.

Mem. 3. Subs. 15.]   *Study, a Cause.*   309

13) in a young divine in Lovain, that was mad, and said [1] *he
had a bible in his head.* Marsilius Ficinus (*de sanit. tuend.
lib. 2. cap.* 1. 3, 4, *et lib. 2. cap.* 10) gives many reasons
[2] *why students dote more often than others:* the first is their
negligence: [3] *other men look to their tools ; a painter will wash
his pensils ; a smith will look to his hammer, anvil, forge ; an
husbandman will mend his plough-irons, and grind his hatchet
if it be dull; a faulkner or huntsman will have an especial care
of his hawks, hounds, horses, dogs, &c.; a musician will string
and unstring his lute, &c.: only scholars neglect that instrument
(their brain and spirits, I mean) which they daily use, and by
which they range over all the world, which by much study is
consumed. Vide* (saith Lucian) *ne, funiculum nimis intendendo,
aliquando abrumpas:* see thou twist not the rope so hard, till at
length it [4] break. Ficinus in his fourth chapter gives some
other reasons: Saturn and Mercury, the patrons of learning,
are both dry planets : and Origanus assigns the same cause,
why Mercurialists are so poor, and most part beggers ; for that
their president Mercury had no better fortune himself. The
Destinies, of old, put poverty upon him as a punishment: since
when, poetry and beggery are *gemelli,* twin-born brats, inseparable companions ;

> [5] And, to this day, is every scholar poor :
> Gross gold from them runs headlong to the boor :

Mercury can help them to knowledge, but not to money.
The second is contemplation, [6] *which dryes the brain, and extinguisheth natural heat ; for, whilst the spirits are intent to
meditation above in the head, the stomach and liver are left
destitute ; and thence come black blood and crudities, by defect of concoction ; and, for want of exercise, the superfluous
vapours cannot exhale, &c.* The same reasons are repeated
by Gomesius (*lib. 4. cap. 1. de sale*), [7] Nymannus (*orat. de
Imag.*) Jo. Voschius (*lib. 2. cap. 5. de peste*): and something

---

[1] Nimiis studiis melancholicus evasit, dicens, se Biblium in capite habere.
[2] Cur melancholiâ assiduâ, crebrisque deliramentis, vexentur eorum animi, ut
desipere cogantur.   [3] Solers quilibet artifex instrumenta sua diligentissime
curat ; penicillos pictor ; malleos incudesque faber ferrarius ; miles equos, arma ;
venator, auceps, aves et canes ; citharam citharœdus, &c. soli Musarum mystæ
tam negligentes sunt, ut instrumentum illud, quo mundum universum metiri
solent, spiritum scilicet, penitus negligere videantur.   [4] Arcus, (et
arma tibi sunt imitanda Dianæ) Si nunquam cesses tendere, mollis erit. Ovid.
[5] Ephemer.   [6] Contemplatio cerebrum exsiccat et extinguit calorem naturalem ; unde cerebrum frigidum et siccum evadit, quod est melancholicum. Accedit ad hoc, quod natura, in contemplatione, cerebro prorsus, cordique intenta,
stomachum heparque destituit ; unde, ex alimentis male coctis, sanguis crassus
et niger efficitur, dum nimio otio membrorum superflui vapores non exhalant.
[7] Cerebrum exsiccatur, corpora sensim gracilescunt.

310   *Causes of Melancholy.*   [Part. 1. Sec. 2.

more they add, that hard students are commonly troubled with
gowts, catarrhes, rheums, *cachexia, bradypepsia*, bad eyes,
stone, and collick, [1] crudities, oppilations, *vertigo*, winds,
consumptions, and all such diseases as come by over-much
sitting: they are most part lean, dry, ill-coloured, spend their
fortunes, lose their wits, and many times their lives; and all
through immoderate pains, and extraordinary studies. If you
will not believe the truth of this, look upon great Tostatus
and Thomas Aquinas works; and tell me whether those men
took pains? peruse Austin, Hierom, &c. and many thousands
besides.

> Qui cupit optatam cursu contingere metam,
> Multa tulit, fecitque puer, sudavit et alsit.

> He that desires this wished goal to gain,
> Must sweat and freeze before he can attain,

and labour hard for it.   So did Seneca, by his own confession
(*ep.* 8): [2] *not a day that I spend idle; part of the night I keep
mine eyes open, tired with waking, and now slumbering, to
their continual task.*   Hear Tully (*pro Archiâ Poëtâ*): *whilst
others loytered, and took their pleasures, he was continually
at his book.*   So they do that will be scholars, and that to the
hazard, (I say) of their healths, fortunes, wits, and lives.   How
much did Aristotle and Ptolemy spend (*unius regni pretium*,
they say—more than a kings ransom) how many crowns *per
annum* to perfect arts, the one about his History of Creatures,
the other on his *Almagest?* How much time did Thebit Ben-
chorat employ, to find out the motion of the eighth sphear?
forty years and more, some write.   How many poor scholars
have lost their wits, or become dizards, neglecting all worldly
affairs, and their own health, wealth, *esse* and *bene esse*, to gain
knowledge! for which, after all their pains, in the worlds esteem
they are accounted ridiculous and silly fools, ideots, asses, and
(as oft they are) rejected, contemned, derided, doting, and mad.
Look for examples in Hildesheim (*spicil.* 2. *de maniâ et delirio*):
read Trincavellius (*l.* 3. *consil.* 36. *et c.* 17), Montanus
(*consil.* 233), [3] Garceus (*de Judic. genit. cap.* 33), Mercurialis
(*consil.* 86. *cap.* 25), Prosper [4] Calenus (in his book *de atrâ
bile*): go to Bedlam, and ask.   Or if they keep their wits, yet

---

[1] Studiosi sunt cachectici, et nunquam bene colorati: propter debilitatem di-
gestivæ facultatis, multiplicantur in iis superfluitates. Jo. Voschius, part. 2.
cap. 5. de peste.   [2] Nullus mihi per otium dies exit; partem noctis studiis
dedico, non vero somno, sed oculos, vigiliâ fatigatos cadentesque, in operâ de-
tineo.   [3] Johannes Hanuschius Bohemus, nat. 1516, eruditus vir, nimiis
studiis in phrenesin incidit. Montanus instanceth in a Frenchman of Tolosa.
[4] Cardinalis Cæcius, ob laborem, vigiliam, et diuturna studia, factus melancholicus.

Mem. 3. Subs. 15.]   *Study, a Cause.*   311

they are esteemed scrubs and fools, [1] by reason of their carriage; *after seven years study,*

> —————————[2] statuâ taciturnius exit
> Plerumque, et risu populum quatit :

because they cannot ride an horse, which every clown can do; salute and court a gentlewoman, carve at table, cringe, and make congies, which every common swasher can do, *hos populus ridet :* they are laughed to scorn, and accounted silly fools, by our gallants. Yea, many times, such is their misery, they deserve it : a meer scholar, a meer ass.

> [3] Obstipo capite, et figentes lumine terram,
> Murmura cum secum et rabiosa silentia rodunt,
> Atque exporrecto trutinantur verba labello,
> Ægroti veteris meditantes somnia, gigni
> De nihilo nihilum ; in nihilum nil posse reverti.

> [4] —————————who do lean awry
> Their heads, piercing the earth with a fixt eye :
> When, by themselves, they gnaw their murmuring,
> And furious silence, as 'twere ballancing
> Each word upon their out-stretcht lip, and when
> They meditate the dreams of old sick men,
> As, *out of nothing nothing can be brought,*
> *And that which is, can ne'er be turn'd to nought.*

Thus they go commonly meditating unto themselves, thus they sit, such is their action and gesture. Fulgosus (*l. 8. c. 7.*) makes mention how Th. Aquinas, supping with king Lewis of France, upon a sudden knocked his fist upon the table, and cryed, *conclusum est contra Manichæos :* his wits were a woolgathering (as they say), and his head busied about other matters : when he perceived his error, he was much [5] abashed. Such a story there is of Archimedes in Vitruvius, that, having found out the means to know how much gold was mingled with the silver in king Hierons crown, ran naked forth of the bath and cryed, εὑρηκα, I have found; [6] *and was commonly so intent to his studies, that he never perceived what was done about him; when the city was taken, and the souldiers now ready to rifle his house, he took no notice of it.* [7] S[t]. Bernard rode all day long by the Lemnian lake, and asked at last where

---

[1] Pers. Sat. 3. They cannot fiddle; but, as Themistocles said, he could make a small town become a great city.   [2] Ingenium, sibi quod vanas desumpsit Athenas, Et septem studiis annos dedit, insenuitque Libris et curis, statuâ taciturnius exit Plerumque, et risu populum quatit. Hor. ep. 2. lib. 2.   [3] Pers. Sat.   [4] Translated by M. B. Holiday.   [5] Thomas, rubore confusus, dixit se de argumento cogitâsse.   [6] Plutarch vitâ Marcelli. Nec sensit urbem captam, nec milites in domum irruentes, adeo intentus studiis, &c.   [7] Lib. 2. cap. 18.

312   *Causes of Melancholy.*   [Part. 1. Sec. 2.

he was (Marullus, *lib. 2. cap. 4.*)   It was Democritus carriage
alone that made the Abderites suppose him to have been mad,
and send for Hippocrates to cure him ; if he had been in any
solemn company, he would upon all occasions fall a laughing.
Theophrastus saith as much of Heraclitus, for that he continually wept, and Laërtius of Menedemus Lampsacenus, because he ran like a mad man, [1] *saying, he came from hell as a
spie, to tell the devils what mortal men did.*   Your greatest
students are commonly no better—silly, soft fellows in their
outward behaviour, absurd, ridiculous to others, and no whit
experienced in worldly business : they can measure the heavens, range over the world, teach others wisdom ; and yet, in
bargains and contracts, they are circumvented by every base
tradesman.   Are not these men fools ? and how should they
be otherwise, *but as so many sots in schools, when* (as [2] he
well observed) *they neither hear nor see such things as are
commonly practised abroad ?* how should they get experience ?
by what means ? [3] *I knew in my time many scholars*, saith
Æneas Sylvius (in an epistle of his to Gasper Scitick, chan-
cellor to the emperour) *excellent well learned, but so rude, so
silly, that they had no common civility, nor knew how to
manage their domestick or public affairs.   Paglarensis was
amazed, and said his farmer had surely cozened him, when he
heard him tell that his sow had eleven pigs, and his ass had
but one foal.*   To say the best of this profession, I can give
no other testimony of them in general, than that of [4] Pliny
of Isæus—*he is yet a scholar; than which kind of men there is
nothing so simple, so sincere, none better ;* they are, most part,
harmless, honest, *upright, innocent*, plain dealing men.

Now, because they are commonly subject to such hazards
and inconveniences, as dotage, madness, simplicity, &c. Jo.
Voschius would have good scholars to be highly rewarded, and
had in some extraordinary respect above other men, [5] *to have
greater privileges than the rest, that adventure themselves and
abbreviate their lives for the publick good.*   But our patrons
of learning are so far, now a dayes, from respecting the
Muses, and giving that honour to scholars, or reward, which
they deserve, and are allowed by those indulgent privileges of

---

[1] Sub Furiæ larvâ circumivit urbem, dictitans se exploratorem ab inferis venisse, delaturum dæmonibus mortalium peccata.   [2] Petronius. Ego arbitror
in scholis stultissimos fieri, quia nihil eorum, quæ in usu habemus, aut audiunt
aut vident.   [3] Novi, meis diebus, plerosque studiis literarum deditos, qui
disciplinis admodum abundabant; sed hi nihil civilitatis habebant, nec rem publ.
nec domesticam regere nôrant. Stupuit Paglarensis, et furti villicum accusavit,
qui suem fetam undecim porcellos, asinam unum duntaxat pullum, enixam retu-
lerat.   [4] Lib. 1. Epist. 3. Adhuc scholasticus tantum est; quo genere
hominum, nihil aut est simplicius, aut sincerius, aut melius.   [5] Jure pri-
vilegiandi, qui ob commune bonum abbreviant sibi vitam.

many noble princes, that, after all their pains taken in the universities, cost and charge, expences, irksom hours, laborious tasks, wearisome dayes, dangers, hazards (barred *interim* from all pleasures which other men have, mewed up like hawks all their lives) if they chance to wade through them, they shall in the end be rejected, contemned, and (which is their greatest misery) driven to their shifts, exposed to want, poverty and beggery. Their familiar attendants are,

[1] Pallentes Morbi, Luctus, Curæque, Laborque,
Et Metus, et malesuada Fames, et turpis Egestas,
Terribiles visu formæ——

Grief, Labour, Care, pale Sickness, Miseries,
Fear, filthy Poverty, Hunger that cryes;
Terrible monsters to be seen with eyes.

If there were nothing else to trouble them, the conceit of this alone were enough to make them all melancholy. Most other trades and professions, after some seven years prenticeship, are enabled by their craft to live of themselves. A merchant adventures his goods at sea; and, though his hazard be great, yet, if one ship return of four, he likely makes a saving voyage. An husbandmans gains are almost certain : *quibus ipse Jupiter nocere non potest* ('tis [2] Catos hyperbole, a great husband himself); only scholars, methinks, are most uncertain, unrespected, subject to all casualties, and hazards: for, first, not one of a many proves to be a scholar; all are not capable and docile ; *ex omni ligno non fit Mercurius :* [3] we can make majors and officers every year, but not scholars ; kings can invest knights and barons, as Sigismond the emperour confessed : universities can give degrees; and

Tu quod es, e populo quilibet esse potest :

but he, nor they, nor all the world, can give learning, make philosophers, artists, oratours, poets. We can soon say, (as Seneca well notes) *O virum bonum! o divitem!* point at a rich man, a good, an happy man, a proper man, *sumtuose vestitum, calamistratum, bene olentem : magno temporis impendio constat hæc laudatio, o virum literatum!* but 'tis not so easily performed to find out a learned man. Learning is not so quickly got: though they may be willing to take pains and to that end sufficiently informed and liberally maintained by their patrons and parents, yet few can compass it : or, if they be docile, yet all mens wills are not answerable to their wits ; they can apprehend, but will not take pains; they

---

[1] Virg. Æn. lib. 6.   [2] Plutarch vitâ ejus. Certum agricolationis lucrum, &c.
[3] Quotannis fiunt consules et proconsules : rex et poëta quotannis non nascitur.

314 *Causes of Melancholy.* [Part. 1. Sec. 2.

are either seduced by bad companions, *vel in puellam impingunt, vel in poculum,* and so spend their time to their friends grief and their own undoings. Or, put case they be studious, industrious, of ripe wits, and perhaps good capacities, then how many diseases of body and mind must they encounter? No labour in the world like unto study. It may be, their temperature will not endure it: but, striving to be excellent, to know all, they lose health, wealth, wit, life, and all. Let him yet happily escape all these hazards, *æreis intestinis,* with a body of brass, and is now consummate and ripe; he hath profited in his studies, and proceeded with all applause: after many expences, he is fit for preferment: where shall he have it? he is as far to seek it, as he was (after twenty years standing) at the first day of his coming to the university. For, what course shall he take, being now capable and ready? The most parable and easie, and about which many are employed, is to teach a school, turn lecturer or curat; and, for that he shall have faulkners wages, ten pound *per annum,* and his diet, or some small stipend, so long as he can please his patron or the parish; if they approve him not (for usually they do but a year or two—as inconstant, as [1] they that cried, " Hosanna" one day, and " Crucifie him" the other), serving-man like, he must go look a new master: if they do, what is his reward?

[2] Hoc quoque te manet, ut pueros elementa docentem
Occupet extremis in vicis balba senectus

Like an ass, he wears out his time for provender, and can shew a stum rod, *togam tritam et laceram,* saith [3] Hædus, an old torn gown, an ensign of his infelicity; he hath his labour for his pain, a *modicum* to keep him till he be decrepit; and that is all. *Grammaticus non est felix, &c.* If he be a trencher chaplain in a gentlemans house, (as it befel [4] Euphormio) after some seven years service, he may perchance have a living to the halves, or some small rectory with the mother of the maids at length, a poor kinswoman, or a crackt chamber-maid, to have and to hold during the time of his life. But, if he offend his good patron, or displease his lady mistres in the mean time,

[5] Ducetur plantâ, velut ictus ab Hercule Cacus,
Poneturque foras, si quid tentaverit unquam
Hiscere————

as Hercules did by Cacus, he shall be dragged forth of doors by the heels, away with him. If he bend his forces to some

[1] Mat. 21. [2] Hor. ep. 20. l. 1. [3] Lib. 1. de contem. amor. [4] Satyricon.
[5] Juv. Sat. 5.

other studies, with an intent to be *a secretis* to some noble man, or in such a place with an ambassadour, he shall find that these persons rise, like prentises, one under another : and so, in many tradesmens shops, when the master is dead, the foreman of the shop commonly steps in his place. Now for poets, rhetoricians, historians, philosophers, [1] mathematicians, sophisters, &c. they are like grashoppers : sing they must in summer, and pine in the winter; for there is no preferment for them. Even so they were at first, if you will believe that pleasant tale of Socrates which he told fair Phædrus under a plane-tree, at the banks of the river Ismenus. About noon, when it was hot, and the grashoppers made a noise, he took that sweet occasion to tell him a tale, how grashoppers were once scholars, musicians, poets, &c. before the Muses were born, and lived without meat and drink, and for that cause were turned by Jupiter into grashoppers : and may be turned again, *in Tithoni cicadas, aut Lyciorum ranas*, for any reward I see they are like to have : or else, in the mean time, I would they could live, as they did, without any viaticum, like so many [2] *manucodiatæ*, those Indian birds of Paradise, as we commonly call them— those, I mean, that live with the air and dew of heaven, and need no other food: for, being as they are, their [3] *rhetorick only serves them to curse their bad fortunes;* and many of them, for want of means, are driven to hard shifts; from grashoppers, they turn humble-bees and wasps, plain parasites, and make the Muses mules, to satisfie their hunger-starved panches, and get a meals meat : To say truth, 'tis the common fortune of most scholars, to be servile and poor, to complain pitifully, and lay open their wants to their respectless patrons as [4] Cardan doth, as [5] Xylander, and many others ; and (which is too common in those dedicatory epistles) for hope of gain, to lye, flatter, and with hyperbolical elogiums and commendations, to magnifie and extol an illiterate unworthy idiot, for his excellent vertues, whom they should rather (as [6] Machiavel observes) vilifie, and rail at downright for his most notorious villanies and vices. So they prostitute themselves, as fidlers or mercenary tradesmen, to serve great mens turns for a small reward. They are like [7] Indians; they have store of gold, but know not the worth of it; for I am of Synesius opinion, [8] *King Hieron got more by Simonides acquaintance, than Simonides did by his :* they have

---

[1] Ars colit astra.   [2] Aldrovandus, de Avibus, l. 12. Gesner, &c.   [3] Literas habent, queis sibi et fortunæ suæ maledicant. Sat. Menip.   [4] Lib. de libris propriis, fol. 24.   [5] Præfat. translat. Plutarch.   [6] Polit. disput. Laudibus extollunt eos, ac si virtutibus pollerent, quos, ob infinita scelera, potius vituperare oporteret.   [7] Or, as horses know not their strength, they consider not their own worth.   [8] Plura ex Simonidis familiaritate Hieron consequutus est, quam ex Hieronis Simonides.

2

316   *Causes of Melancholy.*   [Part. 1. Sec. 2.

their best education, good institution, sole qualification from
us; and, when they have done well, their honour and immortality from us; we are the living tombs, registers, and as so many
trumpetours of their fames: what was Achilles, without Homer? Alexander, without Arrian and Curtius? who had known
the Cæsars, but for Suetonius and Dion?

> [1] Vixerunt fortes ante Agamemnona
> Multi: sed omnes illacrymabiles
> Urgentur, ignotique, longâ
> Nocte, carent quia vate sacro.

They are more beholden to scholars, than scholars to them; but
they under-value themselves, and so, by those great men, are
kept down. Let them have all that Encyclopædia, all the learning in the world; they must keep it to themselves, [2] *live in base
esteem, and starve, except they will submit* (as Budæus well
hath it) *so many good parts, so many ensigns of arts, vertues,
and be slavishly obnoxious to some illiterate potentate, and live
under his insolent worship, or honour, like parasites, qui tamquam mures, alienum panem comedunt.* For, to say truth, *artes
hæ non sunt lucrativæ* (as Guido Bonat, that great astrologer
could foresee) they be not gainful arts these, *sed esurientes et
famelicæ,* but poor and hungry.

> [3] Dat Galenus opes; dat Justinianus honores;
> Sed genus et species cogitur ire pedes:

> The rich physician, honour'd lawyers, ride,
> Whil'st the poor scholar foots it by their side,

Poverty is the Muses patrimony; and, as that poetical divinity
teacheth us, when Jupiters daughters were each of them married to the Gods, the Muses alone were left solitary, Helicon
forsaken of all suters; and I believe it was, because they had
no portion.

> Calliope longum cœlebs cur vixit in ævum?
> Nempe nihil dotis, quod numeraret, erat.

> Why did Calliope live so long a maid?
> Because she had no dowry to be paid.

Ever since, all their followers are poor, forsaken, and left unto
themselves; in so much that, as [4] Petronius argues, you shall

---

[1] Hor. lib. 4. od. 9.   [2] Inter inertes et plebeios fere jacet, ultimum locum
habens, nisi tot artis virtutisque insignia, turpiter, obnoxie, supparasitando fas-
cibus subjecerit protervæ insolentisque potentiæ.   Lib. 1. de contemt. rerum fortuitarum.   [3] Buchanan. eleg. lib.   [4] In Satyrico. Intrat senex, sed cultu
non ita speciosus, ut facile appareret eum hâc notâ literatum esse; quos divites
odisse solent. Ego, inquit, poëta sum. Quare ergo tam male vestitus es? Propter
hoc ipsum; amor ingenii neminem unquam divitem fecit.

Mem. 3. Subs. 15.] *Why the Muses are Melancholy.* 317

likely know them by their cloaths. *There came,* saith he, *by chance into my company, a fellow, not very spruce to look on, that I could perceive, by that note alone, he was a scholar, whom commonly rich men hate. I asked him what he was : he answered a poet. I demanded again why he was so ragged : he told me, this kind of learning never made any man rich.*

> [1] Qui pelago credit, magno se fœnore tollit ;
> Qui pugnas et castra petit, præcingitur auro;
> Vilis adulator picto jacet ebrius ostro ;
> Sola pruinosis horret facundia pannis.

> A merchants gain is great, that goes to sea :
>   A souldier embossed all in gold ;
> A flatterer lyes fox'd in brave array,
>   A scholar only ragged to behold.

All which our ordinary students right well perceiving in the universities—how unprofitable these poetical, mathematical, and philosophical studies are, how little respected, how few patrons—apply themselves in all haste to those three commodious professions of law, physick, and divinity, sharing themselves between them, [2] rejecting these arts in the mean time, history, philosophy, philology, or lightly passing them over, as pleasant toyes, fitting only table talk, and to furnish them with discourse. They are not so behoveful : he that can tell his money, hath arithmetick enough ; he is a true geometrician, can measure out a good fortune to himself ; a perfect astrologer, that can cast the rise and fall of others, and mark their errant motions to his own use. The best opticks are, to reflect the beams of some great mens favour and grace to shine upon him. He is a good engineer, that alone can make an instrument to get preferment. This was the common tenent and practice of Poland, as Cromerus observed, not long since, in the first book of his history : their universities were generally base ; not a philosopher, a mathematician, an antiquary, &c. to be found of any note amongst them, because they had no set reward or stipend ; but every man betook himself to divinity, *hoc solum in votis habens, opimum sacerdotium ;* a good personage was their aim. This was the practice of some of our neer neighbours, as [3] Lipsius inveighs ; *they thrust their children to the study of law and divinity, before they be informed aright, or capable of such studies. Scilicet omnibus*

---

[1] Petronius Arbiter.   [2] Oppressus paupertate animus nihil eximium aut sublime cogitare potest. Amœnitates literarum, aut elegantiam, quoniam nihil præsidii in his ad vitæ commodum videt, primo negligere, mox odisse, incipit. Heins.   [3] Epistol. quæst. lib. 4. ep. 21.

318   *Causes of Melancholy.*   [Part. 1. Sec. 2.

artibus antistat spes lucri; et formosior est cumulus auri, quam quidquid Græci Latinique delirantes scripserunt. Ex hoc numero deinde veniunt ad gubernacula reipub. intersunt et præsunt consiliis regum; o pater! o patria! so he complained; and so many others: for even so we find, to serve a great man, to get an office in some bishops court (to practise in some good town), or compass a benefice, is the mark we shoot at, as being so advantagious, the high way to preferment.

Although, many times, for ought I can see, these men fail as often as the rest in their projects, and are as usually frustrate of their hopes : for, let him be a doctor of the law, an excellent civilian of good worth, where shall he practise and expatiate? Their fields are so scant, the civil law with us so contracted with prohibitions, so few causes, by reason of those all-devouring municipal laws, (*quibus nihil illiteratius*, saith [1] Erasmus— an illiterate and a barbarous study ; for, though they be never so well learned in it, I can hardly vouchsafe them the name of scholars, except they be otherwise qualified) and so few courts are left to that profession, such slender offices, and those commonly to be compassed at such dear rates, that I know not how an ingenious man should thrive amongst them. Now, for physicians, there are in every village so many mountebanks, emperericks, quack-salvers, Paracelsians (as they call themselves), *causifici et sanicidæ* (so [2] Clenard terms them), wisards, alcumists, poor vicars, cast apothecaries, physicians men, barbers, and good wives, professing great skill, that I make great doubt how they shall be maintained, or who shall be their patients. Besides, there are so many of both sorts, and some of them such harpyes, so covetous, so clamorous, so impudent, and (as [3] he said) litigious idiots,

> Quibus loquacis affatim arrogantiæ est,
>   Peritiæ parum aut nihil,
> Nec ulla mica literarii salis ;
>   Crumenimulga natio,
> Loquutuleia turba, litium strophæ,
>   Maligna litigantium
> Cohors, togati vultures,
>   Lavernæ alumni, agyrtæ, &c.

> Which have no skill, but prating arrogance,
>   No learning, such a purse-milking nation,
> Gown'd vultures, thieves, and a litigious rout
>   Of couseners, that haunt this occupation.

that they cannot well tell how to live one by another, but, as he jested (in the comedy) of clocks, they were so many, [4] *major pars populi aridâ reptat fame,* they are almost starved a

---

[1] Ciceron. dial.   [2] Epist. lib. 2.   [3] Ja. Dousa, Epodon lib. 2. car. 2.   [4] Plautus.

Mem. 3. Subs. 15.] *Why the Muses are Melancholy.* 319

great part of them, and ready to devour their fellows, [1] *et noxiâ
calliditate se corripere;* such a multitude of pettifoggers and
empericks, such imposters, that an honest man knows not in
what sort to compose and behave himself in their society, to
carry himself with credit in so vile a rout; *scientiæ nomen, tot
sumtibus partum et vigiliis, profiteri dispudeat, postquam, &c.*

Last of all, to come to our divines, the most noble profession
and worthy of double honour, but of all others the most distressed and miserable. If you will not believe me, hear a brief
of it, as it was, not many years since, publicly preached at Pauls
cross, [2] by a grave minister then, and now a reverend bishop of
this land. *We, that are bred up in learning, and destinated by
our parents to this end, we suffer our childhood in the grammar
school, which Austin calls* magnam tyrannidem, et grave malum, *and compares it to the torments of martyrdom; when we
come to the university, if we live of the college allowance, as
Phalaris objected to the Leontines,* παντων ενδεεις, πλην λιμου
και φοβου, *needy of all things but hunger and fear; or, if we be
maintained but partly by our parents cost, to expend in* [un] *necessary maintenance, books, and degrees, before we come to any
perfection, five hundreth pounds, or a thousand marks. If, by
this price of the expence of time, our bodies and spirits, our substance and patrimonies, we cannot purchase those small rewards, which are ours by law, and the right of inheritance, a
poor personage, or a vicarage of 50l.* per annum, *but we must
pay to the patron for the lease of a life (a spent and out-worn
life), either in annual pension, or above the rate of a copyhold,
and that with the hazard and loss of our souls, by simony and
perjury, and the forfeiture of all our spiritual preferments,* in
esse and posse, *both present and to come; what father after a
while will be so improvident, to bring up his son, to his great
charge, to this necessary beggery? What Christian will be so
irreligious, to bring up his son in that course of life, which, by
all probability and necessity,* cogit ad turpia, *enforcing to sin,
will entangle him in simony and perjury, when as the poet saith,*

Invitatus ad hæc aliquis de ponte negabit—

*a beggers brat, taken from the bridge where he sits a begging,
if he knew the inconvenience, had cause to refuse it.* This being thus, have not we finished fair all this while, that are in-
itiate divines, to find no better fruits of our labours?

[3] Hoc est, cur palles? cur quis non prandeat, hoc est?

Do we macerate our selves for this? is it for this we rise so
early all the year long, [4] *leaping* (as he saith) *out of our beds,
when we hear the bell ring, as if we had heard a thunder clap?*

---

[1] Barc. Argenis. lib. 3.   [2] Joh. Howson, 4 Novembris, 1597.   The sermon was printed by Arnold Hartfield.   [3] Pers. Sat. 3.   [4] E lecto exsi-
lientes, ad subitum tintinnabuli plausum, quasi fulmine territi. 1.

320   *Causes of Melancholy.*   [Part. 1. Sec. 2.

If this be all the respect, reward, and honour, we shall have,

> [1] Frange leves calamos, et scinde, Thalia, libellos :

let us give over our books, and betake our selves to some
other course of life.   To what end should we study?

> [2] Quid me literulas stulti docuere parentes?

what did our parents mean to make us scholars, to be as far to
seek for preferment after twenty years study, as we were at
first? why do we take such pains?

> Quid tantum insanis juvat impallescere chartis?

If there be no more hope of reward, no better encouragement,
I say again,

> Frange leves calamos, et scinde, Thalia, libellos :

let's turn souldiers, sell our books, and buy swords, guns, and
pikes, or stop bottles with them, turn our philosophers gowns
(as Cleanthes once did) unto millers coats, leave all, and rather betake our selves to any other course of life, than to continue longer in this misery.   [3] *Præstat dentiscalpia radere,
quam literariis monumentis magnatum favorem emendicare.*
   Yea, but me thinks I hear some man except at these words,
that (though this be true which I have said of the estate of
scholars, and especially of divines, that it is miserable and
distressed at this time, that the church suffers shipwrack of
her goods, and that they have just cause to complain) there is
a fault; but whence proceeds it? if the cause were justly examined, it would be retorted upon our selves; if we were cited
at that tribunal of truth, we should be found guilty, and not
able to excuse it.   That there is a fault among us, I confess;
and, were there not a buyer, there would not be a seller: but
to him that will consider better of it, it will more than manifestly appear, that the fountain of these miseries proceeds from
these griping patrons.   In accusing them, I do not altogether
excuse us : both are faulty, they and we : yet, in my judgement,
theirs is the greater fault, more apparent causes, and more to
be condemned.   For my part, if it be not with me as I would,
or as it should, I do ascribe the cause (as [4] Cardan did in the
like case) *meo infortunio potius quam illorum sceleri*, to
[5] mine own infelicity, rather than their naughtiness, (although
I have been baffled in my time by some of them, and have as
just cause to complain as another) or rather indeed to mine

----

[1] Mart.   [2] Mart.   [3] Sat. Menip.   [4] Lib. 3. de cons.   [5] I had
no money : I wanted impudence : I could not scamble, temporize, dissemble : non
pranderet olus, &c.—Vis, dicam? ad palpandum et adulandum penitus insulsus,
recudi non possum, jam senior, ut sim talis ; et fingi nolo, utcunque male cedat in
rem meam, et obscurus inde delitescam.

own negligence; for I was ever like that Alexander (in [1] Plutarch) Crassus his tutor in philosophy, who, though he lived many years familiarly with rich Crassus, was even as poor when from, (which many wondered at) as when he came first to him. He never asked; the other never gave him any thing; when he travelled with Crassus, he borrowed an hat of him; at his return restored it again. I have had some such noble friends, acquaintance, and scholars; but, most part, (common courtesies and ordinary respects excepted) they and I parted as we met: they gave me as much as I requested, and that was——And as Alexander ab Alexandro (*Genial. dier. l.* 6. *c.* 16) made answer to Hieronymus Massainus, that wondred, *quum plures ignavos et ignobiles ad dignitates et sacerdotia promotos quotidie videret,* when other men rose, still he was in the same state, *eodem tenore et fortunâ, cui mercedem laborum studiorumque deberi putaret,* whom he thought to deserve as well as the rest —he made answer, that he was content with his present estate, was not ambitious: and, although *objurgabundus suam segnitiem accusaret, cum obscuræ sortis homines ad sacerdotia et pontificatus evectos, &c.* he chid him for his backwardness, yet he was still the same: and for my part (though I be not worthy perhaps to carry Alexanders books) yet, by some overweening and well wishing friends, the like speeches have been used to me; but I replied still, with Alexander, that I had enough, and more peradventure than I deserved; and, with Libanius Sophista, that rather chose (when honours and offices by the emperour were offered unto him) to be *talis sophista, quam talis magistratus,* I had as lieve be still Democritus junior, and *privus privatus, si mihi jam daretur optio, quam talis fortasse doctor, talis dominus.*——*Sed quorsum hæc?* For the rest, 'tis, on both sides, *facinus detestandum* to buy and sell livings, to detain from the church that which Gods and mens laws have bestowed on it; but in them most, and that from the covetousness and ignorance of such as are interested in this business. I name covetousness in the first place, as the root of all these mischiefs, which (Achan like) compels them to commit sacrilege, and to make simoniacal compacts, (and what not?) to their own ends, [2] and that kindles Gods wrath, brings a plague, vengeance, and an heavy visitation upon themselves and others. Some, out of that insatiable desire of filthy lucre, to be enriched, care not how they come by it, *per fas et nefas,* hook or crook, so they have it. And others, when they have, with riot and prodigality, imbezelled their estates, to recover

---

[1] Vit. Crassi. Nec facile judicari potest, utrum pauperior cum primo ad Crassum, &c.   [2] Deum habent iratum; sibique mortem æternam acquirunt, aliis miserabilem ruinam. Serrarius, in Josuam, 7. Euripides.

322   *Causes of Melancholy.*   [Part. 1. Sec. 2.

themselves, make a prey of the church, (robbing it, as
[1] Julian the Apostate did) spoile parsons of their revenues (in
keeping half back, [2] as a great man amongst us observes) *and
that maintenance on which they should live;* by means whereof,
barbarism is increased, and a great decay of Christian profes-
sours: for who will apply himself to these divine studies, his
son, or friend, when, after great pains taken, they shall have
nothing whereupon to live? But with what event do they ·
these things?

> [3] Opesque totis viribus venamini :
> At inde messis accidit miserrima.

They toyle and moyle, but what reap they? They are commonly unfortunate families that use it, accursed in their progeny,
and, as common experience evinceth, accursed themselves in
all their proceedings. *With what face* (as [4] he quotes out of
Austin) *can they expect a blessing or inheritance from Christ
in heaven, that defraud Christ of his inheritance here on earth?*
I would all our simoniacal patrons, and such as detain tithes,
would read those judicious tracts of S[r] Henry Spelman, and S[r]
James Sempill, knights; those late elaborate and learned treatises of D[r] Tilslye and M[r] Montague, which they have written
of that subject. But, though they should read, it would be
to small purpose; *clames, licet, et mare cœlo confundas;*
thunder, lighten, preach hell and damnation, tell them 'tis a
sin; they will not believe it; denounce and terrifie; they
have [5] cauterized consciences; they do not attend; as the inchanted adder, they stop their ears. Call them base, irreligious,
prophane, barbarous, pagans, atheists, epicures, (as some of
them surely are) with the bawd in Plautus, *Euge! optime!*
they cry: and applaud themselves with that miser, [6] *simul ac
nummos contemplor in arcâ :* say what you will, *quocunque
modo rem :* as a dog barks at the moon, to no purpose are your
sayings: take your heaven, let them have money—a base, prophane, epicurean, hypocritical rout. For my part, let them
pretend what zeal they will, counterfeit religion, blear the
worlds eyes, bumbast themselves, and stuffe out their greatness
with church spoils, shine like so many peacocks—so cold is my
charity, so defective in this behalf, that I shall never think
better of them, than that they are rotten at core, their bones
are full of epicurean hypocrisie, and atheistical marrow; they
are worse than heathens. For, as Dionysius Halicarnasseus
observes (*Antiq. Rom. lib.* 7) [7] *Primum locum, &c. Greeks and*

---

[1] Nicephorus, lib. 10. cap. 5.   [2] Lord Cook, in his Reports, second part,
fol. 44.   [3] Euripides.   [4] Sir Henry Spelman, de non temerandis Eccle-
siis.   [5] 1 Tim. 4. 2.   [6] Hor.   [7] Primum locum apud omnes gentes
habet patritius deorum cultus, et geniorum ; nam hunc diutissime custodiunt,
tam Græci quam barbari, &c.

Mem. 3. Subs. 15.]   *Study, a Cause.*   323

*barbarians observe all religious rites, and dare not break them,
for fear of offending their gods :* but our simoniacal contracters,
our senseless Achans, our stupified patrons, fear neither God
nor Devil: they have evasions for it; it is no sin, or not
due *jure divino,* or if a sin, no great sin, &c. And, though they
be daily punished for it, and they do manifestly perceive, that
(as he said) frost and fraud come to foul ends; yet (as [1] Chrysostome follows it) *nulla ex pœná fit correctio; et, quasi adversis
malitia hominum provocetur, crescit quotidie quod puniatur :*
they are rather worse than better :

——iram atque animos a crimine sumunt ;

and the more they are corrected, the more they offend: but let
them take their course, ([2] *Rode, caper, vitem,*) go on still as
they begin, ("'tis no sin!") let them rejoyce secure: Gods
vengeance will overtake them in the end; and these ill gotten
goods, as an eagles feathers, [3] will consume the rest of their
substance: it is [4] *aurum Tolosanum,* and will produce no better
effects. *Let them lay it up safe, and make their conveyances
never so close, lock and shut door,* saith [5] Chrysostome *; yet fraud
and covetousness, two most violent thieves, are still included ; and
a little gain, evil gotten, will subvert the rest of their goods.*
The eagle in Æsop, seeing a piece of flesh, now ready to be
sacrificed, swept it away with her claws, and carried it to her
nest: but there was a burning coal stuck to it by chance, which
unawares consumed her young ones, nest and all together. Let
our simoniacal church-chopping patrons, and sacrilegious harpies, look for no better success.

A second cause is ignorance, and from thence contempt;
successit odium in literas ab ignorantiá vulgi ; which [6] Junius
well perceived: this hatred and contempt of learning proceeds
out of [7] ignorance; as they are themselves barbarous, idiots,
dull, illiterate, and proud, so they esteem of others.

Sint Mæcenates, non deerunt, Flacce, Marones :

let there be bountiful patrons, and there will be painful scholars
in all sciences.   But, when they contemn learning, and think
themselves sufficiently qualified, if they can write and read,
scamble at a piece of evidence, or have so much Latin as that
emperour had, [8] *qui nescit dissimulare, nescit vivere,* they are
unfit to do their countrey service, to perform or undertake

[1] Tom. I. de steril. trium annorum sub Eliâ sermone. [2] Ovid. Fast. [3] De
male quæsitis vix gaudet tertius hæres. [4] Strabo, l. 4. Geog. [5] Nihil
facilius opes evertet, quam avaritia et fraude parta. Etsi enim seram addas tali
arcæ, et exteriore januâ et vecte eam communias, intus tamen fraudem et avaritiam, &c. In 5 Corinth. [6] Acad. cap. 7. [7] Ars neminem habet
inimicum, præter ignorantem. [8] He that cannot dissemble cannot live.

Y 2

324   *Causes of Melancholy.*   [Part. 1. Sec. 2.

any action or employment, which may tend to the good of
a common-wealth, except it be to fight, or to do countrey
justice, with common sense, which every yeoman can likewise do. And so they bring up their children, rude as they are
themselves, unqualified, untaught, uncivil most part. ¹ *Quis
e nostrâ juventute legitime instituitur literis? quis oratores
aut philosophos tangit? quis historiam legit, illam rerum
agendarum quasi animam? Præcipitant parentes vota sua, &c.*
'twas Lipsius complaint to his illiterate countrey-men: it may
be ours. Now shall these men judge of a scholars worth, that
have no worth, that know not what belongs to a students labours,
that cannot distinguish between a true scholar and a drone? or
him that by reason of a voluble tongue, a strong voice, a
pleasing tone, and some trivantly Polyanthean helps, steals
and gleans a few notes from other mens harvests, and so makes
a fairer shew, than he that is truly learned indeed; that thinks
it no more to preach, than to speak, ² *or to run away with
an empty cart* (as a grave man said); and thereupon vilifie
us, and our pains; scorn us, and all learning. ³ Because
they are rich, and have other means to live, they think
it concerns them not to know, or to trouble themselves with
it; a fitter task for younger brothers, or poor mens sons,
to be pen and inkhorn men, pedantical slaves, and no whit be-
seeming the calling of a gentleman, as Frenchmen and Germans commonly do, neglecting therefore all humane learning;
what have they to do with it? Let marriners learn astronomy;
merchants factors study arithmetick; surveyors get them geometry; spectacle-makers opticks: landleapers geography; town-
clarks rhetorick; what should he do with a spade, that hath no
ground to dig? or they with learning, that have no use of it?
Thus they reason, and are not ashamed to let marriners, prentises, and the basest servants, be better qualified than themselves.
In former times, kings, princes, and emperours were the only
scholars, excellent in all faculties.

Julius Cæsar mended the year, and writ his own Commentaries:

————————⁴ media inter prœlia, semper
Stellarum cœlique plagis, superisque vacavit.

⁵ Antoninus, Adrian, Nero, Severus, Julian, &c. ⁶ Michael the
emperour, and Isacius, were so much given to their studies, that

---

¹ Epist. quæst. lib. 4. epist. 21. Lipsius.   ² Dr. King, in his last lecture
on Jonah, sometimes right reverend lord bishop of London.   ³ Quibus opes
et otium, hi barbaro fastu literas contemnunt.   ⁴ Lucan. lib. 8.   ⁵ Spartian.
Soliciti de rebus nimis.   ⁶ Nicet. 1. Anal. Fumis lucubrationum sordebant.

Mem. 3. Subs. 15.]　　　*Study, a Cause.*　　　**325**

no base fellow would take so much pains: Orion, Perseus, Alphonsus, Ptólemæus, famous astronomers : Sabor, Mithridates, Lysimachus, admired physicians—Platos kings, all ; Evax, that Arabian prince, a most expert jueller, and an exquisite philosopher ; the kings of Ægypt were priests of old, and chosen from thence : *Idem rex hominum, Phœbique sacerdos :* but those heorical times are past ; the Muses are now banished, in this bastard age, *ad sordida tuguriola*, to meaner persons, and confined alone almost to universities. In those dayes, scholars were highly beloved, [1] honoured, esteemed, as old Ennius by Scipio Africanus, Virgil by Augustus, Horace by Mæcenas; princes companions ; dear to them, as Anacreon to Polycrates, Philoxenus to Dionysius, and highly rewarded. Alexander sent Xenocrates the philosopher fifty talents, because he was poor, *visu rerum aut eruditione præstantes viri mensis olim regum adhibiti*, as Philostratus relates of Adrian, and Lampridius of Alexander Severus. Famous clarks came to these princes courts, *velut in Lycæum*, as to an university, and were admitted to their tables, *quasi divûm epulis accumbentes ;* Archelaüs, that Macedonian king, would not willingly sup without Euripides, (amongst the rest he drank to him at supper one night, and gave him a cup of gold for his pains) *delectatus poëtæ suavi sermone :* and it was fit it should be so, because (as [2] Plato in his Protagoras well saith) a good philosopher as much excells other men, as a great king doth the commons of his countrey ; and again, [3] *quoniam illis nihil deest, et minime egere solent, et disciplinas, quas profitentur, soli a contemptu vindicare possunt;* they needed not to beg so basely, as they compell [4] scholars in our times to complain of poverty, or crouch to rich chuff for a meals meat, but could vindicate themselves, and those arts which they professed. Now they would and cannot ; for it is held by some of them, as an axiom, that to keep them poor, will make them study ; they must be dieted, as horses to a race, not pampered ; [5] *alendos volunt, non saginandos, ne melioris mentis flammula extinguatur ;* a fat bird will not sing, a fat dog cannot hunt ; and so, by this depression of theirs, [6] some want means, others will, all want [7] incouragement, as being forsaken almost, and generally contemned. 'Tis an old saying,

Sint Mæcenates, non deerunt, Flacce, Marones ;

[1] Grammaticis olim et dialecticis jurisque professoribus, qui specimen eruditionis dedissent, eadem dignitatis insignia decreverunt imperatores, quibus ornabant heroas. Erasm. ep. Jo. Fabio epis. Vien.　[2] Probus vir et philosophus magis præstat, inter alios homines, quam rex inclytus inter plebeios.　[3] Heinsius, præfat. Poëmatum.　[4] Servile nomen scholaris jam.　[5] Seneca.　[6] Haud facile emergunt, &c.　[7] Mediâ quod noctis ab horâ Sedisti, quâ nemo faber, quâ nemo sedebat, Qui docet obliquo lanam diducere ferro ; Rara tamen merces. Juv. Sat. 7.

326   *Causes of Melancholy.*   [Part. 1. Sec. 2.

and 'tis a true saying still. Yet oftentimes, I may not deny it,
the main fault is in ourselves. Our academicks too frequently
offend in neglecting patrons (as [1] Erasmus well taxeth), or
making ill choice of them; *negligimus oblatos, aut amplecti-
mur parum aptos;* or, if we get a good one, *non studemus
mutuis officiis favorem ejus alere,* we do not plye and follow
him as we should. *Idem mihi accidet adolescenti* (saith Erasmus, acknowledging his fault); *et gravissime peccavi :* and so
may [2] I say my self, I have offended in this, and so peradventure
have many others : we did not *respondere magnatum favoribus,
qui cœperunt nos amplecti,* apply our selves with that readiness we should : idleness, love of liberty, (*immodicus amor
libertatis effecit, ut diu cum perfidis amicis,* as he confesseth, *et
pertinaci paupertate, colluctarer*) bashfulness, melancholy, timorousness, cause many of us to be too backward and remiss. So
some offend in one extream, but too many on the other : we
are, most part, too forward, too solicitous, too ambitious, too
impudent : we commonly complain *deesse Mæcenates,* want
of encouragement, want of means, when as the true defect is
our want of worth, our insufficiency. Did Mæcenas take
notice of Horace or Virgil, till they had shewed themselves
first ? or had Bavius and Mævius any patrons ? *Egregium specimen dent,* saith Erasmus : let them approve themselves worthy
first, sufficiently qualified for learning and manners, before they
presume or impudently intrude and put themselves on great
men, as too many do, with such base flattery, parasitical
colloguing, such hyperbolical elogies they do usually insinuate,
that it is a shame to hear and see. *Immodicæ laudes conciliant
invidiam, potius quam laudem ;* and vain commendations derogate from truth ; and we think, in conclusion, *non melius de
laudato, pejus de laudante,* ill of both, the commender and
commended. So we offend ; but the main fault is in their
harshness, defect of patrons. How beloved of old, and how
much respected, was Plato of Dionysius ! How dear to Alexander was Aristotle, Demaratus to Philip, Solon to Crœsus,
Anaxarchus and Trebatius to Augustus, Cassius to Vespasian,
Plutarch to Trajan, Seneca to Nero, Simonides to Hieron !
how honoured !

> [3] Sed hæc prius fuere ; nunc recondita
> Senent quiete :

those dayes are gone ;

> Et spes et ratio studiorum in Cæsare tantum :

---

[1] Chil. 4. cent. 1. adag. 1.   [2] Had I done as others did, put my self forward, I might have haply been as great a man as many of my equals.   [3] Catullus, Juven.

as he said of old, we may truly say now : he is our amulet, our [1] sun, our sole comfort and refuge, our Ptolemy, our common Mæcenas, *Jacobus munificus, Jacobus pacificus, mysta Musarum, rex Platonicus : grande decus, columenque nostrum ;* a famous scholar himself, and the sole patron, pillar, and sustainer of learning : but his worth in this kind is so well known, that (as Paterculus, of Cato) *jam ipsum laudare nefas sit ;* and (which [2] Pliny to Trajan) *seria te carmina, honorque æternus annalium, non hæc brevis et pudenda prædicatio, colet.* But he is now gone, the sun of ours set ; and yet no night follows,

———— Sol occubuit ; nox nulla sequuta est.

We have such another in his room—

———— Aureus [3] alter
Avulsus simili frondescit virgo metallo ;

and long may he reign and flourish amongst us.

Let me not be malitious, and lye against my genius ; I may not deny, but that we have a sprinkling of our gentry, here and there one, excellently well learned, like those Fuggerii in Germany, Dubartas, Du Plessis, Sadael in France, Picus Mirandula, Schottus, Barotius in Italy :

Apparent rari nantes in gurgite vasto :

but they are but few in respect of the multitude : the major part (and some again excepted, that are indifferent) are wholly bent for hawks and hounds, and carried away many times with intemperate lust, gaming, and drinking. If they read a book at any time, (*si quid est interim otii a venatu, poculis, aleâ, scortis*) 'tis an English chronicle, S[r]. Huon of Bordeaux, Amadis de Gaul, &c. a play-book, or some pamphlet of news, and that at such seasons only, when they cannot stir abroad, to drive away time : [4] their sole discourse is dogs, hawks, horses, and what news ? If some one have been a traveller in Italy, or as far as the emperours court, wintered in Orleance, and can court his mistris in broken French, wear his clothes neatly in the newest fashion, sing some choice outlandish tunes, discourse of lords, ladies, towns, palaces, and cities, he is compleat, and to be admired : [5] otherwise he and they are much at one ; no difference betwixt the master and the man, but worshipful titles :—wink, and choose betwixt

---

[1] Nemo est quem non Phœbus hic noster solo intuitu lubentiorem reddat. [2] Panegyr. [3] Virgil. [4] Rarus enim ferme me sensus communis in illâ Fortunâ. Juv. Sat. 8. [5] Quis enim generosum dixerit hunc, qui Indignus genere, et præclaro nomine tantum Insignis ? Juv. Sat. 8.

328   *Causes of Melancholy.*   [Part. 1. Sec. 2.

him that sits down (clothes excepted) and him that holds the
trencher behind him. Yet these men must be our patrons,
our governours too sometimes, statesmen, magistrates, noble,
great and wise by inheritance.

Mistake me not (I say again) *vos, o patricius sanguis!* you
that are worthy senators, gentlemen, I honour your names and
persons, and, with all submissness, prostrate myself to your
censure and service. There are amongst you, I do ingenuously
confess, many well deserving patrons, and true patriots, of my
knowledge, besides many hundreds which I never saw, no
doubt, or heard of—pillars of our common-wealth, [1] whose
worth, bounty, learning, forwardness, true zeal in religion,
and good esteem of all scholars, ought to be consecrated to all
posterity: but, of your rank, there are a deboshed, corrupt, covetous, illiterate crew again, no better than stocks, *merum pecus* (testor Deum, non mihi videri dignos ingenui hominis ap-
pellatione) barbarous Thracians, (*et quis ille Thrax qui hoc
neget?*) a sordid, prophane, pernicious company, irreligious,
impudent, and stupid, (I know not what epithets to give them)
enemies to learning, confounders of the church, and the ruine
of a common-wealth. Patrons they are by right of inheritance,
and put in trust freely to dispose of such livings to the churches
good; but (hard task-masters they prove) they take away their
straw, and compel them to make their number of brick: they
commonly respect their own ends; commodity is the steer of
all their actions; and him they present, in conclusion, as a man
of greatest gifts, that will give most; no penny, [2] no *Pater-
noster,* as the saying is. *Nisi preces auro fulcias, amplius
irritas; ut Cerberus offâ,* their attendants and officers must be
bribed, fed, and made, as Cerberus is by a sop by him that
goes to hell. It was an old saying, *omnia Romæ venalia;* 'tis
a rag of popery, which will never be rooted out; there is no
hope, no good to be done, without money. A clark may offer
himself, approve his [3] worth, learning, honesty, religion, zeal;
they will commend him for it; but

————[4] probitas laudatur, et alget.

If he be a man of extraordinary parts, they will flock afar off
to hear him, as they did, in Apuleius, to see Psyche: *multi
mortales confluebant ad videndum sæculi decus, speculum*

---

[1] I have often met with my self, and conferred with, divers worthy gentlemen in
the countrey, no whit inferiour, if not to be preferred for divers kind of learning
to, many of our academicks.   [2] Ipse, licet Musis venias comitatus, Homere, Si
nihil attuleris, ibis, Homere, foras.   [3] Et legat historicos, auctores noverit
omnes, Tamquam ungues digitosque suos. Juv. Sat. 7.   [4] Juvenal.

gloriosum: laudatur ab omnibus: spectatur ab omnibus; nec quisquam, non rex, non regius, cupiens ejus nuptiarum, petitor accedit; mirantur quidem divinam speciem omnes ; sed, ut simulacrum fabre politum, mirantur : many mortal men came to see fair Psyche, the glory of her age : they did admire her, commend, desire her for her divine beauty, and gaze upon her, but, as on a picture: none would marry her, *quod indotata :* fair Psyche had no money. [1] So they do by learning :

> ——— [2] didicit jam dives avarus
> Tantum admirari, tantum laudare, disertos,
> Ut pueri Junonis avem———

> Your rich men have now learn'd of latter dayes
>   T' admire, commend, and come together
> To hear and see a worthy scholar speak,
>   As children do a peacocks feather.

He shall have all the good words that may be given, " [3] a proper man, and 'tis pity he hath no preferment," all good wishes; but, inexorable, indurate as he is, he will not prefer him, though it be in his power, because he is *indotatus*, he hath no money. Or, if he do give him entertainment, let him be never so well qualified, plead affinity, consanguinity, sufficiency, he shall serve seven years, as Jacob did for Rachel, before he shall have it. [4] If he will enter at first, he must get in at that simoniacal gate, come off soundly, and put in good security to perform all covenants; else he will not deal with, or admit him. But, if some poor scholar, some parson chaff, will offer himself; some trencher chaplain, that will take it to the halves, thirds, or accept of what he will give, he is welcom; be comfortable, preach as he will have him, he likes him before a million of others; for the best is alwayes best cheap : and then (as Hierom said to Cromatius) *patellâ dignum operculum :* such a patron, such a clark; the cure is well supplyed, and all parties pleased. So that is still verified in our age, which [5] Chrysostome complained of in his time: *qui opulentiores sunt, in ordinem parasitorum cogunt eos, et ipsos tamquam canes ad mensas suas enutriunt, eorumque impudentes ventres iniquorum cœnarum reliquiis differciunt, iisdem pro arbitrio abutentes :* rich men keep these lecturers, and fawning parasites, like so many dogs, at their tables; and, filling their hungry guts with the offals of

---

[1] Tu vero licet Orpheus sis, saxa sono testudinis emolliens, nisi plumbea eorum corda auri vel argenti malleo emollias, &c.   Salisburiensis, Polycrat. lib. 5. c. 10. [2] Juven. Sat. 7.   [3] Euge! bene ! no need. Dousa epod. 1. 3. Dos ipsa scientia, sibique congiarium est.   [4] Quatuor ad portas ecclesias itur ad omnes ; Sanguinis, aut Simonis, præsulis, atque Dei. Holcot.   [5] Lib. contra Gentiles, de Babilâ martyre.

330 *Causes of Melancholy.* [Part. 1. Sec. 2.

their meat, they abuse them at their pleasure, and make them say what they propose. [1] *As children do by a bird or a butterflye in a string, pull in and let him out as they list, do they by their trencher chaplains, prescribe, command their wits, let in and out, as to them it seems best.* If the patron be precise, so must his chaplain be ; if he be papistical, his clark must be so too, or else be turned out. These are those clarks which serve the turn, whom they commonly entertain, and present to church-livings, whilst in the mean time we, that are university-men, like so many hide-bound calves in a pasture, tarry out our time, wither away as a flower ungathered in a garden, and are never used ; or, as too many candles, illuminate our selves alone, obscuring one anothers light, and are not discerned here at all; the least of which, translated to a dark room, or to some countrey benefice, where it might shine apart, would give a fair light, and be seen over all. Whilst we lye waiting here (as those sick men did at the pool of [2] Bethesda, till the angel stirred the water) expecting a good hour, they step between, and beguile us of our preferment. I have not yet said. If, after long expectation, much expence, travel, earnest suit of our selves and friends, we obtain a small benefice at last, our misery begins afresh ; we are suddenly encountered with the flesh, world, and devil, with a new onset: we change a quiet life for an ocean of troubles ; we come to a ruinous house, which, before it be habitable, must be necessarily (to our great damage) repaired : we are compelled to sue for dilapidations, or else sued our selves ; and, scarce yet settled, we are called upon for our predecessors arrereages : first fruits, tenths, subsidies, are instantly to be paid, benevolence, procurations, &c. and (which is most to be feared) we light upon a crackt title, as it befell Clenard of Brabant, for his rectory and charge of his Beginæ: he was no sooner inducted, but instantly sued, *cœpimusque* ([3] saith he) *strenue litigare, et implacabili bello confligere :* at length, after ten years suit, (as long as Troyes siege) when he had tired himself, and spent his money, he was fain to leave all for quietness sake, and give it up to his adversary. Or else we are insulted over, and trampled on by domineering officers, fleeced by those greedy harpyes to get more fees, we stand in fear of some precedent lapse ; we fall amongst refractory, seditious sectaries, peevish puritans, perverse papists, a lascivious rout of atheistical Epicures, that will not be

---

[1] Præscribunt, imperant, in ordinem cogunt; ingenium nostrum, prout ipsis videbitur, astringunt et relaxant, ut papilionem pueri aut bruchum filo demittunt aut attrahunt, nos a libidine suâ pendere æquum censentes. Heinsius. [2] John 5. [3] Epist. l. 2. Jam suffectus in locum demortui...protinus exortus est adversarius, &c. post multos labores, sumtus, &c.

2

Mem. 3. Subs. 15.]   *Study, a Cause.*   331

reformed, or some litigious people, (those wild beasts of Ephesus must be fought with) that will not pay their dues without
much repining, or compelled by long suit; *laïci clericis op-*
pido infesti, an old axiom; all they think well gotten that is
had from the church; and by such uncivil harsh dealings, they
make their poor minister weary of his place, if not his life:
and put case they be quiet honest men, make the best of it, as
often it falls out, from a polite and terse academick, he must
turn rustick, rude, melancholise alone, learn to forget, or else,
as many do, become malsters, grasiers, chapmen, &c. (now
banished from the academy, all commerce of the Muses, and
confined to a countrey village, as Ovid was from Rome to
Pontus) and daily converse with a company of idiots and
clowns.

Nos interim quod attinet (nec enim immunes ab hac noxâ
sumus) idem reatus manet; idem nobis, et si non multo gra-
vius, crimen objici potest: nostrâ enim culpâ fit, nostrâ
incuriâ, nostrâ avaritiâ, quod tam frequentes, fœdæque fiant
in ecclesiâ nundinationes, (templum est venale, Deusque) *tot*
sordes invehantur, tanta grassetur impietas, tanta nequitia,
tam insanus miseriarum Euripus, et turbarum æstuarium,
nostro, inquam, omnium (academicorum imprimis) vitio fit.
Quod tot resp. malis afficiatur, a nobis seminarium; ultro
malum hoc accersimus, et quâvis contumeliâ, quâvis interim
miseriâ digni, qui pro virili non occurrimus.   Quid enim
fieri posse speramus, quum tot indies sine delectu pauperes
alumni, terræ filii, et cujuscunque ordinis homunciones, ad gra-
dus certatim admittantur? qui si definitionem, distinctionemque
unam aut alteram memoriter edidicerint, et pro more tot annos
in dialecticâ posuerint, non refert quo profectu, quales demum
sint, idiotæ, nugatores, otiatores, aleatores, compotores, indigni,
libidinis voluptatumque administri,

Sponsi Penelopes, nebulones, Alcinoique,

modo tot annos in academiâ insumpserint, et se pro togatis
venditârint; lucri caussâ, et amicorum intercessu præsentantur:
addo etiam, et magnificis nonnunquam elogiis morum et sci-
entiæ; et, jam valedicturi, testimonialibus hisce literis, am-
plissime conscriptis in eorum gratiam, honorantur, ab iis,
qui fidei suæ et existimationis jacturam proculdubio faciunt.
Doctores enim et professores *(quod ait* [1] *ille)* id unum curant,
ut ex professionibus frequentibus, et tumultuariis potius quam
legitimis, commoda sua promoveant, et ex dispendio publico

[1] Jun. Acad. cap. 6.

332   *Causes of Melancholy.*   [Part. 1. Sec. 2.

suum faciant incrementum. *Id solum in votis habent annui plerumque magistratus, ut ab incipientium numero* [1] *pecunias emungant; nec multum interest, qui sint, literatores an literati, modo pingues, nitidi, ad aspectum speciosi, et (quod verbo dicam) pecuniosi sint.* [2] *Philosophastri licentiantur in artibus, artem qui non habent;* [3] *eosque sapientes esse jubent, qui nullâ præditi sunt sapientiâ, et nihil ad gradum, præterquam velle, adferunt. Theologastri, (solvant modo) satis superque docti, per omnes honorum gradus evehuntur et ascendunt. Atque hinc fit quod tam viles scurræ, tot passim idiotæ, literarum crepusculo positi, larvæ pastorum, circumforanei, vagi, bardi, fungi, crassi, asini, merum pecus, in sacrosanctos theologiæ aditus illotis pedibus irrumpant, præter inverecundam frontem adferentes nihil, vulgares quasdam quisquilias et scholariam quædam nugamenta, indigna quæ vel recipiantur in triviis. Hoc illud indignum genus hominum et famelicum, indignum, vagum, ventris mancipium, ad stivam potius relegandum, ad haras aptius quam ad aras, quod divinas hasce literas turpiter prostituit—hi sunt qui pulpita complent, in ædes nobilium irrepunt, et, quum reliquis vitæ destituantur subsidiis, ob corporis et animi egestatem, aliarum in repub. partium minime capaces sint, ad sacram hanc anchoram confugiunt, sacerdotium quovis modo captantes, non ex sinceritate, (quod* [4] *Paulus ait)* sed cauponantes verbum Dei. *Ne quis interim viris bonis detractum quid putet, quos habet ecclesia Anglicana quamplurimos, egregie doctos, illustres, intactæ famæ homines, et plures forsan quam quævis Europæ provincia; ne quis a florentissimis academiis, quæ viros undequaque doctissimos, omni virtutum genere suspiciendos, abunde producunt; et multo plures utraque habitura, multo splendidior futura, si non hæ sordes splendidum lumen ejus obfuscarent, obstaret corruptio, et cauponantes quædam Harpyiæ, proletariique, bonum hoc nobis non inviderent. Nemo enim tam cæcâ mente, qui non hoc ipsum videat; nemo tam stolido ingenio, qui non intelligat; tam pertinaci judicio, cui non agnoscat, ab his idiotis circumforaneis sacram pollui theologiam, ac cœlestes Musas, quasi profanum quiddam, prostitui.* Viles animæ et affrontes (*sic enim Lutherus* [5] *alicubi vocat*) lucelli caussâ, ut muscæ ad mulctra, ad nobilium et heroum mensas advolant: in spem sacerdotii, *cujuslibet honoris, officii, in quamvis aulam, urbem se ingerunt, ad quodvis se ministerium componunt.*

---

[1] Accipiamus pecuniam, demittamus asinum, ut apud Patavinos Italos.
[2] Hos non ita pridem perstrinxi, in Philosophastro, Comœdiâ Latinâ, in Æde Christi Oxon. publice habitâ, anno 1617. Feb. 16.   [3] Sat. Menip.   [4] 1 Cor. 7. 17.   [5] Comment. in Gal.

——— Ut nervis alienis mobile lignum
Ducitur,

[1]offam sequentes, psittacorum more, in prædæ spem quidvis effutiunt: *obsecundantes parasiti* ([2]Erasmus *ait*) quidvis docent, dicunt, scribunt, suadent, et contra conscientiam probant, non ut salutarem reddant gregem, sed ut magnificam sibi parent fortunam. [3]Opiniones quasvis et decreta contra verbum Dei astruunt, ne offendant patronum, sed ut retineant favorem procerum et populi plausum sibique ipsis opes accumulent. *Eo etenim plerumque animo ad theologiam accedunt, non ut rem divinam, sed ut suam, faciant ; non ad ecclesiæ bonum promovendum, sed expilandum; quærentes (quod Paulus ait)* non quæ Jesu Christi, sed quæ sua, *non Domini thesaurum, sed ut sibi suisque thesaurizent. Nec tantum iis, qui vilioris fortunæ, et abjectæ sortis sunt, hoc in usu est ; sed et medios, summos, elatos, ne dicam episcopos, hoc malum invasit.*

[4]Dicite, pontifices, in sacris quid facit aurum ?

[5]summos sæpe viros transversos agit avaritia ; *et qui reliquis morum probitate prælucerent, hi facem præferunt ad simoniam, et in corruptionis hunc scopulum impingentes, non tondent pecus, sed deglubunt, et, quocunque se conferunt, expilant, exhauriunt, abradunt, magnum famæ suæ, si non animæ, naufragium facientes; ut non ab infimis ad summos, sed a summis ad infimos, malum promanásse videatur, et illud verum sit, quod ille olim lusit,*

Emerat ille prius, vendere jure potest :

Simoniacus enim (*quod cum* Leone *dicam*) gratiam non accipit; si non accipit, non habet, et si non habet, nec gratus potest esse, nec gratis dare : *tantum enim absunt istorum nonnulli, qui ad clavum sedent, a promovendo reliquos, ut penitus impediant, probe sibi conscii, quibus artibus illic pervenerint :* [6]nam qui ob literas emersisse illos credat, desipit ; qui vero ingenii, eruditionis, experientiæ, probitatis, pietatis, et Musarum id esse pretium putat *(quod olim re verá fuit, hodie promittitur)* planissime insanit. *Utcunque vel undecunque malum hoc originem ducat, (non ultra quæram) ex his primordiis cœpit vitiorum colluvies ; omnis calamitas, omne miseriarum agmen, in ecclesiam invehitur. Hinc tam frequens simonia ; hinc ortæ querelæ, fraudes, imposturæ; ab hoc fonte se derivárunt omnes nequitiæ,—ne quid obiter dicam de ambitione, adulatione plusquam aulicá, ne tristi domicœnio laborent, de luxu, de fœdo nonnunquam vitæ exemplo, quo nonnullos offendunt, de*

[1] Heinsius.   [2] Ecclesiast.   [3] Luth. in Gal.   [4] Pers. Sat. 2.
[5] Sallust.   [6] Sat. Menip.

334   *Causes of Melancholy.*   [Part. 1. Sec. 2.

compotatione Sybariticá, &c.   Hinc ille squalor academicus,
tristes hac tempestate Camœnœ, *quum quivis homunculus, ar-*
tium ignarus, his artibus assurgat, hunc in modum promovea-
tur et ditescat, ambitiosis appellationibus insignis, et multis
dignitatibus augustus, vulgi oculos perstringat, bene se habeat,
et grandia gradiens, majestatem quamdam ac amplitudinem
præ se ferens, miramque solicitudinem, barbá reverendus, togá
nitidus, purpurá coruscus, supellectilis splendore et famulorum
numero maxime conspicuus.   Quales statuæ (*quod ait* [1] *ille*)
quæ sacris in ædibus columnis imponuntur, velut oneri ceden-
tes videntur, ac si insudarent, quum re verâ sensu sint carentes, et nihil saxeam adjuvent firmitatem; *Atlantes videri vo-*
lunt, quum sint statuæ lapideæ, umbratiles re verá homuncio-
nes, fungi forsan et bardi, nihil a saxo differentes ; quum in-
terim docti viri, et vitæ sanctioris ornamentis præditi, qui æs-
tum diei sustinent, his iniquá sorte serviant, minimo forsan
salario contenti, puris nominibus nuncupati, humiles, obscuri ;
multoque digniores licet, egentes, inhonorati, vitam privam pri-
vatam agant ; tenuique sepulti sacerdotio, vel in collegiis suis
in æternum incarcerati, inglorie delitescant :—sed nolo diutius
hanc movere sentinam.   Hinc illæ lacrymæ, lugubris Musa-
rum habitus ; [2] *hinc ipsa religio (quod cum Secellio dicam)* in
ludibrium et contemtum adducitur, *abjectum sacerdotium,*
(*atque hæc ubi fiunt, ausim dicere, et putidum* [3] *putidi dicte-*
rium de clero usurpare) putidum vulgus, *inops, rude, sordidum,*
melancholicum, miserum, despicabile, contemnendum.

MEMB. IV. SUBSECT. I.

Non-necessary, remote, outward, adventitious, or accidental
causes: as first from the Nurse.

OF those remote, outward, ambient *necessary* causes, I
have sufficiently discoursed in the precedent member. The
non-necessary follow; of which (saith [4] Fuchsius) no art can
be made, by reason of their uncertainty, casualty, and multitude ; so called *not necessary,* because (according to [5] Fernelius) *they may be avoided, and used without necessity.*
Many of these accidental causes, which I shall entreat of here,
might have well been reduced to the former, because they
cannot be avoided, but fatally happen to us, though accidentally, and unawares, at some time or other ; the rest are con-

---

[1] Budæus, de Asse, lib. 5.   [2] Lib. de rep. Gallorum.   [3] Campian.
[4] Procem. lib. 2. Nulla ars constitui potest.   [5] Lib. 1. c. 19. de morborum
caussis. Quas declinare licet, aut nullâ necessitate utimur.

Mem. 4. Subs. 1.] *Nurse, a Cause.*

tingent and evitable, and more properly inserted in this rank of causes. To reckon up all, is a thing unpossible ; of some therefore most remarkable of these contingent causes which produce melancholy, I will briefly speak, and in their order.

From a childs nativity, the first ill accident that can likely befall him in this kind, is a bad nurse, by whose means alone he may be tainted with this [1] malady from his cradle. Aulus Gellius (*l. 12. c. 1.*) brings in Phavorinus, that eloquent philosopher, proving this at large, [2] *that there is the same vertue and property in the milk as in the seed, and not in men alone, but in all other creatures. He gives instance in a kid and lamb: if either of them suck of the others milk, the lamb of the goates, or the kid of the ewes, the wool of the one will be hard, and the hair of the other soft.* Giraldus Cambrensis (*Itinerar. Cambriæ, l. 1. c. 2.*) confirms this by a notable example, which happened in his time. A sow-pig by chance sucked a brach, and, when she was grown, [3] *would miraculously hunt all manner of deer, and that as well, or rather better, than any ordinary hound.* His conclusion is, [4] *that men and beasts participate of her nature and conditions, by whose milk they are fed.* Phavorinus urgeth it farther, and demonstrates it more evidently, that if a nurse be [5] *mis-shapen, unchaste, unhonest, impudent, drunk,* [6] *cruel,* or the like, the child that sucks upon her breast will be so too ; all other affections of the mind, and diseases, are almost ingraffed, as it were, and imprinted in the temperature of the infant, by the nurses milk, as pox, leprosie, melancholy, &c. Cato, for some such reason, would make his servants children suck upon his wives breast, because, by that means, they would love him and his the better, and in all likelihood agree with them. A more evident example that the minds are altered by milk, cannot be given, than that of [7] Dion, which he relates of Caligulas cruelty; it could neither be imputed to father nor mother, but to his cruel nurse alone, that anointed her paps with blood still when he sucked, which made him such a murderer, and to express her cruelty to an hair; and that of Tiberius, who was a common drunkard, because his nurse was such a one.

---

[1] Quo semel est imbuta recens, servabit odorem Testa diu. Hor.   [2] Sicut valet ad fingendas corporis atque animi similitudines vis et natura seminis, sic quoque lactis proprietas. Neque id in hominibus solum, sed in pecudibus, animadversum : nam si ovium lacte hœdi, aut caprarum agni alerentur, constat fieri in his lanam duriorem, in illis capillum gigni teneriorem.   [3] Adulta in ferarum persequutione ad miraculum usque sagax.   [4] Tam animal quodlibet, quam homo, ab illâ, cujus lacte nutritur, naturam contrahit.   [5] Improba, informis, impudica, temulenta nutrix, &c. quoniam in moribus efformandis magnam sæpe partem ingenium altricis et natura lactis tenet.   [6] Hyrcanæque admorunt ubera tigres. Virg.   [7] Lib. 2. de Cæsaribus.

336   *Causes of Melancholy.*   [Part. 1. Sec. 2.

Et, si delira fuerit, ([1] one observes) *infantulum delirum faciet;*
if she be a fool or dolt, the child she nurseth will take after
her, or otherwise be misaffected; which Franciscus Barbarus
(*l. 2. c. ult. de re uxoriâ*) proves at full, and Ant. Guivarra
(*lib. 2. de Marco Aurelio*): the child will surely participate.
For bodily sickness, there is no doubt to be made. Titus,
Vespasians son, was therefore sickly, because the nurse was so
(Lampridius): and, if we may believe physicians, many times
children catch the pox from a bad nurse, (Botaldus, *cap.* 61.
de. lue Vener.) Besides evil attendance, negligence, and
many gross inconveniences, which are incident to nurses, much
danger may so come to the child. [2] For these causes Aristotle
(*Polit. lib.* 7. *c.* 17), Phavorinus, and Marcus Aurelius, would
not have a child put to nurse at all, but every mother to
bring up her own, of what condition soever she be; for a
sound and able mother to put out her child to nurse, is
naturæ intemperies (so [3] Guatso calls it): 'tis fit therefore she
should be nurse her self; the mother will be more careful,
loving and attendant, than any servile woman, or such hired
creatures; this all the world acknowledgeth: *convenientissimum
est* (as Rod. a Castro, *de nat. mulierum, lib.* 4. *c.* 12, in many
words confesseth) *matrem ipsam lactare infantem,* (who
denies that it should be so?) and which some women most
curiously observe; amongst the rest, [4] that queen of France, a
Spaniard by birth, that was so precise and zealous in this behalf, that when, in her absence, a strange nurse had suckled her
child, she was never quiet till she had made the infant vomit
it up again. But she was too jealous. If it be so, as many
times it is, they must be put forth, the mother be not fit or
well able to be a nurse, I would then advise such mothers, (as
[5] Plutarch doth in his book *de liberis educandis,* and [6] S. Hierome, *lib.* 2. *epist.* 27. *Lætæ de institut. fil.* Magninus, *part.* 2.
Reg. sanit. cap. 7, and the said Rodericus) that they make
choice of a sound woman, of a good complexion, honest, free
from bodily diseases, if it be possible, and all passions, and perturbations of the mind, as sorrow, fear, grief, [7] folly, melancholy : for such passions corrupt the milk, and alter the temperature of the child, which, now being [8] *udum et molle lutum,*
is easily seasoned and perverted. And if such a nurse may
be found out, that will be diligent and careful withall, let Phavorinus and M. Aurelius plead how they can against it, I had
rather accept of her in some cases than the mother her

---

[1] Beda, c. 27. l. 1. Eccles. hist.   [2] Ne insitivo lactis alimento degeneret corpus, et animus corrumpatur.   [3] Lib. 3. de civ. conserv.   [4] Stephanus.
[5] To. 2. Nutrices non quasvis, sed maxime probas, deligamus.   [6] Nutrix non sit
lasciva aut temulenta. Hier.   [7] Prohibendum ne stolida lactet.   [8] Pers.

Mem. 4. Subs. 2.]   *Education, a Cause.*   337

self; and (which Bonacialus the physician, Nic. Biesius the politician, *lib. 4. de repub. cap.* 8. approves) [1] *some nurses are much to be preferred to some mothers.* For why may not the mother be naught, a peevish drunken flurt, a waspish cholerick slut, a crazed piece, a fool, (as many mothers are) unsound, as soon as the nurse? There is more choice of nurses than mothers; and therefore, except the mother be most vertuous, staid, a woman of excellent good parts, and of a sound complexion, I would have all children, in such cases, committed to discreet strangers. And 'tis the only way (as by marriage they are engrafted to other families) to alter the breed, or, if any thing be amiss in the mother, (as Ludovicus Mercatus contends, *Tom. 2. lib. de morb. hæred.*) to prevent diseases and future maladies, to correct and qualifie the childs ill-disposed temperature, which he had from his parents. This is an excellent remedy, if good choice be made of such a nurse.

SUBSECT. II.

Education, a Cause of Melancholy.

EDUCATION, of these accidental causes of melancholy, may justly challenge the next place; for, if a man escape a bad nurse, he may be undone by evil bringing up. [2] Jason Pratensis puts this of education for a principal cause : bad parents, step-mothers, tutors, masters, teachers, too rigorous, too severe, too remiss or indulgent on the other side, are often fountains and furtherers of this disease. Parents, and such as have the tuition and oversight of children, offend many times in that they are too stern, alway threatning, chiding, brawling, whipping, or striking; by means of which, their poor children are so disheartned and cowed, that they never after have any courage, a merry hour in their lives, or take pleasure in any thing. There is a great moderation to be had in such things, as matters of so great moment to the making or marring of a child. Some fright their children with beggars, bugbears and hobgoblins, if they cry or be otherwayes unruly : but they are much to blame in it, many times, saith Lavater (*de spectris, part.* 1. *cap.* 5) : *ex metu in morbos graves incidunt, et noctu dormientes clamant ;* for fear they fall into many diseases, and cry out in their sleep, and are much the worse for it all their lives : these things ought not at all, or to be sparingly

---

[1] Nutrices interdum matribus sunt meliores.   [2] Lib. de morbis capitis, cap. de maniâ. Haud postrema caussa supputatur educatio, inter has mentis abalienationis caussas.—Injusta noverca.

VOL. I.   z

338   *Causes of Melancholy.*   [Part. 1. Sec. 2.

done, and upon just occasion. Tyrannical, impatient, hair-brain'd school-masters, *aridi magistri*, so [1] Fabius terms them, *Ajaces flagelliferi*, are in this kind, as bad as hangmen and executioners: they make many children endure a martyrdom all the while they are at school: with bad diet, if they boord in their houses, too much severity and ill usage, they quite pervert their temperature of body and mind—still chiding, rayling, frowning, lashing, tasking, keeping, that they are *fracti animis*, moped many times, weary of their lives, [2] *nimiâ severitate deficiunt et desperant*, and think no slavery in the world (as once I did myself) like to that of a grammar scholar. *Præceptorum ineptiis discruciantur ingenia puerorum*, saith Erasmus: they tremble at his voice, looks, coming in. St. Austin, in the first book of his *confess.* and 4. *ca.* calls this schooling *meticulosam necessitatem*, and elsewhere a martyrdom, and confesseth of himself, how cruelly he was tortured in mind for learning Greek ; *nulla verba noveram : et sævis terroribus et pœnis, ut nóssem, instabatur mihi vehementer:* I knew nothing: and with cruel terrours and punishment I was daily compel'd. [3] Beza complains in like case of a rigorous schoolmaster in Paris, that made him, by his continual thunder and threats, once in a mind to drown himself, had he not met by the way with an uncle of his that vindicated him from that misery for the time, by taking him to his house. Trincavellius (*lib.* 1. *consil.* 16.) had a patient nineteen years of age, extreamly melancholy, *ob nimium studium Tarvitii et præceptoris minas*, by reason of overmuch study, and his [4] tutors threats. Many masters are hard hearted, and bitter to their servants, and by that means do so deject, with terrible speeches and hard usage so crucifie them, that they become desperate, and can never be recalled.

Others again, in that opposite extream, do as great harm by their too much remissness ; they give them no bringing up, no calling to busie themselves about, or to live in, teach them no trade, or set them in any good course ; by means of which, their servants, children, scholars, are carried away with that stream of drunkenness, idleness, gaming, and many such irregular courses, that in the end they rue it, curse their parents, and mischief themselves. Too much indulgence causeth the like, [5] *inepta patris lenitas et facilitas prava*, when as Miciolike, with too much liberty and too great allowance, they feed their childrens humours, let them revel, wench, riot, swagger,

---

[1] Lib. 2. cap. 4.   [2] Idem. Et, quod maxime nocet, dum in teñeris ita timent, nihil conantur.   [3] Præfat. ad Testam.   [4] Plus mentis pædagogico supercilio abstulit, quam unquam præceptis suis sapientiæ instillavit.
[5] Ter. Adel. 3. 4.

Mem. 4. Subs. 2.]   *Education, a Cause.*   339

and do what they will themselves, and then punish them with a noise of musicians.

> [1] Obsonet, potet, oleat unguenta ; de meo.
> Amat ? dabitur a me argentum, dum erit commodum.
> Fores effregit ? restituentur : discidit
> Vestem ? resarcietur.——Faciat quod lubet,
> Sumat, consumat, perdat : decretum est pati.

But, as Demea told him, *tu illum corrumpi sinis,* your lenity will be his undoing ; *prævidere videor jam diem illum, quum hic egens profugiet aliquo militatum ;* I foresee his ruine. So parents often err : many fond mothers, especially, dote so much upon their children, like [2] Æsops ape, till in the end they crush them to death. *Corporum nutrices, animarum novercæ,* pampering up their bodies to the undoing of their souls, they will not let them be [3] corrected or controled, but still soothed up in every thing they do, that, in conclusion, *they bring sorrow, shame, heaviness, to their parents,* (*Ecclus. cap.* 30. 8. 9) *become wanton, stubborn, wilful, and disobedient ; rude, untaught, head-strong, incorrigible, and graceless. They love them so foolishly,* (saith [4] Cardan) *that they rather seem to hate them, bringing them not up to vertue, but injury, not to learning, but to riot, not to sober life and conversation, but to all pleasure and licentious behaviour.* Who is he of so little experience that knows not this of Fabius to be true ? [5] *Education is another nature, altering the mind and will, and I would to God* (saith he) *we our selves did not spoile our childrens manners, by our overmuch cockering and nice education, and weaken the strength of their bodies and minds. That causeth custom, custom nature,* &c. For these causes, Plutarch (in his book *de lib. educ.*) and Hierom, (*epist. lib.* 1. *epist.* 17. to *Læta de institut. filiæ*) gives a most especial charge to all parents, and many good cautions about bringing up of children, that they be not committed to undiscreet, passionate, Bedlam tutors, light, giddy-headed, or covetous persons, and spare for no cost, that they may be well nurtured and taught ; it being a matter of so great consequence. For, such parents as do otherwise, Plutarch esteems like them [6] *that are more careful*

---

[1] Ter. Adel. act. 1. sc. 2.   [2] Camerarius, em. 77. cent. 2. hath elegantly expressed it in an embleme : perdit amando, &c.   [3] Prov. 13. 24. He that spareth the rod hates his son.   [4] Lib. 2. de consol. Tam stulte pueros diligimus, ut odisse potius videamur : illos non ad virtutem sed ad injuriam, non ad eruditionem sed ad luxum, non ad vitam sed voluptatem educantes.   [5] Lib. 1. c. 3. Educatio altera natura ; alterat animos et voluntatem : atque utinam (inquit) liberorum nostrorum mores non ipsi perderemus, quum infantiam statim deliciis solvimus ; mollior ista educatio, quam indulgentiam vocamus, nervos omnes, et mentis et corporis, frangit : fit ex his consuetudo, inde natura.   [6] Perinde agit ac siquis de calceo sit solicitus, pedem nihil curet. Juven. Nil patri minus est quam filius.

z 2

340   *Causes of Melancholy.*   [Part. 1. Sec. 2.

of their shooes than of their feet, that rate their wealth above their children. And he (saith [1] Cardan) *that leaves his son to a covetous schoolmaster to be informed, or to a close abby to fast and learn wisdom together, doth no other, than that he be a learned fool, or a sickly wise man.*

SUBSECT. III.

Terrours and Affrights, Causes of Melancholy.

TULLY (in the fourth of his Tusculans) distinguisheth these terrours which arise from the apprehension of some terrible object heard or seen, from other fears: and so doth Patritius (*lib. 5. tit. 4. de regis institut.*). Of all fears, they are most pernicious and violent, and so suddainly alter the whole temperature of the body, move the soul and spirits, strike such a deep impression, that the parties can never be recovered, causing more grievous and fiercer melancholy, (as Felix Plater, *c. 3 de mentis alienat.* [2]speaks out of his experience) than any inward cause whatsoever ; *and imprints it self so forcibly in the spirits, brain, humours, that, if all the mass of blood were let out of the body, it could hardly be extracted. This horrible kind of melancholy* (for so he terms it) *had been often brought before him, and troubles and affrights commonly men and women, young and old, of all sorts.* [3] Hercules de Saxoniâ calls this kind of melancholy (*ab agitatione spirituum*) by a peculiar name ; it comes from the agitation, motion, contraction, dilatation of spirits, not from any distemperature of humours, and produceth strong effects. This terrour is most usually caused (as [4] Plutarch will have) *from some imminent danger, when a terrible object is at hand,* heard, seen, or conceived, [5] *truly appearing, or in a* [6] *dream :* and many times, the more sudden the accident, it is the more violent.

> [7] Stat terror animis, et cor attonitum salit,
> Pavidumque trepidis palpitat venis jecur.

---

[1] Lib. 3. de sapient. Qui avaris pædagogis pueros alendos dant, vel clausos in cœnobiis jejunare simul et sapere, nihil aliud agunt, nisi ut sint vel non sine stultitiâ eruditi, vel non integrâ vitâ sapientes.   [2] Terror et metus, maxime ex improviso accidentes, ita animum commovent, ut spiritus nunquam recuperent: gravioremque melancholiam terror facit, quam quæ ab internâ caussâ fit. Impressio tam fortis in spiritibus humoribusque cerebri, ut, extractâ totâ sanguineâ massâ, ægre exprimatur ; et hæc horrenda species melancholiæ frequenter oblata mihi, omnes exercens, viros, juvenes, senes.   [3] Tract. de melan. cap. 7. et 8. Non ab intemperie, sed agitatione, dilatatione, contractione, motu spirituum. [4] Lib. de fort. et virtut. Alex. Præsertim ineunte periculo, ubi res prope adsunt terribiles.   [5] Fit a visione horrendâ, revera apparente, vel per insomnia. Platerus.   [6] A painters wife in Basil, 1600, somniavit filium bello mortuum : inde melancholica consolari noluit.   [7] Senec. Herc. Œt.

Their soul's affright, their heart amazed quakes,
The trembling liver pants ith' veins, and akes.

Artemidorus the grammarian lost his wits by the unexpected sight of a crocodile (*Laurentius, 7. de melan*). [1] The massacre at Lions, in 1572, in the reign of Charles the ninth, was so terrible and fearful, that many ran mad, some died, great-bellied women were brought to bed before their time, generally all affrighted and agast. Many lose their wits [2] *by the sudden sight of some spectrum or devil, a thing very common in all ages,* (saith Lavater, *part. 1. cap.* 9) as Orestes did at the sight of the Furies, which appeared to him in black (as [3] Pausanias records). The Greeks call them μορμολυκεια, which so terrific their souls. Or if they be but affrighted by some counterfeit devils in jest,

(————[4] ut pueri trepidant, atque omnia cæcis
In tenebris metuunt————

as children in the dark conceive hobgoblins, and are sore afraid) they are the worse for it all their lives: some, by sudden fires, earthquakes, inundations, or any such dismal objects. Themison the physician fell into an hydrophobia by seeing one sick of that disease (Dioscorides, *l.* 6. *c.* 33): or by the sight of a monster, a carcase, they are disquieted many months following, and cannot endure the room where a coarse hath been, for a world would not be alone with a dead man, or lye in that bed many years after, in which a man hath died. At [5] Basil, a many little children, in the spring time, went to gather flowers in a meadow at the towns end, where a malefactor hung in gibbets: all gazing at it, one by chance flung a stone, and made it stir; by which accident the children affrighted ran away: one, slower than the rest, looking back, and seeing the stirred carcase wag towards her, cried out it came after, and was so terribly affrighted, that for many dayes she could not rest, eat, or sleep; she could not be pacified, but melancholy died. [6] In the same town, another child, beyond the Rhine, saw a grave opened, and, upon the sight of a carcase, was so troubled in mind, that she could not be comforted, but a little after departed, and was buried by it (Platerus, *observat. l.* 1). A gentlewoman of the same city saw a fat hog cut up, when the

---

[1] Quarta pars comment. de statu religionis in Galliâ sub Carolo ix. 1572.
[2] Ex occursu dæmonum aliqui furore corripiuntur, ut experientiâ notum est.
[3] Lib. 8. in Arcad.   [4] Lucret.   [5] Puellæ extra urbem in prato concurrentes, &c. mœsta et melancholica domum rediit; per dies aliquot vexata, dum mortua est. Plater.   [6] Altera trans-Rhenana, ingressa sepulcrum recens apertum, vidit cadaver, et domum subito reversa putavit eam vocare: post paucos dies obiit, proximo sepulcro collocata. Altera, patibulum sero præteriens, metuebat ne urbe exclusa illic pernoctaret; unde melancholica facta, per multos annos laboravit. Platerus.

342 *Causes of Melancholy.* [Part. 1. Sec. 2.

intrals were opened, and a noysome savour offended her nose, she much misliked, and would not longer abide: a physician, in presence, told her, as that hog, so was she, full of filthy excrements, and aggravated the matter by some other loathsome instances, in so much, this nice gentlewoman apprehended it so deeply, that she fell forthwith a vomiting, was so mightily distempered in mind and body, that, with all his art and perswasions, for some months after, he could not restore her to her self again; she could not forget it, or remove the object out of her sight (*Idem*). Many cannot endure to see a wound opened, but they are offended; a man executed, or labour of any fearful disease, as possession, apoplexies, one bewitched: [1] or, if they read by chance of some terrible thing, the symptomes alone of such a disease, or that which they dislike, they are instantly troubled in mind, agast, ready to apply it to themselves; they are as much disquieted, as if they had seen it, or were so affected themselves. *Hecatas sibi videntur somniare;* they dream and continually think of it. As lamentable effects are caused by such terrible objects heard, read, or seen: *auditus maximos motus in corpore facit,* as [2] Plutarch holds; no sense makes greater alteration of body and mind: sudden speech sometimes, unexpected news, be they good or bad, *prævisa minus oratio,* will move as much, (*animum obruere, et de sede suâ dejicere,* as a [3] philosopher observes) will take away our sleep, and appetite, disturb and quite overturn us. Let them bear witness, that have heard those tragical alarums, out-cryes, hideous noises, which are many times suddenly heard in the dead of the night by irruption of enemies and accidental fires, &c. those [4] panick fears, which often drive men out of their wits, bereave them of sense, understanding, and all, some for a time, some for their whole lives; they never recover it. The [5] Midianites were so affrighted by Gideons souldiers, they breaking but every one a pitcher; and [6] Hannibals army, by such a panick fear, was discomfited at the walls of Rome. Augusta Livia, hearing a few tragical verses recited out of Virgil, (*Tu Marcellus eris, &c.*) fell down dead in a swoon. Edinus, king of Denmark, by a sudden sound which he heard, [7] *was turned into fury, with all his men* (*Cranzius, l. 5. Dan. hist. et Alexander ab Alexandro, l. 3. c. 5*). Amatus Lusitanus had a patient, that, by reason of bad tidings, became *epilepticus* (*cen. 2. cura 90*). Cardan (*subtil. l. 18*) saw one that lost his wits by mistaking of

---

[1] Subitus occursus, inopinata lectio.   [2] Lib. de auditione.   [3] Theod. Prodromus, lib. 7 Amorum.   [4] Effuso cernens fugientes agmine turmas, Quis mea nunc inflat cornua? Faunus ait. Alciat. embl. 122.   [5] Jud. 6. 19.   [6] Plutarchus, vitâ ejus.   [7] In furorem cum sociis versus.

Mem. 4. Subs. 3.]   *Terrours and Affrights, Causes.*   343

an echo. If one sense alone can cause such violent commotions of the mind, what may we think, when hearing, sight, and those other senses, are all troubled at once, as by some earthquakes, thunder, lightning, tempests, &c? At Bologne in Italy, *anno* 1504, there was such a fearful earthquake about eleven o'clock in the night, (as [1] Beroaldus, in his book *de terræ motu*, hath commended to posterity) that all the city trembled, the people thought the world was at an end, *actum de mortalibus;* such a fearful noise it made, such a detestable smell, the inhabitants were infinitely affrighted, and some ran mad. *Audi rem atrocem, et annalibus memorandam,* (mine author adds) : hear a strange story, and worthy to be chronicled: I had a servant at the same time, called Fulco Argelanus, a bold and proper man, so grievously terrified with it, [2] that he was first melancholy, after doted, at last mad, and made away himself. At [3] Fuscinum in Japona, *there was such an earthquake and darkness on a sudden, that many men were offended with headach, many overwhelmed with sorrow and melancholy. At Meacum, whole streets and goodly palaces were overturned at the same time; and there was such an hideous noise withal, like thunder, and filthy smell, that their hair stared for fear, and their hearts quaked; men and beasts were incredibly terrified. In Sacai, another city, the same earthquake was so terrible unto them, that many were bereft of their senses; and others, by that horrible spectacle, so much amazed, that they knew not what they did.* Blasius, a Christian, the reporter of the news, was so affrighted for his part, that, though it were two moneths after, he was scarce his own man, neither could he drive the remembrance of it out of his mind. Many times, some years following, they will tremble afresh at the [4] remembrance or conceit of such a terrible object; even all their lives long, if mention be made of it. Cornelius Agrippa relates (out of Gulielmus Parisiensis) a story of one, that, after a distasteful purge which a physician had prescribed unto him, was so much moved, [5] *that, at the very sight of physick, he would be distempered:* though he never so much as smelled to it, the box of physick long after would give him a purge; nay the very remembrance of it did

---

[1] Subitaneus terræ motus.   [2] Cœpit inde desipere cum dispendio sanitatis, inde adeo dementans, ut sibi ipsi mortem inferret.   [3] Historica relatio de rebus Japonicis, tract. 2. de legat. regis Chinensis, a Lodovico Frois Jesuitâ, A. 1596. Fuscini derepente tanta aëris caligo et terræ motus, ut multi capite dolerent, plurimis cor mœrore et melancholiâ obrueretur. Tantum fremitum edebat, ut tonitru fragorem imitari videretur, tantamque, &c. In urbe Sacai tam horrificus fuit, ut homines vix sui compotes essent, a sensibus abalienati, mœrore oppressi tam horrendo spectaculo, &c.   [4] Quum subit illius tristissima noctis imago.   [5] Qui solo aspectu medicinæ movebatur ad purgandum.

344   *Causes of Melancholy.*   [Part. 1. Sec. 2.

effect it; [1] *like travellers and seamen,* (saith Plutarch) *that, when they have been sanded, or dashed on a rock, for ever after fear not that mischance only, but all such dangers whatsoever.*

SUBSECT. IV.

Scoffs, Calumnies, bitter Jests, how they cause Melancholy.

IT is an old saying, [2] *a blow with a word strikes deeper than a blow with a sword:* and many men are as much gauled with a calumny, [3] a scurril and bitter jest, a libel, a pasquil, satyre, apologe, epigram, stage-playes, or the like, as with any misfortune whatsoever. Princes and potentates, that are otherwise happy, and have all at command, secure and free, *quibus potentia sceleris impunitatem fecit,* are grievously vexed with these pasquelling libells and satyrs: they fear a railing [4]Aretine, more than an enemy in the field: which made most princes of his time (as some relate) *allow him a liberal pension, that he should not tax them in his satyrs.* The gods had their Momus, Homer his Zoïlus, Achilles his Thersites, Philip his Demades: the Cæsars themselves in Rome were commonly taunted. There was never wanting a Petronius, a Lucian, in those times; nor will be a Rabelais, an Euphormio, a Boccalinus, in ours. Adrian the sixth, pope, [5] was so highly offended and grievously vexed with pasquils at Rome, he gave command that his statue should be demolished and burned, the ashes flung into the river Tiber, and had done it forthwith, had not Ludovicus Suessanus, a facete companion, disswaded him to the contrary, by telling him, that Pasquils ashes would turn to frogs in the bottom of the river, and croak worse and lowder than before. *Genus irritabile vatum;* and therefore [6]Socrates (in Plato) adviseth all his friends, *that respect their credits, to stand in awe of poets, for they are terrible fellows, can praise and dispraise, as they see cause.*

Hinc, quam sit calamus sævior ense, patet.

The prophet David complains (Psal. 123. 4) *that his soul was full of the mocking of the wealthy, and of the despitefulness of the proud; and* (Psal. 55. 4) *for the voice of the wicked,*

---

[1] Sicut viatores, si ad saxum impegerint, aut nautæ, memores sui casûs, non ista modo quæ offendunt, sed et similia, horrent perpetuo et tremunt.   [2] Leviter volant, graviter vulnerant. Bernardus.   [3] Ensis sauciat corpus, mentem sermo. [4] Sciatis eum esse qui a nemine fere ævi sui magnate non illustre stipendium habuit, ne mores ipsorum satyris suis notaret. Gasp. Barthius, præfat. parnodid. [5] Jovius, in vitâ ejus. Gravissime tulit famosis libellis nomen suum ad Pasquilli statuam fuisse laceratum; decrevitque ideo statuam demoliri, &c.   [6] Plato, lib. 13. de legibus. Qui existimationem curant, poëtas vereantur, quia magnam vim habent ad laudandum et vituperandum.

&c. and their hate, his heart trembled within him, and the terrors of death came upon him: fear and horrible fear, *&c.* and (Psal. 69. 20) *Rebuke hath broken my heart; and I am full of heaviness.* Who hath not like cause to complain, and is not so troubled, that shall fall into the mouths of such men? for many are of so [1] petulant a spleen, and have that figure *sarcasmus* so often in their mouths, so bitter, so foolish, (as [2] Balthasar Castilio notes of them) that *they cannot speak, but they must bite;* they had rather lose a friend than a jest: and what company soever they come in, they will be scoffing, insulting over their inferiours, especially over such as any way depend upon them, humoring, misusing, or putting gulleries on some or other, till they have made, by their humoring or gulling, [3] *ex stulto insanum,* a mope or a noddy, and all to make themselves merry:

---------------------------------[4]dummodo risum
Excutiat sibi, non hic cuiquam parcit amico:

friends, neuters, enemies, all are as one; to make a fool a madman, is their sport; and they have no greater felicity than to scoff and deride others; they must sacrifice to the god of laughter (with them in [5] Apuleius) once a day, or else they shall be melancholy themselves: they care not how they grinde and misuse others, so they may exhilarate their own persons. Their wits indeed serve them to that sole purpose, to make sport, to break a scurrile jest; which is *levissimus ingenii fructus,* the froth of wit (as [6] Tully holds); and for this they are often applauded. In all other discourse, dry, barren, stramineous, dull and heavy, here lyes their genius; in this they alone excell, please themselves and others. Leo Decimus, that scoffing pope, (as Jovius hath registred in the fourth book of his life) took an extraordinary delight in humoring of silly fellows, and to put gulleries upon them; [7] *by commending some, perswading others* to this or that, he made *ex stolidis stultissimos et maxime ridiculos, ex stultis insanos*—soft fellows, stark noddies; and such as were foolish, quite mad—before he left them. One memorable example he recites there, of Tarascomus of Parma, a musician, that was so humored by Leo Decimus, and Bibiena his second in this business, that he thought himself to be a man of most excellent skill, (who was indeed a ninny): they [8] *made him set foolish songs, and in-*

---

[1] Petulanti splene cachinno. [2] Curial. lib. 2. Ea quorumdam est inscitia, ut, quoties loqui, toties mordere licere sibi putent. [3] Ter. Eunuch. [4] Hor. Ser. l. 2. Sat. 4. [5] Lib. 2. [6] De orat. [7] Laudando, et mira iis persuadendo. [8] Et vanâ inflatus opinione, incredibilia ac ridenda quædam musices præcepta commentaretur, &c.

346   *Causes of Melancholy.*   [Part. 1. Sec. 2.

vent new ridiculous precepts, which they did highly commend, as
to tye his arm that played on the lute, to make him strike a
sweeter stroke, [1] *and to pull down the Arras hangings, because
the voice would be clearer, by reason of the reverberation of
the wall.* In the like manner they perswaded one Barabal-
lius of Caieta, that he was as good a poet as Petrarch; would
have him to be made a laureat poet, and invite all his friends to
his instalment; and had so possessed the poor man with a conceit of his excellent poetry, that, when some of his more discreet friends told him of his folly, he was very angry with
them, and said [2] *they envyed his honour and prosperity.* It was
strange (saith Jovius) to see an old man of sixty years, a vene-
rable and grave old man, so gulled. But what cannot such
scoffers do, especially if they find a soft creature, on whom they
may work? Nay, to say truth, who is so wise, or so discreet,
that may not be humored in this kind, especially if some excellent wits shall set upon him? He that mads others, if he were
so humored, would be as mad himself, as much grieved and
tormented; he might cry with him in the comedy, *Proh Jupiter!
tu homo me adigis ad insaniam :* for all is in these things as they
are taken : if he be a silly soul, and do not perceive it, 'tis well ;
he may happily make others sport, and be no whit troubled
himself : but if he be apprehensive of his folly, and take it to
heart, then it torments him worse than any lash. A bitter jest,
a slander, a calumny, pierceth deeper than any loss, danger,
bodily pain, or injury whatsoever; *leviter enim volat,* (as Bernard, of an arrow) *sed graviter vulnerat ;* especially, if it shall
proceed from a virulent tongue, it cuts (saith David) *like a two-
edged sword.   They shoot bitter words as arrows* (Psal. 64. 3) ;
and they smote with their tongues (Jer. 18. 18), and that so hard,
that they leave an incurable wound behind them. Many men
are undone by this means, moped, and so dejected, that they
are never to be recovered ; and, of all other men living, those
which are actually melancholy, or inclined to it, are most sensible, (as being suspicious, cholerick, apt to mistake) and impatient of an injury in that kind ; they aggravate, and so meditate continually of it, that it is a perpetual corrosive, not to
be removed, till time wear it out. Although they, peradventure, that so scoff, do it alone in mirth and merriment, and
hold it *optimum alienâ frui insaniâ,* an excellent thing to enjoy
another mans madness ; yet they must know that it is a mortal
sin, (as [3] Thomas holds), and (as the prophet [4] David denounceth)
they *that use it shall never dwell in Gods tabernacle.*

---

[1] Ut voces, nudis parietibus illisæ, suavius ac acutius resilirent.   [2] Immor-
talitati et gloriæ suæ prorsus invidentes.   [3] 2. 2dæ quæst. 75. Irrisio mortale
peccatum.   [4] Psal. 15. 3.

2

Such scurrile jests, flouts, and sarcasms, therefore, ought not at all to be used, especially to our betters, to those that are in misery, or any way distressed: for, to such, *ærumnarum incrementa sunt*, they multiply grief; and (as [1] he perceived) *in multis pudor, in multis iracundia, &c.* many are ashamed, many vexed, angred; and there is no greater cause or furtherer of melancholy. Martin Cromerus, in the sixth book of his history, hath a pretty story to this purpose, of Vladislaus the Second, king of Poland, and Peter Dunnius, earl of Shrine; they had been hunting late, and were enforced to lodge in a poor cottage. When they went to bed, Vladislaus told the earl in jest, that his wife lay softer with the abbot of Shrine: he, not able to contain, replyed, *Et tua cum Dabesso,* and yours with Dabessus, a gallant young gentleman in the court, whom Christina the queen loved. *Tetigit id dictum principis animum;* these words of his so galled the prince, that he was long after *tristis et cogitabundus,* very sad and melancholy for many moneths: but they were the earls utter undoing; for when Christina heard of it, she persecuted him to death. Sophia the empress, Justinians wife, broke a bitter jest upon Narses the eunuch, (a famous captain, then disquieted for an overthrow which he lately had) that he was fitter for a distaff, and keep women company, than to wield a sword, or to be general of an army: but it cost her dear; for he so far distasted it, that he went forthwith to the adverse part, much troubled in his thoughts, caused the Lumbards to rebell, and thence procured many miseries to the common-wealth. Tiberius the emperour withheld a legacy from the people of Rome, which his predecessor Augustus had lately given, and perceiving a fellow sound a dead coarse in the ear, would needs know wherefore he did so: the fellow replyed, that he wished the departed soul to signifie to Augustus, the commons of Rome were yet unpaid: for this bitter jest the emperour caused him forthwith to be slain, and carry the news himself. For this reason, all those that otherwise approve of jests in some cases, and facete companions, (as who doth not?) let them laugh and be merry, *rumpantur et ilia Codro;* 'tis laudable and fit; those yet will by no means admit them in their companies, that are any way inclined to this malady; *non jocandum cum iis qui miseri sunt et ærumnosi:* no jesting with a discontented person. 'Tis Castilios caveat, [2] Jo. Pontanus, and [3] Galateus, and every good mans:

> Play with me, but hurt me not;
> Jest with me, but shame me not.

Comitas is a vertue betwixt *rusticity* and *scurrility*, two extreams, as *affability* is betwixt *flattery* and *contention:* it must not ex-

---

[1] Balthasar Castilio, lib. 2. de aulico.   [2] De sermone, lib. 4. cap. 3.
[3] Fol. 55. Galateus.

348　　　　　*Causes of Melancholy.*　　　[Part. 1. Sec. 2.

ceed; but be still accompanied with that [1] αβλαβεια or inno-
cency, *quæ nemini nocet, omnem injuriæ oblationem abhorrens,*
hurts no man, abhors all offer of injury.　Though a man be
liable to such a jest or obloquy, have been overseen, or committed a foul fact, yet it is no good manners or humanity, to upbraid, to hit him in the teeth with his offence, or to scoff at such
a one; 'tis an old axiom, *turpis in reum omnis exprobratio.*　I
speak not of such as generally tax vice, Barclay, Gentilis, Erasmus, Agrippa, Fishcartus, &c. the Varronists and Lucians of
our time, satyrists, epigrammatists, comœdians, apologists, &c.
but such as personate, rail, scoff, calumniate, perstringe by
name, or in presence offend :

> [2] Ludit qui stolidâ procacitate,
> Non est Sestius ille, sed caballus;

'tis horse-play this; and those jests (as he [3] saith) *are no better
than injuries,* biting jests, *mordentes et aculeati;* they are poysoned jests, leave a sting behind them, and ought not to be
used.

> [4] Set not thy foot to make the blind to fall,
> Nor willfully offend thy weaker brother ;
> Nor wound the dead with thy tongues bitter gall ;
> Neither rejoice thou in the fall of other.

If these rules could be kept, we should have much more ease
and quietness than we have, less melancholy: whereas, on the
contrary, we study to misuse each other, how to sting and
gaul, like two fighting boars, bending all our force and wit,
friends, fortunes, to crucifie [5] one anothers souls; by means of
which, there is little content and charity, much virulency,
hatred, malice, and disquietness among us.

---

[1] Tully, Tusc. quæst.　　　[2] Mart. lib. 1. epig. 35.　　　[3] Tales joci ab in-
juriis non possint discerni.　Galateus, fo. 55.　　　[4] Pybrac, in his Quatrains,
37. [5] Ego hujus miserâ fatuitate et dementiâ conflictor. Tull. ad Attic. lib. 11.

SUBSECT. V.

Loss of Liberty, Servitude, Imprisonment, how they cause Melancholy.

To this catalogue of causes, I may well annex loss of liberty, servitude, or imprisonment, which to some persons is as great a torture as any of the rest. Though they have all things convenient, sumptuous houses to their use, fair walks and gardens, delicious bowers, galleries, good fare and dyet, and all things correspondent, yet they are not content, because they are confined, may not come and go at their pleasure; have and do what they will, but live [1] *aliená quadrá*, at another mans table and command. As it is [2] in meats, so is it in all other things, places, societies, sports; let them be never so pleasant, commodious, wholesom, so good; yet *omnium rerum est satietas* there is a lothing satiety of all things (the children of Israel were tired with *manna*): it is irksome to them so to live, as to a bird in a cage, or a dog in his kennel; they are weary of it. They are happy, it is true, and have all things (to another mans judgment) that heart can wish, or that they themselves can desire *bona si sua nórint*: yet they lothe it, and are tired with the present. *Est natura hominum novitatis avida;* mens nature is still desirous of news, variety, delights; and our wandering affections are so irregular in this kind, that they must change, though it be to the worst. Bachelors must be married, and married men would be bachelors; they do not love their own wives, though otherwise fair, wise, vertuous, and well qualified, because they are theirs: our present estate is still the worst; we cannot endure one course of life long (*et quod modo voverat, odit*), one calling long (*esse in honore juvat, mox displicet*), one place long,

[3] Romæ Tibur amo, ventosus, Tibure Romam:

that which we earnestly sought, we now contemn. *Hoc quosdam agit ad mortem* ([4] saith Seneca) *quod proposita sæpe mutando in eadem revolvuntur, et non relinquunt novitati locum. Fastidio cœpit esse vita, et ipse mundus; et subit illud rapidissimarum deliciarum, Quousque eadem?* this alone kills many a man, that they are tyed to the same still; as a horse in a mill, a dog in a wheel, they run round, without alteration or news; their life groweth odious, the world loathsome, and that which crosseth their furious delights, *What? still the same?* Marcus Aurelius and Solomon, that had experience of

---

[1] Miserum est alienâ vivere quadrâ. Juv.   [2] Crambe bis cocta.—Vitæ me redde priori.   [3] Hor.   [4] De tranquil. animæ.

350   *Causes of Melancholy.*   [Part. 1. Sec. 2.

all worldly delights and pleasure, confessed as much of themselves : what they most desired, was tedious at last, and that their lust could never be satisfied : all was vanity and affliction of mind.

Now, if it be death it self, another hell, to be glutted with one kind of sport, dieted with one dish, tyed to one place, though they have all things otherwise as they can desire, and are in heaven to another mans opinion—what misery and discontent shall they have, that live in slavery, or in prison itself? *Quod tristius morte, in servitute vivendum,* as Hermolaüs told Alexander in [1] Curtius ; worse than death is bondage : [2] *hoc animo scito omnes fortes, ut mortem servituti anteponant;* all brave men at arms (Tully holds) are so affected. [3] *Equidem ego is sum, qui servitutem extremum omnium malorum esse arbitror :* I am he (saith Boterus) that account servitude the extremity of misery. And what calamity do they endure, that live with those hard task-masters, in gold-mines (like those thirty thousand [4] Indian slaves at Potosa in Peru), tin-mines, lead-mines, stone-quarries, cole-pits, like so many mouldwarps under ground, condemned to the gallies, to perpetual drudgery, hunger, thirst, and stripes, without all hope of delivery? How are those women in Turkie affected, that most part of the year come not abroad; those Italian and Spanish dames that are mewed up like hawks, and lockt up by their jealous husbands? how tedious is it to them that live in stoves and caves half a year together? as in Island, Moscovy, or under the [5] pole it self, where they have six moneths perpetual night. Nay, what misery and discontent do they endure, that are in prison? They want all those six non-natural things at once, good air, good dyet, exercise, company, sleep, rest, ease, &c. that are bound in chains all day long, suffer hunger, and (as [6] Lucian describes it) *must abide that filthy stink, and ratling of chains, howlings, pitiful out-cryes, that prisoners usually make : these things are not only troublesome, but intolerable.* They lye nastily among toads and frogs in a dark dungeon, in their own dung, in pain of body, in pain of soul, as Joseph did (Psal. 105. 18, *They hurt his feet in the stocks; the iron entred his soul*): they live solitarily, alone, sequestred from all company but heart-eating melancholy : and, for want of meat, must eat that bread of affliction, prey upon themselves. Well might [7] Arculanus put long imprisonment for a cause, especially to such as, having lived jovially in all

---

[1] Lib. 8.   [2] Tullius Lepido, Fam. 10. 27.   [3] Boterus, l. 1. polit. cap. 4.
[4] Laet. descrip. Americæ.   [5] If there be any inhabitants.   [6] In Toxari.
Interdiu quidem collum vinctum est, et manus constricta ; noctu vero totum corpus vincitur : ad has miserias accedit corporis fœtor, strepitus ejulantium, somni brevitas : hæc omnia plane molesta et intolerabilia.   [7] In 9 Rhasis.

Mem. 4. Subs. 6.]   *Poverty and Want, Causes.*   351

sensuality and lust, upon a sudden are estranged and debarred
from all manner of pleasures ; as were Hunniades, Edward
and Richard the Second, Valerian the emperour, Bajazet the
Turk.   If it be irksome to miss our ordinary companions and
repast for once a day, or an hour, what shall it be to lose
them for ever? If it be so great a delight to live at liberty, and
to enjoy that variety of objects the world affords, what misery
and discontent must it needs bring to him, that shall be now
cast headlong into that Spanish inquisition, to fall from heaven to hell, to be cubbed up upon a sudden ? how shall he be
perplexed ? what shall become of him ? [1] Robert, duke of Normandy, being imprisoned by his youngest brother Henry the
First, *ab illo die inconsolabili dolore in carcere contabuit*
(saith Matthew Paris), from that day forward pined away with
grief.   [2] Jugurth, that generous captain, *brought to Rome in
triumph, and after imprisoned, through anguish of his soul,
and melancholy, dyed.*   [3] Roger, bishop of Salisbury, the second man from king Stephen, (he that built that famous castle of [4] Devises in Wiltshire) was so tortured in prison with
hunger, and all those calamities accompanying such men,
[5] *ut vivere noluerit, mori nescierit,* he would not live, and
could not dye, betwixt fear of death and torments of life.
Francis, king of France, was taken prisoner by Charles the
Fifth, *ad mortem fere melancholicus,* saith Guicciardine, melancholy almost to death, and that in an instant.   But this is
as clear as the sun, and needs no further illustration.

SUBSECT. VI.

Poverty and Want, Causes of Melancholy.

Poverty and want are so violent oppugners, so unwel-
come guests, so much abhorred of all men, that I may not
omit to speak of them apart.   Poverty, although (if considered aright, to a wise understanding, truly regenerate, and
contented man) it be *donum Dei,* a blessed estate, the way to
heaven (as [6] Chrysostome calls it), Gods gift, the mother of
modesty, and much to be preferred before riches, (as shall be
shewed in his [7] place), yet, as it is esteemed in the worlds censure, it is a most odious calling, vile and base, a severe torture,
summum scelus, a most intolerable burthen.   We [8] shun it all,

---

[1] William the Conquerors eldest son.   [2] Sallust. Romam triumpho ductus,
tandemque in carcerem conjectus, animi dolore periit.   [3] Camden. in Wiltsh.
Miserum senem ita fame et calamitatibus in carcere fregit, inter mortis metum et
vitæ tormenta, &c.   [4] Vies hodie.   [5] Seneca.   [6] Com. ad Hebræos.
[7] Part. 2. sect. 3. memb. 3.   [8] Quem, ut difficilem morbum, pueris tradere
formidamus. Plut.

352   *Causes of Melancholy.*   [Part. 1. Sec. 2.

cane pejus et angue : we abhor the name of it,

   ([1] Paupertas fugitur : totoque arcessitur orbe . . . . .)

as being the fountain of all other miseries, cares, woes, labours
and grievances whatsoever. To avoid which, we will take any
pains;

   (————extremos currit mercator ad Indos)

we will leave no haven, no coast, no creek of the world un-
searched, though it be to the hazard of our lives; we will dive
to the bottom of the sea, and to the bowels of the earth, [2] five,
six, seven, eight, nine hundred fathom deep, through all the
five zones, and both extreams of heat and cold : we will turn
parasites and slaves, prostitute ourselves, swear and lye, damn
our bodies and souls, forsake God, abjure religion, steal, rob,
murder, rather than endure this unsufferable yoke of poverty,
which doth so tyrannize, crucifie, and generally depress us.

   For, look into the world, and you shall see men, most part,
esteemed according to their means, and happy as they are
rich : [3] *ubique tanti quisque, quantum habuit, fuit.* If he be
likely to thrive, and in the way of preferment, who but he?
In the vulgar opinion, if a man be wealthy, no matter how he
gets it, of what parentage, how qualified, how vertuously endowed, or villanously inclined; let him be a bawd, a gripe,
an usurer, a villain, a pagan, a barbarian, a wretch, [4] Lucians
tyrant *on whom you may look with less security, than on the
sun*—so that he be rich (and liberal withall) he shall be honoured, admired, adored, reverenced, and highly [5] magnified.
The rich is had in reputation, because of his goods (Eccles.
10. 31) : he shall be befriended: *for riches gather many
friends (Prov.* 19. 4) :——*multos numerabit amicos ;* all
[6] happiness ebbs and flows with his money. He shall be accounted a gracious lord, a Mæcenas, a benefactor, a wise,
discreet, a proper, a valiant, a fortunate man, of a generous
spirit, *pullus Jovis, et gallinæ filius albæ,* a hopeful, a good
man, a vertuous honest man. *Quando ego te Junonium
puerum, et matris partum vere aureum,* as [7] Tully said of
Octavianus, while he was adopted Cæsar, and an [8] heir apparent of so great a monarchy; he was a golden child. All
[9] honour, offices, applause, grand titles, and turgent epithets,
are put upon him; *omnes omnia bona dicere ;* all mens eyes

---

[1] Lucan. l. 1.   [2] As in the silver mines in Friburgh in Germany. Fines
Morison.   [3] Euripides.   [4] Tom. 4. dial.   Minore periculo solem quam
hunc defixis oculis licet intueri.   [5] Omnis enim res, Virtus, fama, decus, divina
humanaque, pulchris Divitiis parent. Hor. Ser. l. 2. Sat. 3. Clarus erit, fortis, justus, sapiens, etiam rex, Et quidquid volet. Hor.   [6] Et genus, et formam, regina Pecunia donat.   Money adds spirits, courage, &c.   [7] Epist. ult. ad Atticum.   [8] Our young master, a fine towardly gentlemen, (God bless him !)
and hopeful.   Why ? he is heir apparent to the right worshipful, to the right
honourable, &c.   [9] O nummi, nummi ! vobis hunc præstat honorem.

are upon him, "God bless his good worship! his honour!"
[1] every man speaks well of him; every man presents him, seeks
and sues to him for his love, favour, and protection, to serve
him, belong unto him; every man riseth to him, as to Themistocles in the Olympicks; if he speak, (as of Herod) *vox Dei*,
non hominis! the voice of God, not of man! All the graces,
Veneres, pleasures, elegances attend him: [2] golden Fortune
accompanies and lodgeth with him, and (as to those Roman
emperours) is placed in his chamber.

> ———[3] Securâ naviget aurâ,
> Fortunamque suo temperet arbitrio:

he may sail as he will himself, and temper his estate at his
pleasure: jovial days, splendor and magnificence, sweet musick, dainty fare, the good things and fat of the land, fine
clothes, rich attires, soft beds, down pillows, are at his command; all the world labours for him; thousands of artificers
are his slaves, to drudge for him, run, ride, and post for him:
[4] divines (for *Pythia philippizat*), lawyers, physicians, philosophers, scholars, are his, wholly devote to his service. Every
man seeks his acquaintance, his kindred, to match with him:
[5] though he be an aufe, a ninny, a monster, a goos-cap, *uxorem
ducat Danaën*, when and whom he will; *hunc optant generum
rex et regina*—he is an excellent [6] match for my son, my
daughter, my niece, &c. *Quidquid calcaverit hic, rosa fiet;*
let him go whither he will, trumpets sound, bells ring, &c. all
happiness attends him; every man is willing to entertain him;
he sups in [7] Apollo wheresoever he comes: what preparation
is made for his [8] entertainment! fish and fowl, spices and perfumes, all that sea and land affords. What cookery, masking,
mirth, to exhilarate his person!

> [9] Da Trebio; pone ad Trebium; vis, frater, ab illis
> Ilibus?———

What dish will your good worship eat of?

> ———————[10] dulcia poma,
> Et quoscunque feret cultus tibi fundus honores,
> Ante Larem gustet venerabilior Lare dives.

> Sweet apples, and what e'er thy fields afford,
> Before the Gods be serv'd, let serve thy Lord.

---

[1] Exinde sapere eum omnes dicimus, ac quisque fortunam habet. Plaut. Pseud.
[2] Aurea Fortuna principum cubiculis reponi solita. Julius Capitolinus, vitâ Anto-
nini.　　[3] Petronius.　　[4] Theologi opulentis adhærent, jurisperiti pecuniosis,
literati numinosis, liberalibus artifices.　　[5] Multi illum juvenes, multæ petiere
puellæ.　　[6] Dummodo sit dives, barbarus ille placet.　　[7] Plut. in Lucullo.
A rich chamber so called.　　[8] Panis pane melior.　　[9] Juv. Sat. 5.　　[10] Hor.
Sat. 5. lib. 2.

VOL. 1.　　　　　　　　　A a

354   *Causes of Melancholy.*   [Part. 1. Sec. 2.

What sport will your honour have? hawking, hunting, fishing, fowling, bulls, bears, cards, dice, cocks, players, tumblers, fidlers, jesters, &c. they are at your good worships command. Fair houses, gardens, orchards, tarrasses, galleries, cabinets, pleasant walks, delightsom places, they are at hand; [1] *in
aureis lac, vinum in argenteis, adolescentulæ ad nutum speci-
osæ,* wine, wenches, &c. a Turkie paradise, an heaven upon earth.
Though he be a silly soft fellow, and scarce have common sense,
yet if he be born to fortunes, (as I have said) [2] *jure hæreditario sapere jubetur,* he must have honour and office in his
course; [3] *nemo, nisi dives, honore dignus* (Ambros. *offic.* 21);
none so worthy as himself: he shall have it; *atque esto quidquid Servius aut Labeo.* Get money enough, and command
[4] kingdoms, provinces, armies, hearts, hands, and affections;
thou shalt have popes, patriarks, to be thy chaplains and parasites; thou shalt have (Tamberlain-like) kings to draw thy
coach, queens to be thy landresses, emperours thy foot stools,
build more towns and cities than great Alexander, Babel
towers, pyramids, and Mausolean tombs, &c. command heaven and earth, and tell the world it is thy vassal; *auro emitur
diadema, argento cœlum panditur, denarius philosophum conducit, nummus jus cogit, obolus literatum pascit, metallum
sanitatem conciliat, æs amicos conglutinat.* And therefore,
not without good cause, John Medices, that rich Florentine,
when he lay upon his death-bed, calling his sons Cosmus
and Laurence before him, amongst other sober sayings, repeated
this, *Animo quieto digredior, quod vos sanos et divites post
me relinquam;* it doth me good to think yet, though I be
dying, that I shall leave you, my children, *sound and rich:*
for wealth sways all. It is not with us, as amongst those
Lacedæmonian senators of Lycurgus in Plutarch—*he preferred,
that deserved best, was most virtuous and worthy of the place;*
[5] *not swiftness, or strength, or wealth, or friends, carryed it
in those dayes;* but *inter optimos optimus, inter temperantes
temperantissimus,* the most temperate and best. We have no
aristocracies but in contemplation, all *oligarchies* wherein a
few rich men domineer, do what they list, and are privi-
leged by their greatness. [6] They may freely trespass, and do
as they please; no man dare accuse them, no not so much
as mutter against them; there is no notice taken of it; they
may securely do it, live after their own laws, and, for their mo-

---

[1] Bohemus, de Turcis; et Bredenbach.   [2] Euphormio.   [3] Qui
pecuniam habent, elati sunt animis, lofty spirits, brave men at arms: all rich men
are generous, couragious, &c.   [4] Nummus ait, Pro me nubat Cornubia
Romæ.   [5] Non fuit apud mortales ullum excellentius certamen; non
inter celeres celerrimo, non inter robustos robustissimo, &c.   [6] Quidquid
libet licet.

ney, get pardons, indulgencies, redeem their souls from purgatory and hell it self,—*clausum possidet arca Jovem.* Let them be Epicures, or atheists, libertines, Machiavelians, (as often they are)

> [1] Et quamvis perjurus erit, sine gente, cruentus,

they may go to heaven through the eye of a needle; if they will themselves, they may be canonized for saints, they shall be [2] honourably interred in Mausolean tombs, commended by poets, registered in histories, have temples and statues erected to their names——*e manibus illis nascentur violæ.*——If he be bountiful in his life, and liberal at his death, he shall have one to swear (as he did by Claudius emperour in Tacitus), he saw his soul go to the heaven, and be miserably lamented at his funeral. *Ambubaiarum collegia, &c.* Trimalchionis Topanta, in Petronius, *rectâ in cœlum abiit*, went right to heaven; (a base queen; [3] *thou wouldst have scorned once in thy misery to have a penny from her*) and why? *modo nummos metiit*, she measured her money by the bushel. These prerogatives do not usually belong to rich men, but to such as are most part seeming rich; let him have but a good [4] outside, he carries it, and shall be adored for a God, as [5] Cyrus was amongst the Persians, *ob splendidum apparatum*, for his gay tyres. Now most men are esteemed according to their cloaths: in our gullish times, whom you peradventure in modesty would give place to, as being deceived by his habit, and presuming him some great worshipful man, believe it, if you shall examine his estate, he will likely be proved a serving man of no great note, my ladies taylor, his lordships barber, or some such gull, a Fastidius Brisk, Sir Petronell Flash, a meer out-side. Only this respect is given him, that wheresoever he comes, he may call for what he will, and take place by reason of his outward habit.

But on the contrary, if he be poor, (*Prov.* 15. 15) *all his dayes are miserable;* he is under hatches, dejected, rejected, and forsaken, poor in purse, poor in spirit: [6] *prout res nobis fluit, ita et animus se habet;* [7] money gives life and soul. Though he be honest, wise, learned, well deserving, noble by birth, and of excellent good parts; yet, in that he is poor, unlikely to rise, come to honour, office, or good means, he is contemned, neglected; *frustra sapit, inter literas esurit, amicus*

---

[1] Hor. Sat. 5. lib. 2.   [2] Cum moritur dives, concurrunt undique cives : Pauperis ad funus vix est ex millibus unus.   [3] Et modo quid fuit? ignoscat mihi genius tuus! noluisses de manu ejus nummos accipere.   [4] He that wears silk, sattin, velvet, and gold lace, must needs be a gentleman.   [5] Est sanguis atque spiritus pecunia mortalibus.   [6] Euripides.   [7] Xenophon, Cyropæd. l. 8.

356   *Causes of Melancholy.*   [Part. 1. Sec. 2.

molestus. [1] *If he speak, what babler is this?* (Ecclus.) his nobility without wealth his [2] *projectâ vilior algâ*, and he not esteemed.

Nos viles pulli, nati infelicibus ovis ;

if once poor, we are metamorphosed in an instant, base slaves, villains, and vile drudges; [3] for to be poor, is to be a knave, a fool, a wretch, a wicked, an odious fellow, a common eye-sore: say poor, and say all : they are born to labour, to misery, to carry burdens like juments, *pistum stercus comedere*, with Ulysses companions, and (as Chremylus objected in Aristophanes) [4] *salem lingere*, lick salt, to empty jakes, fay channels, [5] carry out dirt and dunghils, sweep chimneys, rub horse-heels, &c. I say nothing of Turks galley-slaves, which are bought [6] and sold like juments, or those African negroes, or poor [7] Indian drudges, *qui indies hinc inde deferendis oneribus occumbunt ; nam quod apud nos boves et asini vehunt, trahunt, &c. id omne misellis Indis, &c.* they are ugly to behold, and, though earst spruce, now rusty and squalid, because poor: [8] *immundas fortunas æquum est squalorem sequi ;* it is ordinarily so. [9] *Others eat to live, but they live to drudge;* [10] *servilis et misera gens nihil recusare audet ;* a servile generation, that dare refuse no task.

———————————[11] Heus tu, Dore,
Cape hoc flabellum, ventulum huic facito, dum lavamus,

sirrah, blow wind upon us while we wash; and bid your fellow get him up betimes in the morning; be it fair or foul, he shall run fifty miles a foot to morrow, to carry me a letter to my mistress: *Sosia ad pistrinam ;* Sosia shall tarry at home, and grind mault all day long; Tristan thresh. Thus are they commanded, being indeed, some of them, as so many foot-stools for rich men to tread on, blocks for them to get on horseback, or as [12] *walls for them to piss on.* They are commonly such people, rude, silly, superstitious ideots, nasty, unclean, lowsie, poor, dejected, slavishly humble ; and as [13] Leo Afer observes of the commonalty of Africk, *naturâ viliores sunt, nec apud suos duces majore in pretio quam si canes essent:* base by nature, and no more esteemed than dogs; [14] *miseram, laboriosam, calamitosam vitam agunt, et inopem, infelicem ;*

---

[1] In tenui rara est facundia panno. Juv.   [2] Hor.   [3] Egere est offendere ; et indigere scelestum esse. Sat. Menip.   [4] Plaut. act. 4. [5] Nullum tam barbarum, tam vile munus est, quod non lubentissime obire velit gens vilissima.   [6] Lausius, orat. in Hispaniam.   [7] Laet. descrip. Americæ.   [8] Plautus.   [9] Leo Afer, ca. ult. l. 1. Edunt, non ut bene vivant, sed ut fortiter laborent. Heinsius.   [10] Munster de rusticis Germaniæ, Cosmog. cap. 27. lib. 3.   [11] Ter. Eunuch.   [12] Pauper paries factus, quem caniculæ commingant.   [13] Lib. 1. cap. ult.   [14] Deos omnes illis infensos diceres; tam pannosi, fame fracti, tot assidue malis afficiuntur, tamquam pecora quibus splendor rationis emortuus.

rudiores asinis, ut e brutis plane natos dicas : no learning, no knowledge, no civility, scarce common sense, nought but barbarism amongst them; *belluino more vivunt, neque calceos gestant, neque vestes;* like rogues and vagabonds, they go bare-footed and bare-legged, the soals of their feet being as hard as horse hoofs, (as [1] Radzivilius observed at Damiata in Egypt) leading a laborious, miserable, wretched, unhappy life, [2] *like beasts and juments, if not worse* (for a [3] Spaniard in Iucatan sold three Indian boyes for a cheese, and an hundred negro slaves for an horse): their discourse is scurrility, their *summum bonum* a pot of ale. There is not any slavery which these villains will not undergo: *inter illos plerique latrinas evacuant: alii culinariam curant; alii stabularios agunt, urinatores; et id genus similia exercent, &c.* like those people that dwell in the [4] Alps, chimney-sweepers, jakes-farmers, dirt-daubers, vagrant rogues, they labour hard some, and yet cannot get clothes to put on, or bread to eat: for what can filthy poverty give else, but [5] beggery, fulsome nastiness, squalor, contempt, drudgery, labour, ugliness, hunger and thirst, *pediculorum et pulicum numerum* (as [6] he well followed it in Aristophanes) fleas and lice? *pro pallio vestem laceram, et pro pulvinari lapidem bene magnum ad caput,* rags for his rayment, and a stone for his pillow, *pro cathedrâ, ruptæ caput urnæ,* he sits in a broken pitcher, or on a block, for a chair, *et malvæ ramos pro panibus comedit,* he drinks water, and lives on wort leaves, pulse, like a hogg, or scraps like a dog: *ut nunc nobis vita afficitur, quis non putabit insaniam esse, infelicitatemque?* (as Chremylus concludes his speech) as we poor men live now adayes, who will not take our life to be [7] infelicity, misery, and madness?

If they be of little better condition than those base villains, hunger-starved beggars, wandring rogues, those ordinary slaves, and day-labouring drudges, yet they are commonly so preyed upon by [8] poling officers for breaking laws, by their tyrannizing landlords, so flead and fleeced by perpetual [9] exactions, that though they do drudge, fare hard, and starve their Genius, they cannot live in some [10] countries: but what they have is instantly taken from them; the very care they take to live, to be drudges, to maintain their poor families, their trouble and anxiety, *takes*

---

[1] Peregrin. Hieros.   [2] Nihil omnino meliorem vitam degunt, quam feræ in silvis, jumenta in terris. Leo Afer.   [3] Bartholomæus a Casa.   [4] Ortelius, in Helvetiâ. Qui habitant in Cæsiâ valle ut plurimum latomi, in Oscellâ valle cultrorum fabri, fumarii in Vigetiâ, sordidum genus hominum, quod repurgandis caminis victum parat.   [5] I write not this, any wayes to upbraid, or scoffe at, or misuse poor men, but rather to condole and pity them, by expressing, &c.   [6] Chremylus, act. 4. Plut.   [7] Paupertas durum onus miseris mortalibus.   [8] Vexat censura columbas.   [9] *Deux ace* non possunt, et *six cinque* solvere nolunt: Omnibus est notum *quatre tre* solvere totum. [10] Scandia, Africa, Lituania.

358   *Causes of Melancholy.*   [Part. 1. Sec. 2.

away their sleep (*Sirac.* 31. 1); it makes them weary of their lives: when they have taken all pains, done their utmost and honest endeavours, if they be cast behind by sickness, or overtaken with years, no man pities them; hard-hearted, and merciless, uncharitable as they are, they leave them so distressed, to beg, steal, murmur, and [1] rebel, or else starve. The feeling and fear of this misery compelled those old Romans, whom Menenius Agrippa pacified, to resist their governours—outlaws, and rebels in most places, to take up seditious armes; and in all ages hath caused uproars, murmurings, seditions, rebellions, thefts, murders, mutinies, jarrs and contentions in every commonwealth, grudging, repining, complaining, discontent in each private family, because they want means to live according to their callings, bring up their children; it breaks their hearts, they cannot do as they would. No greater misery than for a lord to have a knights living, a gentleman a yeomans, not to be able to live as his birth and place requires. Poverty and want are generally corrosive to all kinds of men, especially to such as have been in good and flourishing estate, are suddenly distressed, [2] nobly born, liberally brought up, and, by some disaster, and casualty, miserably dejected. For the rest, as they have base fortunes, so they have base minds correspondent—like beetles, *e stercore orti, e stercore victus, in stercore delicium*—as they were obscurely born and bred, so they delight and live in obscenity; they are not so thoroughly touched with it.

> Angustas animas angusto in pectore versant.

Yea (that which is no small cause of their torments) if once they come to be in distress, they are forsaken of their fellows, most part neglected, and left unto themselves; as poor [3] Terence in Rome was by Scipio, Lælius, and Furius, his great and noble friends,

> ————————Nihil Publius
> Scipio profuit, nil ei Lælius, nil Furius,
> Tres per idem tempus qui agitabant nobiles facillime.
> Horum ille operâ ne domum quidem habuit conductitiam.

'Tis generally so:

> Tempora si fuerint nubila, solus eris;

he is left cold and comfortless;

> Nullus ad amissas ibit amicus opes;

all flee from him, as from a rotten wall, now ready to fall on

---

[1] Montaigne, in his Essayes, speaks of certain Indians in France, that being asked how they liked the countrey, wondered how a few rich men could keep so many poor men in subjection, that they did not cut their throats.   [2] Angustas animas animoso in pectore versans.   [3] Donatus, vit. ejus.

their heads. Prov. 19. 4. *Poverty separates them from their* [1] *neighbours.*

[2] Dum fortuna favet, vultum servatis, amici:
Cum cecidit, turpi vertitis ora fugâ.

Whil'st fortune favour'd, friends, you smil'd on me :
But, when she fled, a friend I could not see.

Which is worse yet, if he be poor, [3] every man contemns him, insults over him, oppresseth him, scoffs at, aggravates his misery.

[4] Quum cœpit quassata domus subsidere, partes
In proclinatas omne recumbit onus.

When once the tottering house begins to shrink,
Thither comes all the weight by an instinct.

Nay, they are odious to their own brethren, and dearest friends : (Prov. 19. 7.) *his brethren hate him, if he be poor:* [5] *omnes vicini oderunt,* his neighbours hate him (Prov. 14. 20) : [6] *omnes me noti ac ignoti deserunt,* (as he complained in the comedy) friends and strangers all forsake me. Which is most grievous, poverty makes men ridiculous :

Nil habet infelix paupertas durius in se,
Quam quod ridiculos homines facit :

they must endure [7] jests, taunts, flouts, blows of their betters, and take all in good part to get a meals meat :

[8] Magnum pauperies opprobrium jubet
Quidvis et facere et pati.

He must turn parasite, jester, fool, (*cum desipientibus desipere,* saith [9] Euripides), slave, villain, drudge, to get a poor living, apply himself to each mans humours, to win and please, &c. and be buffeted, when he hath all done (as Ulysses was by Melanthius [10] in Homer), be reviled, baffled, insulted over, for [11] *potentiorum stultitia perferenda est,* and may not so much as mutter against it. He must turn rogue and villain; for, as the saying is, *necessitas cogit ad turpia:* poverty alone makes men thieves, rebels, murderers, tratours, assassinates, (*because of poverty, we have sinned, Ecclus.* 27. 1.) swear and forswear, bear false witness, lye, dissemble, any thing, as I say, to advantage themselves, and to relieve their necessites : [12] *culpæ scelerisque magistra est:* when a man is driven to his shifts, what will he not do ?

————si miserum fortuna Sinonem
Finxit, vanum etiam mendacemque improba finget :

---

[1] Prov. 19. 7. Though he be instant, yet they will not.   [2] Petronius.
[3] Non est, qui doleat vicem : ut Petrus Christum, jurant se hominem non novisse.
[4] Ovid. in Trist.   [5] Horat.   [6] Ter. Eunuchus, act. 2.   [7] Quid quod materiam præbet caussamque jocandi, Si toga sordida sit ? Juv. Sat. 2.   [8] Hor.
[9] In Phœnis.   [10] Odyss. 17.   [11] Idem.   [12] Mantuan.

360 *Causes of Melancholy.* [Part. 1. Sec. 2.

he will betray his father, prince and countrey, turn Turk, forsake religion, abjure God and all: *nulla tam horrenda proditio, quam illi lucri caussâ* (saith [1] Leo Afer) *perpetrare nolint.*
[2] Plato therefore calls poverty *thievish, sacrilegious, filthy, wicked, and mischievous;* and well he might; for it makes many an upright man otherwise (had he not been in want) to take bribes, to be corrupt, to do against his conscience, to sell his tongue, heart, hand, &c. to be churlish, hard, unmerciful, uncivil, to use indirect means to help his present estate. It makes princes to exact upon their subjects, great men tyrannize, landlords oppress, justice mercenary, lawyers vultures, physicians harpyes, friends importunate, tradesmen lyars, honest men thieves, devout assassinates, great men to prostitute their wives, daughters, and themselves, middle sort to repine, commons to mutiny, all to grudge, murmur, and complain. A great temptation to all mischief, it compels some miserable wretches to counterfeit several diseases, to dismember, make themselves blind, lame, to have a more plausible cause to beg, and lose their limbs to recover their present wants. Jodocus Damhoderius, a lawyer of Bruges, (*praxi rerum criminal. c.* 112) hath some notable examples of such counterfeit cranks; and every village almost will yield abundant testimonies amongst us; we have dummerers, Abraham men, &c. And (that which is the extent of misery) it enforceth them, through anguish and wearisomness of their lives, to make away themselves: they had rather be hanged, drowned, &c. than to live without means.

[3] In mare cetiferum, ne te premat aspera egestas,
Desili, et a celsis corrue, Cyrne, jugis.

Much better 'tis to break thy neck,
Or drown thy self i'th' sea,
Than suffer irksome poverty :—
Go make thy self away.

A Sybarite of old (as I find it registred in [4] Athenæus), supping *in Phiditiis* in Sparta, and observing their hard fare, said it was no marvel if 'the Lacedæmonians were valiant men; *for his part he would rather run upon a swords point (and so would any man in his wits), than live with such base diet, or lead so wretched a life.* [5] In Japonia, 'tis a common thing to stifle their children if they be poor, or to make an abort; which

---

[1] De Africâ, lib. 1. cap. ult.   [2] 4. de legibus. Furacissima paupertas, sacrilega, turpis, flagitiosa, omnium malorum opifex.   [3] Theognis.
[4] Dipnosophist. lib. 12. Millies potius moriturum (si quis sibi mente constaret) quam tam vilis et ærumnosi victûs communionem habere.   [5] Gasper Vilela Jesuita, epist. Japon. lib.

Aristotle commends. In that civil commonwealth of China, [1] the mother strangles her child, if she be not able to bring it up, and had rather lose than sell it, or have it endure such misery as poor men do. Arnobius (*lib. 7. adversus gentes*), [2] Lactantius (*lib. 5. cap. 9*), objects as much to those ancient Greeks and Romans: *they did expose their children to wild beasts, strangle, or knock out their brains against a stone*, in such cases. If we may give credit to [3] Munster, amongst us Christians, in Lituania they voluntarily mancipate and sell themselves, their wives, and children, to rich men, to avoid hunger and beggery: [4] many make away themselves in this extremity. Apicius, the Roman, when he cast up his accounts, and found but 100,000 crowns left, murdered himself, for fear he should be famished to death. P. Forestus, in his medicinal observations, hath a memorable example of two brothers of Lovain, that, being destitute of means, became both melancholy, and, in a discontented humour, massacred themselves; another of a merchant, learned, wise otherwise and discreet, but, out of a deep apprehension he had of loss at seas, would not be per-swaded but (as [5] Ventidius, in the poet) he should die a begger. In a word, thus much I may conclude of poor men, that, though they have good [6] parts, they cannot shew or make use of them: [7] *ab inopiâ ad virtutem obsepta est via:* 'tis hard for a poor man to [8] rise;

> Haud facile emergunt, quorum virtutibus obstat
> Res angusta domi:

the wisdom of the poor is despised, and his words are not heard. (Eccles. 6. 19): his works are rejected, contemned for the base-ness and obscurity of the author; though laudable and good in themselves, they will not likely take.

> Nulla placere diu, neque vivere, carmina possunt,
> Quæ scribuntur aquæ potoribus.

Poor men cannot please: their actions, counsels, consultations, projects, are vilified in the worlds esteem: *amittunt consilium in re*, which Gnatho long since observed. [9] *Sapiens crepidas sibi nunquam, Nec soleas, fecit:* a wise man never cobled shoes; as he said of old; but how doth he prove it? I am sure we find it otherwise in our dayes; [10] *pruinosis horret facundia pannis.* Homer himself must beg, if he want means, and (as

---

[1] Mat Riccius, expedit. in Sinas, lib. 1. c. 3.   [2] Vos Romani procreatos filios feris et canibus exponitis, nunc strangulatis, vel in saxum eliditis, &c. [3] Cosmog. 4. lib. cap. 22. Vendunt liberos victu carentes, tamquam pecora, inter-dum et seipsos, ut apud divites saturentur cibis.   [4] Vel bonorum despera-tione vel malorum perpessione fracti et fatigati, plures violentas manus sibi infe-runt.   [5] Hor.   [6] Ingenio poteram superas volitare per arces: Ut me pluma levat, sic grave mergit onus.   [7] Terent.   [8] Juvenal. Sat. 3. [9] Hor. Sat. 3. lib. 1.   [10] Petronius.

362   *Causes of Melancholy.*   [Part. 1. Sec. 2.

by report, sometimes he did) [1] *go from door to door, and sing
ballads, with a company of boyes about him.* This common
misery of theirs must needs distract, make them discontent and
melancholy, as ordinarily they are, wayward, pievish, like a
weary travailer, (for

> [2] Fames et mora bilem in nares conciunt)

still murmuring and repining. *Ob inopiam morosi sunt, quibus
est male,* as Plutarch quotes out of Euripides, and that comical
poet well seconds—

> [3] Omnes, quibus res sunt minus secundæ, nescio quomodo
> Suspiciosi, ad contumeliam omnia accipiunt magis;
> Propter suam impotentiam se credunt negligi:

if they be in adversity, they are more suspicious and apt to mistake; they think themselves scorned by reason of their misery;
and therefore many generous spirits, in such cases, withdraw
themselves from all company, as that comedian [4] Terence is said
to have done; when he perceived himself to be forsaken and
poor, he voluntarily banished himself to Stymphalus, a base
town in Arcadia, and there miserably dyed:

> —— ad summam inopiam redactus:
> Itaque e conspectu omnium abiit, Græciæ in terram ultimam.

Neither is it without cause; for we see men commonly respected according to their means, (*[5] an dives sit, omnes quærunt;
nemo, an bonus*) and vilified if they be in bad clothes. [6] Philo-
pœmen the orator was set to cut wood, because he was so
homely attired. [7] Terentius was placed at the lower end of
Cæcilius table, because of his homely outside. [8] Dante, that
famous Italian poet, by reason his clothes were but mean, could
not be admitted to sit down at a feast. Gnatho scorned his
old familiar friend, because of his apparel; [9] *hominem video
pannis annisque obsitum; hic ego illum contempsi præ me.*
King Perseus, overcome, sent a letter to [10] Paullus Æmilius
the Roman general, "*Perseus P. Consuli S.*" but he scorned
him any answer, *tacite exprobrans fortunam suam* (saith mine
author), upbraiding him with a present fortune. [11] Carolus
Pugnax, that great duke of Burgundy, made H. Holland, late
duke of Exeter, exil'd, run after his horse like a lacky, and

---

[1] Herodotus, vitâ ejus. Scaliger, in poët. Potentiorum ædes ostiatim adiens,
aliquid accipiebat, canens carmina sua, concomitante eum puerorum choro.
[2] Plautus, Amph.   [3] Ter. Act. 4. Scen. 3. Adelph. Hegio.   [4] Donat.
vitâ ejus.   [5] Euripides.   [6] Plutarch. vitâ ejus.   [7] Vit. Ter.
[8] Gomesius, lib. 3. c. 21. de sale.   [9] Ter. Eunuch. Act. 2. Scen. 2.   [10] Liv.
dec. 9. l. 2.   [11] Comineus.

Mem. 4. Subs. 7.] *Other Accidents and Grievances.* 363

would take no notice of him: [1] 'tis the common fashion of the world : so that such men as are poor may justly be discontent, melancholy, and complain of their present misery; and all may pray with [2] Solomon, *Give me, O Lord, neither riches nor poverty ; feed me with food convenient for me.*

SUBSECT. VII.

An heap of other Accidents causing Melancholy, Death of Friends, Losses, &c.

In this labyrinth of accidental causes, the farther I wander, the more intricate I find the passage; *multæ ambages :* and new causes, as so many by-paths, offer themselves to be discussed. To search out all, were an Herculean work, and fitter for Theseus: I will follow mine intended thred, and point only at some few of the chiefest ;

Death of friends.] amongst which, loss and death of friends may challenge a first place. *Multi tristantur* (as [3] Vives well observes) *post delicias, convivia, dies festos ;* many are melancholy after a feast, holy-day, merry-meeting, or some pleasing sport, if they be solitary by chance, left alone to themselves, without employment, sport, or want their ordinary companions; some, at the departure of friends only whom they shall shortly see again, weep and howl, and look after them as a cow lows after her calf, or a child takes on, that goes to school after holidayes. *Ut me levârat tuus adventus, sic discessus afflixit,* (which [4] Tully writ to Atticus) thy coming was not so welcome to me as thy departure was harsh. Montanus (*consil.* 132) makes mention of a countrey-woman, that, parting with her friends and native place, became grievously melancholy for many years ; and Trallianus, of another, so caused for the absence of her husband; which is an ordinary passion amongst our good wives; if their husband tarry out a day longer than his appointed time, or break his hour, they take on presently with sighs and tears ; " he is either robbed or dead ; some mischance or other is surely befaln him :" they cannot eat, drink, sleep, or be quiet in mind, till they see him again. If parting of friends, absence alone, can work such violent effects, what shall death do, when they must eternally be separated, never in this world to meet again? This is so grievous a torment for the time, that it takes away their appetite, desire of life,

---

[1] He that hath 5*l.* per annum coming in more than others, scorns him that hath less, and is a better man.   [2] Prov. 30. 8.   [3] De animâ, cap. de mœrore.
[4] Lib. 12. epist.

364 *Causes of Melancholy.* [Part. 1. Sec. 2.

extinguisheth all delights, it causeth deep sighs and groans,
tears, exclamations,

(O dulce germen matris ! o sanguis meus !
Eheu ; tepentes, &c.———o flos tener !)

howling, roaring, many bitter pangs,

[1] (Lamentis gemituque et femineo ululatu.
Tecta fremunt)

and by frequent meditation extends so far sometimes, [2] *they
think they see their dead friends continually in their eyes, ob-
versantes imagines*, as Conciliator confesseth he saw his mothers
ghost presenting herself still before him. *Quod nimis miseri
volunt, hoc facile credunt;* still, still, still, that good father, that
good son, that good wife, that dear friend, runs in their minds :
totus animus hac unâ cogitatione defixus est, all the year long
as [3] Pliny complains to Romanus, *methinks I see Virginius,
I hear Virginius, I talk with Virginius, &c.*

[4] Te sine, væ misero mihi, lilia nigra videntur,
Pallentesque rosæ, nec dulce rubens hyacinthus ;
Nullos nec myrtus, nec laurus, spirat odores.

They that are most staid and patient, are so furiously carryed
headlong by the passion of sorrow in this case, that brave discreet men otherwise, oftentimes forget themselves, and weep
like children many moneths together, as [5] *if that they to water
would*, and will not be comforted. They are gone ! they are
gone !

Abstulit atra dies, et funere mersit acerbo !

what shall I do ?

Quis dabit in lacrymas fontem mihi? quis satis altos
Accendet gemitus, et acerbo verba dolori ?
Exhaurit pietas oculos, et hiantia frangit
Pectora, nec plenos avido sinit edere questus ;
Magna adeo jactura premit, &c.

Fountains of tears who gives? who lends me groans,
Deep sighs, sufficient to express my moans ;
Mine eyes are dry, my breast in pieces torn ;
My loss so great, I cannot enough mourn.

So Stroza filius, that elegant Italian poet, in his Epicedium,
bewails his fathers death ; he could moderate his passions in
other matters (as he confesseth), but not in this ; he yields
wholly to sorrow.

Nunc, fateor, do terga malis ; mens illa fatiscit,
Indomitus quondam vigor et constantia mentis.

---

[1] Virg. 4. Æn. [2] Patres mortuos coram astantes, et filios, &c. Marcellus
Donatus. [3] Epist. l. 2. Virginium video, audio ; defunctum cogito, allo-
quor. [4] Calphurnius Græcus. [5] Chaucer.

Mem. 4. Subs. 7.] *Other Accidents and Grievances.* 365

How doth [1] Quintilian complain for the loss of his son, to despair almost! Cardan lament his only child, in his book *de libris propriis*, and elsewhere, in many other of his tracts,[2] St. Ambrose his brothers death! (*an ego possum non cogitare de te, aut sine lacrymis cogitare? O amari dies! o flebiles noctes!*) *&c.* Gregory Nazianzen, that noble Pulcheria! (*O decorem, &c. flos recens, pullulans, &c.*) Alexander, a man of a most invincible courage, after Hephæstions death (as Curtius relates), *triduum jacuit ad moriendum obstinatus,* lay three dayes together upon the ground, obstinate to dye with him, and would neither eat, drink, nor sleep. The woman that communed with Esdras (*lib.* 2. *cap.* 10), when her son fell down dead, *fled into the field, and would not return into the city, but there resolved to remain, neither to eat nor drink, but mourn and fast until she dyed. Rachel wept for her children, and would not be comforted, because thay were not* (Matt. 2. 18). So did Adrian the emperour bewail his Antinoüs; Hercules, Hylas; Orpheus, Eurydice; David, Absolon (O my dear son Absolon); Austin, his mother Monica; Niobe, her children, insomuch, that the [3] poets feigned her to be turned into a stone, as being stupified through the extremity of grief. [4] *Ægeus, signo lugubri filii consternatus, in mare se præcipitem dedit,* impatient of sorrow for his sons death, drowned himself. Our late physicians are full of such examples. Montanus (*consil.* 242) [5] had a patient troubled with this infirmity, by reason of her husbands death, many years together: Trincavellius (*l.* 1. *c.* 14) hath such another, almost in despair, after his [6] mothers departure, *ut se ferme præcipitem daret,* and ready through distraction to make away himself; and (in his fifteenth counsel) tells a story of one fifty years of age, *that grew desperate upon his mothers death;* and, cured by Phalopius, fell many years after into a relapse, by the sudden death of a daughter which he had, and could never after be recovered. The fury of this passion is so violent sometimes, that it daunts whole kingdoms and cities. Vespasians death was pittifully lamented all over the Roman empire; *totus orbis lugebat,* saith Aurelius Victor. Alexander commanded the battlements of houses to be pulled down, mules and horses to have their manes shorn off, and many common souldiers to be slain, to accompany his dear Hephæstions death; which is now practised amongst the Tartars: when [7] a great Cham dyeth, ten or twelve thousand must be slain, men and horses,

---

[1] Præfat. lib. 6.   [2] Lib. de obitu Satyri fratris.   [3] Ovid. Met.   [4] Plut. vitâ ejus.   [5] Nobilis matrona melancholica ob mortem mariti.   [6] Ex matris obitu in desperationem incidit.   [7] Mathias a Michou. Boter. Amphitheat.

366 *Causes of Melancholy.* [Part. 1. Sec. 2.

all they meet: and, among those [1] pagan Indians, their wives
and servants voluntarily dye with them. Leo Decimus was
so much bewailed in Rome after his departure, that (as Jovius
gives out) [2] *communis salus, publica hilaritas,* the common
safety, all good fellowship, peace, mirth, and plenty, died with
him; *tamquam eodem sepulcro cum Leone condita lugebantur;*
for it was a golden age whilst he lived; [3] but after his decease,
an iron season succeeded, *barbara vis, et fœda vastitas, et dira
malorum omnium incommoda,* wars, plagues, vastity, discontent.
When Augustus Cæsar dyed, saith Paterculus, *orbis ruinam
timueramus,* we were all afraid, as if heaven had fallen upon
our heads. [4] Budæus records, how that, at *Lewis the twelfth
his death, tam subita mutatio, ut qui prius digito cœlum attin-
gere videbantur, nunc humi derepente serpere, sideratos esse
diceres,* they that were erst in heaven, upon a sudden, as if
they had been planet strucken, lay groveling on the ground;

> [5] Concussis cecidere animis, ceu frondibus ingens
> Sylva dolet lapsis————

they look't like cropt trees.
    [6] At Nancy in Lorain, when Claudia Valesia, Henry the
second French kings sister, and the duke's wife, deceased, the
temples for forty dayes were all shut up, no prayers nor
masses, but in that room where she was; the senators all seen
in black; *and for a twelve moneths space throughout the city,
they were forbid to sing or dance.*

> ————————[7] Non ulli pastos illis egere diebus
> Frigida, Daphni, boves ad flumina; nulla nec amnem
> Libavit quadrupes, nec graminis attigit herbam.

How were we affected here in England for our Titus, *deliciæ
humani generis,* Prince Henries immature death, as if all our
dearest friends lives had exhaled with his! [8] Scanderbegs death
was not so much lamented in Epirus. In a word, as [9] he saith
of Edward the First at the news of Edward of Caernarvan his
sons birth, *immortaliter gavisus,* he was immortally glad,
may we say on the contrary of friends deaths, *immortaliter
gementes,* we are, divers of us, as so many turtles, eternally
dejected with it.

---

[1] Lo. Vertoman. M. Polus Venetus, lib. 1. c. 54. Perimunt eos quos in viâ ob-
vios habent, dicentes, Ite, et domino nostro regi servite in aliâ vitâ. Nec tam in
homines insaniunt, sed in equos, &c.   [2] Vit. ejus.   [3] Lib. 4. vitæ ejus.
Auream ætatem condiderat ad humani generis salutem, quum nos statim ab optimi
principis excessu vere ferream pateremur, famem, pestem, &c.   [4] Lib. 5. de
asse.   [5] Maph.   [6] Ortelius, Itinerario. Ob annum integrum a cantu, tripudiis, et saltationibus, tota civitas abstinere jubetur.   [7] Virg.   [8] See
Barletius, de vitâ et ob. Scanderbeg. lib. 13. hist.   [9] Matth. Paris.

Mem. 4. Subs. 7.]   *Other Accidents and Grievances.*   367

There is another sorrow, which ariseth from the loss of temporal goods and fortunes, which equally afflicteth, and may go hand in hand with the precedent.   Loss of time, loss of honour, office, of good name, of labour, frustrate hopes will much torment; but, in my judgment, there is no torment like unto it, or that sooner procureth this malady and mischief:

> [1] Ploratur lacrymis amissa pecunia veris:

it wrings true tears from our eyes, many sighs, much sorrow from our hearts, and often causeth habitual melancholy it self. Guianerius (*tract.* 15. 5) repeats this for an especial cause ; [2] *loss of friends, and loss of goods, make many men melancholy (as I have often seen), by continual meditation of such things.* The same causes Arnoldus Villanovanus inculcates (*Breviar. l.* 1. *c.* 18), *ex rerum amissione, damno, amicorum morte, &c.* Want alone will make a man mad; to be *sans argent*, will cause a deep and grievous melancholy.   Many persons are affected like [3] Irishmen in this behalf, who, if they have a good scimiter, had rather have a blow on their arm, than their weapon hurt : they will sooner lose their life, than their goods: and the grief that cometh hence, continueth long (saith [4] Plater), *and, out of many dispositions, procureth an habit.*   [5] Montanus and Frisemelica cured a young man of twenty two years of age, that so became melancholy *ob amissam pecuniam*, for a summ of money which he had unhappily lost.   Sckenkius hath such another story of one melancholy, because he overshot himself, and spent his stock in unnecessary building. [6] Roger, that rich bishop of Salisbury, *exutus opibus et castris a rege Stephano*, spoiled of his goods by king Stephen, *vi doloris absorptus, atque in amentiam versus, indecentia fecit*, through grief ran mad, spake and did he knew not what. Nothing so familiar, as for men in such cases, through anguish of mind, to make away themselves.   A poor fellow went to hang himself (which Ausonius hath elegantly expressed in a neat [7] epigram), but, finding by chance a pot of money, flung away the rope, and went merrily home ; but he that hid the gold, when he missed it, hanged himself with that rope which the other man had left, in a discontented humour.

> At qui condiderat, postquam non reperit aurum,
> Aptavit collo, quem reperit, laqueum.

---

[1] Juvenal.   [2] Multi, qui res amatas perdiderant, ut filios, opes, non sperantes recuperare, propter assiduam talium considerationem melancholici fiunt, ut ipse vidi.   [3] Stanihurstus, Hib. Hist.   [4] Cap. 3. Melancholia semper venit ob jacturam pecuniæ, victoriæ repulsam, mortem liberorum, quibus longo post tempore animus torquetur ; et a dispositione fit habitus.   [5] Consil. 26. [6] Nubrigensis.   [7] Epig. 22.

368   *Causes of Melancholy.*   [Part. 1. Sec. 2.

Such feral accidents can want and penury produce. Be it by
suretiship, shipwrack, fire, spoil and pillage of souldiers, or
what loss soever, it boots not ; it will work the like effect, the
same desolation in provinces and cities, as well as private persons. The Romans were miserably dejected after the battel of
Cannæ, the men amazed for fear, the stupid women tore their
hair and cryed ;—the Hungarians, when their king Ladislaus,
and bravest souldiers, were slain by the Turks : *luctus publicus,*
&c.—the Venetians, when their forces were overcome by the
French king Lewis, the French and Spanish kings, pope, emperour, all conspired against them, at Cambray, the French
herald denounced open war in the senate, *Lauredane, Vene-*
torum dux, &c. and they had lost Padua, Brixia, Verona, Forum Julii, their territories in the continent, and had now nothing left but the city of Venice it self, *et urbi quoque ipsi* (saith
[1] Bembus) *timendum putarent,* and the loss of that was likewise to be feared ; *tantus repente dolor omnes tenuit, ut nun-*
quam alias, &c. they were pittifully plunged, never before in
such lamentable distress. Anno 1527, when Rome was sacked
by Burbonius, the common souldiers made such spoil, that
fair [2] churches were turned to stables, old monuments and
books made horse-litter, or burned like straw ; reliques, costly
pictures defaced ; altars demolished, rich hangings, carpets,
&c. trampled in the dirt ; [3] their wives and loveliest daughters
constuprated by every base cullion (as Sejanus daughter was
by the hangman in publick) before their fathers and husbands
faces ; noblemens children, and of the wealthiest citizens, reserved for princes beds, were prostitute to every common souldier, and kept for concubines ; senators and cardinals themselves drag'd along the streets, and put to exquisite torments,
to confess where their money was hid ; the rest, murdered on
heaps, lay stinking in the streets ; infants brains dashed out
before their mothers eyes. A lamentable sight it was to see so
goodly a city so suddenly defaced, rich citizens sent a begging,
to Venice, Naples, Ancona, &c. that erst lived in all manner of
delights. [4] *Those proud palaces, that even now vaunted their*
tops up to heaven, were dejected as low as hell in an instant.
Whom will not such misery make discontent ? Terence the
poet drowned himself (some say) for the loss of his comedies,
which suffered shipwrack. When a poor man hath made many

---

[1] Lib. 8. Venet. hist.   [2] Templa ornamentis nudata, spoliata, in stabula
equorum et asinorum versa, &c. Infulæ humi conculcatæ pedibus, &c.   [3] In
oculis maritorum dilectissimæ conjuges ab Hispanorum lixis constupratæ sunt.
Filiæ magnatum thoris destinatæ, &c.   [4] Ita fastu ante unum mensem turgida
civitas, et cacuminibus cœlum pulsare visa, ad inferos usque paucis diebus dejecta.

Mem. 4. Subs. 7.] *Other Accidents and Grievances.* 369

hungry meals, got together a small summ, which he loseth in
an instant—a scholar spent many an hours study to no purpose, his labours lost, &c.—how should it otherwise be? I
may conclude, with Gregory, *temporalium amor quantum afficit,
cum hæret possessio, tantum, quum subtrahitur, urit dolor;*
riches do not so much exhilarate us with their possession, as
they torment us with their loss.

Fear from ominous accidents, destinies foretold.] Next to
sorrow still I may annex such accidents as procure fear; for,
besides those terrors which I have [1] before touched, and many
other fears (which are infinite), there is a superstitious fear,
(one of the three great causes of fear in Aristotle) commonly
caused by prodigies and dismal accidents, which much trouble
many of us, (*Nescio quid animus mihi præsagit mali,*) as, if a
hare cross the way at our going forth, or a mouse gnaw our
clothes: if they bleed three drops at the nose, the salt falls
towards them, a black spot appear in their nails, &c. with
many such, which Delrio (*Tom. 2. l. 3. sec. 4*), Austin Niphus
(in his book *de Auguriis*), Polydore Virg. (*l. 3. de Prodigiis*)
Sarisburiensis (*Polycrat. l. 1. c.* 13), discuss at large. They
are so much affected, that, with the very strength of imagination, fear, and the devils craft, [2] *they pull those misfortunes
they suspect upon their own heads, and that which they fear,
shall come upon them,* as So!omon foretelleth (Prov. 10, 24)
and I say denounceth (66, 4), which if [3] *they could neglect and
contemn, would not come to pass. Eorum vires nostrâ resident
opinione, ut morbi gravitas ægrotantium cogitatione,* they are
intended and remitted, as our opinion is fixed, more or less.
N. N. dat pœnas, saith [4] Crato of such a one; *utinam non
attraheret:* he is punished, and is the cause of it [5] himself.

[6] Dum fata fugimus, fata stulti incurrimus;

the thing that I feared, saith Job, is faln upon me.
As much we may say of them that are troubled with their
fortunes, or ill destinies fore-seen; *multos angit præscientia
malorum:* the fore-knowledge of what shall come to pass, crucifies many men, fore-told by astrologers, or wizards, *iratum
ob cœlum,* be it ill accident, or death it self; which often falls
out by Gods permission, *quia dæmonem timent* (saith Chrysostom), *Deus ideo permittit accidere.* Severus, Adrian, Domitian, can testifie as much, of whose fear and suspicion,
Sueton, Herodian, and the rest of those writers, tell strange
stories in this behalf. [7] Montanus (*consil.* 31) hath one

---

[1] Sect. 2. Memb. 4. Subs. 3.
vemus, nihil valent. Polydor.
catch.   [6] Geor. Bucha.
melancholicus.

[2] Accersunt sibi malum.   [3] Si non obser-
[4] Consil. 26. l. 2.   [5] Harm watch, harm
[7] Juvenis, solicitus de futuris frustra, factus

VOL. I.   B B

370   *Causes of Melancholy.*   [Part. 1. Sec. 2.

example of a young man, exceeding melancholy upon this occasion. Such fears have still tormented mortal men in all ages, by reason of those lying oracles, and jugling priests. [1] There was a fountain in Greece, near Ceres temple in Achaia, where the event of such diseases was to be known: *a glass let down by a thred, &c.* Amongst those Cyanean rocks at the springs of Lycia, was the oracle of Thrixeus Apollo, *where all fortunes were fore-told, sickness, health, or what they would besides :* so common people have been alwayes deluded with future events. At this day, *metus futurorum maxime torquet Sinas,* this foolish fear mightily crucifies them in China: as [2] Matthew Riccius the Jesuit informeth us, in his Commentaries of those countreys, of all nations they are most superstitious, and much tormented in this kind, attributing so much to their divinators, *ut ipse metus fidem faciat,* that fear it self and conceit cause it to [3] fall out: if he foretell sickness such a day, that very time they will be sick (*vi metûs afflicti in ægritudinem cadunt*), and many times dye as it is fore-told. A true saying, *timor mortis morte pejor,* the fear of death is worse than death it self; and the memory of that sad hour, to some fortunate and rich men, *is as bitter as gaul* (Eccles. 41. 1). *Inquietam nobis vitam facit mortis metus :* a worse plague cannot happen to a man, than to be so troubled in his mind; 'tis *triste divortium,* an heavy separation, to leave their goods, with so much labour got, pleasures of the world, which they have so deliciously enjoyed, friends and companions whom they so dearly love, all at once. Axiochus the philosopher was bold and couragious all his life, and gave good precepts *de contemnendâ morte,* and against the vanity of the world, to others; but, being now ready to dye himself, he was mightily dejected; *hac luce privabor? his orbabor bonis?* he lamented like a child, &c. And though Socrates himself was there to comfort him, *ubi pristina virtutum jactatio, O Axioche?* yet he was very timorous and impatient of death, much troubled in his mind: *imbellis pavor et impatientia, &c. O Clotho!* Megapetus the tyrant in Lucian exclaims, now ready to depart, *let me live a while longer.* [4] *I will give thee a thousand talents of gold, and two boles besides, which I took from Cleocritus, worth an hundred talents apiece. Woe's me!* [5] saith another, *what goodly manors shall I leave! what fertile fields !*

---

[1] Pausanias in Achaïc. lib. 7. Ubi omnium eventus dignoscuntur. Speculum tenui suspensum funiculo demittunt : et ad Cyaneas petras, ad Lyciæ fontes, &c. [2] Expedit. in Sinas, lib. 1. c. 3.   [3] Timendo præoccupat, quod vitat, ultro, provocatque quod fugit, gaudetque mœrens, et lubens miser fuit. Heinsius, Anstriac.   [4] Tom. 4. dial. 8. Cataplo. Auri puri mille talenta me hodie tibi daturum promitto, &c.   [5] Ibidem. Hei mihi! quæ relinquenda prædia! quam fertiles agri ! &c.

Mem. 4. Subs. 7.]   *Other Accidents and Grievances.*   371

*what a fine house ! what pretty children ! how many servants !
Who shall gather my grapes, my corn ? Must I now dye, so
well setled? leave all, so richly and well provided ? Woe's
me! what shall I do?* [1] *Animula vagula, blandula, quæ
nunc abibis in loca?*

To these tortures of fear and sorrow, may well be annexed
curiosity, that irksome, that tyrannizing care, *nimia solicitudo,*
[2] *superfluous industry about unprofitable things, and their qualities,* as Thomas defines it : an itching humour or kind of
longing to see that which is not to be seen, to do that which
ought not to be done; to know that [3] secret, which should
not be known, to eat of the forbidden fruit. We commonly
molest and tire our selves about things unfit and unnecessary,
as Martha troubled her self to little purpose. Be it in religion,
humanity, magick, philosophy, policy, any action or study,
'tis a needless trouble, a meer torment. For what else is
school-divinity? how many doth it puzzle! what fruitless
questions about the Trinity, resurrection, election, predesti-
nation, reprobation, hell-fire, &c. how many shall be saved,
damned ? What else is all superstition, but an endless observation of idle ceremonies, traditions? What is most of our
philosophy, but a labyrinth of opinions, idle questions, pro-
positions, metaphysical terms? Socrates therefore held all
philosophers cavillers and mad men ; *circa subtilia cavillatores
pro insanis habuit, palam eos arguens,* saith [4] Eusebius, because they commonly sought after such things *quæ nec percipi
a nobis neque comprehendi possent;* or, put case they did
understand, yet they were altogether unprofitable: for what
matter is it for us to know how high the Pleiades are, how far
distant Perseus and Cassiopeia from us, how deep the sea, &c. ?
we are neither wiser, as he follows it, nor modester, nor better,
nor richer, nor stronger, for the knowledge of it : *quod supra
nos nihil ad nos.* I may say the same of those genethliacal
studies, what is astrology, but vain elections, predictions ? all
magick, but a troublesome error, a pernicious foppery ? physick, but intricate rules and prescriptions? philology, but vain
criticisms ? logick, needless sophisms ? metaphysicks themselves, but intricate subtilties, and fruitless abstractions?
alcumy, but a bundle of errors? To what end are such great
tomes? why do we spend so many years in their studies?
Much better to know nothing at all, as those barbarous
Indians are wholly ignorant, than, as some of us, to be so sore
vexed about unprofitable toyes; *stultus labor est ineptiarum;*

---

[1] Adrian.   [2] Industria superflua circa res inutiles.   [3] Flavæ secreta
Minervæ ut viderat Aglaurus. Ov. Met. 2.   [4] Contra Philos. cap. 61.

B B 2

372   *Causes of Melancholy.*   [Part. 1. Sec. 2.

to build an house without pins, make a rope of sand; to what end? *cui bono?* He studies on; but, as the boy told S[t]. Austin, when I have laved the sea dry, thou shalt understand the mysterie of the Trinity. He makes observations, keeps times and seasons; (and as [1]Conradus the emperour would not touch his new bride, till an astrologer had told him a masculine hour) but with what success? He travels into Europe, Africk, Asia, searcheth every creek, sea, city, mountain, gulf; to what end? See one promontory (said Socrates of old), one mountain, one sea, one river; and see all. An alchymist spends his fortunes to find out the philosophers stone forsooth, cure all diseases, make men long-lived, victorious, fortunate, invisible, and beggars himself, misled by those seducing impostors (which he shall never attain) to make gold: an antiquary consumes his treasure and time to scrape up a company of old coyns, statues, rolls, edicts, manuscripts, &c. he must know what was done of old in Athens, Rome, what lodging, dyet, houses, they had, and have all the present news at first, though never so remote, before all others, what projects, counsels, consultations, &c. *quid Juno in aurem insusurret Jovi,* what's now decreed in France, what in Italy: who was he, whence comes he, which way, whither goes he, &c. Aristotle must find out the motion of Euripus; Pliny must needs see Vesuvius; but how sped they? One loseth goods, another his life. Pyrrhus will conquer Africk first, and then Asia: he will be a sole monarch, a second immortal, a third rich, a fourth commands. [2]*Turbine magno spes solicitæ in urbibus errant;* we run, ride, take indefatigable pains, all up early, down late, striving to get that which we had better be without: Ardelions, busie-bodies, as we are, it were much fitter for us to be quiet, sit still, and take our ease. His sole study is for words, that they be,

——— Lepide λεξεις compostæ, ut tesserulæ omnes,

not a syllable misplaced, to set out a stramineous subject; as thine is about apparel, to follow the fashion, to be terse and polite; 'tis thy sole business; both with like profit. His only delight is building; he spends himself to get curious pictures, intricate models and plots; another is wholly ceremonious about titles, degrees, inscriptions; a third is over-solicitous about his diet; he must have such and such exquisite sauces, meat so dressed, so far fetched, *peregrini aëris volucres,* so cooked, &c. something to provoke thirst, something anon to quench his thirst. Thus he redeems his appetite with extraordinary charge to his purse, is seldome pleased with any meal, whilst a trivial

---

[1] Mat. Paris.   [2] Seneca.

Mem. 4. Subs. 7.] *Other Accidents and Grievances.* 373

stomach useth all with delight, and is never offended. Another must have roses in winter, *alieni temporis flores,* snow-water in summer, fruits before they can be or are usually ripe, artificial gardens and fish-ponds on the tops of houses, all things opposite to the vulgar sort, intricate and rare, or else they are nothing worth. So busie, nice, curious wits, make that unsupportable in all vocations, trades, actions, employments, which to duller apprehensions is not offensive, earnestly seeking that, which others as scornfully neglect. Thus, through our foolish curiosity, do we macerate our selves, tire our souls, and run headlong, through our indiscretion, perverse will, and want of government, into many needless cares and troubles, vain expences, tedious journeys, painful hours; and, when all is done, *quorsum hæc? cui bono?* to what end?

> [1] Nescire velle quæ Magister maximus
> Docere non vult, erudita inscitia est.

Unfortunate marriage.] Amongst these passions and irksome accidents, unfortunate marriage may be ranked : a condition of life appointed by God himself in Paradise, an honourable and happy estate, and as great a felicity as can befall a man in this world, [2] if the parties can agree as they ought, and live as [3] Seneca lived with his Paullina; but if they be unequally matched, or at discord, a greater misery cannot be expected, to have a scold, a slut, an harlot, a fool, a Fury or a fiend: there can be no such plague. (Eccles. 26. 14) *He that hath her, is as if he held a scorpion;* (and 26. 25) *a wicked wife makes a sorry countenance, an heavy heart; and he had rather dwell with a lyon, than keep house with such a wife.* Her [4] properties Jovianus Pontanus hath described at large (*Ant. Dial. Tom.* 2) under the name of Euphorbia. Or if they be not equal in years, the like mischief happens. Cæcilius (in Agellius, *lib.* 2. *cap.* 23) complains much of an old wife : *dum ejus morti inhio, egomet mortuus vivo inter vivos;* whilst I gape after her death, I live a dead man amongst the living; or, if they dislike upon any occasion,

> [5] Judge, you that are unfortunately wed,
> What 'tis to come into a loathed bed.

The same inconvenience befalls women.

> [5] At vos, o duri, miseram lugete, parentes,
> Si ferro aut laqueo lævâ hac me exsolvere sorte
> Sustineo :———

---

[1] Jos. Scaliger, in Gnomis.   [2] A vertuous woman is the crown of her husband. Prov. 12. 4. but she, &c.   [3] Lib. 17. epist. 105.   [4] Titionatur, candelabratur, &c.   [5] Daniel, in Rosamund.   [6] Chalinorus, lib. 9. de repub. Angl.

374   *Causes of Melancholy.*   [Part. 1. Sec. 2.

Hard hearted parents, both lament my fate,
If self I kill or hang, to ease my state.

[1] A young gentlewoman in Basil was married (saith Felix Plater, *Observat. l.* 1) to an ancient man against her will, whom she could not affect; she was continually melancholy, and pined away for grief; and, though her husband did all he could possibly to give her content, in a discontented humour at length she hanged her self. Many other stories he relates in this kind. Thus men are plagued with women, they again with men, when they are of divers humours and conditions; he a spendthrift, she sparing; one honest, the other dishonest, &c. Parents many times disquiet their children, and they their parents. [2] *A foolish son is an heaviness to his mother. Injusta noverca :* a stepmother often vexeth a whole family, is matter of repentance, exercise of patience, fuel of dissention, which made Catos son expostulate with his father, why he should offer to marry his client Solinius daughter, a young wench—*cujus caussâ novercam induceret?* what offence had he done, that he should marry again?

Unkind, unnatural friends, evil neighbours, bad servants, debts, and debates, &c.—'twas Chilons sentence, *comes æris alieni et litis est miseria,* misery and usury do commonly go together; suretiship is the bane of many families; *sponde, præsto noxa est : he shall be sore vexed that is surety for a stranger* (Prov. 11. 15), *and he that hateth suretiship is sure.* Contention, brawling, law-suits, falling out of neighbours and friends (*discordia demens, Virg. Æn.* 6), are equal to the first, grieve many a man, and vex his soul. *Nihil sane miserabilius eorum mentibus* (as [3] Boter holds): *nothing so miserable as such men, full of cares, griefs, anxieties, as if they were stabbed with a sharp sword : fear, suspicion, desperation, sorrow, are their ordinary companions.* Our Welchmen are noted, by some of their [4] own writers, to consume one another in this kind; but, whosoever they are that use it, these are their common symptomes, especially if they be convict or overcome, [5] cast in a suit. Arius, put out of a bishoprick by Eustathius, turned heretick, and lived after discontented all his life. [6] Every repulse is of like nature; *heu ! quantâ de spe decidi !* Disgrace, infamy, detraction, will almost effect as much, and that

---

[1] Elegans virgo invita cuidam e nostratibus nupsit, &c.   [2] Prov.   [3] De increm. urb. lib. 3. c. 3. Tamquam diro mucrone confossi : his nulla requies, nulla delectatio ; solicitudine, gemitu, furore, desperatione, timore, tamquam ad perpetuam ærumnam infeliciter rapti.   [4] Humfredus Lluyd, epist. ad Abrahamum Ortelium. M. Vaughan, in his Golden Fleece. Litibus et controversiis usque ad omnium bonorum consumptionem contendunt.   [5] Spretæque injuria formæ.
[6] Quæque repulsa gravis.

Mem. 4. Subs. 7.] *Other Accidents and Grievances.* 375

a long time after. Hipponax, a satyrical poet, so vilified, and lashed two painters in his iambicks, *ut ambo laqueo se suffocarent* ([1] Pliny saith), both hanged themselves. All oppositions, dangers, perplexities, discontents, [2] to live in any suspence, are of the same rank: *potes hoc sub casu ducere somnos?* who can be secure in such cases? Ill bestowed benefits, ingratitude, unthankful friends, much disquiet and molest some. Unkind speeches trouble as many: uncivil carriage or dogged answers, weak women above the rest, if they proceed from their surly husbands, are as bitter as gaul, and not to be digested. A glass-mans wife in Basil became melancholy, because her husband said he would marry again if she dyed. *No cut, to unkindness,* as the saying is: a frown and hard speech, ill respect, a brow-beating, or bad-look, especially to courtiers, or such as attend upon great persons, is present death.

Ingenium vultu statque caditque suo;

they ebb and flow with their masters favours. Some persons are at their wits ends, if by chance they overshoot themselves in their ordinary speeches or actions, which may after turn to their disadvantage or disgrace, or have any secret disclosed. Ronseus (*epist. miscel.* 3) reports of a gentlewoman twenty five years old, that, falling foul with one of her gossips, was upbraided with a secret infirmity (no matter what), in publick, and so much grieved with it, that she did thereupon *solitudines quærere, omnes ab se ablegare, ac tandem in gravissimam incidens melancholiam, contabescere*—forsake all company, quite moped, and in a melancholy humour pine away. Others are much tortured to see themselves rejected, contemned, scorned, disabled, diffamed, detracted, undervalued, or [3] *left behind their fellows.* Lucian brings in Ætamocles a philosopher in his *Lapith. convivio,* much discontented that he was not invited amongst the rest, expostulating the matter, in a long epistle, with Aristænetus their host. Prætextatus, a robed gentleman iu Plutarch, would not sit down at a feast, because he might not sit highest, but went his wayes all in a chafe. We see the common quarrellings that are ordinary with us, for taking of the wall, precedency, and the like, which though toyes in themselves, and things of no moment, yet they cause many distempers, much heart-burning amongst us. Nothing pierceth deeper than a contempt or disgrace; [4] especially if they be generous spirits, scarce any thing affects them more than to

---

[1] Lib. 36. c. 5.   [2] Nihil æque amarum, quam diu pendere: æquiore quidam animo ferunt præcidi spem suam, quam trahi. Seneca, cap. 5. lib. 2. de Ben.—Virg.—Plater. observat. l. 1.   [3] Turpe relinqui est. Hor.   [4] Scimus enim generosas naturas nullâ re citius moveri, aut gravius affici, quam contemtu ac despicientiâ.

376   *Causes of Melancholy.*   [Part. 1. Sec. 2.

be despised or vilified. Crato (*consil.* 16. *l.* 2) exemplifies it,
and common experience confirms it. Of the same nature is
oppression ; (*Eccles.* 77.) *surely oppression makes a man mad ;*
loss of liberty, which made Brutus venture his life, Cato kill
himself, and [1]Tully complain, *omnem hilaritatem in perpetuum
amisi*, mine heart's broken, I shall never look up, or be merry
again ; [2]*hæc jactura intolerabilis ;* to some parties 'tis a most
intolerable loss. Banishment, a great misery, as Tyrtæus describes it in an epigram of his,

> Nam miserum est, patriâ amissâ, Laribusque, vagari
>   Mendicum, et timidâ voce rogare cibos.
> Omnibus invisus, quocumque accesserit, exsul
>   Semper erit ; semper spretus egensque jacet, &c.

> A miserable thing 'tis so to wander,
>   And like a beggar for to whine at door.
> Contemn'd of all the world an exile is,
>   Hated, rejected, needy still, and poor.

Polynices, in his conference with Iocasta, in [3]Euripides,
reckons up five miseries of a banished man, the least of
which alone were enough to deject some pusillanimous creatures. Oftentimes a too great feeling of our own infirmities
or imperfections of body or mind will rivel us up ; as, if we be
long sick,

> (O beata sanitas ! te præsente, amœnum
> Ver floret gratiis ; absque te nemo beatus :

O blessed health ! *thou art above all gold and treasure* (*Ecclus.*
30. 15), the poor mans riches, the rich mans bliss : without
thee, there can be no happiness) or visited with some loathsome disease, offensive to others, or troublesome to our selves,
as a stinking breath, deformity of our limbs, crookedness,
loss of an eye, leg, hand, paleness, leanness, redness, baldness,
loss or want of hair, &c. *hic ubi fluere cœpit, diros ictus cordi
infert* (saith [4]Synesius, he himself troubled not a little *ob
comæ defectum*), the loss of hair alone strikes a cruel stroke to
the heart. Acco, an old woman, seeing by chance her face in
a true glass (for she used false flattering glasses, belike, at other
times, as most gentlewomen do) *animi dolore in insaniam delapsa
est* (Cœlius Rhodoginus, *l.* 17. *c.* 2) ran mad. [5]Broteas, the
son of Vulcan, because he was ridiculous for his imperfections,
flung himself into the fire. Laïs of Corinth, now grown old,
gave up her glass to Venus ; for she could not abide to look
upon it.

> [6]Qualis sum, nolo ; qualis eram, nequeo.

---

[1] Ad Atticum epist. lib. 12.   [2] Epist. ad Brutum.   [3] In Phœniss.
[4] In laudem calvit.   [5] Ovid.   [6] E Cret.

Mem. 4. Subs. 7.] *Other Accidents and Grievances.* 377

Generally, to fair nice pieces, old age and foul linnen are two odious things, a torment of torments ; they may not abide the thought of it.

> —————————————[1] ô Deorum
> Siquis hæc audis, utinam inter errem
> Nuda leones !
> Antequam turpis macies decentes
> Occupet malas, teneræque succus
> Defluat prædæ, speciosa quæro
> Pascere tigres.

To be foul, ugly, and deformed ! much better to be buried alive. Some are fair, but barren ; and that gauls them. Hannah *wept sore, did not eat, and was troubled in spirit, and all for her barrenness* (1 Sam. 1), and (Gen. 30) Rachel said *in the anguish of her soul, give me a child, or I shall dye:* another hath too many : one was never married, and that's his hell ; another is, and that's his plague. Some are troubled in that they are obscure ; others by being traduced, slandered, abused, disgraced, vilified, or any way injured : *minime miror eos* (as he said) *qui insanire occipiunt ex injuriâ ;* I marvel not at all if offences make men mad. Seventeen particular causes of anger and offence Aristotle reckons them up, which, for brevities sake, I must omit. No tydings troubles one ; ill reports, rumors, bad tidings, or news, hard hap, ill success, cast in a sute, vain hopes, or hope deferred, another : expectation, *adeo omnibus in rebus molesta semper est expectatio* (as [2] Polybius observes) : one is too eminent, another too base born ; and that alone tortures him as much as the rest : one is out of action, company, imployment ; another overcome and tormented with worldly cares, and onerous business. But what [3] tongue can suffice to speak of all ?

Many men catch this malady by eating certain meats, herbs, roots, at unawares, as henbane, nightshade, cicuta, mandrakes, &c. [4] A company of young men at Agrigentum, in Sicily, came into a tavern ; where after they had freely taken their liquor, whether it were the wine it self, or something mixt with it, 'tis not yet known, [5] but upon a sudden they began to be so troubled in their brains, and their phantasie so crazed, that they thought they were in a ship at sea, and now ready to be cast away by reason of a tempest. Wherefore, to avoid

---

[1] Hor. 3. Car. Ode 27.   [2] Hist. 1. 6.   [3] Non, mihi si centum linguæ sint, oraque centum, Omnia *caussarum* percurrere nomina possim.   [4] Cœlius, l. 17. c. 2.   [5] Ita mente exagitati sunt, ut in triremi se constitutos putarent, marique vagabundo tempestate jactatos : proinde naufragium veriti, egestis undique rebus, vasa omnia in viam e fenestris, ceu in mare, præcipitârunt : postridie, &c.

378   *Causes of Melancholy.*   [Part. 1. Sec. 2.

shipwreck and present drowning, they flung all the goods in the house out of the windows into the street, or into the sea, as they supposed. Thus they continued mad a pretty season ; and, being brought before the magistrate, to give an account of this their fact, they told him (not yet recovered of their madness) that what was done they did for fear of death, and to avoid eminent danger. The spectators were all amazed at this their stupidity, and gazed on them still, whilst one of the antientest of the company, in a grave tone, excused himself to the magistrate upon his knees. *O viri Tritones, ego in imo jacui ;* I beseech your deities, &c. for I was in the bottom of the ship all the while : another besought them, as so many sea gods, to be good unto them; and, if ever he and his fellows came to land again, [1] he would build an altar to their service. The magistrate could not sufficiently laugh at this their madness, bid them sleep it out, and so went his wayes. Many such accidents frequently happen upon these unknown occasions. Some are so caused by philters, wandring in the sun, biting of a mad dog, a blow on the head, stinging with that kind of spider called tarantula—an ordinary thing (if we may believe Skenck. *l. 6. de Venenis*) in Calabria and Apulia in Italy (Cardan, *subtil. l. 9.* Scaliger, *exercitat.* 185). Their symptomes are merrily described by Jovianus Pontanus (*Ant. dial.*) how they dance altogether, and are cured by musick. [2] Cardan speaks of certain stones, if they be carried about one, which will cause melancholy and madness ; he calls them unhappy, as an [3] *adamant, selenites, &c. which dry up the body, increase cares, diminish sleep.* Ctesias (in Persicis) makes mention of a well in those parts, of which if any man drink, [4] *he is mad for four and twenty hours.* Some lose their wits by terrible objects (as elsewhere I have more [5] copiously dilated), and life it self many times, as Hippolytus affrighted by Neptunes seahorses, Athamas by Junos Furies: but these relations are common in all writers.

> [6] Hic alias poteram et plures subnectere caussas :
> Sed jumenta vocant, et Sol inclinat. Eundum est.

> Many such causes, much more could I say,
> But that for provender my cattle stay,
> The sun declines, and I must needs away.

These causes, if they be considered, and come alone, I do easily yield, can do little of themselves, seldome, or apart (an old oak is not felled at a blow), though many times they are all sufficient

---

[1] Aram vobis servatoribus Diis erigemus.   [2] Lib. de gemmis.   [3] Quæ gestatæ infelicem et tristem reddunt, curas augent, corpus siccant, somnum minuunt.   [4] Ad unum diem mente alienatus.   [5] Part. 1. Sect. 2. Subsect. 3.
[6] Juven. Sat. 3.

Mem. 5. Subs. 1.] *Other Accidents and Grievances.* 379

every one : yet, if they concurr, as often they do, *vis unita fortior :*

> Et quæ non obsunt singula, multa nocent ;

they may batter a strong constitution; as [1] Austin said, *many grains and small sands sink a ship, many small drops make a flood, &c.* Often reiterated, many .dispositions produce an habit.

MEMB. V. SUBSECT. I.

Continent, inward, antecedent, next Causes, and how the Body works on the Mind.

As a purly hunter, I have hitherto beaten about the circuit of the forrest of this microcosm, and followed only those outward adventitious causes. I will now break into the inner rooms, and rip up the antecedent immediate causes which are there to be found. For, as the distraction of the mind, amongst other outward causes, and perturbations, alters the temperature of the body, so the distraction and distemper of the body will cause a distemperature of the soul; and 'tis hard to decide which of these two do more harm to the other. Plato, Cyprian, and some others (as I have formerly said), lay the greatest fault upon the soul, excusing the body; others again, accusing the body, excuse the soul, as a principal agent. Their reasons are, because [2] *the manners do follow the temperature of the body,* as Galen proves in his book of that subject, Prosper Galenius, *de Atrâ Bile,* Jason Pratensis, *c. de Maniâ,* Lemnius, *l. 4. c.* 16, and many others. And that which Gualter hath commented (*hom.* 10. *in epist. Johannis*) is most true ; concupiscence and original sin, inclinations, and bad humours, are [3] radical in every one of us, causing these perturbations, affections, and several distempers, offering many times violence unto the soul. *Every man is tempted by his own concupiscence* (James 1. 14); *the spirit is willing ; but the flesh is weak, and rebelleth against the spirit,* as our [4] apostle teacheth us : that methinks the soul hath the better plea against the body, which so forcibly inclines us, that we cannot resist ;

> Nec nos obniti contra, nec tendere tantum,
> Sufficimus.

How the body, being material, worketh upon the immaterial soul, by meditation of humours and spirits which participate of both, and ill disposed organs, Cornelius Agrippa hath discoursed, *lib.* 1. *de occult. Philos. cap.* 63, 64, 65. Levinus

---

[1] Intus bestiæ minutæ multæ necant. Numquid minutissima sunt grana arenæ ? sed si arena amplius in navem mittatur, mergit illam. Quam minutæ guttæ pluviæ ! et tamen implent flumina, domus ejiciunt : timenda ergo ruina multitudinis, si non magnitudinis.   [2] Mores sequuntur temperaturam corporis.   [3] Scintillæ latent in corporibus.   [4] Gal. 5.

380 *Causes of Melancholy.* [Part. 1. Sec. 2.

Lemnius, *lib.* 1. *de occult. nat. mir. cap.* 12. *et* 16. *et* 21. *institut. ad opt. vit.* Perkins, *lib.* 1. *Cases of Cons. cap.* 12. T. Bright, *c.* 10, 11, 12. *in his Treatise of Melancholy.* For, as [1] anger, fear, sorrow, obtrectation, emulation, &c. *si mentes intimos recessus occupárint* (saith [2] Lemnius), *corpori quoque infesta sunt, et illi teterrimos morbos inferunt,* cause grievous diseases in the body, so bodily diseases affect the soul by consent. Now the chiefest causes proceed from the [3] heart, humours, spirits: as they are purer, or impurer, so is the mind, and equally suffers, as a lute out of tune; if one string or one organ be distempered, all the rest miscarry:

$$\text{---------------------}^4 \text{ Corpus, onustum}$$
Hesternis vitiis, animum quoque prægravat unà.

The body is *domicilium animæ,* her house, abode, and stay; and, as a torch gives a better light, a sweeter smell, according to the matter it is made of, so doth our soul perform all her actions better or worse, as her organs are disposed; or as wine savours of the cask wherein it is kept, the soul receives a tincture from the body, through which it works. We see this in old men, children, Europeans, Asians, hot and cold climes. Sanguin are merry, melancholy sad, phlegmatick dull, by reason of abundance of those humours; and they cannot resist such passions which are inflicted by them: for, in this infirmity of humane nature (as Melancthon declares), the understanding is so tied to and captivated by his inferiour senses, that, without their help, he cannot exercise his functions; and the will, being weakened, hath but a small power to restrain those outward parts, but suffers herself to be overruled by them; that I must needs conclude with Lemnius, *spiritus et humores maximum nocumentum obtinent,* spirits and humours do most harm in [5] troubling the soul. How should a man choose but be cholerick and angry, that hath his body so clogged with abundance of gross humours? or melancholy, that is so inwardly disposed? That thence comes then this malady, madness, apoplexies, lethargies, &c. it may not be denied.

Now this body of ours is, most part, distempered by some precedent diseases, which molest his inward organs and instruments, and so, *per consequens,* cause melancholy, according to the consent of the most approved physicians. [6] *This humour* (as Avicenna, *l.* 3. *Fen.* 1. *Tract.* 4. *c.* 18. Arnoldus, *breviar. l.* 1. *c.* 18. Jacchinus, *comment. in.* 9. Rhasis. *c.* 15. Montaltus,

---

[1] Sicut ex animi affectionibus corpus languescit, sic ex corporis vitiis et morborum plerisque cruciatibus animum videmus hebetari. Galenus.   [2] Lib. 1. c. 16.   [3] Corporis itidem morbi animam per consensum, a lege consortii, afficiunt; et, quanquam objecta multos motus turbulentos in homine concitent, præcipua tamen caussa in corde, et humoribus, spiritibusque, consistit, &c. [4] Hor.   [5] Humores pravi mentem obnubilant.   [6] Hic humor vel a partis intemperie generatur, vel relinquitur post inflammationes, vel crassior in venis conclusus vel torpidus malignam qualitatem contrahit.

Mem. 5. Subs. 2.] *Other Accidents and Grievances.* **381**

c. 10. Nicholas Piso, *c. de Melan. &c.* suppose) *is begotten by the distemperature of some inward part, innate, or left after some inflammation, or else included in the blood after an* [1] *ague, or some other malignant disease.* This opinion of theirs concurrs with that of Galen, *l.* 3. *c.* 6. *de locis affect.* Guianerius gives an instance in one so caused by a quartan ague; and Montanus (*consil.* 32), in a young man of twenty eight years of age, so distempered after a quartan, which had molested him for five years together. Hildesheim (*spicil.* 2. *de Maniâ*) relates of a Dutch baron, grievously tormented with melancholy after a long [2] ague. Galen (*l. de atrâ bile, c.* 4) puts the plague a cause; Botaldus (in his book *de lue vener. c.* 2) the French pox for a cause: others, phrensie, epilepsie, apoplexie, because those diseases do often degenerate into this. Of suppression of hæmrods, hæmorrhagia, or bleeding at nose, menstruous retentions (although they deserve a larger explication, as being the sole cause of a proper kind of melancholy, in more ancient maids, nuns, and widows, handled apart by Rodericus a Castro, and Mercatus, as I have elsewhere signified), or any other evacuation stopped, I have already spoken. Only this I will add, that this melancholy, which shall be caused by such infirmities, deserves to be pittied of all men, and to be respected with a more tender compassion (according to Laurentius), as coming from a more inevitable cause.

SUBSECT. II.

Distemperature of particular Parts, Causes.

THERE is almost no part of the body, which, being distempered, doth not cause this malady, as the brain and his parts, heart, liver, spleen, stomach, matrix or womb, pylorus, myrache, mesentery, hypochondries, mesaraïck veins; and, in a word (saith [3] Arculanus), *there is no part which causeth not melancholy, either because it is adust, or doth not expel the superfluity of the nutriment.* Savanarola (*Pract. Major. rubric.* 11. *Tract.* 6. *cap.* 1) is of the same opinion, that melancholy is ingendred in each particular part; and [4] Crato (*in*

---

[1] Sæpe constat in febre hominem melancholicum vel post febrem reddi, aut alium morbum. Calida intemperies innata, vel a febre contracta.   [2] Raro quis diuturno morbo laborat, qui non sit melancholicus. Mercurialis, de affect. capitis, lib. 1. c. 10. de Melanc.   [3] Ad nonum lib. Rhasis ad Almansor. c. 16. Universaliter a quâcunque parte potest fieri melancholicus; vel quia aduritur, vel quia non expellit superfluitatem excrementi.   [4] A liene, jecinore, utero, et aliis partibus, oritur.

382   *Causes of Melancholy.*   [Part. 1. Sec. 2.

consil. 17. *lib.* 2). Gordonius who is *instar omnium* (*lib. med. partic.* 2. *cap.* 19). confirms as much, putting the [1] *matter of melancholy sometimes in the stomach, liver, heart, brain, spleen, myrach, hypochondries, whenas the melancholy humour resides there, or the liver is not well cleansed from melancholy blood.*

The brain is a familiar and frequent cause, too hot, or too cold, [2] *through adust blood so caused* (as Mercurialis will have it) *within or without the head;* the brain it self being distempered. Those are most apt to this disease, [3] *that have a hot heart and moist brain:* which Montaltus (*cap.* 11. *de Melanch.*) approves out of Halyabbas, Rhasis, and Avicenna. Mercurialis (*consil.* 11) assigns the coldness of the brain a cause; and Sallustius Salvianus (*med. lect.* 2. *c.* 1) [4] *will have it arise from a cold and dry distemperature of the brain.* Piso, Benedictus, Victorius Faventinus, will have it proceed from a [5] *hot distemperature of the brain;* and [6] Montaltus (*cap.* 10) from the brains heat scorching the blood. The brain is still distempered by himself, or by consent; by himself or his proper affection (as Faventinus calls it), [7] *or by vapours which arise from the other parts, and fume up into the head, altering the animal faculties.*

Hildesheim (*spicil.* 2. *de Maniâ*) thinks it may be caused from a [8] *distemperature of the heart, sometimes hot, sometimes cold.* A hot liver and a cold stomach are put for usual causes of melancholy. Mercurialis (*consil.* 11. *et consil.* 6. *consil.* 86) assignes a hot liver and cold stomach for ordinary causes. [9] Monavius (in an epistle of his to Crato, in Scoltzius) is of opinion that hypochondriacal melancholy may arise from a cold liver. The question is there discussed. Most agree that a hot liver is in fault. [10] *The liver is the shop of humours, and especially causeth melancholy by his hot and dry distemperature.* [11] *The stomach, and mesaraïck veins do often concurr, by reason of their obstructions; and thence their heat cannot be avoided; and many times the matter is so adust and inflamed in those parts, that it degenerates into hypochondriacal melancholy.* Guianerius (*c.* 2. *Tract.* 15) holds the mesaraïck veins

---

[1] Materia melancholiæ aliquando in corde, in stomacho, hepate, hypochondriis, myrache, splene, cum ibi remanet humor melancholicus.   [2] Ex sanguine adusto, intra vel extra caput.   [3] Qui calidum cor habent, cerebrum humidum, facile melancholici.   [4] Sequitur melancholia malam intemperiem frigidam et siccam ipsius cerebri.   [5] Sæpe fit ex calidiore cerebro, aut corpore colligente melancholiam. Piso.   [6] Vel per propriam affectionem, vel per consensum, cum vapores exhalant in cerebrum. Montalt. cap. 14.   [7] Aut ibi gignitur melancholicus fumus, aut aliunde vehitur, alterando animales facultates.   [8] Ab intemperie cordis, modo calidiore, modo frigidiore.   [9] Epist. 239. Scoltzii.   [10] Officina humorum hepar concurrit, &c.   [11] Ventriculus et venæ mesaraïcæ concurrunt, quod hæ partes obstructæ sunt, &c.

Mem. 5. Subs. 3.]   *Causes of Head-Melancholy.*   383

to be a sufficient [1] cause alone. The spleen concurrs to this
malady (by all their consents), and suppression of hæmrods :
dum non expurgat, altera causa, lien, saith Montaltus : if it be
[2] *too cold and dry, and do not purge the other parts as it ought*
(*Consil. 23*). Montanus puts the [3] *spleen stopped* for a great
cause. [4] Christophorus a Vega reports, of his knowledge, that
he hath known melancholy caused from putrified blood in
those seed veins and womb : [5] Arculanus *from that menstruous
blood turned into melancholy, and seed too long detained* (as
I have already declared) *by putrefaction or adustion.*

The *mesenterium,* or midriffe, *diaphragma,* is a cause (which
the [6] Greeks called φρεναç) because, by his inflammation, the
mind is much troubled with convulsions and dotage. All
these, most part, offend by inflammation, corrupting humours
and spirits, in this non-natural melancholy ; for from these are
ingendred fuliginous and black spirits. And, for that reason,
[7] Montaltus (*cap.* 10. *de caussis melan.*) will have *the efficient
cause of melancholy to be hot and dry, not a cold and dry distemperature, as some hold, from the heat of the brain, rosting
the blood, immoderate heat of the liver and bowels, and inflammation of the pylorus : and so much the rather, because that*
(as Galen holds) *all spices inflame the blood, solitariness,
waking, agues, study, meditation, all which heat ; and therefore
he concludes that this distemperature causing adventitious melancholy, is not cold and dry, but hot and dry.* But of this
I have sufficiently treated in the matter of melancholy, and
hold that this may be true in non-natural melancholy which
produceth madness, but not in that natural, which is more
cold, and, being immoderate, produceth a gentle dotage ;
[8] which opinion Geraldus de Solo maintains in his comment
upon Rhasis.

SUBSECT. III.

Causes of Head-Melancholy.

AFTER a tedious discourse of the general causes of melancholy, I am now returned at last to treat in brief of the
three particular species, and such causes as properly appertain

---

[1] Per se sanguinem adurentes.   [2] Lien frigidus et siccus, c. 13.   [3] Splen
obstructus.   [4] De arte med. lib. 3. cap. 24.   [5] A sanguinis putredine in
vasis seminariis et utero, et quandoque a spermate diu retento, vel sanguine men-
struo in melancholiam verso per putrefactionem, vel adustionem.   [6] Magirus.
[7] Ergo efficiens caussa melancholiæ est calida et sicca intemperies, non frigida et
sicca, quod multi opinati sunt ; oritur enim a calore cerebri assante sanguinem,
&c. tum quod aromata sanguinem incendunt, solitudo, vigiliæ, febris præcedens,
meditatio, studium ; et hæc omnia calefaciunt : ergo ratum sit.   [8] Lib. 1.
cap. 13. de Melanch.

384   Causes of Melancholy.   [Part. 1. Sec. 2.

unto them. Although these causes promiscuously concur to
each and every particular kind, and commonly produce their
effects in that part which is most weak, ill-disposed, and least
able to resist, and so cause all three species, yet many of them
are proper to some one kind, and seldom found in the rest :
as, for example, head-melancholy is commonly caused by a
cold or hot distemperature of the brain, according to Laurentius (*cap.* 5. *de melan.*), but, as [1] Hercules de Saxoniâ contends, from that agitation or distemperature of the animal spirits alone. Sallust. Salvianus, before mentioned (*lib.* 2, *cap.* 3.
de re med.) will have it proceed from cold; but that I take of
natural melancholy, such as are fools, and dote : for (as Galen
writes, *lib.* 4. *de puls.* 8. and Avicenna) [2] *a cold and moist
brain is an unseparable companion of folly.* But this adventitious melancholy, which is here meant, is caused of an hot
and dry distemperature, as [3] Damascen the Arabian *lib.* 3.
cap. 22) thinks, and most writers. Altomarus and Piso call
it [4] *an innate burning untemperateness, turning blood and
choler into melancholy.* Both these opinions may stand good,
as Bruel maintains, and Capivaccius, *si cerebrum sit calidius,*
[5] *if the brain be hot, the animal spirits will be hot, and thence
comes madness : if cold, folly.* David Crusius (*Theat. morb.
Hermet. lib.* 2. *cap.* 6. *de atrâ bile*) grants melancholy to be a
disease of an inflamed brain, and cold notwithstanding of itself:
calida per accidens, frigida per se, hot by accident only. I
am of Capivaccius mind, for my part. Now this humour,
according to Salvianus, is sometimes in the substance of the
brain, sometimes contained in the membranes and tunicles that
cover the brain, sometimes in the passages of the ventricles of
the brain, or veins of those ventricles. It follows many times
[6] *phrensie, long diseases, agues, long abode in hot places, or
under the sun, a blow on the head,* as Rhasis informeth us :
Piso adds solitariness, waking, inflammations of the head, proceeding most part [7] from much use of spices, hot wines, hot
meats (all which Montanus reckons up, *consil* 22. for a melancholy Jew ; and Heurnius repeats, *cap.* 12. *de Maniâ*), hot
baths, garlick, onions (saith Guianerius), bad aire, corrupt,
much [8] waking, &c. retention of seed, or abundance, stopping
of *hæmorrhagia,* the midriffe misaffected : and (according to

_____

[1] Lib. 3. Tract. posthum. de melan.   [2] A fatuitate inseparabilis cerebri fri-
giditas.   [3] Ab interno calore assatur.   [4] Intemperies innata exurens,
flavam bilem ac sanguinem in melancholiam convertens.   [5] Si cerebrum sit
calidius, fiet spiritus animalis calidior, et delirium maniacum ; si frigidior, fiet fa-
tuitas.   [6] Melancholia capitis accedit post phrenesim aut longam moram sub
sole, aut percussionem in capite. cap. 13. lib. I.   [7] Qui bibunt vina potentia, et sæpe sunt sub sole.   [8] Curæ validæ, largioris vini et aromatum
usus.

Mem. 5. Subs. 4.]   *Other Accidents and Grievances.*   385

Trallianus, *l.* 1. 16) immoderate cares, troubles, griefs, discontents, study, meditation, and, in a word, the abuse of all those six non-natural things.   Hercules de Saxoniâ (*cap.* 16. *lib.* 1) will have it caused from a [1] cautery, or boyl dried up, or any issue.   Amatus Lusitanus (*cent.* 2. *cura* 67) gives instance, in a fellow that had a boyl in his arm, and, [2] *after that was healed, ran mad ; and when the wound was open, he was cured again.* Trincavellius (*consil.* 13. *lib.* 1) hath an example of a melancholy man so caused by overmuch continuance in the sun, frequent use of venery, and immoderate exercise ; and (in his *cons.* 49. *lib.* 3) from an [3] headpiece overheated, which caused head-melancholy.   Prosper Calenus brings in Cardinal Cæsius for a pattern of such as are so melancholy by long study : but examples are infinite.

SUBSECT. IV.

Causes of Hypochondriacal, or Windy Melancholy.

In repeating of these causes, I must *cramben bis coctam apponere,* say that again which I have formerly said, in applying them to their proper species.   Hypochondriacal or flatuous melancholy is that which the Arabians call myrachial, and is, in my judgement, the most grievous and frequent, though Bruel and Laurentius make it least dangerous, and not so hard to be known or cured.   His causes are inward or outward :—inward from divers parts or organs, as midriffe, spleen, stomach, liver, pylorus, womb, diaphragma, mesaraick veins, stopping of issues, &c.   Montaltus (*cap.* 15. out of Galen) recites [4] *heat and obstruction of those mesaraick veins, as an immediate cause, by which means the passage of the chylus to the liver is detained, stopped, or corrupted, and turned into rumbling and wind.*   Montanus (*consil.* 233) hath an evident demonstration, Trincavellius another (*lib.* 1. *cap.* 12), and Plater a third (*observat. lib.* 1) for a doctour of the law visited with this infirmity, from the said obstruction and heat of these mesaraick veins, and bowels ; *quoniam inter ventriculum et jecur venæ effervescunt,* the veins are inflamed about the liver and stomach.   Sometimes those other parts are together misaffected, and concurr to the production of this malady—a hot liver or cold stomach or cold belly.   Look for instances in Hollerius,

---

[1] A cauterio et ulcere exsiccato.   [2] Ab ulcere curato incidit in insaniam ; aperto vulnere, curatur.   [3] A galeâ nimis calefactâ.   [4] Exuritur sanguis, et venæ obstruuntur, quibus obstructis prohibetur transitus chyli ad jecur, corrumpitur, et in rugitus et flatus vertitur.

VOL. I.   C C

386 *Causes of Melancholy.* [Part. 1. Sec. 2.

Victor, Trincavellius, *consil.* 35. *l.* 3. Hildesheim, *spicil.* 2. *fol.* 132. Solenander, *consil.* 9. *pro cive Lugdunensi*, Montanus, *consil.* 229. for the Earl of Montfort in Germany, 1549, and Frisimelica in the 233 consultation of the said Montanus. I. Cæsar Claudinus gives instance of a cold stomach and over-hot liver, almost in every consultation, *con.* 89, for a certain count, and *con.* 106, for a Polonian baron: by reason of heat, the blood is inflamed, and gross vapours sent to the heart and brain. Mercurialis subscribes to them, (*cons.* 89) [1] *the stomach being misaffected*, which he calls the king of the belly, because, if he be distempered, all the rest suffer with him, as being deprived of their nutriment or fed with bad nourishment; by means of which, come crudities, obstructions, wind, rumbling, griping, &c. Hercules de Saxoniâ, besides heat, will have the weakness of the liver and his obstruction a cause, *facultatem debilem jecinoris*, which he calls [2] the mineral of melancholy. Laurentius assigns this reason, because the liver overhot draws the meat undigested out of the stomach, and burneth the humours. Montanus (*cons.* 244) proves that sometimes a cold liver may be a cause. Laurentius (*c.* 12), Trincavellius (*lib.* 12. *consil.*) and Gualter Bruel, seem to lay the greatest fault upon the spleen, that doth not his duty in purging the liver as he ought, being too great, or too little, in drawing too much blood sometimes to it, and not expelling it, as P. Cnemiandrus in a [3] consultation of his noted: *tumorem lienis*, he names it, and the fountain of melancholy. Diocles supposed the ground of this kind of melancholy to proceed from the inflammation of the pylorus, which is the nether mouth of the ventricle. Others assign the mesenterium or midriffe distempered by heat, the womb misaffected, stopping of hæmrods, with many such: all which Laurentius (*cap.* 12) reduceth to three, mesentery, liver, and spleen; from whence he denominates hepatick, splenetick, and mesaraïck melancholy. Outward causes are bad diet, care, griefs, discontents, and, in a word, all those six non-natural things, as Montanus found by his experience (*consil.* 244). Solenander (*consil.* 9. for a citizen of Lyons in France) gives his reader to understand, that he knew this mischief procured by a medicine of cantharides, which an unskilful physician ministered his patient to drink, *ad venerem excitandam*. But most commonly fear, grief, and some sudden commotion or perturbation of the mind, begin it, in such bodies especially as are ill disposed. Melancthon (*tract.* 14. *cap.* 2. *de animâ*) will have it as common to men, as the mother to women, upon some grievous trouble, dislike, passion, or discontent: for, as

---

[1] Stomacho læso, robur corporis imminuitur; et reliqua membra alimento orbata, &c.   [2] Cap. 12.   [3] Hildesheim.

Camerarius records in his life, Melancthon himself was much troubled with it, and therefore could speak out of experience. Montanus (*consil. 22. pro delirante Judæo*) confirms it : [1] grievous symptomes of the mind brought him to it. Randolotius relates of himself, that, being one day very intent to write out a physicians notes, molested by an occasion, he fell into an hypochondriacal fit, to avoid which he drank the decoction of wormwood, and was freed. [2] Melancthon (*being the disease is so troublesome and frequent*) *holds it a most necessary and profitable study, for every man to know the accidents of it, and a dangerous thing to be ignorant,* and would therefore have all men, in some sort, to understand the causes, symptomes, and cures of it.

SUBSECT. V.

Causes of Melancholy from the whole Body.

As before, the cause of this kind of melancholy is inward or outward:—inward, [3] *when the liver is apt to ingender such a humour, or the spleen weak by nature, and not able to discharge his office.* A melancholy temperature, retention of hæmrods, monthly issues, bleeding at nose, long diseases, agues, and all those six non-natural things, increase it ; but especially [4] bad dyet (as Piso thinks), pulse, salt meat, shell-fish, cheese, black wine, &c. Mercurialis (out of Averroës and Avicenna) condemns all herbs ; Galen (*lib. 3. de loc. affect. cap.* 7) especially cabbage :—so likewise fear, sorrow, discontents, &c. but of these before. And thus in brief you have had the general and particular causes of melancholy.

Now go and brag of thy present happiness, whosoever thou art ; brag of thy temperature, of thy good parts ; insult, triumph, and boast ; thou seest in what a brittle state thou art, how soon thou maist be dejected, how many several wayes, by bad diet, bad ayre, a small loss, a little sorrow or discontent, an ague, &c.: how many sudden accidents may procure thy ruine, what a small tenure of happiness thou hast in this life, how weak and silly a creature thou art, *Humble thy self therefore under the mighty hand of God* (1 Pet. 5. 6), know thy self, acknowledge thy present misery, and make right use of it. *Qui stat, videat ne cadat.*

---

[1] Habuit sæva animi symptomata, quæ impediunt concoctionem, &c.   [2] Usitatissimus morbus cum sit, utile est hujus visceris accidentia considerare: nec leve periculum hujus caussas morbi ignorantibus.   [3] Jecur aptum ad generandum talem humorem, splen naturâ imbecillior. Piso, Altomarus, Guianerius. [4] Melancholiam, quæ fit a redundantiâ humoris in toto corpore, victus imprimis generat, qui eum humorem parit.

388   *Causes of Melancholy.*   [Part. 1. Sec. 3.

Thou dost now flourish, and hast *bona animi, corporis, et for-tunæ,* goods of body, mind, and fortune: *nescis quid serus sécum vesper ferat,* thou knowest not what storms and tempests the late evening may bring with it.   Be not secure then ; *be sober and watch ;* [1]*fortunam reverenter habe,* if fortunate and rich; if sick and poor, moderate thy self.   I have said.

SECT. III.

MEMB. I. SUBSECT. I.

Symptomes, or signs of Melancholy in the Body.

PARRHASIUS, a painter of Athens, amongst those Olynthian captives Philip of Macedon brought home to sell, [2]bought one very old man ; and, when he had him at Athens, put him to extream torture and torment, the better, by his example, to express the pains and passions of his Prometheus, whom he was then about to paint.   I need not be so barbarous, inhumane, curious, or cruel, for this purpose to torture any poor melancholy man : their symptomes are plain, obvious, and familiar : there needs no such accurate observation or far fetcht object ; they delineate themselves ; they voluntarily bewray themselves ; they are too frequent in all places ; I meet them still as I go ; they cannot conceal it ; their grievances are too well known ; I need not seek far to describe them.

Symptomes therefore are either [3]universal or particular, (saith Gordonius, *lib. med. cap.* 19. *part.* 2) to persons, to species.   *Some signs are secret, some manifest; some in the body, some in the mind ; and diversly vary, according to the in-ward or outward causes* (Capivaccius), or from stars (according to Jovianus Pontanus, *de reb. cœlest. lib.* 10. *cap.* 13) and cœlestial influences, or from the humours diversly mixt (Ficinus, *lib.* 1. *cap.* 4. *de sanit. tuendâ*).   As they are hot, cold, natural, unnatural, intended, or remitted, so will Aëtius have *melan-cholica deliria multiformia,* diversity of melancholy signs. Laurentius ascribes them to their several temperatures, delights, natures, inclinations, continuance of time, as they are simple or mixt with other diseases; as the causes are divers, so must the signs be almost infinite, (Altomarus, *cap.* 7. *art. med.*) and as wine produceth divers effects, or that herb tortocolla (in [4]*Lau-*

---

[1] Ausonius.   [2] Seneca, cont. lib. 10. cont. 5.   [3] Quædam universalia, particularia quædam ; manifesta quædam in corpore, quædam in cogitatione et animo ; quædam a stellis, quædam ab humoribus, quæ, ut vinum corpus varie disponit, &c.   Diversa phantasmata pro varietate caussæ externæ, internæ. [4] Lib. 1. de risu. fol. 17.   Ad ejus esum alii sudant; alii vomunt, flent, bibunt, saltant; alii rident, tremunt, dormiunt, &c.

Mem. 1. Subs. 1.] *Symptomes of Melancholy.* 389

rentius), *which makes some laugh, some weep, some sleep, some dance, some sing, some howle, some drink, &c.* so doth this our melancholy humour work several signs in several parties.

But to confine them, these general symptomes may be reduced to those of the body or the mind. Those usual signs, appearing in the bodies of such as are melancholy, be these, cold and dry, or they are hot and dry, as the humour is more or less adust. From [1] these first qualities, arise many other second, as that of [2] colour, black, swarthy, pale, ruddy, &c. some are *impense rubri,* (as Montaltus, *cap.* 16. observes out of Galen, *lib.* 3. *de locis affectis*) very red and high coloured. Hippocrates, in his book, [3] *de insaniá et melan.* reckons up these signs, that they are [4] *lean, withered, hollow-eyed, look old, wrinkled, harsh, much troubled with wind, and a griping in their bellies, or belly-ake, belch often, dry bellies and hard, dejected looks, flaggy beards, singing of the ears, vertigo, light-headed, little or no sleep, and that interrupt, terrible fearful dreams:*

[5] *Anna soror, quæ me suspensam insomnia terrent?*

The same symptomes are repeated by Melanelius (in his book of melancholy collected out of Galen, Ruffus, Aëtius), by Rhasis, Gordonius, and all the juniors—[6] *continual, sharp, and stinking belchings, as if their meat in their stomach were putrified, or that they had eaten fish, dry bellies, absurd and interrupt dreams, and many phantastical visions about their eyes, vertiginous, apt to tremble, and prone to venery.* [7] Some add palpitation of the heart, cold sweat, as usual symptomes, and a leaping in many parts of the body, *saltum in multis corporis partibus,* a kind of itching (saith Laurentius) on the superficies of the skin, like a flea-biting sometimes. [8] Montaltus (*c.* 21) puts fixed eyes and much twinkling of their eyes for a sign; and so doth Avicenna, *oculos habentes palpitantes, trauli, vehementer rubicundi, &c.* (*l.* 3. *Fen.* 1. *Tract.* 4. *c.* 18.) They stut most part, which he took out of Hippocrates Aphorisms. [9] Rhasis makes *head-ach and a binding heaviness*

---

[1] T. Bright, cap. 20. [2] Nigrescit hic humor aliquando supercalefactus, aliquando superfrigefactus. Melanel. e Gal. [3] Interprete F. Calvo. [4] Oculi his excavantur, venti gignuntur circum præcordia, et acidi ructus, sicci fere ventres, vertigo, tinnitus aurium, somni pusilli, somnia terribilia et interrupta. [5] Virg. Æn. [6] Assiduæ eæque acidæ ructationes, quæ cibum virulentum pisculentumque nidorem (etsi nil tale ingestum sit) referant, ob cruditatem. Ventres hisce aridi, somnus plerumque parcus et interruptus, somnia absurdissima, turbulenta, corporis tremor, capitis gravedo, strepitus circa aures, et visiones ante oculos, ad venerem prodigi. [7] Altomarus, Bruel, Piso, Montaltus. [8] Frequentes habent oculorum nictationes; aliqui tamen fixis oculis plerumque sunt. [9] Cent. lib. 1. tract. 9. Signa hujus morbi sunt plurimus saltus, sonitus aurium, capitis gravedo, lingua titubat, oculi excavantur &c.

390   *Symptomes of Melancholy.*   [Part. 1. Sec. 3.

for a principal token, *much leaping of wind about the skin,
as well as stutting or tripping in speech, &c. hollow eyes,
gross veins, and broad lips.* To some too, if they be far
gone, mimical gestures are too familiar, laughing, grinning,
fleering, murmuring, talking to themselves, with strange
mouths and faces, inarticulate voices, exclamations, &c. And,
although they be commonly lean, hirsute, unchearful in
countenance, withered, and not so pleasant to behold, by
reason of those continual fears, griefs, and vexations, dull,
heavy, lazy, restless, unapt to go about any business; yet their
memories are most part good, they have happy wits, and excellent apprehensions. Their hot and dry brains make them
they cannot sleep: *ingentes habent et crebras vigilias* (Aretæus),
mighty and often watchings, sometimes waking for a moneth,
a year together. [1] Hercules de Saxoniâ faithfully averreth,
that he hath heard his mother swear, she slept not for seven
months together. Trincavellius (*Tom. 2. cons.* 16) speaks of
one that waked fifty days; and Skenkius hath examples of two
years; and all without offence. In natural actions, their appetite is greater than their concoction: *multa appetunt, pauca
digerunt* (as Rhasis hath it); they covet to eat, but cannot digest. And, although they [2] *do eat much, yet they are lean, ill
liking* (saith Aretæus), *withered and hard, much troubled with
costiveness*, crudities, oppilations, spitting, belchings, &c.
Their pulse is rare and slow, except it be of the [3] *carotides*,
which is very strong; but that varies according to their intended passions or perturbations, as Struthius hath proved at
large (*Spigmaticæ artis. l.* 4. *c.* 13). To say truth, in such
chronick diseases the pulse is not much to be respected, there
being so much superstition in it, as [4] Crato notes, and so many
differences in Galen, that he dares say they may not be observed, or understood of any man.

Their urine is most part pale and low coloured; *urina pauca,
acris, biliosa* (Aretæus), not much in quantity. But this, in my
judgement, is all out as uncertain as the other, varying so often
according to several persons, habits, and other occasions not to
be respected in chronick diseases. [5] *Their melancholy excrements, in some very much, in others little, as the spleen plays his
part;* and thence proceeds wind, palpitation of the heart, short
breath, plenty of humidity in the stomach, heaviness of heart and
heartake, and intolerable stupidity and dulness of spirits; their
excrements or stool hard, black to some, and little. If the

---

[1] In Pantheon, cap. de Melancholiâ.   [2] Alvus arida nihil dejiciens; cibi
capaces, nihilo minus tamen extenuati sunt.   [3] Nic. Piso. Inflatio carotidum,
&c.   [4] Andreas Dudith Rahamo. ep. lib. 3. Crat. epist. Multa in pulsibus
superstitio; ausim etiam dicere, tot differentias, quæ describuntur a Galeno, neque intelligi a quoquam nec observari posse.   [5] T. Bright, cap. 20.

Mem. 1. Subs. 2.] *Symptomes in the Mind.* 391

heart, brain, liver, spleen, be misaffected, as usually they are, many inconveniences proceed from them, many diseases accompany, as incubus, [1] apoplexy, epilepsie, vertigo, those frequent wakings and terrible dreams, [2] intempestive laughing, weeping, sighing, sobbing, bashfulness, blushing, trembling, sweating, swouning, &c. [3] All their senses are troubled : they think they see, hear, smell, and touch that which they do not, as shall be proved in the following discourse.

SUBSECT. II.

Symptomes or signes in the Mind.

Fear.] Arculanus (*in* 9 *Rhasis ad Almansor. cap.* 16) will have these symptomes to be infinite, as indeed they are, varying according to the parties ; *for scarce is there one of a thousand that dotes alike* ([4] Laurentius, *c.* 16). Some few of greater note I will point at; and, amongst the rest, fear and sorrow, which as they are frequent causes, so if they persevere long, according to Hippocrates [5] and Galens Aphorismes, they are most assured signes, inseperable companions, and characters of melancholy; of present melancholy, and habituated, saith Montaltus (*c.* 11), and common to them all, as the said Hippocrates, Galen, Avicenna, and all neotericks, hold. But, as hounds many times run away with a false cry, never perceiving themselves to be at a fault, so do they; for Diocles of old, (whom Galen confutes) and, amongst the juniors, [6] Hercules de Saxoniâ, with Lod. Mercatus, (*cap.* 17. *l.* 1. *de melan.*) take just exceptions at this aphorism of Hippocrates : 'tis not alwayes true, or so generally to be understood : fear and sorrow are no common symptomes to all melancholy : *upon more serious consideration, I find some* (saith he) *that are not so at all. Some indeed are sad, and not fearful : some fearful, and not sad ; some neither fearful nor sad ; some both.* Four kinds he excepts, fanatical persons, such as were Cassandra, Manto, Nicostrata, Mopsus, Proteus, the Sibylls, whom [7] Aristole confesseth to have been deeply melancholy. Baptista Porta seconds him

---

[1] Post 40. ætat. annum, saith Jacchinus, in 15. 9. Rhasis. Idem Mercurialis, consil. 86. Trincavellius, tom. 2. cons. 1. [2] Gordonius. Modo rident, modo flent, silent, &c. [3] Fernelius, consil. 43. et 45. Montanus, consil. 230. Galen. de locis affectis, lib. 3. cap. 6. [4] Aphorism. et lib. de Melan. [5] Lib. 2. cap. 6. de locis affect. Timor et mœstitia, si diutius perseverent, &c. [6] Tract. postumo de Melan. edit. Venetiis 1620, per Bolzuttam bibliop. Mihi diligentius hanc rem consideranti, patet quosdam esse, qui non laborant mœrore et timore. [7] Prob. lib. 3.

392   *Symptomes of Melancholy.*   [Part. 1. Sec. 3.

(*Physiog. lib.* 1. *cap.* 8) : they were *atrá bile perciti.* Dæmoniacal persons, and such as speak strange languages, are of this rank : some poets; such as laugh alwayes, and think themselves kings, cardinals, &c. sanguine they are, pleasantly disposed most part, and so continue.   [1] Baptista Porta confines fear and sorrow to them that are cold ; but lovers, Sibylls, enthusiasts, he wholly excludes. So that I think I may truly conclude, they are not alwayes sad and fearful, but usually so, and that [2] *without a cause : timent de non timendis* (Gordonius), *quæque momenti non sunt : although not all alike,* (saith Altomarus) [3] *yet all likely fear,* [4] *some with an extraordinary and a mighty fear* (Aretæus). [5] *Many fear death, and yet, in a contrary humour, make away themselves* (Galen, *lib.* 3. *de loc. affect. cap.* 7). Some are afraid that heaven will fall on their heads; some, they are damned, or shall be.   [6] *They are troubled with scruples of conscience, distrusting Gods mercies, think they shall go certainly to hell, the devil will have them, and make great lamentation* (Jason Pratensis).   Fear of devils, death, that they shall be so sick of some such or such disease, ready to tremble at every object, they shall dye themselves forthwith, or that some of their dear friends or near allies are certainly dead; imminent danger, loss, disgrace, still torment others, &c. that they are all glass, and therefore will suffer no man to come near them; that they are all cork, as light as feathers; others as heavy as lead ; some are afraid their heads will fall off their shoulders: that they have frogs in their bellies, &c.   [7] Montanus (*consil.* 23) speaks of one *that durst not walk alone from home, for fear he should swoon, or die.*   A second [8] *fears every man he meets will rob him, quarrel with him, or kill him.*   A third dares not venture to walk alone, for fear he should meet the devil, a thief, be sick ; fears all old women as witches: and every black dog or cat he sees, he suspecteth to be a devil; every person comes near him is malificiated; every creature, all intend to hurt him, seek his ruine: another dares not go over a bridge, come near a pool, rock, steep hill, lye in a chamber where cross beams are, for fear he be tempted to hang, drown, or precipitate himself. If he be in a silent auditory, as at a sermon, he is afraid he shall speak aloud, at unawares, some

---

[1] Physiog. lib. 1. c. 8.   Quibus multa frigida bilis atra, stolidi et timidi ; at qui calidi, ingeniosi, amasii, divinosi, spiritu instigati, &c.   [2] Omnes exercent metus et tristitia, et sine caussâ.   [3] Omnes timent, licet non omnibus idem timendi modus.   Aëtius, Tetrab. lib. 2. sect. c. 9.   [4] Ingenti pavore trepidant.   [5] Multi mortem timent, et tamen sibi ipsis mortem consciscunt: alii cœli ruinam timent.   [6] Affligit eos plena scrupulis conscientia ; divinæ misericordiæ diffidentes, Orco se destinant fœdâ lamentatione deplorantes. [7] Non ausus egredi domo, ne deficeret.   [8] Multi dæmones timent, latrones, insidias. Avicenna.

Mem. 1. Subs. 2.] *Symptomes in the Mind.* 393

thing undecent, unfit to be said. If he be locked in a close
room, he is afraid of being stifled for want of air, and still carries
bisket, aquavitæ, or some strong waters about him, for fear of
deliquiums, or being sick; or, if he be in a throng, middle of
a church, multitude, where he may not well get out, though
he sit at ease, he is so misaffected. He will freely promise,
undertake any business beforehand; but when it comes to be
performed, he dare not adventure, but fears an infinite number
of dangers, disasters, &c. Some are [1] *afraid to be burned, or
that the* [2] *ground will sink under them, or* [3] *swallow them
quick, or that the king will call them in question for some fact
they never did (Rhasis, cont.) and that they shall surely be
executed.* The terror of such a death troubles them; and
they fear as much, and are equally tormented in mind, [4] *as
they that have committed a murder; and are pensive without
a cause, as if they were now presently to be put to death.*
(Plater, *cap. 3. de mentis alienat.*) They are afraid of some
loss, danger, that they shall surely lose their lives, goods, and
all they have; but why, they know not. Trincavellius (*consil. 13. lib. 1.*) had a patient that would needs make away
himself, for fear of being hanged, and could not be perswaded,
for three years together, but that he had killed a man. Plater
(*observat. lib. 1.*) hath two other examples of such as feared to
be executed without a cause. If they come in a place where a
robbery, theft, or any such offence, hath been done, they presently fear they are suspected, and many times betray themselves without a cause. Lewis the eleventh, the French king,
suspected every man a traitour that came about him, durst
trust no officer. *Alii formidolosi omnium, alii quorumdam,*
(Fracastorius, *lib. 2. de Intellect.*) [5] *some fear all alike, some
certain men,* and cannot endure their companies, are sick in
them, or if they be from home. Some suspect [6] treason still;
others *are afraid of their* [7] *dearest and nearest friends* (Melanelius e Galeno, Ruffo, Aëtio), and dare not be alone in the
dark, for fear of hobgoblins and devils: he suspects every thing
he hears or sees to be a devil, or enchanted, and imagineth
a thousand chimeras and visions, which to his thinking he
certainly sees, bugbears, talks with black men, ghosts, goblins, &c.

[8] Omnes se terrent auræ, sonus excitat omnis.

---

[1] Alii comburi, alii de rege. Rhasis.
tus. [3] Ne terra dehiscat. Gordon.
malâ gratiâ principum; putant se aliquid commisisse, et ad supplicium requiri.
[5] Alius domesticos timet, alius omnes. Aëtius.
Aurel. lib. 1. de morb. chron. c. 6.
citra discrimen, timet. [8] Virgil.
[2] Ne terrâ absorbeantur. Fores-
[4] Alii timore mortis tenentur, et
[6] Alii timent insidias.
[7] Ille carissimos, hic omnes homines

394   *Symptomes of Melancholy.* [Part. 1. Sec. 3.

Another, through bashfulness, suspicion, and timorousness, will not be seen abroad, [1] *loves darkness as life, and cannot endure the light,* or to sit in lightsome places; his hat still in his eyes, he will neither see, nor be seen by his good will (Hippocrates, *lib. de insaniá et melancholiá*). He dare not come in company, for fear he should be misused, disgraced, overshoot himself in gesture or speeches, or be sick; he thinks every man observes him, aims at him, derides him, owes him malice. Most part, [2] *they are afraid they are bewitched, possessed or poisoned by their enemies;* and sometimes they suspect their nearest friends : *he thinks something speaks or talks within him, or to him; and he belcheth of the poyson.* Christophorus a Vega (*lib. 2. cap. 1*) had a patient so troubled, that by no perswasion or physick he could be reclaimed. Some are afraid that they shall have every fearful disease they see others have, hear of, or read, and dare not therefore hear or read of any such subject, no not of melancholy it self, lest, by applying to themselves that which they hear or read, they should aggravate and increase it. If they see one possessed, bewitched, an epileptick paroxysme, a man shaking with the palsie, or giddy headed, reeling or standing in a dangerous place, &c. for many dayes after it runs in their minds; they are afraid they shall be so too, they are in like danger, as Perk, (*c. 12. se. 2.*) well observes in his *Cases of Cons.* and many times, by violence of imagination, they produce it. They cannot endure to see any terrible object, as a monster, a man executed, a carcase, hear the devil named, or any tragical relation seen, but they quake for fear; *Hecatas somniare sibi videntur* (Lucian); they dream of hobgoblins, and may not get it out of their minds a long time after : they apply (as I have said) all they hear, see, read, to themselves; as [3] Felix Plater notes of some young physicians, that study to cure diseases, catch them themselves, will be sick, and appropriate all symptomes they find related of others, to their own persons. And therefore (*quod iterum moneo, licet nauseam paret lectori; malo decem potius verba, decies repetita licet, abundare, quam unum desiderari*) I would advise him, that is actually melancholy, not to read this tract of symptomes, lest he disquiet or make himself for a time worse and more melancholy than he was before. Generally of them all take this—*de inanibus semper*

---

[1] Hic in lucem prodire timet, tenebrasque quærit ; contra, ille caliginosa fugit.
[2] Quidam larvas et malos spiritus ab inimicis veneficiis et incantationibus sibi putant objectari. Hippocrates.—Potionem se veneficam sumpsisse putat ; et de hac ructare sibi crebro videtur. Idem Montaltus, cap. 21. Aëtius, lib. 2. et alii. Trallianus, l. 1. cap. 16. [3] Observat. l. 1. Quando iis nil nocet, nisi quod mulieribus melancholicis.

Mem. 1. Subs. 2.]   *Symptomes in the Mind.*   395

conqueruntur, et timent, saith Aretæus; they complain of toyes, and fear [1] without a cause, and still think their melancholy to be most grievous; none so bad as they are; though it be nothing in respect, yet never any man sure was so troubled, or in this sort: as really tormented and perplexed, in as great an agony for toyes and trifles (such things as they will after laugh at themselves), as if they were most material and essential matters indeed, worthy to be feared, and will not be satisfied. Pacifie them for one, they are instantly troubled with some other fear; alwayes afraid of something, which they foolishly imagine or conceive to themselves, which never peradventure was, never can be, never likely will be; troubled in mind upon every small occasion, unquiet, still complaining, grieving, vexing, suspecting, grudging, discontent, and cannot be freed so long as melancholy continues. Or, if their minds be more quiet for the present, and they free from forraign fears, outward accidents, yet their bodies are out of tune, they suspect some part or other to be amiss; now their head akes, heart; stomach, spleen, &c. is misaffected; they shall surely have this or that disease; still troubled in body, mind, or both, and through wind, corrupt phantasie, some accidental distemper, continually molested. Yet, for all this, (as [2] Jacchinus notes) *in all other things they are wise, staid, discreet, and do nothing unbesceming their dignity, person, or place, this foolish, ridiculous, and childish fear excepted,* which so much, so continually, tortures and crucifies their souls; like a barking dog that alwayes bawls, but seldom bites, this fear ever molesteth, and, so long as melancholy lasteth, cannot be avoided.

Sorrow is that other character, and inseparable companion, as individual as saint Cosmus and Damian, *fidus Achates,* as all writers witness, a common symptome, a continual; and still, without any evident cause, [3] *mœrent omnes,* and, *si roges eos reddere caussam, non possunt;* grieving still, but why, they cannot tell: *agelasti, mœsti, cogitabundi,* they look as if they had newly come forth of Trophonius den; and though they laugh many times, and seem to be extraordinary merry (as they will by fits), yet extream lumpish again in an instant, dull, and heavy, *semel et simul* merry and sad, but most part sad:

[4] Si qua placent, abeunt; inimica tenacius hærent:

sorrow sticks by them still, continually gnawing, as the vulture

---

[1] —timeo tamen, metusque caussæ nescius caussa est metûs. Heinsius, Austriaco.   [2] Cap. 15. in 9 Rhasis. In multis vidi: præter rationem semper aliquid timent, in cæteris tamen optime se gerunt, neque aliquid præter dignitatem committunt.   [3] Altomarus, cap. 7.—Aretæus. Tristes sunt.   [4] Mant. Ecl. 1.

396   *Symptomes of Melancholy.*   [Part. 1. Sec. 3.

did [1] Tityus bowels : and they cannot avoid it.   No sooner are
their eyes open, but, after terrible and troublesome dreams, their
heavy hearts begin to sigh : they are still fretting, chafing, sighing, grieving, complaining, finding faults, repining, grudging,
weeping, *heautontimorumenoi*, vexing themselves, [2] disquieted
in mind, with restless, unquiet thoughts, discontent, either for
their own, other mens, or public affairs, such as concern them
not, things past, present, or to come : the remembrance of some
disgrace, loss, injury, abuse, &c. troubles them now, being idle,
afresh, as if it were new done ; they are afflicted otherwise for
some danger, loss, want, shame, misery, that will certainly come
as they suspect and mistrust. *Lugubris Ate* frowns upon them,
insomuch that Aretæus well calls it *angorem animi*, a vexation
of the mind, a perpetual agony.   They can hardly be pleased
or eased, though, in other mens opinion, most happy.   Go,
tarry, run, ride,

> [3] ———post equitem sedet atra cura :

they cannot avoid this feral plague, let them come in what
company they will : [4] *hæret lateri letalis arundo ;* as to a
deer that is struck, whether he run, go, rest, with the herd, or
alone, this grief remains ; irresolution, inconstancy, vanity of
mind, their fear, torture, care, jealousie, suspicion, &c. continues, and they cannot be relieved.   So [5] he complained in the
poet,

> Domum revertor mœstus, atque animo fere
> Perturbato atque incerto, præ ægritudine.
> Assido : accurrunt servi ; soccos detrahunt.
> Video alios festinare, lectos sternere,
> Cœnam apparare : pro se quisque sedulo
> Faciebant, quo illam mihi lenirent miseriam.

He came home sorrowfull, and troubled in his mind ; his servants
did all they possibly could to please him ; one pulled off his
socks ; another made ready his bed, a third his supper ; all did
their utmost endeavours to ease his grief, and exhilarate his
person ; he was profoundly melancholy ; he had lost his son ;
illud angebat ; that was his *cordolium*, his pain, his agony, which
could not be removed.   Hence it proceeds many times, that
they are weary of their lives ; and feral thoughts, to offer violence to their own persons, come into their minds.

Tædium vitæ.]   *Tædium vitæ* is a common symptome ; *tarda
fluunt, ingrataque tempora ;* they are soon tired with all things ;
they will now tarry, now be gone ; now in bed they will rise, now

---

[1] Ovid. Met. 4.   [2] Inquies animus.   [3] Hor. l. 3. Od. 1.   [4] Virg.
[5] Mened. Heautont. act. 1. sc. 1.

Mem. 1. Subs. 2.]   *Symptomes in the Mind.*   397

up, then go to bed, now pleased, then again displeased; now they
like, by and by dislike all, weary of all ; *sequitur nunc vivendi,
nunc moriendi, cupido,* saith Aurelianus (*lib.* 1. *cap.* 6), but,
most part, [1]*vitam damnant;* discontented, disquieted, perplexed upon every light or no occasion, object: often tempted, I
say, to make away themselves : [2]*vivere nolunt, mori nesciunt :*
they cannot dye, they will not live: they complain, weep, lament, and think they lead a most miserable life ; never was any
man so bad, or so before; every poor man they see is more fortunate in respect of them ; every beggar that comes to the door
is happier than they are ; they could be contented to change
lives with them; especially if they be alone, idle, and parted
from their ordinary company, molested, displeased, or provoked,
grief, fear, agony, discontent, wearisomness, laziness, suspicion,
or some such passion, forcibly seizeth on them.   Yet by and
by, when they come in company again, which they like, or be
pleased, *suam sententiam rursus damnant, et vitæ solatio delectantur* (as Octavius Horatianus observes, *lib.* 2. *cap.* 5); they
condemn their former dislike, and are well pleased to live. And
so they continue, till with some fresh discontent they be molested again ; and then they are weary of their lives, weary of
all ; they will dye, and shew rather a necessity to live, than a
desire.   Claudius, the emperour, (as [3]Sueton describes him)
had a spice of this disease ; for, when he was tormented with
the pain of his stomach, he had a conceit to make away himself.
Jul. Cæsar Claudinus (*consil.* 84) had a Polonian to his patient,
so affected, that through fear [4]and sorrow, with which he was
still disquieted, hated his own life, wished for death every moment, and to be freed of his misery.   Mercurialis another, and
another that was often minded to dispatch himself, and so continued for many years.

Suspicion, Jealousie.   Anger sine caussâ.] Suspicion and
jealousie are general symptomes : they are commonly distrustful, timorous, apt to mistake, and amplifie, *facile irascibiles,*
[5]testy, pettish, pievish, and ready to snarl upon every [6]small
occasion, *cum amicissimis,* and without a cause, *datum vel non
datum,* it will be *scandalum acceptum.* If they speak in jest,
he takes it in good earnest. If they be not saluted, invited,
consulted with, called to counsel, &c. or that any respect, small
compliment, or ceremony, be omitted, they think themselves

---

[1] Altomarus.   [2] Seneca.   [3] Cap. 31. Quo (stomachi dolore) se correptum etiam de consciscendâ morte cogitâsse dixit.   [4] Luget, et semper
tristatur, solitudinem amat, mortem sibi precatur, vitam propriam odio habet.
[5] Facile in iram incidunt. Aret.   [6] Ira sine caussâ ; velocitas iræ. Savanarola, pract. major. Velocitas iræ signum. Avicenna, l. 3. Fen. 1. tract. 4.
cap. 18.

neglected and contemned; for a time that tortures them. If two talk together, discourse, whisper, jest, or tell a tale in general, he thinks presently they mean him, applyes all to himself, *de se putat omnia dici.* Or if they talk with him, he is ready to misconstrue every word they speak, and interpret it to the worst; he cannot endure any man to look steadily on him, speak to him almost, laugh, jest, or be familiar, or hemm, or point, cough, or spit, or make a noise sometimes, &c. [1] He thinks they laugh or point at him, or do it in disgrace of him, circumvent him, contemn him; every man looks at him, he is pale, red, sweats for fear and anger, lest some body should observe him. He works upon it; and, long after this, this false conceit of an abuse troubles him. Montanus (*consil.* 22) gives instance in a melancholy Jew, that was *iracundior Adriâ*, so waspish and suspicious, *tam facile iratus,* that no man could tell how to carry himself in his company.

Inconstancy.] Inconstant they are in all their actions, vertiginous, restless, unapt to resolve of any business; they will and will not, perswaded to and fro upon every small occasion, or word spoken; and yet, if once they be resolved, obstinate, hard to be reconciled: if they abhor, dislike, or distaste, once setled, though to the better by odds, by no counsel or perswasion to be removed: yet, in most things, wavering, irresolute, unable to deliberate, through fear; *faciunt, et mox facti pœnitet* (Aretæus); *avari, et paullo post prodigi;* now prodigal, and then covetous, they do, and by-and-by repent them of that which they have done; so that both wayes they are troubled, whether they do or do not, want or have, hit or miss, disquieted of all hands, soon weary, and still seeking change; restless, I say, fickle, fugitive, they may not abide to tarry in one place long,

> [2] (Romæ rus optans, absentem rusticus urbem
> Tollit ad astra——)

no company long, or to persevere in any action or business;

> [3] (Et similis regum pueris, pappare minutum
> Poscit, et iratus mammæ lallare recusat)

eftsoons pleased, and anon displeased: as a man that's bitten with fleas, or that cannot sleep, turns to and fro in his bed, their restless minds are tossed and vary; they have no patience to read out a book, to play out a game or two, walk a mile, sit an hour, &c. erected and dejected in an instant; animated to undertake, and, upon a word spoken, again discouraged.

---

[1] Suspicio, diffidentia, symptomata. Crato, Ep. Julio Alexandrino, cons. 185. Scoltzii.   [2] Hor.   [3] Pers. Sat. 3.

Mem. 1. Subs. 2.]   *Symptomes in the Mind.*   399

Passionate.] Extream passionate, *quidquid volunt, valde volunt;* and what they desire, they do most furiously seek; anxious ever and very solicitous, distrustful and timorous, envious, malicious, profuse one while, sparing another, but most part covetous, muttering, repining, discontent, and still complaining, grudging, pievish, *injuriarum tenaces*, prone to revenge, soon troubled, and most violent in all their imaginations, not affable in speech, or apt to vulgar compliment, but surly, dull, sad, austere; *cogitabundi*, still very intent, and as [1] Albertus Durer paints Melancholy, like a sad woman, leaning on her arm, with fixed looks, neglected habit, &c. held therefore by some proud, soft, sottish, or half mad, as the Abderites esteemed of Democritus; and yet of a deep reach, excellent apprehension, judicious, wise, and witty: for I am of that [2] noblemans mind, *melancholy advanceth mens conceits, more than any humour whatsoever,* improves their meditations more than any strong drink or sack.   They are of profound judgement in some things, although, in others, *non recte judicant inquieti,* saith Fracastorius, (*lib. 2. de Intell.*) and, as Arculanus (*c. 16. in 9 Rhasis*) terms it, *judicium plerumque perversum, corrupti, cum judicant honesta inhonesta, et amicitiam habent pro inimicitiâ:* they count honesty dishonesty, friends as enemies; they will abuse their best friends, and dare not offend their enemies.   Cowards most part, *et ad inferendam injuriam timidissimi,* saith Cardan, (*lib. 8. cap. 4. de rerum varietate):* loth to offend; and, if they chance to overshoot themselves in word or deed, or any small business or circumstance be omitted, forgotten, they are miserably tormented, and frame a thousand dangers and inconveniences to themselves, *ex muscâ elephantem,* if once they conceit it: overjoyed with every good humour, tale, or prosperous event, transported beyond themselves; with every small cross again, bad news, misconceived injury, loss, danger, afflicted, beyond measure, in great agony, perplexed, dejected, astonished, impatient, utterly undone; fearful, suspicious of all: yet again, many of them, desperate hare-brains, rash, careless, fit to be assassinates, as being void of all fear and sorrow, according to [3] Hercules de Saxoniâ, *most audacious, and such as dare walk alone in the night, through deserts and dangerous places, fearing none.*

Amorous.] *They are prone to love,* and [4] easie to be taken: *propensi ad amorem et excandescentiam,* (Montaltus, *cap.* 21.) quickly inamored, and dote upon all, love one dearly, till they

_____
[1] In his Dutch-work picture.   [2] Howard, cap. 7. differ.   [3] Tract. de mel. cap. 2. Noctu ambulant per sylvas, et loca periculosa; neminem timent.   [4] Facile amant. Altom.

400   *Symptomes of Melancholy.*   [Part. 1. Sec. 3.

see another, and then dote on her, *et hanc, et hanc, et illam, et omnes;* the present moves most, and the last commonly they love best. Yet some again, *anterotes*, cannot endure the sight of a woman, abhor the sex, as that same melancholy [1] duke of Muscovy, that was instantly sick, if he came but in sight of them; and that [2] anchorite, that fell into a cold palsie, when a woman was brought before him.

Humorous.] Humorous they are beyond all measure, sometimes profusely laughing, extraordinary merry, and then again weeping without a cause, (which is familiar with many gentlewomen) groaning, sighing, pensive, sad, almost distracted: *multa absurda fingunt, et a ratione aliena* (saith [3] Frambesarius): they feign many absurdities, vain, void of reason: one supposeth himself to be a dog, cock, bear, horse, glass, butter, &c. He is a giant, a dwarf, as strong as an hundred men, a lord, duke, prince, &c. And, if he be told he hath a stinking breath, a great nose, that he is sick, or inclined to such or such a disease, he believes it eftsoons, and peradventure, by force of imagination, will work it out. Many of them are immoveable, and fixed in their conceits; others vary, upon every object heard or seen. If they see a stage-play, they run upon that a week after; if they hear musick, or see dancing, they have nought but bag-pipes in their brain: if they see a combat, they are all for arms: [4] if abused, an abuse troubles them long after: if crossed, that cross, &c. Restless in their thoughts and actions, continually meditating,

————velut ægri somnia, vanæ
Finguntur species;

more like dreamers than men awake, they feign a company of antick, fantastical conceits; they have most frivolous thoughts, impossible to be effected; and sometimes think verily they hear and see present before their eyes such phantasms or goblins, they fear, suspect, or conceive, they still talk with, and follow them. In fine, *cogitationes somniantibus similes, id vigilant, quod alii somniant, cogitabundi;* still (saith Avicenna), they wake, as others dream; and such, for the most part, are their imaginations and conceits, [5] absurd, vain, foolish toyes; yet they are [6] most curious and solicitous; continually *et supra modum* (Rhasis, *cont. lib.* 1. *cap.* 9) *præmeditantur de aliquâ re.* As serious in a toy, as if it were a most necessary business, of

[1] Bodine.   [2] Jo. Major vitis patrum, fol. 202. Paullus abbas, eremita, tantâ solitudine perseverat, ut nec vestem nec vultum mulieris ferre possit, &c.   [3] Consult. lib. 1. 17. Cons.   [4] Generally, as they are pleased or displeasing, so are their continual cogitations pleasing or displeasing.   [5] Omnes exercent vanæ intensæque animi cogitationes, (N. Piso. Bruel.) et assiduæ.   [6] Curiosi de rebus minimis. Aretæus.

Mem. 1. Subs. 2.]   *Symptomes in the Mind.*   401

great moment, importance, and still, still, still thinking of it, *sæviunt in se*, macerating themselves. Though they do talk with you, and seem to be otherwise employed, and, to your thinking, very intent and busie, still that toy runs in their mind, that fear, that suspicion, that abuse, that jealousie, that agony, that vexation, that cross, that castle in the air, that crotchet, that whimsie, that fiction, that pleasant waking dream, whatsoever it is. *Nec interrogant* (saith [1] Fracastorius), *nec interrogati recte respondent;* they do not much heed what you say; their mind is on another matter. Ask what you will; they do not attend, or much intend that business they are about, but forget themselves what they are saying, doing, or should otherwise say or do, whither they are going, distracted with their own melancholy thoughts. One laughs upon a sudden, another smiles to himself, a third frowns, calls, his lips go still, he acts with his hand as he walks, &c. 'Tis proper to all melancholy men (saith [2] Mercurialis, *con.* 11), *what conceit they have once entertained, to be most intent, violent, and continually about it. Invitis occurrit;* do what they may, they cannot be rid of it; against their wills they must think of it a thousand times over; *perpetuo molestantur, nec oblivisci possunt;* they are continually troubled with it, in company, out of company: at meat, at exercise, at all times and places, [3] *non desinunt ea, quæ minime volunt, cogitare;* if it be offensive especially, they cannot forget it; they may not rest or sleep for it, but, still tormenting themselves, *Sisyphi saxum volvunt sibi ipsis*, as [4] Brunner observes; *perpetua calamitas, et miserabile flagellum.*

Bashfulness.]   [5] Crato, [6] Laurentius, and Fernelius, put bashfulness for an ordinary symptome; *subrusticus pudor*, or *vitiosus pudor*, is a thing which much haunts and torments them. If they have been misused, derided, disgraced, chidden, &c. or, by any perturbation of mind, misaffected, it so far troubles them, that they become quite moped many times, and so disheartened, dejected, they dare not come abroad, into strange companies especially, or manage their ordinary affairs; so childish, timorous, and bashful, they can look no man in the face. Some are more disquieted in this kind, some less, longer some, others shorter, by fits, &c. though some, on the other side (according to [7] Fracastorius), be *inverecundi et pertinaces*, impudent and pievish. But, most part, they are very shamefac'd; and that makes them (with Pet. Blesensis,

---

[1] Lib. 2. de Intell.   [2] Hoc melancholicis omnibus proprium, ut, quas semel imaginationes valde receperint, non facile rejiciant, sed hæ etiam vel invitis semper occurrant.   [3] Tullius, de Sen.   [4] Consil. med. pro Hypochondriaco.   [5] Consil. 43.   [6] Cap. 5.   [7] Lib. 2. de Intell.

VOL. I.   D D

402   *Symptomes of Melancholy.*   [Part. 1. Sec. 3.

Christopher Urswick, and many such) to refuse honours, offices, and preferments, which sometimes fall into their mouths: they cannot speak, or put forth themselves, as others can; *timor hos, pudor impedit illos;* timorousness and bashfulness hinder their proceedings; they are contented with their present estate, unwilling to undertake any office, and therefore never likely to rise. For that cause, they seldome visit their friends, except some familiars; *pauciloqui*, of few words, and oftentimes wholly silent. [1] Frambesarius, a Frenchman, had two such patients, *omnino taciturnos :* their friends could not get them to speak: Rodericus a Fonseca (*consult. Tom.* 2. 85. *consil.*) gives instance in a young man, of twenty-seven years of age, that was frequently silent, bashful, moped, solitary, that would not eat his meat, or sleep, and yet again by fits apt to be angry, &c.

Solitariness.] Most part they are (as Plater notes), *desides, taciturni, ægre impulsi, nec nisi coacti procedunt, &c.* they will scarce be compelled to do that which concerns them, though it be for their good; so diffident, so dull, of small or no complement, unsociable, hard to be acquainted with, especially of strangers; they had rather write their minds, than speak, and above all things love solitariness. *Ob voluptatem, an ob timorem, soli sunt?* Are they so solitary for pleasure, (one asks), or pain? for both: yet I rather think, for fear and sorrow, &c.

> [2] Hinc metuunt, cupiuntque, dolent, fugiuntque, nec auras
> Respiciunt, clausi tenebris, et carcere cæco.

> Hence 'tis they grieve and fear, avoiding light,
> And shut themselves in prison dark from sight.

As Bellerophon, in [3] Homer,

> Qui miser in sylvis mœrens errabat opacis,
> Ipse suum cor edens, hominum vestigia vitans—

> That wandred in the woods sad all alone,
> Forsaking mens society, making great moan—

they delight in floods and waters, desert places, to walk alone in orchards, gardens, private walks, back-lanes; averse from company, as Diogenes in his tub, or Timon Misanthropus, [4] they abhor all companions at last, even their nearest acquaintance, and most familiar friends; for they have a conceit (I say), every man observes them, will deride, laugh to scorn, or misuse them; confining themselves therefore wholly to their private houses or chambers, *fugiunt homines sine caussâ* (saith

---

[1] Consil. 15. et 16. lib. 1.   [2] Virg. Æn. 6.   [3] Iliad. 6.   [4] Si malum exasperatur, homines odio habent, et solitaria petunt.

Mem. 1. Subs. 2.]   *Symptomes in the Mind.*   403

Rhasis) *et odio habent* (*cont. l.* 1. *c.* 9): they will dyet themselves, feed and live alone.   It was one of the chiefest reasons,
why the citizens of Abdera suspected Democritus to be melancholy and mad, because that (as Hippocrates related in his
epistle to Philopœmenes) [1] *he forsook the city, and lived in
groves and hollow trees, upon a green bank by a brook side,
or confluence of waters, all day long, and all night.   Quæ
quidem* (saith he) *plurimum atrâ bile vexatis et melancholicis
eveniunt; deserta frequentant, hominumque congressum aversantur;* [2] which is an ordinary thing with melancholy men.
The Ægyptians therefore, in their *hieroglyphicks,* expressed a
melancholy man by a hare sitting in her form, as being a most
timorous and solitary creature (Pierius, *Hieroglyph. l.* 12).
But this and all precedent symptomes are more or less apparent, as the humour is intended or remitted, hardly perceived
in some, or not at all, most manifest in others.   Childish in
some, terrible in others; to be derided in one, pitied or admired
in another; to him by fits, to a second continuate; and, howsoever these symptomes be common and incident to all persons,
yet they are the more remarkable, frequent, furious, and violent, in melancholy men.   To speak in a word, there is nothing
so vain, absurd, ridiculous, extravagant, impossible, incredible,
so monstrous a chimæra, so prodigious and strange, [3] such as
painters and poets durst not attempt, which they will not really
fear, fain, suspect, and imagine unto themselves: and that
which [4] Lod. Viv. said in jest of a silly countrey fellow, that
kill'd his ass for drinking up the moon, *ut lunam mundo redderet;* you may truly say of them in earnest: they will act,
conceive all extreams, contrarieties, and contradictions, and
that in infinite varieties.   *Melancholici plane incredibilia sibi
persuadent, ut vix omnibus sæculis duo reperti sint, qui idem
imaginati sint* (Erastus, *de Lamiis*): scarce two of two thousand
that concur in the same symptomes.   The tower of Babel never
yielded such confusion of tongues, as this chaos of melancholy
doth variety of symptomes.   There is in all melancholy *similitudo dissimilis,* like mens faces, a disagreeing likeness still;
and as, in a river, we swim in the same place, though not
in the same numerical water; as the same instrument affords
several lessons, so the same disease yields diversity of symptomes; which howsoever they be diverse, intricate, and hard
to be confined, I will adventure yet, in such a vast confusion

[1] Democritus solet noctes et dies apud se degere, plerumque autem in spe-
luncis, sub amœnis arborum umbris vel in tenebris, et mollibus herbis, vel ad aquarum crebra et quieta fluenta, &c.   [2] Gaudet tenebris, aliturque dolor. Ps. 62.
Vigilavi, et factus sum velut nycticorax in domicilio, passer solitarius in templo.
[3] Et, quæ vix audet fabula, monstra parit.   [4] In cap. 18. l. 10. de civ. Dei.
Lunam ab asino epotam videns.

404   *Symptomes of Melancholy.*   [Part. 1. Sec. 3.

and generality, to bring them into some order ; and so descend
to particulars.

SUBSECT. III.

Particular Symptomes from the influence of Stars ; parts of the
body, and humours.

SOME men have peculiar symptomes, according to their temperament and *crisis,* which they had from the stars and
those celestial influences, variety of wits and dispositions, as
Anthony Zara contends (*Anat. ingen. sect.* 1. *memb.* 11, 12,
13, 14), *plurimum irritant influentiæ cœlestes, unde cientur*
animi ægritudines, et morbi corporum. [1] One saith, diverse
diseases of the body and mind proceed from their influences,
[2] as I have already proved out of Ptolemy, Pontanus, Lemnius, Cardan, and others, as they are principal significators of
manners, diseases, mutually irradiated, or lords of the geniture,
&c. Ptolemæus, in his Centiloquy, (or Hermes, or whosoever
else the author of that tract,) attributes all these symptomes,
which are in melancholy men, to celestial influences ; which
opinion Mercurialis (*de affect. lib.* 1. *cap.* 10) rejects : but, as
I say, [3] Jovianus Pontanus and others stifly defend. That some
are solitary, dull, heavy, churlish; some again blith, buxom,
light and merry, they ascribe wholly to the stars.   As, if
Saturn be predominant in his nativity, and cause melancholy
in his temperature, then [4]he shall be very austere, sullen,
churlish, black of colour, profound in his cogitations, full of
cares, miseries, and discontents, sad and fearful, alwayes
silent, solitary, still delighting in husbandry, in woods, orchards, gardens, rivers, ponds, pools, dark walks and close ;
cogitationes sunt velle ædificare, velle arbores plantare, agros
colere, &c. to catch birds, fishes, &c. still contriving and
musing of such matters.   If Jupiter domineers, they are more
ambitious, still meditating of kingdoms, magistracies, offices,
honours, or that they are princes, potentates, and how they
would carry themselves, &c.—if Mars, they are all for wars,
brave combats, monomachies, testy, cholerick, hare-brain'd,
rash, furious and violent in their actions : they will fain
themselves victors, commanders, are passionate and satyrical
in their speeches, great braggers, ruddy of colour: and though
they be poor in shew, vile and base, yet, like Telephus and
Peleus in the [5] poet,

Ampullas jactant, et sesquipedalia verba ;

[1] Velc. l. 4. c. 5.   [2] Sect. 2. Memb. 1. Subs. 4.   [3] De reb. cœlest.
lib. 10. c. 13.   [4] J. de Indagine Goclenius.   [5] Hor. de Art. Poët.

Mem. 1. Subs. 3.] *Symptomes from the Stars, &c.* 405

their mouths are full of myriades, and tetrarchs at their tongues end:—if the Sun, they will be lords, emperours, in conceit at least, and monarchs, give offices, honours, &c.—if Venus, they are still courting of their mistresses, and most apt to love, amorously given; they seem to hear musick, playes, see fine pictures, dancers, merriments, and the like—ever in love, and dote on all they see. Mercurialists are solitary, much in contemplation, subtile, poets, philosophers, and musing most part about such matters. If the Moon have a hand, they are all for peregrinations, sea-voyages, much affected with travels, to discourse, read, meditate of such things; wandring in their thoughts, divers, much delighting in waters, to fish, fowl, &c.

But the most immediate symptomes proceed from the temperature it self, and organical parts, as head, liver, spleen, mesaraïck veins, heart, womb, stomach, &c. and most especially from distemperature of spirits (which, as [1] Hercules de Saxoniâ contends, are wholly immaterial), or from the four humours in those seats, whether they be hot or cold, natural, unnatural, innate or adventitious, intended or remitted, simple or mixt, their diverse mixtures, and several adustions, combinations, which may be as diversly varied, as those [2] four first qualities in [3] Clavius, and produce as many several symptomes and monstrous fictions as wine doth effects, which (as Andreas Bachius observes, *lib. 3. de vino, cap.* 20) are infinite. Of greater note be these.

If it be natural melancholy (as Lod. Mercatus, *lib. 1. cap.* 17. *de melan.* T. Bright, *c.* 16. hath largely described) either of the spleen, or of the veins, faulty by excess of quantity, or thickness of substance, it is a cold and dry humour, as Montanus affirms (*consil.* 26); the parties are sad, timorous, and fearful. Prosper Calenus, in his book *de atrâ bile*, will have them to be more stupid than ordinary, cold, heavy, dull, solitary, sluggish, *si multam atram bilem et frigidam habent.* Hercules de Saxoniâ (*c.* 19. *l.* 7) [4] *holds these that are naturally melancholy, to be of a leaden colour or black* (and so doth Guianerius, *c. 3. tract.* 15), and such as think themselves dead many times, or that they see, talk with, black men, dead men, spirits and goblins frequently, if it be in excess. These symptomes vary according to the mixture of those four humours adust, which is unnatural melancholy. For (as Trallianus hath written, *cap.* 16. *l.* 7) [5] *there is not one cause of this*

---

[1] Tract. 7. de Melan.   [2] Humidum, calidum, frigidum, siccum.   [3] Com. in 1. c. Johannis de Sacrobosco.   [4] Si residet melancholia naturalis, tales plumbei coloris aut nigri, stupidi, solitarii.   [5] Non una melancholiæ caussa est, nec unus humor vitii parens, sed plures, et alius aliter mutatus; unde non omnes eadem sentiunt symptomata.

406   *Symptomes of Melancholy.*   [Part. 1. Sec. 3.

melancholy, nor one humour which begets it, but divers diversly intermixt; from whence proceeds this variety of symptomes; and those varying again as they are hot or cold. [1] *Cold melancholy* (saith Benedic. Vittorius Faventinus, *prac. mag.) is a cause of dotage, and more mild symptomes; if hot or more adust, of more violent passions, and furies.* Fracastorius (*l. 2. de intellect.*) will have us to consider well of it, [2] *with what kind of melancholy every one is troubled; for it much avails to know it: one is inraged by fervent heat; another is possessed by sad and cold: one is fearful, shamefac't; the other, impudent and bold, as Ajax,*

> Arma rapit, Superosque furens in prælia poscit;

quite mad, or tending to madness; *nunc hos, nunc impetit illos.* Bellerophon, on the other side, *solis errat male sanus in agris,* wanders alone in the woods: one despairs, weeps, and is weary of his life; another laughs, &c. All which variety is produced from the several degrees of heat and cold, which [3] Hercules de Saxoniâ will have wholly proceed from the distemperature of spirits alone, animal especially, and those immaterial, the next and immediate causes of melancholy, as they are hot, cold, dry, moist; and from their agitation proceeds that diversity of symptomes, which he reckons up, in the [4] thirteenth chapter of his Tract of Melancholy, and that largely through every part. Others will have them come from the divers adustion of the four humours, which, in this unnatural melancholy, by corruption of blood, adust choler or melancholy natural, [5] *by excessive distemper of heat, turned, in comparison of the natural, into a sharp lye by force of adustion, cause, according to the diversity of their matter, diverse and strange symptomes,* which T. Bright reckons up in his following chapter. So doth [6] Arculanus, according to the four principal humours adust, and many others.

For example, if it proceed from flegm (which is seldom and not so frequent as the rest) [7] it stirs up dull symptomes, and a kind of stupidity, or impassionate hurt: they are sleepy, saith [8] Savanarola, dull, slow, cold, blockish, ass-like, *asininam melancholiam,* [9] Melancthon calls it, *they are much given to weeping, and delight in waters, ponds, pools, rivers, fishing, fowling, &c.* (Arnoldus, *breviar. lib.* 1. *cap.* 18) they

---

[1] Humor frigidus delirii caussa, humor calidus furoris.   [2] Multum refert quâ quisque melancholiâ teneatur; hunc fervens et accensa agitat; illum tristis et frigens occupat: hi timidi, illi inverecundi, intrepidi, &c.   [3] Cap. 7. et 8. Tract. de Mel.   [4] Signa melancholiæ ex intemperie et agitatione spirituum sine materiâ.   [5] T. Bright, cap. 16. Treat. Mel.   [6] Cap. 16. in 9. Rhasis.   [7] Bright, c. 16.   [8] Pract. major. Somnians, piger, frigidus. [9] De animâ, cap. de humor. Si a phlegmate, semper in aquis fere sunt, et circa fluvios plorant multum, &c.

[1] pale of colour, slothful, apt to sleep, heavy; [2] *much troubled with the head-ach,* continual meditation, and muttering to themselves; they dream of waters, [3] that they are in danger of drowning, and fear such things (Rhasis). They are fatter than others that are melancholy, of a muddy complexion, apter to spit, [4] sleep, more troubled with rheum than the rest, and have their eyes still fixed on the ground. Such a patient had Hercules de Saxoniâ, a widow in Venice, that was fat and very sleepy still, Christophorus a Vega, another affected in the same sort. If it be inveterate or violent, the symptomes are more evident, they plainly dote and are ridiculous to others, in all their gestures, actions, speeches: imagining impossibilities, as he in Christophorus a Vega, that thought he was a tun of wine, [5] and that Siennois, that resolved with himself not to piss, for fear he should drown all the town.

If it proceed from blood adust, or that there be a mixture of blood in it, [6] *such are commonly ruddy of complexion, and high-coloured,* according to Sallust Salvianus, and Hercules de Saxoniâ; and, as Savanarola, Vittorius Faventinus Empir. farther add, [7] *the veins of their eyes be red, as well as their faces.* They are much inclined to laughter, witty and merry, conceited in discourse, pleasant, if they be not far gone, much given to musick, dancing, and to be in womens company. They meditate wholly on such things, and think [8] *they see or hear playes, dancing, and such like sports* (free from all fear and sorrow, as [9] Hercules de Saxoniâ supposeth) if they be more strongly possessed with this kind of melancholy (Arnoldus adds, *Breviar. lib.* 1. *cap.* 18), like him of Argos, in the poet, that sate laughing [10] all day long, as if he had been at a theatre. Such another is mentioned by [11] Aristotle living at Abydos a town of Asia Minor, that would sit after the same fashion, as if he had been upon a stage, and sometimes act himself; now clap his hands, and laugh, as if he had been well pleased with the sight. Wolfius relates of a countrey fellow, called Brunsellius, subject to this humour, [12] *that being by chance at a sermon, saw a woman fall off from a form half asleep; at which object most of the*

---

[1] Pigra nascitur ex colore pallido et albo. Her. de Saxon. [2] Savanarola. [3] Muros cadere in se, aut submergi, timent, cum torpore et segnitie, et fluvios amant tales. Alexand. c. 16. lib. 7. [4] Semper fere dormit somnolenta, c. 16. l. 7. [5] Laurentius. [6] Cap. 6. de mel. Si a sanguine, venit rubedo oculorum et faciei, plurimus risus. [7] Venæ oculorum sunt rubræ; vide an præcesserit vini et aromatum usus, et frequens balneum. Trallian. lib. 1. 16. an præcesserit mora sub sole. [8] Ridet patiens, si a sanguine; putat se videre choreas, musicam audire, ludos, &c. [9] Cap. 2. Tract. de Melan. [10] Hor. ep. lib. 2. Quidam haud ignobilis Argis, &c. [11] Lib. de reb. mir. [12] Cum, inter concionandum, mulier dormiens e subsellio caderet, et omnes reliqui, qui id viderent, riderent, tribus post diebus, &c.

408   *Symptomes of Melancholy.*   [Part. 1. Sec. 3.

company laughed; but he, for his part, was so much moved, that, for three whole daies after, he did nothing but laugh; by which means he was much weakened, and worse a long time following. Such a one was old Sophocles; and Democritus himself had *hilare delirium*, much in this vein. Laurentius (*cap. 3. de melan.*) thinks this kind of melancholy which is a little adust with some mixture of blood, to be that which Aristotle meant, when he said melancholy men of all others are most witty, which causeth many times a divine ravishment, and a kind of *enthusiasmus*, which stirreth them up to be excellent philosophers, poets, prophets, &c. Mercurialis (*consil.* 110) gives instance in a young man his patient, sanguine melancholy, [1] *of a great wit, and excellently learned.*

If it arise from choler adust, they are bold and impudent, and of a more hair-brain disposition, apt to quarrel, and think of such things, battels, combats, and their manhood; furious, impatient in discourse, stiff, irrefragable and prodigious in their tenents; and, if they be moved, most violent, outragious, [2] ready to disgrace, provoke any, to kill themselves and others; Arnoldus adds, stark mad by fits; [3] *they sleep little, their urine is subtle and fiery;* (Guianerius) *in their fits you shall hear them speak all manner of languages, Hebrew, Greek, and Latine, that never were taught or knew them before.* Apponensis (*in com. in Pro. sec.* 30) speaks of a mad woman that spake excellent good Latine; and Rhasis knew another, that could prophesie in her fit, and foretel things truely to come. [4] Guianerius had a patient could make Latine verses when the moon was combust, otherwise illiterate. Avicenna and some of his adherents will have these symptomes, when they happen, to proceed from the devil, and that they are rather *dæmoniaci*, possessed, than mad or melancholy, or both together, as Jason Pratensis thinks; *immiscent se mali genii, &c.* but most ascribe it to the humour; which opinion Montaltus (*cap.* 21.) stifly maintains, confuting Avicenna and the rest, referring it wholly to the quality and disposition of the humour and subject. Cardan (*de rerum var. lib.* 8. *cap.* 10) holds these men, of all others, fit to be assassinates, bold, hardy, fierce, and adventurous, to undertake any thing by reason of their choler adust. [5] *This humour,* saith he, *prepares them to endure death itself, and all manner of torments, with invincible courage; and*

---

[1] Juvenis, et non vulgaris eruditionis.   [2] Si a cholerâ, furibundi interficiunt se et alios; putant se videre pugnas.   [3] Urina subtilis et ignea; parum dormiunt.   [4] Tract. 15. c. 4.   [5] Ad hæc perpetranda furore rapti ducuntur; cruciatus quosvis tolerant, et mortem; et furore exacerbato audent, et ad supplicia plus irritantur; mirum est, quantam habeant in tormentis patientiam.

Mem. 1. Subs. 3.] *Symptomes from the Stars, &c.* 409

'tis a wonder to see with what alacrity they will undergo such tortures, *ut supra naturam res videatur :* he ascribes this generosity, fury, or rather stupidity, to this adustion of choler and melancholy : but I take these rather to be mad or desperate, than properly melancholy : for commonly this humour, so adust and hot, degenerates into madness.

If it come from melancholy it self adust, those men (saith Avicenna [1]) *are usually sad and solitary, and that continually, and in excess, more than ordinary suspicious, more fearful, and have long, sore, and most corrupt imaginations;* cold and black, bashful, and so solitary, that (as [2] Arnoldus writes) *they will endure no company ; they dream of graves still, and dead men, and think themselves bewitched or dead :* if it be extream, they think they hear hideous noyses, see and talk [3] *with black men, and converse familiarly with devils ; and such strange chimeras and visions* (Gordonius), or that they are possessed by them, that some body talks to them, or within them. *Tales melancholici plerumque dæmoniaci* (Montaltus, *consil.* 26 *ex* Avicenna.) Valescus de Taranta had such a woman in cure, [4] *that thought she had to do with the devil :* and Gentilis Fulgosus (*quæst.* 55) writes that he had a melancholy friend, that [5] *had a black man in the likeness of a souldier,* still following him wheresoever he was. Laurentius (*cap.* 7) hath many stories of such as have thought themselves bewitched by their enemies; and some that would eat no meat, as being dead. [6] Anno 1550, an advocate of Paris fell into such a melancholy fit, that he believed verily he was dead ; he could not be perswaded otherwise, or to eat or drink, till a kinsman of his, a scholar of Bourges, did eat before him, dressed like a corse. The story (saith Serres) was acted in a comedy before Charles the Ninth. Some think they are beasts, wolves, hogs, and [7] cry like dogs, foxes, bray like asses, and low like kine, as king Prœtus daughters. Hildesheim (*spicil.* 2 *de Maniá*) hath an example of a Dutch baron so affected; and Trincavellius (*lib.* 1. *consil.* 11) another of a noble man in his countrey, [8] *that thought he was certainly a beast, and would imitate most of their voices,* with many such symptomes, which may properly be reduced to this kind.

If it proceed from the several combinations of these four

---

[1] Tales plus cæteris timent, et continue tristantur; valde suspiciosi, solitudinem diligunt; corruptissimas habent imaginationes, &c. [2] Si a melancholiâ adustâ, tristes, de sepulcris somniant, timent ne fascinentur, putant se mortuos, adspici nolunt. [3] Videntur sibi videre monachos nigros et dæmones, et suspensos et mortuos. [4] Quâvis nocte se cum dæmone coire putavit. [5] Semper fere vidisse militem nigrum præsentem. [6] Anthony de Verdeur. [7] Quidam mugitus boum æmulantur, et pecora se putant, ut Prœti filiæ. [8] Baro quidam mugitus boum, et rugitus asinorum, et aliorum animalium voces, effingit.

410   *Symptomes of Melancholy.*   [Part. 1. Sec. 3.

humours, or spirits (Herc. de Saxon. adds hot, cold, dry, moist, dark, confused, setled, constringed, as it participates of matter, or is without matter), the symptomes are likewise mixt. One thinks himself a giant, another a dwarf; one is heavy as lead, another is as light as a feather. Marcellus Donatus (*l. 2. cap.* 41) makes mention, out of Seneca, one of Seneccio, a rich man, [1] *that thought himself and every thing else he had, great—great wife, great horses; could not abide little things, but would have great pots to drink in, great hose, and great shoos bigger than his feet*—like her in [2] Trallianus, *that supposed she could shake all the world with her finger,* and was afraid to clinch her hand together, lest she should crush the world like an apple in pieces—or him in Galen, that thought he was [3] Atlas, and sustained heaven with his shoulders.   Another thinks himself so little, that he can creep into a mousehole: one fears heaven will fall on his head: a second is a cock; and such a one [4] Guianerius saith he saw at Padua, that would clap his hands together, and crow.   [5] Another thinks he is a nightingale, and therefore sings all the night long: another, he is all glass, a pitcher, and will therefore let no body come near him; and such a one [6] Laurentius gives out upon his credit, that he knew in France. Christophorus a Vega (*cap.* 3. *lib.* 14), Skenkius, and Marcellus Donatus (*l. 2. cap.* 1), have many such examples, and one, amongst the rest, of a baker in Ferrara, that thought he was composed of butter, and durst not sit in the sun, or come near the fire, for fear of being melted; of another that thought he was a case of leather, stuffed with wind.   Some laugh, weep; some are mad, some dejected, moped, in much agony, some by fits, others continuate, &c.   Some have a corrupt ear (they think they hear musick, or some hideous noise, as their phantasie conceives), corrupt eyes, some smelling, some one sense, some another. [7] Lewis the eleventh had a conceit every thing did stink about him: all the odoriferous perfumes they could get, would not ease him; but still he smelled a filthy stink.   A melancholy French poet, in [8] Laurentius, being sick of a fever, and troubled with waking, by his physicians was appointed to use *unguentum populeum* to anoint his temples; but he so distasted the smell of it, that, for many years after, all that came near him he imagined to scent of it, and would let no man talk with him but aloof off, or wear any new clothes, because he thought still

---

[1] Omnia magna putabat, uxorem magnam, grandes equos; abhorruit omnia parva : magna pocula, et calceamenta pedibus majora.   [2] Lib. 1. cap. 16. Putavit se uno digito posse totum mundum conterere.   [3] Sustinet humeris cœlum cum Atlante. Alii cœli ruinam timent.   [4] Cap. 1. Tract. 15. Alius se gallum putat, alius lusciniam.   [5] Trallianus.   [6] Cap. 7. de mel.   [7] Anthony de Verdeur.   [8] Cap. 7. de mel.

Mem. 1. Subs. 4.] *Symptomes from Custome.* 411

are they smelled of it; in all other things wise and dicreet, he would talk sensibly, save only in this. A gentleman in Lymosen (saith Anthony Verdeur), was perswaded he had but one legg: affrighted by a wild boar, that by chance stroke him on the legg, he could not be satisfied his legg was sound (in all other things well) until two Franciscans, by chance coming that way, fully removed him from the conceipt. *Sed abunde fabularum audivimus.*

SUBSECT. IV.

Symptomes from education, custome, continuance of time, our condition, mixt with other diseases, by fits, inclination, &c.

ANOTHER great occasion of the variety of these symptomes proceeds from custome, discipline, education, and several inclinations. [1] This humour will imprint in melancholy men the objects most answerable to their condition of life, and ordinary actions, and dispose men according to their several studies and callings. If an ambitious man become melancholy, he forthwith thinks he is a king, an emperour, a monarch, and walks alone, pleasing himself with a vain hope of some future preferment, or present, as he supposeth, and withal acts a lords part, takes upon him to be some statesman, or magnifico, makes congies, gives entertainments, looks big, &c. Francisco Sansovino records of a melancholy man in Cremona, that would not be induced to believe but that he was pope, gave pardons, made cardinals, &c. [2] Christophorus a Vega makes mention of another of his acquaintance, that thought he was a king driven from his kingdom, and was very anxious to recover his estate. A covetous person is still conversant about purchasing of lands and tenements, plotting in his mind how to compass such and such mannors, as if he were already lord of, and able to go through with it; all he sees is his, *re* or *spe ;* he hath devoured it in hope, or else in conceit esteems it his own; like him in [3] Athenæus, that thought all the ships in the haven to be his own. A lascivious *inamorato* plots all the day long to please his mistriss, acts and struts, and carries himself, as if she were in presence, still dreaming of her, as

[1] Laurentius, cap. 6.   [2] Lib. 3. cap. 14. Qui se regem putavit regno expulsum.   [3] Dipnosophist. lib. Thrasylaüs putavit omnes naves in Piræeum portum appellentes suas esse.

412   *Symptomes of Melancholy.*   [Part. 1. Sec. 3.

Pamphilus of his Glycerium, or as some do in their morning sleep. [1] Marcellus Donatus knew such a gentlewoman in Mantua, called Elionora Meliorina, that constantly believed she was married to a king, and [2] would kneel down and talk with him, as if he had been there present with his associates; and if she had found by chance a piece of glass in a muck-hill or in the street, she would say that it was a jewell sent from her lord and husband. If devout and religious, he is all for fasting, prayer, ceremonies, alms, interpretations, visions, prophecies, revelations; [3] he is inspired by the Holy Ghost, full of the spirit; one while he is saved, another while damned, or still troubled in mind for his sins; the devil will surely have him, &c. More of these in the third partition of love-melancholy. [4] A scholars mind is busied about his studies; he applauds himself for that he hath done, or hopes to do, one while fearing to be out in his next exercise, another while contemning all censures; envies one, emulates another; or else, with indefatigable pains and meditation, consumes himself. So of the rest, all which vary according to the more remiss and violent impression of the object, or as the humour it self is intended or remitted: for some are so gently melancholy, that, in all their carriage, and to the outward apprehension of others, it can hardly be discerned, yet to them an intolerable burden, and not to be endured. [5] *Quædam occulta, quædam manifesta;* some signs are manifest and obvious to all at all times, some to few, or seldom, or hardly perceived: let them keep their own counsel, none will take notice or suspect them. *They do not express in outward shew their depraved imaginations* (as [6] Hercules de Saxoniâ observes), *but conceal them wholly to themselves, and are very wise men, as I have often seen; some fear; some do not fear at all, as such as think themselves kings or dead; some have more signs, some fewer, some great, some less;* some vex, fret, still fear, grieve, lament, suspect, laugh, sing, weep, chafe, &c. by fits (as I have said), or more during and permanent. Some dote in one thing, are most childish, and ridiculous, and to be wondered at in that, and yet, for all other matters, most discreet and wise. To some it is in disposition, to another in habit: and, as they write of heat and cold, we may say of this humour, one is *melancholicus ad octo,* a second two degrees less, a third half way. 'Tis super-particular, *sesquialtera, ses-*

---

[1] De hist. Med. mirab. lib. 2. cap. 1.   [2] Genibus flexis loqui cum illo voluit, et adstare jam tum putavit, &c.   [3] Gordonius. Quod sit propheta, et inflatus a Spiritu Sancto.   [4] Qui forensibus caussis insudat, nil nisi arresta cogitat, et supplices libellos; alius non nisi versus facit. P. Forestus.   [5] Gordonius. [6] Verbo non exprimunt, nec opere, sed altâ mente recondunt; et sunt viri prudentissimi, quos ego sæpe novi; cum multi sint sine timore, ut qui se reges et mortuos putant; plura signa quidam habent, pauciora, majora, minora.

Mem. 1. Subs. 4.] *Symptomes from Custome.* 413

quitertia, and *superbipartiens tertias, quintas melancholiæ, &c.*
all those geometrical proportions are too little to express it.
[1] *It comes to many by fits, and goes; to others it is continuate:*
many (saith [2] Faventinus) *in spring and fall only are molested;*
some once a year, as that Roman, [3] Galen speaks of; [4] one,
at the conjunction of the moon alone, or some unfortunate
aspects, at such and such set hours and times, like the sea-
tides; to some women when they be with child, as [5] Plater
notes, never otherwise; to others 'tis settled and fixed: to one,
led about and variable still by that *ignis fatuus* of phantasie,
like an *arthritis*, or running gout, 'tis here and there, and in
every joint, always molesting some part or other; or if the
body be free, in a myriad of forms exercising the mind. A
second, once peradventure in his life, hath a most grievous fit,
once in seven years, once in five years, even to the extremity
of madness, death, or dotage, and that upon some feral accident or perturbation, terrible object, and that for a time, never
perhaps so before, never after. A third is moved upon all
such troublesome objects, cross fortune, disaster, and violent
passions, otherwise free, once troubled in three or four years.
A fourth, if things be to his mind, or he in action, well pleased
in good company, is most jocund, and of a good complexion;
if idle, or alone, *à la mort*, or carryed away wholly with
pleasant dreams and phantasies, but if once crossed and displeased,

> Pectore concipiet nil nisi triste suo:

his countenance is altered on a sudden, his heart heavy: irksome thoughts crucifie his soul, and in an instant he is moped
or weary of his life, he will kill himself. A fifth complains in
his youth, a sixth in his middle age, the last in his old age.

Generally thus much we may conclude of melancholy—that
it is [6] most pleasant at first, I say, *mentis gratissimus error*, a
most delightsome humour, to be alone, dwell alone, walk alone,
meditate, lye in bed whole dayes, dreaming awake as it were,
and frame a thousand phantastical imaginations unto themselves. They are never better pleased than when they are so
doing: they are in Paradise for the time, and cannot well endure to be interrupt; with him in the poet,

> ——————[7] pol! me occidistis, amici,
> Non servâstis, ait——————

you have undone him, he complains, if you trouble him: tell

---

[1] Trallianus, lib. 1. 16. Alii intervalla quædam habent, ut etiam consueta
administrent; alii in continuo delirio sunt, &c.   [2] Prag. mag. Vere tantum et
autumno.   [3] Lib. de humoribus.   [4] Guianerius.   [5] De mentis alienat.
cap. 3.   [6] Levinus Lemnius, Jason Pratensis, Blanda ab initio.   [7] Hor.

414   *Symptomes of Melancholy.*   [Part.1. Sec. 3.

him what inconvenience will follow, what will be the event;
all is one; *canis ad vomitum:* [1] 'tis so pleasant, he cannot refrain.   He may thus continue peradventure many years by
reason of a strong temperature, or some mixture of business,
which may divert his cogitations; but, at the last, *læsa imaginatio,* his phantasie is crazed, and, now habituated to such
toyes, cannot but work still like a fat; the scene alters upon a
sudden; fear and sorrow supplant those pleasing thoughts;
suspicion, discontent, and perpetual anxiety succeed in their
places: so by little and little, by that shooing-horn of idleness, and voluntary solitariness, Melancholy, this feral fiend,
is drawn on; and

[2] Quantum vertice ad auras
Æthereas, tantum radice in Tartara tendit:

it was not so delicious at first, as it is now bittèr and harsh: a
cankered soul macerated with cares and discontents, *tædium
vitæ,* impatience, agony, inconstancy, irresolution, precipitate
them unto unspeakable miseries.   They cannot endure company, light, or life it self, some; unfit for action, and the like.
[3] Their bodies are lean and dryed up, withered, ugly, their
looks harsh, very dull, and their souls tormented, as they are
more or less intangled, as the humour hath been intended, or
according to the continuance of time they have been troubled.
   To discern all which symptomes the better, [4] Rhasis the
Arabian makes three degrees of them.   The first is [5] *falsa cogitatio,* false conceits and idle thoughts: to misconstrue and
amplifie, aggravating every thing they conceive or fear; the
second is *falsò cogitata loqui,* to talk to themselves, or to use
inarticulate, incondite voices, speeches, obsolete gestures, and
plainly to utter their minds and conceits of their hearts by
their words and actions, as to laugh, weep, to be silent, not to
sleep, eat their meat, &c. the third is to put in practice that
which they think or speak. Savanarola (*Rub.* 11. *tract.* 8.
cap. 1. *de ægritudine*) confirms as much: [6] *when he begins to
express that in words, which he conceives in his heart, or talks
idly, or goes from one thing to another* (which [7] Gordonius
cells *nec caput habentia, nec caudam*), he is in the middle way:
[8] *but, when he begins to act it likewise, and to put his fopperies
in execution, he is then in the extent of melancholy or madness*

---

[1] Facilis descensus Averni.   [2] Virg.   [3] Corpus cadaverosum. Psa. 67.
Cariosa est facies mea præ ægritudine animæ.   [4] Lib. 9. ad Almansorem.
[5] Practicâ majore.   [6] Quum ore loquitur quæ corde concepit, quum subito
de unâ re ad aliud transit, neque rationem de aliquo reddit, tunc est in medio: at
quum incipit operari quæ loquitur, in summo gradu est.   [7] Cap. 19. Partic. 2.
Loquitur secum, et ad alios, ac si vere præsentes. Aug. c. 11. lib. de curâ pro
mortuis gerendâ. Rhasis.   [8] Quum res ad hoc devenit, ut ea, quæ cogitare
cœperit, ore promat, atque acta permisceat, tum perfecta melancholia est.

Mem. 1. Subs. 4.] *Symptomes from Custome.* 415

it self. This progress of melancholy you shall easily observe in them that have been so affected : they go smiling to themselves at first, at length they laugh out ; at first solitary, at last they can endure no company : or, if they do, they are now dizards, past sense and shame, quite moped ; they care not what they say or do ; all their actions, words, gestures, are furious or ridiculous. At first his mind is troubled ; he doth not attend what is said ; if you tell him a tale, he cryes at last, what said you ? but in the end he mutters to himself, as old women do many times, or old men when they sit alone ; upon a sudden they laugh, whoop, hollow, or run away, and swear they see or hear players, [1] devils, hobgoblins, ghosts ; strike, or strut, &c. grow humorous in the end. Like him in the poet—*sæpe ducentos, sæpe decem servos*—he will dress himself, and undress, careless at last, grows insensible, stupid, or mad. [2] He howls like a woolf, barks like a dog, and raves like Ajax and Orestes, hears musick and outcryes, which no man else hears ; as [3] he did whom Amatus Lusitanus mentioneth (*cent. 3. cura 55*), or that woman in [4] Springer, that spake many languages, and said she was possessed ; that farmer, in [5] Prosper Calenus, that disputed and discoursed learnedly in philosophy and astronomy, with Alexander Achilles his master, at Boloigne in Italy. But of these I have already spoken.

Who can sufficiently speak of these symptomes, or prescribe rules to comprehend them ? As Echo to the painter in Ausonius, *vane, quid affectas, &c.* foolish fellow, what wilt ? if you must needs paint me, paint a voice, *et similem si vis pingere, pinge sonum :* if you will describe melancholy, describe a phantastical conceit, a corrupt imagination, vain thoughts and different : which who can do ? The four and twenty letters make no more variety of words in divers languages, than melancholy conceits produce diversity of symptomes in several persons. They are irregular, obscure, various : so infinite, Proteus himself is not so divers ; you may as well make the moon a new coat, as a true character of a melancholy man ; as soon find the motion of a bird in the air, as the heart of man, a melancholy man. They are so confused, I say, divers, intermixt with other diseases—as the species be confounded (which [6] I have shewed) so are the symptomes ; sometimes with headach, cachexia, dropsie, stone (as you may perceive by those several examples and illustrations, collected by [7] Hildesheim, *spicil. 2.* Mercurialis, *consil. 118. cap. 6. et 11*), with head-ach,

---

[1] Melancholicus se videre et audire putat dæmones.   Lavater, de spectris, par. **3. cap. 2.**   [2] Wierus, l. 3. c. 31.   [3] Michael, a musician.   [4] Malleo malef.   [5] Lib. de atrâ bile.   [6] Part. 1. Subs. 2. Memb. 2.   [7] De delirio, melancholiâ, et maniâ.

13

416   *Symptomes of Melancholy.*   [Part. 1. Sec. 3.

epilepsie, priapismus (Trincavellius, *consil.* 12. lib. 1. *consil.* 39)
with gout, *caninus appetitus* (Montanus, *consil.* 26. &c. 23. 234.
249), with falling-sickness, head-ach, vertigo, lycanthropia,
&c. (J. Cæsar Claudinus, *consult.* 4. *consult.* 80. et 116) with
gout, agues, hemroids, stone, &c.   Who can distinguish these
melancholy symptomes so intermixt with others, or apply
them to their several kinds, confine them into method?   'Tis
hard, I confess ; yet I have disposed of them as I could, and
will descend to particularize them according to their species :
for hitherto I have expatiated in more general lists or terms,
speaking promiscuously of such ordinary signs, which occur
amongst writers.   Not that they are all to be found in one
man ; for that were to paint a monster or chimera, not a man ;
but some in one, some in another, and that successively or at
several times.

Which I have been the more curious to express and report,
not to upbraid any miserable man, or by way of derision (I
rather pity them), but the better to discern, to apply remedies
unto them ; and to shew that the best and soundest of us all is
in great danger ; how much we ought to fear our own fickle
estates, remember our miseries and vanities, examine and hu-
miliate our selves, seek to God, and call to him for mercy,
that needs not look for any rods to scourge our selves, since
we carry them in our bowels, and that our souls are in a miserable captivity, if the light of grace and heavenly truth doth
not shine continually upon us; and by our discretion to moderate our selves, to be more circumspect and wary in the
midst of these dangers.

MEMB. II. SUBSECT. I.

Symptomes of Head-Melancholy.

If [1] *no symptomes appear about the stomach, nor the blood be
misaffected, and fear and sorrow continue, it is to be thought
the brain it self is troubled, by reason of a melancholy juyce
bred in it, or otherwayes conveyed into it ; and that evil juyce
is from the distemperature of the part, or left after some inflammation.*   Thus far Piso.   But this is not always true ;
for blood and hypochondries both are often affected even in
head-melancholy.   [2] Hercules de Saxoniâ differs here from
the common current of writers, putting peculiar signs of head-

---

[1] Nicholas Piso.   Si signa circa ventriculum non apparent, nec sanguis male
affectus, et adsunt timor et mœstitia, cerebrum ipsum existimandum est, &c.
[2] Tract. de mel. c. 13, &c.   Ex intemperie spirituum, et cerebri motu et tenebrositate.

Mem. 2. Subs. 1.] *Symptomes of Head-Melancholy.* 417

melancholy, from the sole distemperature of spirits in the brain, as they are hot, cold, dry, moist, *all without matter, from the motion alone, and tenebrosity of spirits.* Of melancholy which proceeds from humours by adustion, he treats apart, with their several symptomes and cures. The common signs, if it be by essence in the head, *are ruddiness of face, high sanguine complexion, most part,* (*rubore saturato,* [1] one calls it) a blewish, and sometimes full of pumples, with red eyes. (Avicenna, *l.* 3. *Fen.* 2. *Tract.* 4. *c.* 18. Duretus, and others out of Galen, *de affect. l.* 3. *c.* 6.) [2] Hercules de Saxoniâ, to this of redness of face, adds *heaviness of the head, fixed and hollow eyes.* [3] *If it proceed from dryness of the brain, then their heads will be light, vertiginous, and they most apt to wake, and to continue whole months together without sleep. Few excrements in their eyes and nostrils; and often bald by reason of excess of dryness,* Montaltus adds (c. 17). If it proceeds from moisture, dulness, drowsiness, head-ach follows; and (as Sallust. Salvianus, *c.* 1. *l.* 2. out of his own experience found) epileptical, with a multitude of humours in the head. They are very bashful, if ruddy, apt to blush, and to be red upon all occasions, *præsertim si metus accesserit.* But the chiefest symptome to discern this species, as I have said, is this, that there be no notable signs in the stomach, hypochondries, or elsewhere, *digna,* as [4] Montaltus terms them, or of greater note, because oftentimes the passions of the stomach concurr with them. Wind is common to all three species, and is not excluded, only that of the hypochondries is [5] *more windy* than the rest, saith Hollerius. Aëtius (*tetrab. l.* 2. *se.* 2. *c.* 9 *et* 10) maintains the same: [6] if there be more signs, and more evident, in the head than elsewhere, the head is primarily affected, and prescribes head-melancholy to be cured by meats (amongst the rest) void of wind, and good juyce, not excluding wind, or corrupt blood, even in head-melancholy itself: but these species are often confounded, and so are their symptomes, as I have already proved. The symptomes of the mind are superfluous and continual cogitations; [7] *for, when the head is heated, it scorcheth*

---

[1] Facie sunt rubente et livescente, quibus etiam aliquando adsunt pustulæ. [2] Jo. Pantheon, cap. de Mel. Si cerebrum primario afficiatur, adsunt capitis gravitas, fixi oculi, &c. [3] Laurent. cap. 5. Si a cerebro, ex siccitate, tum capitis erit levitas, sitis, vigilia, paucitas superfluitatum in oculis et naribus. [4] Si nulla digna læsio ventriculo, quoniam, in hac melancholiâ capitis, exigua nonnunquam ventriculi pathemata coëunt; duo enim hæc membra sibi invicem affectionem transmittunt. [5] Postrema magis flatuosa. [6] Si minus molestiæ circa ventriculum aut ventrem, in iis cerebrum primario afficitur; et curare oportet hunc affectum, per cibos flatûs exsortes, et bonæ concoctionis, &c. raro cerebrum afficitur sine ventriculo. [7] Sanguinem adurit caput calidius; et inde fumi melancholici adusti animum exagitant.

VOL. I.   E E

418   *Symptomes of Melancholy.* [Part. 1. Sec. 3.

the blood; and from thence proceed melancholy fumes, which trouble the mind (Avicenna). They are very cholerick, and soon hot, solitary, sad, often silent, watchful, discontent (*Montaltus, cap.* 24). If any thing trouble them, they cannot sleep, but fret themselves still, till another object mitigate, or time wear it out. They have grievous passions, and immoderate perturbations of the mind, fear, sorrow, &c. yet not so continuate, but that they are sometimes merry, apt to profuse laughter (which is more to be wondred at), and that by the authority of [1] Galen himself, by areason of mixture of blood; *prærubri jocosis delectantur, et irrisores plerumque sunt :* if they be ruddy, they are delighted in jests, and oftentimes scoffers themselves, conceited, and (as Rodericus a Vega comments on that place of Galen) merry, witty, of a pleasant disposition, and yet grievously melancholy anon after. *Omnia discunt sine doctore,* saith Aretæus : they learn without a teacher : and, as [2] Laurentius supposeth, those feral passions and symptomes of such as think themselves glass, pitchers, feathers, &c. speak strange languages, proceed *a calore cerebri* (if it be in excess), from the brain's distempered heat.

SUBSECT. II.

Symptomes of Windy Hypochondriacal Melancholy.

In this hypochondriacal or flatuous melancholy, the symptomes are so ambiguous, (saith [3] Crato, in a counsel of his for a noblewoman) *that the most exquisite physicians cannot determine of the part affected.* Matthew Flaccius, consulted about a noble matron, confessed as much, that in this maladie, he, with Hollerius, Fracastorius, Falopius, and others, being to give their sentence of a party labouring of hypochondriacal melancholy, could not find out by the symptomes, which part was most especially affected : some said the womb, some heart, some stomach, &c. and therefore Crato (*consil.* 24. *lib.* 1) boldly avers, that, in this diversity of symptomes which commonly accompany this disease [4] *no physician can truly say what part is affected.* Galen (*lib.* 3. *de loc. affect.*) reckons up these ordinary symptomes (which all the neotericks repeat) out of Diocles; only this fault he finds with him, that he puts not *fear* and *sorrow* amongst the other signs.

---

[1] Lib. de loc. affect. cap. 6.   [2] Cap. 6.   [3] Hildesheim, spicil. 1. de mel. In hypochondriacâ melancholiâ, adeo ambigua sunt symptomata, ut etiam exercitatissimi medici de loco affecto statuere non possint.   [4] Medici de loco affecto nequeunt statuere.

Mem. 2. Subs. 2.] *Symptomes of windy Melancholy.* 419

Trincavellius excuseth Diocles (*lib. 3. consil.* 35), because that oftentimes, in a strong head and constitution, a generous spirit, and a valiant, these symptomes appear not, by reason of his valour and courage. [1] Hercules de Saxoniâ (to whom I subscribe) is of the same mind (which I have before touched) that *fear* and *sorrow* are not general symptomes: some fear, and are not sad; some be sad, and fear not; some neither fear nor grieve. The rest are these, beside fear and sorrow, [2] *sharp belchings, fulsome crudities, heat in the bowels, wind and rumbling in the guts, vehement gripings, pain in the belly and stomach sometimes, after meat that is hard of concoction, much watering of the stomach, and moist spittle, cold sweat,* importunus sudor, *unseasonable sweat all over the body,* (as Octavius Horatianus, lib. 2. cap. 5. calls it) *cold joynts, indigestion;* [3] *they cannot endure their own fulsome belchings; continual wind about their hypochrondries, heat and griping in their bowels;* præcordia sursum convelluntur, *midriff, and bowels are pulled up; the veins about their eyes look red, and swell from vapours and wind.* Their ears sing now and then; vertigo and giddiness come by fits, turbulent dreams, driness, leanness; apt they are to sweat upon all occasions, of all colours and complexions. Many of them are high coloured, especially after meals; which symptome Cardinal Cæsius was much troubled with, and of which he complained to Prosper Calenus his Physician, he could not eat, or drink a cup of wine, but he was as red in the face, as if he had been at a maior's feast. That symptome alone vexeth many. [4] Some again are black, pale, ruddy; sometime their shoulders and shoulder-blades ake; there is a leaping all over their bodies, sudden trembling, a palpitation of the heart, and that *cardiaca passio,* grief in the mouth of the stomach, which maketh the patient think his heart it self aketh, and sometimes suffocation, *difficultas anhelitûs,* short breath, hard wind, strong pulse, swooning. Montanus (*consil.* 55), Trincavellius (*lib. 3. consil.* 36 *et* 37), Fernelius (*cons.* 43), Frambesarius (*consult. lib.* 1. *consil.* 17), Hildesheim, Claudinus, &c. give instance of every particular. The peculiar symptomes, which properly belong to each part, be these. If it proceed from the stomach, saith

---

[1] Tract. postumo de mel. Patavii edit. 1620. per Bozettum Bibliop. cap. 2.
[2] Acidi ructus, cruditates, æstus in præcordiis, flatus, interdum ventriculi dolores vehementes, sumtoque cibo concoctu difficili, sputum humidum idque multum sequetur, &c. Hip. lib. de mel. Galenus, Melanelius e Ruffo et Aëtio, Altomarus, Piso, Montaltus, Bruel, Wecker, &c. [3] Circa præcordia de assiduâ inflatione queruntur; et, cum sudore totius corporis importuno, frigidos articulos sæpe patiuntur, indigestione laborant, ructus suos insuaves perhorrescunt, viscerum dolores habent. [4] Montaltus, c. 13. Wecker, Fuchsius, c. 13. Altomarus, c. 7. Laurentius, c. 73. Bruel, Gordon.

E E 2

420 *Symptomes of Melancholy.* [Part. 1. Sec. 3.

[1] Savanarola, 'tis full of pain, wind. Guianerius adds, *vertigo, nausea,* much spitting, &c. If from the myrache, a swelling and wind in the hypochondries, a loathing, and appetite to vomit, pulling upward. If from the heart, aking and trembling of it, much heaviness. If from the liver, there is usually a pain in the right hypochondry. If from the spleen, hardness and grief in the left hypochondry, a rumbling, much appetite and small digestion (Avicenna). If from the mesaraïck veins and liver on the other side, little or no appetite (Herc. de Saxoniâ). If from the hypochondries, a rumbling inflation, concoction is hindred, often belching, &c. And from these crudities, windy vapours ascend up to the brain, which trouble the imagination, and cause fear, sorrow, dulness, heaviness, many terrible conceits and chimeras, as Lemnius well observes (*l.* 1. *c.* 16): *as* [2] *a black and thick cloud covers the sun, and intercepts his beams and light, so doth this melancholy vapour obnubilate the mind, inforce it to many absurd thoughts and imaginations,* and compel good, wise, honest, discreet men (arising to the brain from the [3] lower parts, *as smoak out of a chimney*) to dote, speak, and do that which becomes them not, their persons, callings, wisdoms. One, by reason of those ascending vapours and gripings rumbling beneath, will not be persuaded but that he hath a serpent in his guts, a viper: another, frogs. Trallianus relates a story of a woman, that imagined she had swallowed an eel, or a serpent; and Felix Platerus (*observat. lib.* 1) hath a most memorable example of a countreyman of his, that by chance falling into a pit where frogs and frogs spawn was, and a little of that water swallowed, began to suspect that he had likewise swallowed frogs spawn ; and, with that conceit and fear, his phantasie wrought so far, that he verily thought he had young live frogs in his belly, *qui vivebant ex alimento suo,* that lived by his nourishment, and was so certainly perswaded of it, that, for many years following, he could not be rectified in his conceit; he studied physick seven years together, to cure himself, travelled into Italy, France, and Germany, to conferr with the best physicians about it, and, *anno* 1609, asked his counsel amongst the rest. He told him it was wind, his conceipt, &c. but *mordicus contradicere, et ore et scriptis probare nitebatur :* no saying would serve : it was no wind, but real frogs *: and do you not hear them croak ?* Platerus would have deceived him, by putting live frogs into his excrements: but he, being a physician himself, would not be deceived, *vir prudens alias, et*

---

[1] Pract. major. Dolor in eo et ventositas, nausea. [2] Ut atra densaque nubes, soli offusa, radios et lumen ejus intercipit et offuscat : sic, &c. [3] Ut fumus e camino.

Mem. 2. Subs. 3.] *Symptomes of Windy Melancholy.* 421

doctus a wise and learned man otherwise, a doctor of physick; and after seven years dotage in this kind, *a phantasiâ liberatus est,* he was cured. Laurentius and Goulart have many such examples, if you be desirous to read them. One commodity, above the rest which are melancholy, these windy flatuous have —*lucida intervalla :* their symptomes and pains are not usually so continuate as the rest, but come by fits, fear and sorrow and the rest: yet, in another, they exceed all others ; and that is, [1] they are luxurious, incontinent, and prone to venery, by reason of wind, *et facile amant, et quamlibet fere amant* (Jason Pratensis).   [2] Rhasis is of opinion, that Venus doth many of them much good ; the other symptomes of the mind be common with the rest.

SUBSECT. III.

Symptomes of Melancholy abounding in the whole body.

THEIR bodies, that are affected with this universal melancholy, are most part black; [3] *the melancholy juyce is redundant all over;* hirsute they are, and lean ; they have broad veins, their blood is gross and thick.   [4] *Their spleen is weak,* and a liver apt to ingender the humour ; they have kept bad diet or have had some evacuation stopped, as hæmroids, or months in women, which [5] Trallianus, in the cure, would have carefully to be inquired, and withal to observe of what complexion the party is, black or red.   For, as Forrestus and Hollerius contend, if [6] they be black, it proceeds from abundance of natural melancholy ; if it proceed from cares, agony, discontents, diet, exercise, &c. they may be as well of any other colour, red, yellow, pale, as black, and yet their whole blood corrupt ; *prærubri colore sæpe sunt tales, sæpe flavi* (saith [7] Montaltus, *cap.* 22). The best way to discern this species, is to let them bleed ; if the blood be corrupt, thick, and black, and they withal free from those hypochondriacal symptomes, and not so grievously troubled with them, or those of the head, it argues they are melancholy *a toto corpore.*   The fumes which arise from this

---

[1] Hypochondriaci maxime affectant coire, et multiplicatur coitus in ipsis, eo quod ventositates multiplicantur in hypochondriis, et coitus sæpe allevat has ventositates.   [2] Cont. lib. 1. tract. 9.   [3] Wecker. Melancholicus succus toto corpore redundans.   [4] Splen. naturâ imbecillior. Montaltus, cap. 22. [5] Lib. 1. cap. 16. Interrogare convenit, an aliqua evacuationis retentio obvenerit, viri in hæmorrhoïd. mulierum menstruis ; et vide faciem similiter, an sit rubicunda.   [6] Naturales nigri acquisiti a toto corpore, sæpe rubicundi.   [7] Montaltus, cap. 22. Piso. Ex colore sanguinis, si minuas venam, si fluat niger, &c.

422   *Symptomes of Melancholy.*   [Part. 1. Sec. 3.

corrupt blood, disturb the mind and make them fearful and sorrowful, heavy-hearted, as the rest, dejected, discontented, solitary, silent, weary of their lives, dull and heavy, or merry, &c. and, if far gone, that which Apuleius wished to his enemy, by way of imprecation, is true in them : [1] *dead mens bones, hobgoblins, ghosts, are ever in their minds, and meet them still in every turn: all the bugbears of the night, and terrours and fairybabes of tombs and graves, are before their eyes and in their thoughts, as to women and children, if they be in the dark alone.* If they hear, or read, or see, any tragical object, it sticks by them ; they are afraid of death, and yet weary of their lives; in their discontented humours, they quarrel with all the world, bitterly inveigh, tax satyrically ; and because they cannot otherwise vent their passions, or redress what is amiss, as they mean, they will, by violent death, at last be revenged on themselves.

SUBSECT. IV.

Symptomes of Maids, Nuns, and Widows Melancholy.

BECAUSE Ludovicus Mercatus (in his second book *de mulier. affect. c.* 4), and Rodericus a Castro (*de morb. mulier. c.* 3. *l.* 2), two famous physicians in Spain, Daniel Sennertus of Wittenberg (*lib.* 1. *part.* 2. *cap.* 13), with others, have vouchsafed, in their works not long since published, to write two just treatises *de Melancholiâ Virginum, Monialium, et Viduarum,* as a peculiar species of melancholy (which I have already specified) distinct from the rest, ([2] for it much differs from that which commonly befals men and other women, as having one only cause proper to women alone) I may not omit, in this generall survey of melancholy symptomes, to set down the particular signs of such parties so misaffected.

The causes are assigned out of Hippocrates, Cleopatra, Moschion, and those old *gynæciorum scriptores,* of this feral malady, in more ancient maids, widows, and barren women, *ob septum transversum violatum* (saith Mercatus), by reason of the midriffe or *diaphragma,* heart and brain offended with those vicious vapours which come from menstruous blood : *inflammationem arteriæ circa dorsum ;* Rodericus adds, an inflammation of

---

[1] Apul. l. 1. Semper obviæ species mortuorum : quidquid umbrarum est uspiam, quidquid lemurum et larvarum, oculis suis aggerunt : sibi fingunt omnia noctium occursacula, omnia bustorum formidamina ; omnia sepulcrorum terriculamenta.   [2] Differt enim ab eâ quæ viris et reliquis feminis communiter contingit, propriam habens caussam.

the back, which with the rest is offended by [1] that fuliginous exhalation of corrupt seed, troubling the brain, heart and mind; the brain I say, not in essence, but by consent; *universa enim hujus affectús causa ab utero pendet, et a sanguinis menstrui malitiá;* for, in a word, the whole malady proceeds from that inflammation, putredity, black smoky vapours, &c., from thence comes care, sorrow, and anxiety, obfuscation of spirits, agony, desperation, and the like, which are intended or remitted, *si amatorius accesserit ardor,* or any other violent object or perturbation of mind. This melancholy may happen to widows, with much care and sorrow, as frequently it doth, by reason of a sudden alteration of their accustomed course of life, &c. To such as lye in childe-bed, *ob suppressam purgationem;* but to nunnes and more ancient maids, and some barren women, for the causes abovesaid, 'tis more familiar; *crebrius his quam reliquis accidet, inquit Rodericus;* the rest are not altogether excluded.

Out of these causes Rodericus defines it, with Aretæus, to be *angorem animi,* a vexation of the mind, a sudden sorrow from a small, light, or no occasion, [2] with a kind of still dotage and grief of some part or other, head, heart, breasts, sides, back, belly, &c. with much solitariness, weeping, distraction, &c. from which they are sometimes suddenly delivered, because it comes and goes by fits, and is not so permanent as other melancholy.

But, to leave this brief description, the most ordinary symptomes be these: *pulsatio juxta dorsum,* a beating about the back, which is almost perpetual; the skin is many times rough, squalid, especially (as Aretæus observes) about the arms, knees, and knuckles. The midriffe and heart-strings do burn and beat very fearfully; and, when this vapour or fume is stirred, flyeth upward, the heart it self beats, is sore grieved, and faints; *fauces siccitate præcluduntur, ut difficulter possit ab uteri strangulatione discerni,* like fits of the mother; *alvus plerisque nil reddit, aliis exiguum, acre, biliosum; lotium flavum.* They complain many times, saith Mercatus, of a great pain in their heads, about their hearts, and hypochondries, and so likewise in their breasts, which are often sore; sometimes ready to swoon, their faces are inflamed and red, they are dry, thirsty, suddenly hot, much

---

[1] Ex menstrui sanguinis tetrâ ad cor et cerebrum exhalatione: vitiatum semen, mentem perturbat, &c. non per essentiam, sed per consensum. Animus mœrens et anxius inde malum trahit, et spiritus cerebri obfuscantur; quæ cuncta augentur, &c.   [2] Cum tacito delirio ac dolore alicujus partis internæ, dorsi, hypochondrii, cordis regionem et universam mammam interdum occupantis, &c. Cutis aliquando squalida, aspera, rugosa, præcipue cubitis, genibus, et digitorum articulis; præcordia ingenti sæpe terrore æstuant et pulsant; cumque vapor excitatus sursum evolat, cor palpitat aut premitur, animus deficit, &c.

424   *Symptomes of Melancholy.*   [Part. 1. Sec. 3.

troubled with wind, cannot sleep, &c. And from hence proceed *ferina deliramenta,* a brutish kind of dotage, troublesome sleep, terrible dreams in the night, *subrusticus pudor, et verecundia ignava,* a foolishly kind of bashfulness to some, perverse conceites and opinions, [1] dejection of mind, much discontent, preposterous judgement. They are apt to loath, dislike, disdain, to be weary of every object, &c. each thing almost is tedious to them; they pine away, void of counsel, apt to weep, and tremble, timorous, fearful, sad, and out of all hopes of better fortunes. They take delight in nothing for the time, but love to be alone and solitary, though that do them more harm. And thus they are affected so long as this vapour lasteth; but, by and by, as pleasant and merry as ever they were in their lives, they sing, discourse and laugh in any good company, upon all occasions; and so by fits it takes them now and then, except the malady be inveterate; and then 'tis more frequent, vehement, and continuate. Many of them cannot tell how to express themselves in words, how it holds them, what ails them; you cannot understand them, or well tell what to make of their sayings; so far gone sometimes, so stupified and distracted, they think themselves bewitched; they are in despair, *aptæ ad fletum, desperationem, dolores mammis et hypochondriis.* Mercatus therefore adds, now their breasts, now their hypochondries, belly and sides, then their heart and head akes; now heat, then wind, now this, now that offends; they are weary of all: [2] and yet will not, cannot again tell how, where or what offends them, though they be in great pain, agony, and frequently complain, grieving, sighing, weeping and discontented still, *sine caussâ manifestâ,* most part; yet, I say, they will complain, grudge, lament, and not be perswaded but that they are troubled with an evil spirit; which is frequent in Germany (saith Rodericus), amongst the common sort, and to such as are most grievously affected; (for he makes three degrees of this disease in women) they are in despair, surely forespoken or bewitched, and in extremity of their dotage, (weary of their lives) some of them will attempt to make away themselves. Some think they see visions, confer with spirits and devils; they shall surely be damned, are afraid of some treachery, imminent danger, and the like; they will not speak, make answer to any question, but are almost distracted,

---

[1] Animi dejectio, perversa rerum existimatio, præposterum judicium. Fastidiosæ, languentes, tædiosæ, consilii inopes, lacrymosæ, timentes, mœstæ, cum summâ rerum meliorum desperatione, nullâ re delectantur, solitudinem amant, &c.   [2] Nolunt aperire molestiam quam patiuntur; sed conqueruntur tamen de capite, corde, mammis, &c. In puteos fere maniaci prosilire, ac strangulari cupiunt, nullâ orationis suavitate ad spem salutis recuperandam erigi, &c. Familiares non curant; non loquuntur, non respondent, &c. et hæc graviora, si, &c.

Mem. 2. Subs. 4.] *Symptomes of Women's Melancholy.* 425

mad, or stupid for the time, and by fits : and thus it holds them, as they are more or less affected and as the inner humour is intended or remitted, or by outward objects and perturbations aggravated, solitariness, idleness, &c.

Many other maladies there are, incident to young women, out of that one and only cause above specified, many feral diseases. I will not so much as mention their names : melancholy alone is the subject of my present discourse, from which I will not swerve. The several cures of this infirmity, concerning diet, which must be very sparing, phlebotomy, physick, internal, external remedies, are at large in great variety in [1] Rodericus a Castro, Sennertus, and Mercatus, which who so will, as occasion serves, may make use of. But the best and surest remedy of all, is to see them well placed, and married to good husbands in due time ; *hinc illæ lacrymæ,* that's the primary cause, and this is the ready cure, to give them content to their desires. I write not this to patronize any wanton, idle flurt, lascivious or light huswives, which are too forward many times, unruly, and apt to cast away themselves on him that comes next, without all care, counsel, circumspection, and judgement. If religion, good discipline, honest education, wholsome exhortation, fair promises, fame and loss of good name, cannot inhibit and deterr such, (which, to chaste and sober maids, cannot chuse but avail much) labour and exercise, strict diet, rigour, and threats, may more opportunely be used, and are able of themselves to qualifie and divert an ill disposed temperament. For seldome shall you see an hired servant, a poor handmaid, though antient, that is kept hard to her work and bodily labour, a coarse countrey wench, troubled in this kind ; but noble virgins, nice gentlewomen, such as are solitary and idle, live at ease, lead a life out of action and employment, that fare well, in great houses, and jovial companies, ill disposed peradventure of themselves, and not willing to make any resistance, discontented otherwise, of weak judgement, able bodies, and subject to passions (*grandiores virgines,* saith Mercatus, *steriles, et viduæ, plerumque melancholicæ*) such for the most part are misaffected, and prone to this disease. I do not so much pity them that may otherwise be eased ; but those alone, that, out of a strong temperament, innate constitution, are violently carryed away with this torrent of inward humours, and, though very modest of themselves, sober, religious, vertuous, and well given (as many so distressed maids are), yet cannot make resistance ; these grievances will appear, this malady will take place, and now manifestly shews it self, and may not other-

[1] Clysteres et helleborismum Matthioli summe laudat.

426 *Symptomes of Melancholy.* [Part. 1. Sec. 3.

wise be helped. But where am I? Into what subject have I rushed? What have I to do with nunns, maids, virgins, widows? I am a bachelor my self, and lead a monastick life in a college : *næ ego sane ineptus, qui hæc dixerim;* I confess 'tis an indecorum : and as Pallas a virgin blushed, when Jupiter by chance spake of love matters in her presence, and turn'd away her face ; *me reprimam;* though my subject necessarily require it, I will say no more.

And yet I must and will say something more, add a word or two *in gratiam virginum et viduarum,* in favour of all such distressed parties, in commiseration of their present estate. And, as I cannot chuse but condole their mishap that labour of this infirmity, and are destitute of help in this case, so must I needs inveigh against them that are in fault, more than manifest causes, and as bitterly tax those tyrannizing pseudopoliticians, superstitious orders, rash vows, hard-hearted parents, guardians, unnatural friends, allies, (call them how you will) those careless and stupid overseers, that, out of worldly respects, covetousness, supine negligence, their own private ends, *(cum sibi sit interim bene)* can so severely reject, stubbornly neglect, and impiously contemn, without all remorse and pity, the tears, sighs, groans, and grievous miseries, of such poor souls committed to their charge. How odious and abominable are those superstitious and rash vows of popish monasteries, so to bind and inforce men and women to vow virginity, to lead a single life against the laws of nature, opposite to religion, policy, and humanity ! so to starve, to offer violence, to suppress the vigour of youth, by rigorous statutes, severe laws, vain perswasions, to debar them of that, to which by their innate temperature they are so furiously inclined, urgently carried, and sometimes precipitated, even irresistibly led, to the prejudice of their souls health, and good estate of body and mind ! and all for base and private respects, to maintain their gross superstition, to inrich themselves and their territories (as they falsly suppose) by hindering some marriages, that the world be not full of beggers, and their parishes pestered with orphans. Stupid politicians ! *hæccine fieri flagitia?* ought these things so to be carried? *Better marry than burn,* saith the apostle ; but they are otherwise perswaded. They will by all means quench their neighbours house, if it be on fire; but that fire of lust, which breaks out into such lamentable flames, they will not take notice of; their own bowels oftentimes, flesh and blood, shall so rage and burn ; and they will not see it. *Miserum est,* saith Austin, *seipsum non miserescere ;* and they are miserable in the mean time, that cannot pity themselves, the common good of all, and, *per consequens,* their own estates. For, let them but consider

Mem. 3.]   *Causes of these Symptomes.*   427

what fearful maladies, feral diseases, gross inconveniencies come to both sexes by this enforced temperance. It troubles me to think of, much more to relate, those frequent aborts and murdering of infants in their nunneries (read [1] Kemnitius and others), their notorious fornications, those spintrias, tribadas, ambubaias, &c. those rapes, incests, adulteries, mastuprations, sodomies, buggeries, of monks and friers. (See Bales Visitation of Abbies, [2] Mercurialis, Rodericus a Castro, Peter Forestus, and divers physicians.) I know their ordinary apologies and excuses for these things ; *sed viderint politici, medici, theologi:* I shall more opportunely meet with them [3] elsewhere.

> Illius viduæ, aut patronum virginis hujus,
> Ne me forte putes, verbum non amplius addam.

MEMB. III.

Immediate Cause of these precedent Symptomes.

To give some satisfaction to melancholy men that are troubled with these symptomes, a better means, in my judgement, cannot be taken, than to shew them the causes whence they proceed ; not from devils, as they suppose, or that they are bewitched or forsaken of God, hear or see, &c. as many of them think, but from natural and inward causes; that, so knowing them, they may better avoid the effects, or at least endure them with more patience. The most grievous and common symptomes are fear and sorrow, and that without a cause, to the wisest and discreetest men, in this malady not to be avoided. The reason why they are so, Aëtius discusseth at large, Tetrabib. 2. 2. in his first problem out of Galen, *lib. 2. de caussis sympt.* 1. For Galen imputeth all to the cold that is black, and thinks that the spirits being darkned, and the substance of the brain cloudy and dark, all the objects thereof appear terrible, and the [4] mind it self, by those dark, obscure, gross fumes, ascending from black humours, is in continual darkness, fear, and sorrow; divers terrible monstrous fictions in a thousand shapes and apparitions occurr, with violent passions, by which the brain and phantasie are troubled and eclipsed. [5] Fracastorius (*lib. 2. de intellect.*)

---

[1] Examen conc. Trident. de cœlibatu sacerd.   [2] Cap. de Satyr. et Priapis. [3] Part. 3. sect. 2. Mem. 5. Subs. 5.   [4] Vapores crassi et nigri a ventriculo in cerebrum exhalant. Fel. Platerus.   [5] Calidi hilares, frigidi indispositi ad lætitiam, et ideo solitarii, taciturni, non ob tenebras internas, ut medici volunt, sed ob frigus : multi melancholici nocte ambulant intrepidi. Vapores melancholici, spiritibus mixti, tenebrarum caussæ sunt. Cap. 1.

428   *Symptomes of Melancholy.*   [Part. 1. Sec. 3.

*will have cold to be the cause of fear and sorrow; for such as
are cold, are ill disposed to mirth, dull and heavy, by nature solitary, silent; and not for any inward darkness (as
physicians think); for many melancholy men dare boldly be,
continue, and walk in the dark, and delight in it: solum frigidi timidi:* if they be hot, they are merry; and the more hot,
the more furious, and void of fear, as we see in mad men: but
this reason holds not; for then no melancholy, proceeding from
choler adust, should fear. Averroës scoffs at Galen for his reasons, and brings five arguments to refell them: so doth Herc.
de Saxoniâ (*Tract. de melan. cap.* 3) assigning other causes,
which are copiously censured and confuted by Ælianus Montaltus, *cap.* 5 *et* 6. Lod. Mercatus, *de inter. morb. cur. lib.* 1.
cap. 17. Altomarus, *cap.* 7. *de mel.* Guianerius, *tract.* 15.
c. 1. Bright, *cap.* 17. Laurentius, *cap.* 5. Valesius, *med.
cont. lib.* 5. *cont.* 1. [1] *Distemperature* (they conclude) *makes
black juice; blackness obscures the spirits; the spirits, obscured, cause fear and sorrow.* Laurentius (*cap.* 13) supposeth
these black fumes offend especially the diaphragma or midriff,
and so, *per consequens,* the mind, which is obscured, as [2] the
sun by a cloud. To this opinion of Galen, almost all the
Greeks and Arabians subscribe, the Latines new and old; *internæ tenebræ offuscant animum, ut externæ nocent pueris:*
as children are affrighted in the dark, so are melancholy men at
all times, [3] as having the inward cause with them, and still carrying it about. Which black vapours, whether they proceed
from the black blood about the heart, (as T. W. Jes. thinks, in
his Treatise of the passions of the mind) or stomach, spleen,
midriff, or all the misaffected parts together, it boots not;
they keep the mind in a perpetual dungeon, and oppress it
with continual fears, anxieties, sorrows, &c. It is an ordinary thing for such as are sound, to laugh at this dejected
pusillanimity, and those other symptomes of melancholy, to
make themselves merry with them, and to wonder at such,
as toyes and trifles, which may be resisted and withstood, if
they will themselves: but let him that so wonders, consider
with himself, that, if a man should tell him on a sudden,
some of his especial friends were dead, could he choose but
grieve? or set him upon a steep rock, where he should be
in danger to be precipitated, could he be secure? his heart
would tremble for fear, and his head be giddy. P. Byarus

---

[1] Intemperies facit succum nigrum; nigrities obscurat spiritum; obscuratio
spiritûs facit metum et tristitiam.   [2] Ut nubecula solem offuscat. Constantinus, lib. de melanch.   [3] Altomarus, c. 7. Caussam timoris circumfert.
Ater humor passionis materia; et atri spiritus perpetuam animæ domicilio offun-
dunt noctem.

Mem. 3.] *Causes of these Symptomes.* 429

(*Tract. de pest.*) gives instance (as I have said) [1] *and put case* (saith he) *in one that walks upon a plank; if it lye on the ground, he can safely do it; but if the same plank be laid over some deep water, instead of a bridge, he is vehemently moved; and 'tis nothing but his imagination,* formâ cadendi impressâ, *to which his other members and faculties obey.* Yea, but you infer, that such men have a just cause to fear, a true object of fear: so have melancholy men an inward cause, a perpetual fume and darkness, causing fear, grief, suspicion, which they carry with them—an object which cannot be removed, but sticks as close, and is as inseparable, as a shadow to a body; and who can expel, or over-run his shadow: remove heat of the liver, a cold stomach, weak spleen: remove those adust humours and vapours arising from them, black blood from the heart, all outward perturbations; take away the cause; and then bid them not grieve nor fear, or be heavy, dull, lumpish *:* otherwise counsel can do little good; you may as well bid him that is sick of an ague, not to be adry; or him that is wounded, not to feel pain.

Suspicion follows fear and sorrow at heels, arising out of the same fountain; so thinks [2] Fracastorius, *that fear is the cause of suspicion, and still they suspect some treachery, or some secret machinations to be framed against them;* still they distrust. Restlessness proceeds from the same spring; variety of fumes makes them like and dislike. Solitariness, avoiding of light, that they are weary of their lives, hate the world, arise from the same causes; for their spirits and humours are opposite to light; fear makes them avoid company, and absent themselves, lest they should be misused, hissed at, or overshoot themselves; which still they suspect. They are prone to venery, by reason of wind; angry, waspish, and fretting still, out of abundance of choler, which causeth fearful dreams, and violent perturbations to them, both sleeping and waking. That they suppose they have no heads, flye, sink, they are pots, glasses, &c. is wind in their heads. [3] Herc. de Saxoniâ doth ascribe this to the several motions in the animal spirits, *their dilatation, contraction, confusion, alteration, tenebrosity, hot or cold distemperature,* excluding all material humours. [4] Fra-

---

[1] Pone exemplum, quod quis potest ambulare super trabem quæ est in viâ: sed si sit super aquam profundam, loco pontis, non ambulabit super eam, eo quod imaginatur in animo et timet vehementer, formâ cadendi impressâ, cui obediunt membra omnia, et facultates reliquæ.   [2] Lib. 2. de intellectione. Suspiciosi ob timorem et obliquum discursum; et semper inde putant sibi fieri insidias. Lauren. 5.   [3] Tract. de mel. cap. 7. Ex dilatatione, contractione, confusione, tenebrositate spirituum, calidâ, frigidâ intemperie, &c.   [4] Illud inquisitione dignum, cur tam falsa recipiant, habere se cornua, esse mortuos, nasutos, esse aves, &c.

430   *Symptomes of Melancholy.*   [Part. 1. Sec. 3.

castorius *accounts it a thing worthy of inquisition, why they should entertain such false conceits, as that they have horns, great noses, that they are birds, beasts, &c.* why they should think themselves kings, lords, cardinals. For the first, [1] Fracastorius gives two reasons : *one is the disposition of the body ; the other, the occasion of the phantasie,* as if their eyes be purblind, their ears sing by reason of some cold and rheume, &c. To the second, Laurentius answers, the imagination, inwardly or outwardly moved, represents to the understanding, not inticements only, to favour the passion, or dislike : but a very intensive pleasure follows the passion, or displeasure ; and the will and reason are captivated by delighting in it.

Why students and lovers are so often melancholy and mad, the philosopher of [2] Conimbra assigns this reason, *because by a vehement and continual meditation of that wherewith they are affected, they fetch up the spirits into the brain ; and, with the heat brought with them, they incend it beyond measure ; and the cells of the inner senses dissolve their temperature ; which being dissolved, they cannot perform their offices as they ought.*

Why melancholy men are witty, (which Aristotle hath long since maintained in his problems ; and that [3] all learned men, famous philosophers, and law-givers, *ad unum fere omnes melancholici,* have still been melancholy) is a problem much controverted. Jason Pratensis will have it understood of natural. melancholy ; which opinion Melancthon inclines to, in his book *de Animâ,* and Marcilius Ficinus, (*de san. tuen. lib.* 1. *cap.* 5) but not simple; for that makes men stupid, heavy, dull, being cold and dry, fearful, fools, and solitary, but mixt with the other humours, flegm only excepted; and they not adust, [4] but so mixt, as that blood be half, with little or no adustion, that they be neither too hot nor too cold.   Aponensis (cited by Melancthon) thinks it proceeds from melancholy adust, excluding all natural melancholy, as too cold. Laurentius condemns his tenent, because adustion of humours makes men mad, as lime burns when water is cast on it. It must be mixt with blood, and somewhat adust ; and so that old aphorism of Aristotle may be verified: *nullum magnum ingenium sine mixturâ dementiæ,* no excellent wit without a mixture of madness. Fracastorius shall decide the controversie ;

---

[1] 1. Dispositio corporis.   2. Occasio imaginationis.   [2] In pro. li. de cœlo. Vehemens et assidua cogitatio rei erga quam afficitur, spiritus in cerebrum evocat.
[3] Melancholici ingeniosi omnes, summi viri in artibus et disciplinis, sive circum imperatoriam aut reip. disciplinam, omnes fere melancholici.   Aristoteles.
[4] Adeo miscentur, ut sit duplum sanguinis ad reliqua duo.

[1] *phlegmatick are dull: sanguine, lively, pleasant, acceptable and merry, but not witty: cholerick are too swift in motion, and furious, impatient of contemplation, deceitful wits: melancholy men have the most excellent wits, but not all: this humour may be hot or cold, thick or thin; if too hot, they are furious and mad; if too cold, dull, stupid, timorous and sad: if temperate, excellent, rather inclining to that extream of heat, than cold.* This sentence of his will agree with that of Heraclitus; a dry light makes a wise mind; temperate heat and driness are the chief causes of a good wit; therefore, saith Ælian, an elephant is the wisest of all bruit beasts, because his brain is dryest, *et ob atræ bilis copiam:* this reason Cardan approves (*subtil. l.* 12). Jo. Baptista Silvaticus, a physician of Milan, (in his first controversie) hath copiously handled this question; Rulandus, in his problems, Cælius Rhodoginus, *lib.* 17. Valleriola, 6to *narrat. med.* Herc. de Saxoniâ, *Tract. post. de mel. cap.* 3. Lodovicus Mercatus, *de inter. morb. cur. lib. cap.* 17. Baptista Porta, *Physiog. lib.* 1. *c.* 13. and many others.

Weeping, sighing, laughing, itching, trembling, sweating, blushing, hearing and seeing strange noises, visions, wind, crudity, are motions of the body, depending upon these precedent motions of the mind. Neither are tears affections, but actions (as Scaliger holds): [2] *the voice of such as are afraid trembles, because the heart is shaken.* (Conimb. *prob.* 6. *sec.* 3. *de som.*) Why they stut or faulter in their speech, Mercurialis and Montaltus (*cap.* 17) give like reasons out of Hippocrates, [3] *driness, which makes the nerves of the tongue torpid.* Fast speaking, (which is a symptome of some few) Aëtius will have caused [4] *from abundance of wind, and swiftness of imagination:* [5] *baldness comes from excess of dryness;* hirsuteness, from a dry temperature. The cause of much waking is a dry brain, continual meditation, discontent, fears, and cares, that suffer not the mind to be at rest: incontinency is from wind, and an hot liver (Montanus, *cons.* 26). Rumbling in the guts is caused from wind, and wind from ill concoction, weakness of natural heat, or a distempered heat and cold; [6] palpitation of the heart, from vapours; heaviness and aking, from the same cause. That the belly is hard, wind is a cause, and of that leaping in many parts. Redness of the face, and

---

[1] Lib. 2. de intellectione. Pingui sunt Minervâ phlegmatici: sanguinei amabiles, grati, hilares, at non ingeniosi; cholerici celeres motu, et ob id contemplationis impatientes: melancholici solum excellentes, &c. [2] Trepidantium vox tremula, quia cor quatitur. [3] Ob ariditatem quæ reddit nervos linguæ torpidos. [4] Incontinentia linguæ ex copiâ flatuum, et velocitate imaginationis. [5] Calvities ob siccitatis excessum. [6] Aëtius.

432   *Symptomes of Melancholy.*   [Part. 1. Sec. 3.

itching, as if they were flea-bitten, or stung with pis-mires, from a sharp subtile wind : [1] cold sweat, from vapours arising from the hypochondries, which pitch upon the skin ; leanness for want of good nourishment. Why their appetite is so great, [2] Aëtius answers: *os ventris frigescit,* cold in those inner parts, cold belly and hot liver, causeth crudity ; and intention proceeds from perturbations; [3] our soul, for want of spirits, cannot attend exactly to so many intentive operations; being exhaust, and overswayed by passion, she cannot consider the reasons which may disswade her from such affections.

[4] Bashfulness and blushing is a passion proper to men alone, and is not only caused for [5] some shame and ignominy, or that they are guilty unto themselves of some foul fact committed, but (as [6] Fracastorius well determines) *ob defectum proprium, et timorem, from fear, and a conceit of our defects. The face labours and is troubled at his presence that sees our defects; and nature, willing to help, sends thither heat; heat draws the subtilest blood; and so we blush. They that are bold, arrogant, and careless, seldome or never blush, but such as are fearful.* Anthonius Lodovicus, in his book *de pudore,* will have this subtil blood to arise in the face, not so much for the reverence of our betters in presence [7], *but for joy and pleasure, or if any thing at unawares shall pass from us, a sudden accident, occurse, or meeting* (which Disarius, in [8] Macrobius, confirms) any object heard or seen (for blind men never blush, as Dandinus observes ; the night and darkness make men impudent)—or that we be staid before our betters, or in company we like not, or if any thing molest and offend us—*erubescentia* turns to *rubor,* blushing to a continuate redness. [9] Sometimes the extremity of the ears tingle, and are red, sometimes the whole face, *et si nihil vitiosum commiseris,* as Lodovicus holds : though Aristotle is of opinion, *omnis pudor ex vitio commisso,* all shame for some offence. But we find otherwise ; it may as well proceed [10] from fear, from force, and inexperience, (so [11] Dandinus holds) as vice ; a hot liver, saith Duretus (*notis in Hollerium*) *; from a hot brain, from wind, the lungs*

[1] Lauren. c. 13.   [2] Tetrab. 2. ser. 2. c. 10.   [3] Ant. Lodovicus prob. lib. 1. sec. 5. de atrabilariis.   [4] Subrusticus pudor, vitiosus pudor.   [5] Ob ignominiam aut turpedinem facti, &c.   [6] De symp. et antip. cap. 12. Laborat facies ob præsentiam ejus qui defectum nostrum videt; et natura, quasi opem latura, calorem illuc mittit; calor sanguinem trahit : unde rubor. Audaces non rubent, &c.   [7] Ob gaudium et voluptatem, foras exit sanguis, aut ob melioris reverentiam, aut ob subitum occursum, aut si quid incautius exciderit.   [8] Com. in Arist. de animâ. Cæci ut plurimum impudentes. Nox facit impudentes. [9] Alexander Aphrodisiensis makes all bashfulness a vertue ; eamque se refert in seipso experiri solitum, etsi esset admodum senex.   [10] Sæpe post cibum apti ad ruborem, ex potu vini, ex timore sæpe, et ab hepate calido, cerebro calido, &c. [11] Com. in Arist. de animâ. Tam a vi et inexperientiâ quam a vitio.

Mem. 3.]   *Causes of these Symptomes.*   433

heated, or after drinking of wine, strong drink, perturbations, &c.

Laughter, what is it, saith [1] Tully, *how caused, where, and so suddenly breaks out, that, desirous to stay it, we cannot, how it comes to possess and stir our face, veins, eyes, countenance, mouth, sides, let Democritus determine.* The cause, that it often affects melancholy men so much, is given by Gomesius (*l. 3. de sale genial. cap.* 18)—abundance of pleasant vapours, which, in sanguine melancholy especially, break from the heart, [2] *and tickle the midriff, because it is transverse and full of nerves; by which titillation the sense being moved, and the arteries distended, or pulled, the spirits from thence move and possess the sides, veins, countenance, eyes.* See more in Jossius, *de risu, et fletu,* Vives, 3. *de Animâ.* Tears, as Scaliger defines, proceed from grief and pity, [3] *or from the heating of a moist brain; for a dry cannot weep.*

That they see and hear so many phantasms, chimeras, noises, visions, &c. (as Fienus hath discoursed at large in his book of imagination, and [4] Lavater, *de spectris, part.* 1. *cap.* 2, 3, 4) their corrupt phantasie makes them see and hear that which indeed is neither heard nor seen. *Qui multum jejunant, aut noctes ducunt insomnes,* they that much fast, or want sleep, as melancholy or sick men commonly do, see visions, or such as are weak-sighted, very timorous by nature, mad, distracted, or earnestly seek. *Sabini, quod volunt, somniant,* as the saying is; they dream of that they desire. Like Sarmiento the Spaniard, who, when he was sent to discover the Streights of Magellan, and confine places, by the prorex of Peru, standing on the top of an hill, *amœnissimam planitiem despicere sibi visus fuit, ædificia magnifica, quamplurimos pagos, altas turres, splendida templa,* and brave cities, built like ours in Europe; not (saith mine [5] author) that there was any such thing, but that he was *vanissimus et nimis credulus,* and would fain have had it so. Or (as [6] Lod. Mercatus proves), by reason of inward vapours, and humours from blood, choler, &c. diversly mixt, they apprehend and see outwardly, as they suppose, divers images, which indeed are not. As they that drink wine think all runs round, when it is their own brain; so is it with these men; the fault and cause is inward, as Galen affirms; [7] mad men and such as are near death, *quas extra se*

---

[1] De oratore. Quid ipse risus, quo pacto concitetur, ubi sit, &c.   [2] Diaphragma titillant, quia transversum et nervosum, quâ titillatione moto sensu atque arteriis distentis, spiritus inde latera, venas, os, oculos occupant.   [3] Ex calefactione humidi cerebri; nam ex sicco lacrymæ non fluunt.   [4] Res mirandas imaginantur; et putant se videre quæ nec vident, nec audiunt.   [5] Laët. lib. 13. cap. 2. descript. Indiæ Occident.   [6] Lib. 1. cap. 17. cap. de mel.   [7] Insani, et qui morti vicini sunt, res, quas extra se videre putant, intra oculos habent.

VOL. I.   F F

434   *Symptomes of Melancholy.*   [Part. 1. Sec. 3.

videre putant imagines, intra oculos habent; 'tis in their brain,
which seems to be before them; the brain, as a concave glass,
reflects solid bodies. *Senes etiam decrepiti cerebrum habent
concavum et aridum, ut imaginentur se videre* (saith [1] Boissardus)
quæ non sunt; old men are too frequently mistaken, and dote
in like case: or, as he that looketh through a piece of red glass,
judgeth every thing he sees to be red; corrupt vapours mount-
ing from the body to the head, and distilling again from thence
to the eyes, when they have mingled themselves with the
watery crystal which receiveth the shadows of things to be seen,
make all things appear of the same colour, which remains in
the humour that overspreads our sight, as to melancholy men
all is black, to phelgmatick all white, &c.   Or else, as before,
the organs, corrupt by a corrupt phantasie, (as Lemnius, *lib.* 1.
cap. 16. well quotes) [2] *cause a great agitation of spirits and
humours, which wander to and fro in all the creeks of the brain,
and cause such apparitions before their eyes.*   One thinks he
reads something written in the moon, as Pythagoras is said to
have done of old; another smells brimstone, hears Cerberus
bark: Orestes, now mad, supposed he saw the Furies tormenting him, and his mother still ready to run upon him.

> O mater! obsecro, noli me persequi
> His Furiis, adspectu anguineis, horribilibus!
> Ecce! ecce! in me jam ruunt!

but Electra told him, thus raving in his mad fit, he saw no such
sights at all; it was but his crazed imagination.

> Quiesce, quiesce, miser, in linteis tuis:
> Non cernis etenim, quæ videre te putas.

So Pentheus (*in Bacchis Euripidis*) saw two suns, two
Thebes: his brain alone was troubled. Sickness is an ordinary
cause of such sights.   Cardan, *subtil.* 8: *mens ægra, laboribus
et jejuniis fracta, facit eos videre, audire, &c.*   And. Osiander
beheld strange visions, and Alexander ab Alexandro, both
in their sickness, which he relates (*de rerum varietat. lib.* 8.
cap. 44).   Albategnius, that noble Arabian, on his death-bed,
saw a ship ascending and descending; which Fracastorius records of his friend Baptista Turrianus. Weak sight, and a vain
perswasion withall, may effect as much, and second causes
concurring, as an oare in water makes a refraction, and seems
bigger, bended double, &c. The thickness of the aire may
cause such effects: or any object not well discerned in the dark,

---

[1] Cap. 10. de spirit. apparitione.   [2] De occult. nat. mirac.

Mem. 3.] *Causes of these Symptomes.* 435

fear and phantasie will suspect to be a ghost, a devil, &c.
[1] *Quod nimis miseri timent, hoc facile credunt:* we are apt to
believe, and mistake in such cases. Marcellus Donatus (*lib. 2.
cap. 2.*) brings in a story out of Aristotle, of one Antepheron,
which likely saw, wheresoever he was, his own image in the
aire, as in a glass. Vitellio (*lib.* 10. *perspect.*) hath such another instance of a familiar acquaintance of his, that after the
want of three or four nights sleep, as he was riding by a river
side, saw another riding with him, and using all such gestures
as he did; but, when more light appeared, it vanished. Ere-
mites and anachorites have frequently such absurd visions, revelations, by reason of much fasting, and bad diet: many are
deceived by legerdemain, as Scot hath well shewed in his
book of the discovery of witchcraft, and Cardan, *subtil.* 18.
Suffites, perfumes, suffumigations, mixt candles, perspective
glasses, and such natural causes, make men look as if they
were dead, or with horse-heads, bulls-horns, and such like
bruitish shapes, the room full of snakes, adders, dark, light,
green, red, of all colours, as you may perceive in Baptista
Porta, Alexis, Albertus, and others:—glow-worms, fire-drakes,
meteors, *ignis fatuus,* (which Plinius *lib.* 2. *cap.* 37. calls
Castor and Pollux) with many such as appear in moorish
grounds, about church-yards, moist valleys, or where battels
have been fought; the causes of which read in Goclenius,
Velcurius, Finkius, &c. Such feats are often done, to frighten
children, with squibs, rotten wood, &c. to make folks look as
if they were dead, [2] *solito majores,* bigger, lesser, fairer,
fouler, *ut astantes sine capitibus videantur, aut toti igniti, aut
formâ dæmonum. Accipe pilos canis nigri, &c.* saith Albertus;
and so 'tis ordinary to see strange uncouth sights by catoptricks;
who knows not that if, in a dark room, the light be admitted
at one only little hole, and a paper or glass put upon it, the
sun shining, will represent, on the opposite wall, all such
objects as are illuminated by his rays? With concave and
cylinder glasses, we may reflect any shape of men, devils,
anticks, (as magicians most part do, to gull a silly spectator in
a dark room) we will our selves, and that hanging in the air,
when 'tis nothing but such an horrible image (as [3] Agrippa
demonstrates) placed in another room. Roger Bacon of old is
said to have represented his own image walking in the aire by
this art, though no such thing appear in his perspectives. But,

---

[1] Seneca. Quod metuunt nimis, nunquam amoveri posse nec tolli putant.
[2] Sanguis upupæ cum melle compositus et centaureâ, &c. Albertus.   [3] Lib.
1. occult. philos. Imperiti homines dæmonum et umbrarum imagines videre se
putant, quum nihil sint aliud, quam simulacra animæ expertia.

436 *Symptomes of Melancholy.* [Part. 1. Sec. 3.

most part, it is in the brain that deceives them; although I may not deny, but that oftentimes the devil deludes them, takes his opportunity to suggest and represent vain objects to melancholy men, and such as are ill affected. To these you may add the knavish impostures of juglers, exorcists, mass-priests, and mountebanks, of whom Roger Bacon speaks, &c. *de miraculis naturæ et artis, cap.* 1. [1] They can counterfeit the voices of all birds and bruit beasts almost, all tones and tunes of men, and speak within their throats, as if they spoke afar off, that they make their auditors believe they hear spirits, and are thence much astonished and affrighted with it. Besides, those artificial devices to overhear their confessions, like that whispering place of Glocester with us, or like the Dukes place at Mantua in Italy, where the sound is reverberated by a concave wall; a reason of which Blancanus in his Echometria gives, and mathematically demonstrates.

So that the hearing is as frequently deluded as the sight, from the same causes almost, as he that hears bells, will make them sound what he list. *As the fool thinketh, so the bell clinketh.* Theophilus (in Galen) thought he heard musick, from vapours which made his ears sound, &c. Some are deceived by echoes, some by roaring of waters, or concaves and reverberation of aire in the ground, hollow places and walls. [2] At Cadurcum in Aquitany, words and sentences are repeated by a strange echo to the full, or whatsoever you shall play upon a musical instrument, more distinctly and louder, than they are spoken at first. Some echoes repeat a thing spoken seven times, as at Olympus in Macedonia (as Pliny relates, *lib.* 36. *cap.* 15) some twelve times, as at Charenton, a village near Paris in France. At Delphos in Greece heretofore was a miraculous echo, and so in many other places. Cardan (*subtil.* l. 18) hath wonderful stories of such as have been deluded by these echoes. Blancanus the Jesuite (in his Echometria) hath variety of examples, and gives his reader full satisfaction of all such sounds, by way of demonstration. [3] At Barrey, an isle in the Severn mouth, they seem to hear a smith's forge: so at Lipara, and those sulphureous isles, and many such like which Olaus speaks of in the continent of Scandia, and those northern countries. Cardan (*de rerum var. l.* 15. *c.* 84) mentioneth a woman, that still supposed she heard the devil call her, and speaking to her, (she was a painter's wife in Milan)

---

[1] Pythonissæ, vocum varietatem in ventre et gutture fingentes, formant voces humanas a longe vel prope, prout volunt, ac si spiritus cum homine loqueretur; et sonos brutorum fingunt, &c. [2] Tam clare et articulate audies repetitum, ut perfectior sit Echo quam ipse dixeris. [3] Blowing of bellows, and knocking of hammers, if they apply their ear to the cliff.

Sec. 4. Mem. 1.]   *Prognosticks of Melancholy.*   437

and many such illusions and voices, which proceed most part
from a corrupt imagination.

Whence it comes to pass, that they prophesie, speak several
languages, talk of astronomy, and other unknown sciences to
them, (of which they have ever been ignorant) [1] I have in brief
touched; only this I will here add, that Arculanus, Bodin,
(*lib.* 3. *cap.* 6. *dæmon.*) and some others, [2] hold as a manifest
token that such persons are possessed with the devil, (so doth
[3] Hercules de Saxoniâ, and Apponensis) and fit only to be cured
by a priest.   But [4] Guianerius, [5] Montaltus, Pomponatius of
Padua, and Lemnius (*lib.* 2. *cap.* 2), refer it wholly to the
ill disposition of the [6] humour, and that out of the authority of
Aristotle, *prob.* 30. 1, because such symptomes are cured by
purging; and as, by the striking of a flint, fire is inforced, so, by
the vehement motions of spirits, they do *elicere voces inauditas*,
compel strange speeches to be spoken.   Another argument he
hath from Plato's *reminiscentia*, which is, all out, as likely as
that which [7] Marsilius Ficinus speaks of his friend Pierleonus;
by a divine kind of infusion, he understood the secrets of nature,
and tenents of Græcian and barbarian philosophers, before
ever he heard of, saw, or read their works: but in this I should
rather hold, with Avicenna and his associates, that such symptomes proceed from evil spirits, which take all opportunities of
humours decayed, or otherwise, to pervert the soul of man;
and besides, the humour it self is *balneum diaboli*, the devil's
bath, and (as Agrippa proves) doth intice him to seize upon
them.

SECT. IV.   MEMB. I.

Prognosticks of Melancholy.

PROGNOSTICKS, or signs of things to come, are either good
or bad.   If this malady be not hereditary, and taken at the
beginning, there is good hope of cure; *recens curationem
non habet difficilem,* saith Avicenna (*l.* 3. *Fen.* 1. *Tract.* 4.
c. 18).   That which is with laughter, of all others, is most
secure, gentle and remiss (Hercules de Saxoniâ).   [8] *If that
evacuation of hæmrods, or varices which they call the water*

---

[1] Memb. 1. Sub. 3. of this partition, cap. 16. in 9 Rhasis.   [2] Signa dæmonis nulla sunt, nisi quod loquantur ea quæ ante nesciebant, ut Teutonicum aut
aliud idioma, &c.   [3] Cap. 12. tract. de mel.   [4] Tract. 15. c. 4.
[5] Cap. 9.   [6] Mira vis concitat humores, ardorque vehemens mentem exagi-
tat, quum, &c.   [7] Præfat. Jamblici mysteriis.   [8] Si melancholicis
hæmorrhoïdes supervenerint, varices, vel (ut quibusdam placet) aqua inter cutem, solvitur malum.

438   *Prognosticks of Melancholy.*   [Part. 1. Sec. 4.

*between the skin, shall happen to a melancholy man, his misery
is ended* (Hippocrates, *Aphor.* 6. 11). Galen (*l.* 6. *de morbis
vulgar. com.* 8) confirms the same; and to this aphorism of
Hippocrates all the Arabians, new and old Latines, subscribe
(Montaltus, *c.* 25. Hercules de Saxoniâ, Mercurialis, Vittorius,
Faventinus, &c.) Skenkius (*l.* 1. *observat. med. c. de Maniâ*)
illustrates this aphorism, with an example of one Daniel Federer
a coppersmith, that was long melancholy, and in the end mad
about the twenty-seventh year of his age: these *varices* or
water began to arise in his thighs; and he was freed from his
madness. Marius the Roman was so cured, some say, though
with great pain. Skenkius hath some other instances of women that have been helped by flowing of their moneths,
which before were stopped. That the opening of the hæmrods
will do as much for men, all physicians joyntly signifie, so they
be voluntary, some say, and not by compulsion. All melancholy men are better after a quartane. [1] Jobertus saith,
scarce any man hath that ague twice. But, whether it free
him from this malady, 'tis a question; for many physicians
ascribe all along agues for especial causes, and a quartane ague
amongst the rest. [2] Rhasis, *cont. lib.* 1. *tract.* 9. *When melancholy gets out at the superficies of the skin, or settles,
breaking out in scabs, leprosie, morphew, or is purged by
stools, or by the urine, or that the spleen is enlarged, and
those varices appear, the disease is dissolved.* Guianerius
(*cap.* 5. *tract.* 15.) adds dropsie, jaundise, dysentery, leprosie,
as good signs, to these scabs, morphews, and breaking out,
and proves it, out of the sixth of Hippocrates Aphorismes.

Evil prognosticks, on the other part. *Inveterata melancholia incurabilis;* if it be inveterate, it is [3] incurable (a common
axiome), *aut difficulter curabilis,* (as they say that make the
best) hardly cured. This Galen witnesseth (*l.* 3. *de loc. affect.
cap.* 6): [4] *be it in whom it will, or from what cause soever,
it is ever long, wayward, tedious, and hard to be cured, if
once it be habituated.* As Lucian said of the gout, she was [5] *the
queen of the diseases, and inexorable,* may we say of melancholy. Yet Paracelsus will have all diseases whatsoever cu-
rable, and laughs at them which think otherwise, as T. Erastus
(*part.* 3) objects to him; although, in another place, hereditary
diseases he accounts incurable, and by no art to be [6] removed.

---

[1] Cap. 10. de quartanâ.   [2] Cum sanguis exit per superficiem, et residet
melancholia per scabiem, morpheam nigram, vel expurgatur per inferiores partes,
vel urinam, &c. non erit, &c. splen magnificatur, et varices apparent.   [3] Quia
jam conversa in naturam.   [4] In quocunque sit, a quâcunque caussâ, hypochon.
præsertim, semper est longa, morosa, nec facile curari potest.   [5] Regina
morborum et inexorabilis.   [6] Omne delirium, quod oritur a paucitate cerebri,
incurabile. Hildesheim. spicil. de maniâ.

Hildesheim (*spicil. 2. de mel.*) holds it less dangerous, if only [1]*imagination be hurt, and not reason:* [2]*the gentlest is from blood, worse from choler adust, but the worst of all from melancholy putrified.* [3]Bruel esteems hypochondriacal least dangerous, and the other two species (opposite to Galen) hardest to be cured. [4]The cure is hard in man, but much more difficult in women. And both men and women must take notice of that saying of Montanus, (*pro Abbate Italo*): [5]*this malady doth commonly accompany them to their grave; physicians may ease, and it may lye hid for a time; but they cannot quite cure it, but it will return again more violent and sharp than at first, and that upon every small occasion or errour:* as in Mercuries weather-beaten statue, that was once all over gilt, the open parts were clean, yet there was *in fimbriis aurum*, in the chinks a remnant of gold—there will be some reliques of melancholy left in the purest bodies (if once tainted), not so easily to be rooted out. [6]Oftentimes it degenerates into epilepsy, apoplexy, convulsions, and blindness, (by the authority of Hippocrates and Galen) [7]all averr, if once it possess the ventricles of the brain—Frambesarius, and Sallust Salvianus [8]adds, if it get into the optick nerves, blindness. Mercurialis (*consil. 20*) had a woman to his patient, that from melancholy, became epileptick and blind. [9]If it come from a cold cause, or so continue cold, or increase, epilepsie, convulsions follow, and blindness; or else, in the end, they are moped, sottish, and, in all their actions, speeches, gestures, ridiculous. [10]If it come from a hot cause, they are more furious and boisterous, and in conclusion mad. *Calescentem melancholiam sæpius sequitur mania.* [11]If it heat and increase, that is the common event: *per circuitus, aut semper, insanit;* he is mad by fits, or altogether: for (as [12]Sennertus contends out of Crato) there is *seminarium ignis* in this humour, the very seeds of fire. If it come from melancholy natural adust, and in excess, they are often dæmoniacal. (Montanus.)

[13]Seldom this malady procures death, except (which is the greatest, most grievous calamity, and the misery of all miseries)

---

[1] Si sola imaginatio lædatur, et non ratio.   [2] Mala a sanguine fervente, deterior a bile assatâ, pessima ab atrâ bile putrefactâ.   [3] Difficilior cura ejus quæ fit vitio corporis totius et cerebri.   [4] Difficilis curatu in viris, multo difficilior in feminis.   [5] Ad interitum plerumque homines comitatur : licet medici levent plerumque, tamen non tollunt unquam, sed recidet acerbior quam antea, minimâ occasione, aut errore.   [6] Periculum est, ne degeneret in epilepsiam, apoplexiam, convulsionem, cæcitatem.   [7] Montal. c. 25. Laurentius. Nic. Piso.   [8] Her. de Saxoniâ, Aristotle, Capivaccius.   [9] Favent. Humor frigidus sola delirii caussa, furoris vero humor calidus.   [10] Heurnius calls madness sobolem melancholiæ.   [11] Alexander, l. 1. c. 18.   [12] Lib. 1. part. 2. c. 11.   [13] Montalt. c. 15. Raro mors aut nunquam, nisi sibi ipsis inferant.

440 · *Prognosticks of Melancholy.* [Part. 1. Sec. 4.

they make away themselves; which is a frequent thing, and familiar amongst them. 'Tis [1] Hippocrates observation, Galens sentence, (*etsi mortem timent, tamen plerumque sibi ipsis mortem consciscunt, l. 3. de locis affect. cap.* 7) the doom of all physicians. 'Tis Rabbi Moses aphorism, the prognosticon of Avicenna, Rhasis, Aëtius, Gordonius, Valescus, Altomarus, Sallust Salvianus, Capivaccius, Mercatus, Hercules de Saxoniâ, Piso, Bruel, Fuchsius, all, &c.

> [2] Et sæpe usque adeo, mortis formidine, vitæ
> Percipit infelix odium, lucisque videndæ,
> Ut sibi consciscat mœrenti pectore letum.

> And so far forth deaths terrour doth affright,
> He makes away himself, and hates the light:
> To make an end of fear and grief of heart,
> He voluntary dies, to ease his smart.

In such sort doth the torture and extremity of his misery torment him, that he can take no pleasure in his life, but is in a manner inforced to offer violence unto himself, to be freed from his present insufferable pains. So some (saith [3] Fracastorius) *in fury, but most in despair, sorrow, fear, and out of the anguish and vexation of their souls, offer violence to themselves; for their life is unhappy and miserable. They can take no rest in the night, nor sleep : or, if they do slumber, fearful dreams astonish them.* In the day time, they are affrighted still by some terrible object, and torn in pieces with suspicion, fear, sorrow, discontents, cares, shame, anguish, &c. as so many wild horses, that they cannot be quiet an hour, a minute of time, but, even against their wills, they are intent, and still thinking of it; they cannot forget it; it grinds their souls day and night; they are perpetually tormented, a burden to themselves, as Job was; they can neither eat, drink, or sleep. Psal. 107. 18. *Their soul abhorreth all meat, and they are brought to deaths door,* [4] *being bound in misery and iron:* [5] they curse their stars (with Job), [6] *and day of their birth, and wish for death* (for, as Pineda and most interpreters hold, Job was even melancholy, to despair, and almost [7] madness it self) : they murmur many times against the world, friends, allies, all mankind, even against God himself in the bitterness of their passion : [8] *vivere nolunt, mori nesciunt;* live they will not, die they cannot. And, in

[1] Lib. de insan. Fabio Calvo interprete. Nonnulli violentas manus sibi inferunt. [2] Lucret. l. 3. [3] Lib. 2. de Intell. Sæpe mortem sibi consciscunt ob timorem et tristitiam, tædio vitæ affecti ob furorem et desperationem. Est enim infera, &c. Ergo sic perpetuo afflictati vitam oderunt, se præcipitant, his malis carituri, aut interficiunt se, aut tale quid committunt. [4] Psal. 107. 10. [5] Job. 33. [6] Job, 6. 8. [7] Vi doloris et tristitiæ ad insaniam pæne redactus. [8] Seneca.

the midst of these squalid, ugly, and such irksome dayes, they seek at last, (finding no comfort, [1] no remedy in this wretched life) to be eased of all by death. *Omnia appetunt bonum;* all creatures seek the best, and for their good, as they hope, *sub specie*, in shew at least, *vel quia mori pulchrum putant*, (saith [2] Hippocrates) *vel quia putant inde se majoribus malis liberari*, to be freed as they wish. Though, many times, as Æsops fishes, they leap from the frying-pan into the fire it self, yet they hope to be eased by this means; and therefore, (saith Felix [3] Platerus) *after many tedious dayes, at last, either by drowning, hanging, or some such fearful end,* they precipitate or make away themselves : *many lamentable examples are daily seen amongst us : alius ante fores se laqueo suspendit,* (as Seneca notes) *alius se præcipitavit a tecto, ne dominum stomachantem audiret; alius, ne reduceretur a fugâ, ferrum adegit in viscera :* so many causes there are

————His amor exitio est, furor his————

love, grief, anger, madness; and shame, &c. 'Tis a common calamity, [4] a fatal end to this disease : they are condemned to a violent death, by a jury of physicians, furiously disposed, carried headlong by their tyrannizing wills, inforced by miseries ; and there remains no more to such persons, if that heavenly physician, by his assisting grace and mercy alone, do not prevent, (for no humane perswasion or art can help) but to be their own butchers, and execute themselves. Socrates his *cicuta,* Lucretias dagger, Timons halter are yet to be had ; Catoes knife, and Neroes sword are left behind them, as so many fatal engines, bequeathed to posterity, and will be used, to the worlds end, by such distressed souls : so intolerable, unsufferable, grievous and violent is their pain, [5] so unspeakable, and continuate. One day of grief is an hundred years, as Cardan observes : 'tis *carnificina hominum, angor animi,* as well saith Aretæus, a plague of the soul, the cramp and convulsion of the soul, an epitome of hell ; and, if there be an hell upon earth, it is to be found in a melancholy mans heart :

> For that deep torture may be call'd an hell,
> When more is felt, than one hath power to tell.

Yea, that which scoffing Lucian said of the gout in jest, I may truly affirm of melancholy in earnest.

---

[1] In salutis suæ desperatione proponunt sibi mortis desiderium. Oct. Horat. l. 2. c. 5. [2] Lib. de insaniâ. Sic sic juvat ire per umbras. [3] Cap. 3. de mentis alienat. Mœsti degunt, dum tandem mortem, quam timent, suspendio aut submersione, aut aliquâ aliâ vi, ut multa tristia exempla vidimus. [4] Arculanus, in 9 Rhasis, c. 16. Cavendum, ne ex alto se præcipitent, aut alias lædant. [5] O omnium opinionibus incogitabile malum! Lucian. Mortesque mille, mille, dum vivit, neces, gerit, peritque. Heinsius, Austriaco.

442   *Prognosticks of Melancholy.*   [Part. 1. Sec. 4.

O triste nomen! O Diis odibile,
[1] Melancholia lacrymosa, Cocyti filia!
Tu tartari specubus opacis edita
Erinnys, utero quam Megæra suo tulit,
Et ab uberibus aluit, cuique parvulæ
Amarulentum in os lac Alecto dedit.
Omnes abominabilem te dæmones
Produxere in lucem, exitio mortalium.

Et paullo post—

Non Jupiter fert tale telum fulminis,
Non ulla sic procella sævit æquoris,
Non impetuosi tanta vis est turbinis.
An asperos sustineo morsus Cerberi?
Num virus Echidnæ membra mea depascitur?
Aut tunica sanie tincta Nessi sanguinis?
Illacrymabile et immedicabile malum hoc.

O sad and odious name! a name so fell,
Is this of melancholy, brat of hell.
There born in hellish darkness doth it dwell.
The Furies brought it up, Megæra's teat,
Alecto gave it bitter milk to eat:
And all conspir'd a bane to mortal men,
To bring this devil out of that black den.

Jupiters thunderbolt, nor storm at sea,
Nor whirl-wind, doth our hearts so much dismay.
What? am I bit by that fierce Cerberus?
Or stung by [2] serpent so pestiferous?
Or put on shirt that's dipt in Nessus blood?
My pain's past cure; physick can do no good.

No torture of body like unto it;

————Siculi non invenere tyranni
Majus tormentum;

no strappados, hot irons, Phalaris bulls,

[3] ————Nec ira Deûm tantum, nec tela, nec hostis,
Quantum sola noces animis illapsa.

Joves wrath, nor devils, can
Do so much harm to th' soul of man.

All fears, griefs, suspicions, discontents, imbonities, insuavities,
are swallowed up and drowned in this Euripus, this Irish sea,
this ocean of misery, as so many small brooks; 'tis *coagulum
omnium ærumnarum*, which [4] Ammianus applied to his distressed Palladius. I say of our melancholy man, he is the
cream of humane adversity, the [5] quintessence, and upshot;

---

[1] Regina morborum, cui famulantur omnes et obediunt. Cardan.   [2] Eheu!
quis intus scorpio, &c. Seneca, Act. 4. Herc. Œt.   [3] Silius Italicus.
[4] Lib. 29.   [5] Hîc omnis imbonitas et insuavitas consistit, ut Tertulliani
verbis utar, orat. ad martyr.

Mem. 1.]   *Prognosticks of Melancholy.*   443

all other diseases whatsoever are but flea-bitings, to melancholy, in extent : 'tis the pith of them all,

> [1] Hospitium est calamitatis.   Quid verbis opus est ?
> Quamcunque malam rem quæris, illic reperies.

> What need more words ? 'tis calamities inn,
> Where seek for any mischief, 'tis within ;

and a melancholy man is that true Prometheus, which is bound to Caucasus ; the true Tityus, whose bowels are still by a vulture devoured (as poets feign); for so doth [2] Lilius Giraldus interpret it of anxieties, and those griping cares ; and so ought it to be understood. In all other maladies we seek for help : if a leg or an arm ake, through any distemperature or wound, or that we have an ordinary disease, above all things whatsoever we desire help and health, a present recovery, if by any means possible it may be procured : we will freely part with all our other fortunes, substance, endure any misery, drink bitter potions, swallow those distasteful pills, suffer our joynts to be seared, to be cut off, any thing for future health ; so sweet, so dear, so precious above all other things in this world is life : 'tis that we chiefly desire, long and happy days; ([3]*multos da, Jupiter, annos!*) increase of years all men wish ; but, to a melancholy man, nothing so tedious, nothing so odious ; that which they so carefully seek to preserve, [4] he abhors, he alone.   So intolerable are his pains, some make a question, *graviores morbi corporis an animi,* whether the diseases of the body or mind be more grievous : but there is no comparison, no doubt to be made of it ; *multo enim sævior longeque est atrocior animi quam corporis cruciatus* (Lem. *l.* 1. *c.* 12): the diseases of the mind are far more grievous.—*Totum hic pro vulnere corpus ;* body and soul is misaffected here, but the soul especially.   So Cardan testifies (*de rerum. var. lib.* 8. 40) : [5] Maximus Tyrius a Platonist, and Plutarch, have made just volumes to prove it.   [6] *Dies adimit ægritudinem hominibus;* in other diseases there is some hope likely ; but these unhappy men are born to misery, past all hope of recovery, incurably sick; the longer they live, the worse they are ; and death alone must ease them.

Another doubt is made by some philosophers, whether it be lawful for a man, in such extremity of pain and grief, to make away himself, and how those men that so do are to be censured.   The Platonists approve of it, that it is lawful in such cases, and upon a necessity.   Plotinus (*l. de beatitud. c.* 7), and Socrates himself defends it, (in Platos Phædon): *if any man labour of an incurable disease, he may dispatch himself, if*

---

[1] Plautus.   [2] Vit. Herculis.   [3] Persius.   [4] Quid est miserius in vitâ, quam velle mori ? Seneca.   [5] Tom. 2. Libello, an graviores passiones, &c.
[6] Ter.

444 *Prognosticks of Melancholy.* [Part. 1. Sec. 4.

it be to his good. Epicurus and his followers, the Cynicks, and Stoicks, in general affirm it, Epictetus and [1] Seneca amongst the rest: *quamcunque veram esse viam ad libertatem;* any way is allowable, that leads to liberty; [2] *let us give God thanks, that no man is compelled to live against his will:* [3] *quid ad hominem claustra, carcer, custodia? liberum ostium habet;* death is always ready and at hand. *Vides illum præcipitem locum, illud flumen?* dost thou see that steep place, that river, that pit, that tree? there is liberty at hand; *effugia servitutis et doloris sunt,* as that Laconian lad cast himself headlong, (*non serviam, aiebat puer*) to be freed of his misery. Every vein in thy body, if these be *nimis operosi exitus,* will set thee free: *quid tua refert, finem facias an accipias?* there's no necessity for a man to live in misery. *Malum est necessitati vivere; sed in necessitate vivere, necessitas nulla est. Ignavus, qui sine caussâ moritur; et stultus, qui cum dolore vivit* (*Idem, epi.* 58). Wherefore hath our mother the earth brought out poisons (saith [4] Pliny) in so great a quantity, but that men in distress might make away themselves? which kings of old had ever in a readiness, *ad incerta fortunæ venenum sub custode promtum* (Livy writes,) and executioners alwayes at hand. Speusippus, being sick, was met by Diogenes; and, carried on his slaves shoulders, he made his moan to the philosopher: but, I pity thee not, quoth Diogenes, *qui cum talis sis, vivere sustines:* thou maist be freed when thou wilt,—meaning by death. [5] Seneca therefore commends Cato, Dido, and Lucretia, for their generous courage in so doing, and others that voluntarily die, to avoid a greater mischief, to free themselves from misery, to save their honour, or vindicate their good name, as Cleopatra did, as Sophonisba (Syphax wife) did, Hannibal did, as Junius Brutus, as Vibius Virius, and those Campanian senatours in Livy (*Dec. 3. lib.* 6), to escape the Roman tyranny, that poisoned themselves. Themistocles drank bulls blood, rather than he would fight against his countrey; and Demosthenes chose rather to drink poyson, Publius *Crassi filius,* Censorius, and Plancus, those heroical Romans, to make away themselves, than to fall into their enemies hands. How many myriads besides in all ages might I remember,

———————— qui sibi letum
Insontes peperere manu, &c.

[6] Rhasis, in the Macchabees, is magnified for it, Sampsons death approved. So did Saul and Jonas sin; and many

---

[1] Patet exitus; si pugnare non vultis, licet fugere: quis vos tenet invitos? De provid. cap. 8.   [2] Agamus Deo gratias, quod nemo invitus in vitâ teneri potest.   [3] Epist. 26. Senec. et de sacra. 2. cap. 15. et Epist. 70. et 12.   [4] Lib. 2. cap. 83. Terra mater nostri miserta.   [5] Epist. 24. 71. 82.   [6] Mac. 14. 42.

Mem. 1.]   *Prognosticks of Melancholy.*   445

worthy men and women, *quorum memoria celebratur in ecclesiá*, saith [1] Leminchus, for killing themselves to save their chastity and honour, when Rome was taken (as Austin instances, *l.* 1. *de Civit. Dei, cap.* 16). Jerome vindicateth the same (*in Jonam*); and Ambrose (*l.* 3. *de virginitate*) commendeth Pelagia for so doing. Eusebius (*lib.* 8. *cap.* 15) admires a Roman matron for the same fact, to save herself from the lust of Maxentius the tyrant. Adelhelmus, abbot of Malmesbury, calls them *beatas virgines, quæ sic, &c.* Titus Pomponius Atticus, that wise, discreet, renowned Roman senator, Tullys dear friend, when he had been long sick, as he supposed of an incurable disease, *vitamque produceret ad augendos dolores, sine spe salutis*, was resolved voluntarily by famine to dispatch himself, to be rid of his pain ; and when as Agrippa and the rest of his weeping friends earnestly besought him, *osculantes obsecrarent, ne id, quod natura cogeret, ipse acceleraret*, not to offer violence to himself—*with a settled resolution he desired again they would approve of his good intent, and not seek to dehort him from it ;* and so constantly died, *precesque eorum taciturná suá obstinatione depressit.* Even so did Corellius Rufus, another grave senator, (by the relation of Plinius Secundus, *epist. lib.* 1. *epist.* 12) famish himself to death ; *pedibus correptus, cum incredibiles cruciatus et indignissima tormenta pateretur, a cibis omnino abstinuit :* neither he nor Hispulla his wife could divert him; but *destinatus mori obstinate magis,* &c. die he would, and die he did. So did Lycurgus, Aristotle, Zeno, Chrysippus, Empedocles, with myriads, &c. In warrs, for a man to run rashly upon imminent danger, and present death, is accounted valour and magnanimity ; [2] to be the cause of his own, and many a thousands ruine besides, to commit wilful murther in a manner, of himself and others, is a glorious thing ; and he shall be crowned for it. The [3] Massagetæ in former times, [4] Barbiccians, and I know not what nations besides, did stifle their old men, after seventy years, to free them from those grievances incident to that age. So did the inhabitants of the island of Choa; because their aire was pure and good, and the people generally long lived, *antevertebant fatum suum, priusquam manci forent, aut imbecillitas accederet, papavere vel cicutá ;* with poppy or hemlock they prevented death. Sr Thomas More, in his Utopia, commends voluntary death, if he be *sibi aut aliis molestus,* troublesome to himself or others: [5] *especially if to live be a*

---

[1] Vindicatio Apoc. lib.   [2] As amongst Turks and others.   [3] Bohemus, de moribus gent.   [4] Ælian. lib. 4. cap. 1. Omnes 70 annum egressos interficiunt.   [5] Lib. 2.   Præsertim cum tormentum ei vita sit, bonâ spe fretus, acerbâ vitâ, velut a carcere, se eximat, vel ab aliis eximi suâ voluntate patiatur.

446 *Prognosticks of Melancholy.* [Part. 1. Sec. 4.

torment to him, let him free himself with his own hands from this tedious life, as from a prison, or suffer himself to be freed by others. [1] And 'tis the same tenent which Laërtius relates of Zeno, of old : *juste sapiens sibi mortem consciscit, si in acerbis doloribus versetur, membrorum mutilatione, aut morbis ægre curandis,* and which Plato (9. *de legibus*) approves, if old age, poverty, ignominy, &c. oppress; and which Fabius expresseth in effect (*Præfat. 7. Institut.*) *nemo, nisi suâ culpâ, diu dolet.* It is an ordinary thing in China, (saith Mat. Riccius the Jesuit) [2] *if they be in despair of better fortunes, or tyred and tortured with misery, to bereave themselves of life, and many times, to spite their enemies the more, to hang at their door.* Tacitus the historian, Plutarch the philosopher, much approve a voluntary departure, and Austin (*de Civ. Dei, l. 1. c. 29*) defends a violent death, so that it be undertaken in a good cause : *nemo sic mortuus, qui non fuerat aliquando moriturus : quid autem interest, quo mortis genere vita ista finiatur, quando ille, cui finitur, iterum mori non cogitur? &c.* no man so voluntarily dies, but *volens nolens,* he must die at last; and our life is subject to innumerable casualties : who knows when they may happen? *utrum satius est, unam perpeti moriendo, an omnes timere vivendo?* [3] rather suffer one, than fear all. *Death is better than a bitter life* (*Ec.* 30. 17) : [4] and a harder choice to live in fear, than, by once dying, to be freed from all. Cleombrotus Ambraciotes perswaded I know not how many hundreds of his auditors, by a luculent oration he made of the miseries of this, and happiness of that other life, to precipitate themselves : and (having read Platos divine tract *de animâ*) for example's sake, led the way first. That neat epigram of Callimachus will tell you as much :

> Jamque vale, Soli cum diceret Ambraciotes,
>   In Stygios fertur desiluisse lacus,
> Morte nihil dignum passus : sed forte Platonis
>   Divini eximium de nece legit opus.

[5] Calenus and his Indians hated of old to die a natural death : the Circumcellians and Donatists, loathing life, compelled others to make them away :—with many such [6] : but these are

---

[1] Nam quis, amphoram exsiccans, fæcem exsorberet? (Seneca, epist. 58.) quis in pœnas et risum viveret? Stulti est manere in vitâ, cum sit miser. [2] Expedit. ad Sinas, l. 1. c. 9. Vel bonorum desperatione, vel malorum perpessione, fracti et fatigati, vel manus violentas sibi inferunt, vel, ut inimicis suis ægre faciant, &c. [3] So did Anthony, Galba, Vitellius, Otho, Aristotle himself, &c. Ajax in despair, Cleopatra to save her honour. [4] Inertius deligitur diu vivere in timore tot morborum, quam, semel moriendo, nullum deinceps formidare. [5] Curtius, l. 16. [6] Laqueus præcisus, cont. 1. l. 5. Quidam, naufragio facto, amissis tribus liberis et uxore, suspendit se; præcidit illi quidam ex prætereuntibus laqueum : a liberato reus fit maleficii. Seneca.

Mem. 1.] *Prognosticks of Melancholy.* 447

false and pagan positions, prophane stoical paradoxes, wicked examples: it boots not what heathen philosophers determine in this kind: they are impious, abominable, and upon a wrong ground. *No evil is to be done, that good may come of it ; reclamat Christus, reclamat scriptura ;* God, and all good men are [1] against it. He that stabs another, can kill his body ; but he that stabs himself, kills his own soul. [2] *Male meretur, qui dat mendico, quod edat; nam et illud quod dat, perit ; et illi producit vitam ad miseriam :* he that gives a beggar an almes (as that comical poet said) doth ill, because he doth but prolong his miseries. But Lactantius (*l. 6. c. 7. de vero cultu*) calls it a detestable opinion, and fully confutes it (*lib. 3. de sap. cap.* 18); and S. Austin (*ep. 52. ad Macedonium, cap. 61. ad Dulcitium Tribunum*): so doth Hierom, to Marcella of Blæsillas death: *non recipio tales animas,* &c. he calls such men *martyres stultæ philosophiæ :* so doth Cyprian (*de duplici martyrio*): *si qui sic moriantur, aut infirmitas, aut ambitio, aut dementia. cogit eos :* 'tis meer madness so to do; [3] *furor est, ne moriare, mori.* To this effect writes Arist. 3. *Ethic.* Lipsius, *Manuduc. ad Stoïcam Philosophiam, lib. 3. dissertat. 23 :* but it needs no confutation. This only let me add, that, in some cases, those [4] hard censures of such as offer violence to their own persons, or in some desperate fit to others, which sometimes they do by stabbing, slashing, &c. are to be mitigated, as in such as are mad, beside themselves for the time, or found to have been long melancholy, and that in extremity : they know not what they do, deprived of reason, judgement, all, [5] as a ship, that is void of a pilot, must needs impinge upon the next rock, or sands, and suffer shipwrack. [6] P. Forestus hath a story of two melancholy brethren, that made away themselves, and, for so foul a fact, were accordingly censured to be infamously buried, as in such cases they use, to terrifie others (as it did the Milesian virgins of old : but, upon further examination of their misery and madness, the censure was [7] revoked, and they were solemnly interred, as Saul was by David (*2 Sam.* 2. 4), and Seneca well adviseth, *irascere interfectori, sed miserere interfecti ;* be justly offended with him, as he was a mur-

---

[1] See Lipsius, Manuduc. ad Stoïcam philosophiam, lib. 3. dissert. 22. D. Kings 14 Lect. on Jonas. D. Abbots 6 Lect. on the same prophet.   [2] Plautus.
[3] Martial.   [4] As to be buried out of Christian burial, with a stake. Idem Plato (9. de legibus) vult separatim sepeliri, qui sibi ipsis mortem consciscunt, &c. lose their goods, &c.   [5] Navis, destituta nauclero, in terribilem aliquem scopulum impingit.   [6] Observat.   [7] Seneca, tract. 1. l. 8. c. 4. Lex, homicida insepultus abjiciatur : contradicitur, eo quod afferre sibi manus coactus sit assiduis malis ; summam infelicitatem suam in hoc removit, quod existimabat licere misero mori.

448   *Prognosticks of Melancholy.*   [Part. 1. Sec. 4.

derer, but pity him now, as a dead man.   Thus of their goods
and bodies we can dispose; but what shall become of their
souls, God alone can tell: his mercy may come *inter pontem
et fontem, inter gladium et jugulum,* betwixt the bridge and
the brook, the knife and the throat.   *Quod cuiquam contigit,
cuivis potest :* who knows how he may be tempted?   It is his
case ; it may be thine :

[1] Quæ sua sors hodie est, cras fore vestra potest.

We ought not to be so rash and rigorous in our censures, as
some are : charity will judge and hope the best: God be mer-
ciful unto us all !.

[1] Buchanan, Eleg. lib.

THE SYNOPSIS
OF THE
SECOND PARTITION.

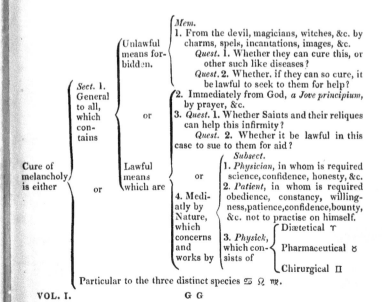

VOL. I. G G

SYNOPSIS OF THE SECOND PARTITION.

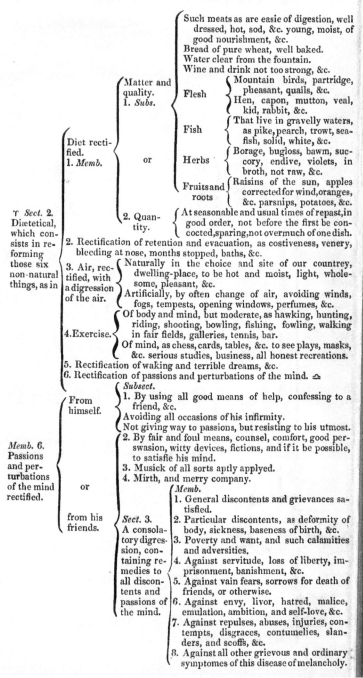

SYNOPSIS OF THE SECOND PARTITION. 451

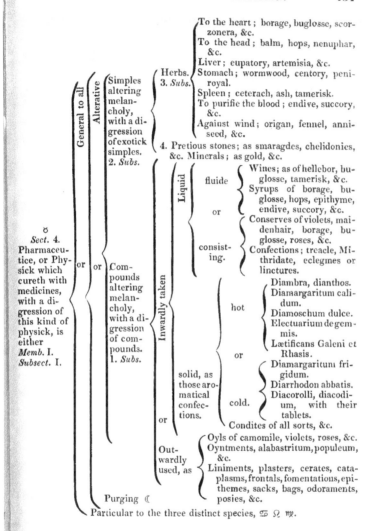

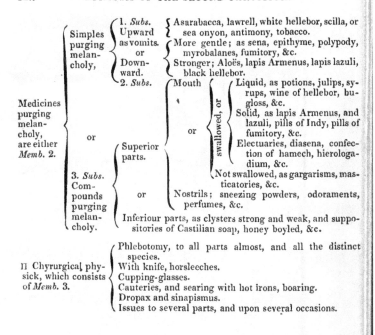

SYNOPSIS OF THE SECOND PARTITION. 453

1. *Subsect.*
Moderate diet, meat of good juice, moistning, easie of digestion.
Good air.
Sleep more than ordinary.
Excrements daily to be voided by art or nature.
Exercise of body and mind not too violent, or too remiss, passions of the mind, and perturbations to be avoided.

2. Blood-letting, if there be need, or that the blood be corrupt, in the arm, forehead, &c. or with cupping-glasses.

℥ *Sect.* 5. Cure of head melancholy. *Memb.* 1.

3. Preparatives and purgers.
{ Preparatives; as syrup of borage, bugloss, epithyme, hops, with their distilled waters, &c.
Purgers; as Montanus and Matthiolus helleborismus, Quercetanus syrup of hellebor, extract of hellebor, pulvis Hali, antimony prepared, *Rulandi aqua mirabilis:* which are used, if gentler medicines will not take place: with Arnoldus *vinum buglossatum,* sena, cassia, myrobalanes, *aurum potabile,* or before Hamech, pil. Indæ. hiera. pil. de lap. Armeno, lazuli.

4. Averters.
{ Cardans nettles, frictions, clysters, suppositories, sneezings, masticatories, nasals, cupping-glasses.
To open the hæmorrhoids with horsleeches, to apply horsleeches to the forehead without scarification, to the shoulders, thighs.
Issues, boaring, cauteries, hot irons in the suture of the crown.

5. Cordials, resolvers, hinderers.
{ A cup of wine or strong drink.
Bezoars stone, amber, spice.
Conserves of borage, bugloss, roses, fumitory.
Confection of alchermes.
Electuarium lætificans Galeni et Rhasis, &c.
Diamargaritum frig. diaboraginatum, &c.

6. Correctors of accidents, as,
{ Odoraments of roses, violets.
Irrigations of the head, with the decoctions of nymphea, lettice, maloes, &c.
Epithemes, oyntments, bags to the heart.
Fomentations of oyl for the belly.
Baths of sweet water, in which were sod mallows, violets, roses, water-lillies, borage flowers, rams heads, &c.

To procure sleep, and are
{ Inwardly taken,
{ Simples { Poppy, nymphea, lettice, roses, purslane, henbane, mandrake, nightshade, opium, &c.
or
Compounds. { Liquid, as syrups of poppy, verbasco, violets, roses.
Solid, as *requies Nicholai, Philonium Romanum, laudanum Paracelsi.*
or
Outwardly used, as,
{ Oyls of nymphea, poppy, violets, roses, mandrake, nutmegs.
Odoraments of vinegar, rose-water, opium.
Frontals of rose-cake, rose-vinegar, nutmeg.
Qyntments, alabastritum, unguentum populeum, simple or mixt with opium.
Irrigations of the head, feet, spunges, musick, murmur and noise of waters.
Frictions of the head, and outward parts, sacculi of henbane, wormwood at his pillow, &c.

Against terrible dreams; not to sup late, or eat pease, cabbage, venison, meats heavy of digestion, use bawm, harts-tongue, &c.
Against ruddiness and blushing, inward and outward remedies.

℥. 2. *Memb.* ⎰ Diet, preparatives, purges, averters, cordials, correctors, as before:
Cure of melan- ⎱ Phlebotomy, in this kind more necessary, and more frequent.
choly over the ⎰ To correct and cleanse the blood with fumitory, sena, succory,
body.　　　 ⎱ 　 dandelion, endive, &c.

Subsect. 1.

Phlebotomy, if need require.

Diet preparatives, averters, cordials, purgers, as before, saving that they must not be so vehement.

Use of peny-royal, wormwood, centaury sod, which alone hath cured many.

To provoke urine with anniseed, daucus, asarum, &c. and stools, if need be, by clysters and suppositories.

To respect the spleen, stomach, liver, hypochondries.

To use treacle now and then in winter.

To vomit after meals sometimes, if it be inveterate.

℞ Cure of Hypochondriacal or windy melancholy. 3. *Memb.*

To expel wind.

Inwardly taken,

or

Simples,

Roots,
{ Galanga, gentian, enula, angelica, calamus aromaticus, zedoary, china, condite ginger, &c.

Herbs,
{ Peniroyal, rue, calamint, bay leaves, and berries, scordium, bettany, lavander, camomile, centaury, wormwood, cumin, broom, orange pills.

Spices,
{ Saffron, cinnamon, mace, nutmeg, pepper, musk, zedoary with wine, &c.

Seeds,
{ Anniseed, fennel-seed, ammi, cari, cumin, nettle, bayes, parsley, grana paradisi.

Compounds, as
Dianisum, diagalanga, diaciminum, diacalaminthes, electuarium de baccis lauri, benedicta laxativa, &c. pulvis carminativus, et pulvis descrip. Antidotario Florentino, aromaticum rosatum, Mithridate.

Outwardly used, as cupping-glasses to the hypochondries without scarification, oyl of camomile, rue, anniseed, their decoctions, &c.

THE

SECOND PARTITION.

THE CURE OF MELANCHOLY.

THE FIRST { SECTION. MEMBER. SUBSECTION.

Unlawful cures rejected.

INVETERATE melancholy, howsoever it may seem to be a continuate, inexorable disease, hard to be cured, accompanying them to their graves most part (as [1] Montanus observes), yet many times it may be helped, even that which is most violent, or at least (according to the same [2] author) *it may be mitigated and much eased. Nil desperandum.* It may be hard to cure, but not impossible for him that is most grievously affected, if he be but willing to be helped.

Upon this good hope I will proceed, using the same method in the cure, which I have formerly used in the rehearsing of the causes; first *general*, then *particular;* and those according to their several species. Of these cures some be *lawful,* some again *unlawful,* which though frequent, familiar, and often used, yet justly censured, and to be controverted: as, first, whether, by these diabolical means, which are commonly practised by the devil and his ministers, sorcerers, witches, magicians, &c. by spells, cabalistical words, charms, characters, images, amulets, ligatures, philtres, incantations, &c. this disease and the like may be cured? and, if they may, whether it be lawful to make use of them, those magnetical cures, or for our good to seek after such means in any case?

[1] Consil. 235. pro Abbate Italo. certe minus afficietur, si volet.

[2] Consil. 223. Aut curabitur, aut

456   *Cure of Melancholy.*   [Part. 2. Sec. 1.

The first, whether they can do any such cures, is questioned
amongst many writers, some affirming, some denying. Valesius, *cont. med. lib. 5. cap.* 6. Malleus Maleficor. Heurnius,
l. 3. *pract. med. cap.* 28. Cœlius, *lib.* 16. *c.* 16. Delrio,
tom. 3. Wierus, *lib.* 2. *de præstig. dæm.* Libanius, Lavater,
de spect. part. 2. *cap.* 7. Holbrenner the Lutheran in *Pisto-
rium,* Polydor Virg. *l.* 1. *de prodig.* Tandlerus, Lemnius,
(Hippocrates, and Avicenna amongst the rest) deny that spirits
or devils have any power over us, and refer all (with Pomponatius of Padua) to natural causes and humours. Of the other
opinion are Bodinus, *Dæmonomantiæ, lib.* 3. *cap.* 2. Arnoldus
Marcellus Empiricus, J. Pistorius, Paracelsus, *Apodix. Magic.*
Agrippa, *lib.* 2. *de. occult. Philos. cap.* 36. 69. 71, 72. *et l.* 3.
c. 23. *et* 10. Marcilius Ficinus, *de vit. cœlit. compar. cap.* 13.
15. 18. 21. &c. Galleottus, *de promiscuâ doct. cap.* 24. Jovianus Pontanus, *Tom.* 2. Plin. *lib.* 28. *c.* 2. Strabo, *lib.* 15.
Geog. Leo Suavius; Goclenius, *de ung. armar.* Oswoldus
Crollius, Ernestus Burgravius, D[r]. Flud, &c.—Cardan (*de
subt.*) brings many proofs out of *Ars Notoria,* and Solomons
decayed works, old Hermes, Artesius, Costaben Luca, Pica-
trix, &c. that such cures may be done. They can make fire it
shall not burn, fetch back thieves or stoln goods, shew their
absent faces in a glass, make serpents lye still, stanch blood,
salve gouts, epilepsies, biting of mad dogs, tooth-ach, melancholy, *et omnia mundi mala,* make men immortal, young
again, as the [1] Spanish marquess is said to have done by one of
his slaves, and some, which juglers in [2] China maintains still (as
Tragaltius writes) that they can do by their extraordinary skill
in physick, and some of our modern chymists by their strange
limbecks, by their spels, philosophers stones and charms.
[3] *Many doubt,* saith Nicholas Taurellus, *whether the devil can cure such diseases he hath not made; and some flatly
deny it: howsoever common experience confirms to our astonishment, that magicians can work such feats, and that the devil without impediment can penetrate through all the parts of
our bodies, and cure such maladies, by means to us unknown.*
Daneus, in his tract *de Sortiariis,* subscribes to this of Taurellus;
Erastus (*de Lamiis*) maintaineth as much; and so do most divines, that, out of their excellent knowledge and long experience,
they can commit [4] *agentes cum patientibus, colligere semina
rerum, eaque materiæ applicare,* as Austin infers (*de Civ. Dei,*

---

[1] Vide Renatum Morey, Anim. in scholam Salernit. c. 38. Si ad 40 annos
possent producere vitam, cur non ad centum? si ad centum, cur non ad mille?
[2] Hist. Chinensium.   [3] Alii dubitant an dæmon possit morbos curare quos non
fecit; alii negant; sed quotidiana experientia confirmat, magos magno multorum
stupore morbos curare, singulas corporis partes citra impedimentum permeare, et
mediis nobis ignotis curare.   [4] Agentia cum patientibus conjungunt.

et de Trinit. lib. 3. cap. 7. et 8): they can work stupend and admirable conclusions; we see the effects only, but not the causes of them. Nothing so familiar as to hear of such cures. Sorcerers are too common; cunning men, wizards, and white-witches (as they call them), in every village, which, if they be sought unto, will help almost all infirmities of body and mind— *servatores* in Latin; and they have commonly S^t. Catherines wheel printed in the roof of their mouth, or in some other part about them; *resistunt incantatorum præstigiis*, ([1] Boissardus writes) *morbos a sagis motos propulsant, &c.* that to doubt of it any longer, [2] *or not to believe, were to run into that other sceptical extreme of incredulity*, saith Taurellus. Leo Suavius (in his comment upon Paracelsus) seems to make it an art, which ought to be approved; Pistorius and others stifly maintain the use of charmes, words, characters, &c. *Ars vera est; sed pauci artifices reperiuntur;* the art is true, but there be but a few that have skill in it. Marcellus Donatus (*lib. 2. de hist. mir. cap.* 1) proves, out of Josephus eight books of anti-quities, that [3] *Solomon so cured all the diseases of the mind by spels, charmes, and drove away devils, and that Eleazar did as much before Vespasian.* Langius (in his *med. epist.*) holds Jupiter Menecrates, that did so many stupend cures in his times, to have used this art, and that he was no other than a magician. Many famous cures are daily done in this kind; the devil is an expert physician (as Godelman calls him, *lib.* 1. *c.* 18): and God permits oftentimes these witches and magicians to pro-duce such effects, as Lavater (*cap.* 3. *lib.* 8. *part.* 3. *cap.* 1), Poly. Virg. (*lib.* 1. *de prodigiis*), Delrio, and others, admit. Such cures may be done; and, as Paracels. (*Tom.* 4. *de morb. ament.*) stifly maintains, [4] *they cannot otherwise be cured but by spells, seals, and spiritual physick.* [5] Arnoldus (*lib. de sigillis*) sets down the making of them; so doth Rulandus, and many others.

Hoc posito, they can effect such cures, the main question is, whether it be lawful, in a desperate case, to crave their help, or ask a wisards advice. 'Tis a common practice of some men to go first to a witch, and then to a physician; if one cannot, the other shall:

Flectere si *nequeunt* Superos, Acheronta *movebunt.*

[6] *It matters not*, saith Paracelsus, *whether it be God or the devil,*

---

[1] Cap. 11. de Servat.   [2] Hæc alii rident: sed vereor, ne, dum nolumus esse creduli, vitium non effugiamus incredulitatis.   [3] Refert Solomonem mentis morbos curâsse, et dæmones abegisse ipsos carminibus, quod et coram Vespasiano fecit Eleazar.   [4] Spirituales morbi spiritualiter curari debent.   [5] Sigil-lum ex auro peculiari ad melancholiam, &c.   [6] Lib. 1. de occult. Philos. Nihil refert, an Deus an diabolus, angeli an immundi spiritus, ægro opem ferant modo morbus curetur.

458 *Cure of Melancholy.* [Part. 2. Sec. 1.

angels, or unclean spirits, cure him, so that he be eased. If a man fall into a ditch, (as he prosecutes it) what matter is it whether a friend or an enemy help him out? and if I be troubled with such a malady, what care I whether the devil himself, or any of his ministers, by Gods permission, redeem me? He calls a [1] magician Gods minister and his vicar, applying that of *vos estis Dii* prophanely to them (for which he is lashed by T. Erastus, *part.* 1. *fol.* 45); and elsewhere he encourageth his patients to have a good faith, [2] *a strong imagination, and they shall find the effects; let divines say to the contrary what they will.* He proves and contends that many diseases cannot otherwise be cured: *incantatione orti, incantatione curari debent;* if they be caused by incantation, [3] they must be cured by incantation. Constantinus (*l.* 4) approves of such remedies: Bartolus the lawyer, Peter Ærodius (*rerum Judic. lib.* 3. *tit.* 7), Salicetus, Godefridus, with others of that sect, allow of them, *modo sint ad sanitatem, quæ a magis fiunt, secus non;* so they be for the parties good, or not at all. But these men are confuted by Remigius, Bodinus (*dæm. lib.* 3. *cap.* 2), Godelmannus (*lib.* 1. *cap.* 8), Wierus, Delrio (*lib.* 6. *quæst.* 2 *Tom.* 3. *mag. inquis.*) Erastus (*de Lamiis*): all [4] our divines, schoolmen, and such as write cases of conscience, are against it; the scripture it self absolutely forbids it as a mortal sin. (*Levit. cap.* 18, 19, 20. *Deut.* 18, *&c. Rom.* 8. 19). *Evil is not to be done, that good may come of it.* Much better it were for such patients that are so troubled, to endure a little misery in this life, than to hazard their souls health for ever! and (as Delrio counselleth) [5] *much better dye, than be so cured.* Some take upon them to expel devils by natural remedies, and magical exorcisms, which they seem to approve out of the practice of the primitive church, as that above cited of Josephus, Eleazar, Irenæus, Tertullian, Austin. Eusebius makes mention of such; and magick it self hath been publickly professed in some universities, as of old in Salamanca in Spain, and Cracovia in Poland: but condemned, *anno* 1318, by the chancellour and university of [6] Paris. Our pontifical writers retain many of these adjurations and forms of exorcisms still in their church; besides those in baptism used, they exorcise meats, and such as are possessed, as they hold, in Christs name. Read Hieron, Mengus, *cap.* 3. Pet. Tyreus, *part.* 3. *cap.* 8. what exorcisms they prescribe,

---

[1] Magus minister et vicarius Dei.   [2] Utere forti imaginatione, et experieris effectum; dicant in adversum quidquid volunt theologi.   [3] Idem Plinius contendit, quosdam esse morbos, qui incantationibus solum curentur.   [4] Qui talibus credunt, aut ad eorum domos euntes, aut suis domibus introducunt, aut interrogant, sciant se fidem Christianam et baptismum prævaricâsse, et apostatas esse. Austin. de superst. observ. Hoc pacto a Deo deficitur ad diabolum. P. Mart.   [5] Mori præstat quam superstitiose sanari, Disquis. mag. l. 2. c. 2. sect. 1. quæst. 1. Tom. 3.   [6] P. Lumbard.

besides those ordinary means of [1]*fire, suffumigations, lights, cutting the air* with swords, *cap.* 57. herbs, odours; of which Tostatas treats, 2 *Reg. cap.* 16. *quæst.* 43. You shall find many vain and frivolous superstitious forms of exorcisms among them, not to be tolerated, or endured.

MEMB. II.

Lawful cures, first from God.

BEING so clearly evinced as it is, all unlawful cures are to be refused, it remains to treat of such as are to be admitted; and those are commonly such which God hath appointed, [2]by vertue of stones, herbs, plants, meats, &c. and the like, which are prepared and applyed to our use, by art and industry of physicians, who are the dispensers of such treasures for our good, and to be [3]*honoured for necessities sake*—Gods intermediate ministers, to whom, in our infirmities, we are to seek for help: yet not so that we rely too much, or wholly, upon them. *A Jove principium;* we must first begin with prayer, and then use physick; not one without the other, but both together. To pray alone, and reject ordinary means, is to do like him in Æsop, that, when his cart was stalled, lay flat on his back, and cried aloud, " Help Hercules ;" but that was to little purpose, except as his friend advised him, *rotis tute ipse annitaris,* he whipt his horses withal, and put his shoulder to the wheel. God works by means, as Christ cured the blind man with clay and spittle.

> Orandum est, ut sit mens sana in corpore sano.

As we must pray for health of body and mind, so we must use our utmost endeavours to preserve and continue it. Some kind of devils are not cast out but by fasting and prayer, and both necessarily required, not one without the other. For all the physick we can use, art, excellent industry, is to no purpose without calling upon God :

> Nil juvat immensos Cratero promittere montes :

it is in vain to seek for help, run, ride, except God bless us.

> —————————— non Siculæ dapes
> [4] Dulcem elaborabunt saporem :
>   Non avium citharæve cantus,———

---

[1] Suffitus, gladiorum ictus, &c.   [2] The Lord hath created medicines of the earth ; and he that is wise will not abhor them, Ecclus. 38. 4.   [3] My son, fail not in thy sickness, but pray unto the Lord ; and he will make thee whole, Ecclus. 38. 9. Huc omne principium, huc refer exitum. Hor. 3. carm. Od. 6.   [4] Musick and fine fare can do no good.

460   *Cure of Melancholy.*   [Part. 2. Sec. 1.

[1] Non domus et fundus, non æris acervus et auri,
    Ægroto possunt domino deducere febres.

[2] With house, with land, with money, and with gold,
    The masters fever will not be control'd.

We must use prayer and physick both together: and so, no
doubt, our prayers will be available, and our physick take
effect. 'Tis that Hezekiah practised (2 Kings 20), Luke the
Evangelist; and which we are enjoynd (Coloss. 4), not the
patient only, but the physician himself. Hippocrates, an heathen, required this in a good practitioner, and so did Galen,
lib. de Plat. et Hipp. dog. lib. 9. c. 15; and in that tract of
his, *an mores sequantur temp. cor. c. 11.* 'tis that which he
doth inculcate, [3] and many others. Hyperius, (in his first book
de sacr. script. lect.) speaking of that happiness and good success which all physicians desire and hope for in their cures,
[4] tells them, *that it is not to be expected, except, with a true
faith, they call upon God, and teach their patients to do the like.*
The council of Lateran (*Canon. 22*) decreed they should do so:
the fathers of the church have still advised as much. Whatsoever thou takest in hand, (saith [5] Gregory) *let God be of thy
counsel: consult with him, that healeth those that are broken
in heart,* (Psal. 147. 3.) *and bindeth up their sores.* Otherwise, as the prophet Jeremy (*cap.* 46. 11) denounced to
Ægypt, in vain shalt thou use many medicines; for thou shalt
have no health. It is the same counsel which [6] Comineus, that
politick historiographer, gives to all Christian princes, upon occasion of that unhappy overthrow of Charles duke of Burgundy,
by means of which he was extreamly melancholy, and sick to
death, in so much that neither physick nor perswasion could
do him any good,—perceiving his preposterous error belike,
adviseth all great men, in such cases, [7] *to pray first to God with
all submission and penitency, to confess their sins, and then to
use physick.* The very same fault it was, which the prophet
reprehends in Asa king of Juda, that he relyed more on physick than on God, and by all means would have him to amend

---

[1] Hor. 1. 1. ep. 2.   [2] Sint Crœsi et Crassi licet, non hos Pactolus, aureas
undas agens, eripiet unquam e miseriis.   [3] Scientia de Deo debet in medico
infixa esse. Mesue Arabs. Sanat omnes languores Deus. For you shall pray to
your Lord, that he would prosper that which is given for ease, and then use physick for the prolonging of life. Ecclus. 38. 4.   [4] Omnes optant quamdam in
medicinâ felicitatem; sed hanc non est quod expectent, nisi Deum verâ fide invo-
cent, atque ægros similiter ad ardentem vocationem excitent.   [5] Lemnius e
Gregor. exhor. ad vitam opt. instit. c. 48. Quidquid meditaris aggredi aut per-
ficere, Deum in consilium adhibeto.   [6] Commentar. lib. 7. Ob infelicem
pugnam contristatus, in ægritudinem incidit, ita ut a medicis curari non posset.
[7] In his animi malis, princeps imprimis ad Deum precetur, et peccatis veniam
exoret; inde ad medicinam, &c.

Mem. 2.] *Patient.* 461

it. And 'tis a fit caution to be observed of all other sorts of
men. The prophet David was so observant of this precept,
that, in his greatest misery and vexation of mind, he put this
rule first in practice : (Psal. 77. 3.) *When I am in heaviness,
I will think on God.* (Psal. 86. 4.) *Comfort the soul of thy
servant, for unto thee I lift up my soul.* (and verse 7.) *In
the day of trouble will I call upon thee, for thou hearest me.*
(Psal. 54. 1) *Save me, O God, by thy name, &c.* (Psal. 82.
Psal. 20.) And 'tis the common practice of all good men :
(Psal. 107. 13.) *when their heart was humbled with heaviness,
they cryed to the Lord in their trouble, and he delivered them
from their distress.* And they have found good success in so
doing, as David confesseth (Psal. 30. 12.) : *Thou hast turned
my mourning into joy ; thou hast loosed my sackcloth, and girded
me with gladness.* Therefore he adviseth all others to do the
like : (Psal. 31. 24.) *All ye that trust in the Lord, be strong,
and he shall establish your heart.* It is reported by [1] Suidas,
speaking of Hezekiah, that there was a great book of old,
of king Solomons writing, which contained medicines for all
manner of diseases, and lay open still as they came into the
temple : but Hezekiah, king of Jerusalem, caused it to be taken
away, because it made the people secure, to neglect their duty
in calling and relying upon God, out of a confidence on those
remedies. [2] Minutius, that worthy consul of Rome, in an oration he made to his souldiers, was much offended with them,
and taxed their ignorance, that, in their misery, called more on
him than upon God. A general fault it is all over the world ;
and Minutius his speech concerns us all : we rely more on physick, and seek oftner to physicians, than to God himself. As
much faulty are they that prescribe, as they that ask, respecting wholly their gain, and trusting more to their ordinary receipts and medicines many times, than to him that made them.
I would wish all patients in this behalf, in the midst of their
melancholy, to remember that of Siracides, (Ecc. 1. 12.)
*The fear of the Lord is glory and gladness, and rejoycing.
The fear of the Lord maketh a merry heart, and giveth gladness, and joy, and long life ;* and all such as prescribe physick, to begin in *nomine Dei*, as [3] Mesue did, to imitate Lælius a Fonte Eugubinus, that, in all his consultations, still concludes with a prayer for the good success of his business ; and

---

[1] Greg. Tholos. To. 2. l. 28. c. 7. Syntax. In vestibulo templi Solomonis liber
remediorum cujusque morbi fuit, quem revulsit Ezechias, quod populus, neglecto
Deo nec invocato, sanitatem inde peteret. [2] Livius, l. 23. Strepunt aures
clamoribus plorantium sociorum, sæpius nos quam Deorum invocantium opem.
[3] Rulandus adjungit optimam orationem ad finem Empiricorum. Mercurialis
(consil. 25) ita concludit. Montanus passim, &c. et plures alii, &c.

462   *Cure of Melancholy.*   [Part. 2. Sec. 1.

to remember that of Crato, one of their predecessors, *fuge avaritiam; et sine oratione et invocatione Dei nihil facias;* avoid
covetousness, and do nothing without invocation upon God.

MEMB. III.

Whether it be lawful to seek to Saints for aid in this disease.

THAT we must pray to God, no man doubts: but, whether
we should pray to saints in such cases, or whether they
can do us any good, it may be lawfully controverted—whether
their images, shrines, reliques, consecrated things, holy water,
medals, benedictions, those divine amulets, holy exorcisms,
and the sign of the cross, be available in this disease. The
papists, on the one side, stifly maintain, how many melancholy, mad, dæmoniacal persons are daily cured at S[t]. Anthonies Church in Padua, at S[t]. Vitus in Germany, by our Lady
of Lauretta in Italy, our Lady of Sichem in the Low Countreys, [1] *quæ et cæcis lumen, ægris salutem, mortuis vitam,
claudis gressum, reddit, omnes morbos corporis, animi, curat, et in ipsos dæmones imperium exercet:* she cures halt,
lame, blind, all diseases of body and mind, and commands
the devil himself, saith Lipsius: 25000 *in a day come thither:* [2] *quis nisi numen in illum locum sic induxit?* who
brought them? *in auribus, in oculis omnium gesta, nova
novitia;* new news lately done; our eyes and ears are full of
her cures; and who can relate them all? They have a proper
saint almost for every peculiar infirmity; for poyson, gouts,
agues, Petronella: S[t]. Romanus for such as are possessed: Va-
lentine for the falling sickness: S[t]. Vitus for mad men, &c.
And as, of old, [3] Pliny reckons up gods for all diseases, (*Febri
fanum dicatum est*) Lilius Giraldus repeats many of her ceremonies: all affections of the mind were heretofore accounted
gods: Love, and Sorrow, Vertue, Honour, Liberty, Contumely, Impudency, had their temples; tempests, seasons, *Cre-
pitus ventris, Dea Vacuna, Dea Cloacina:* there was a goddess
of idleness, a goddess of the draught or jakes, *Prema, Pre-
munda, Priapus,* bawdy gods, and gods for all [4] offices. Varro
reckons up 30000 gods; Lucian makes Podagra (the gout) a
goddess, and assigns her priests and ministers: and Melan-

---

[1] Lipsius.   [2] Cap. 26.   [3] Lib. 2. c. 7. de Deo. Morbisque in genera
descriptis, Deos reperimus. Selden. prolog. c. 3. de Diis Syris. Rosinus.   [4] See
Lilii Giraldi syntagma de Diis, &c.

8

Mem. 3.]   *Saints Cure rejected.*   463

choly comes not behind ; for (as Austin mentioneth, *lib.* 4. *de
Civit. Dei, cap.* 9) there was of old *Angerona dea*, and she
had her chappel and feasts; to whom (saith [1] Macrobius) they
did offer sacrifice yearly, that she might be pacified as well as
the rest.   'Tis no new thing, you see, this of papists; and, in
my judgement, that old doting Lipsius might have fitter dedicated his [2] pen, after all his labours, to this old goddess of
Melancholy, than to his *Virgo Halensis*, and been her chaplain ;
it would have becomed him better.   But he, poor man, thought
no harm in that which he did, and will not be perswaded but
that he doth well; he hath so many patrons, and honourable
precedents in the like kind, that justify as much, as eagerly,
and more than he there saith of his Lady and Mistris : read
but superstitious Coster and Gretsers Tract. *de Cruce Laur.*
Arcturus Fanteus, *de invoc. Sanct.*   Bellarmine, Delrio, *dis.
mag. Tom.* 3. *l.* 6. *quæst.* 2. *sect.* 3.   Greg. Tolosanus, *tom.* 2.
lib. 8. *cap.* 24. *Syntax.* Strozius Cicogna, *lib.* 4. *cap.* 9. Tyreus,
Hieronymus Mengus; and you shall find infinite examples of
cures done in this kind, by holy waters, reliques, crosses, exorcisms, amulets, images, consecrated beads, &c.   Barradius
the Jesuit boldly gives it out, that Christs countenance, and
the Virgin Maries, would cure melancholy, if one had looked
steadfastly on them.   P. Morales the Spaniard (in his book *de
pulch. Jes. et Mar.*) confirms the same out of Carthusianus,
and I know not whom, that it was a common proverb in those
daies, for such as were troubled in mind, to say *Eamus ad
videndum filium Mariæ* (let us see the son of Mary), as they
do now post to S[t]. Anthonies in Padua, or to S[t], Hillaries at
Poictiers in France.   [3] In a closet of that church, there is at
this day S[t]. Hillaries bed to be seen, *to which they bring all the
mad men in the country; and, after some prayers and other
ceremonies, they lay them down there to sleep, and so they recover.*   It is an ordinary thing in those parts, to send all their
mad men to S[t]. Hillaries cradle.   They say the like of S[t]. Tu-
bery in [4] another place.   Giraldus Cambrensis (*Itin. Camb.
c.* 1.) tells strange stories of S. Ciricius staffe, that would cure
this and all other diseases.   Other say as much (as [5] Hospinian observes) of the Three Kings of Colen; their names
written in parchment, and hung about a patients neck, with
the sign of the crosse, will produce like effects.   Read Lipo-
mannus, or that golden legend of Jacobus de Voragine, you shall

---

[1] 12 Cal. Januarii ferias celebrant, ut angores et animi solicitudines propitiata
depellat.   [2] Hanc Divæ pennam consecravi, Lipsius.   [3] Jodocus Sincerus, itin. Galliæ, 1617.   Huc mente captos deducunt, et statis orationibus, sacrisque peractis, in illum lectum dormitum ponunt, &c.   [4] In Gallia Nar-
bonensi.   [5] Lib. de orig. Festorum. Collo suspensa, et pergameno inscripta,
cum signo crucis, &c.

464   *Cure of Melancholy.*   [Part. 2. Sec. 1.

have infinite stories,—or those new relations of our [1] Jesuits
in Japona and China, of Mat. Riccius, Acosta, Loiola, Xave-
rius life, &c. Jasper Belgar, a Jesuit, cured a mad woman by
hanging S[t]. Johns Gospel about her neck, and many such.
Holy water did as much in Japona, &c. Nothing so familiar
in their works, as such examples.

But we, on the other side, seek to God alone. We say with
David, (Ps. 46. 1.) *God is our hope and strength, and help in
trouble, ready to be found.* For their catalogue of examples,
we make no other answer, but that they are false fictions, or
diabolical illusions, counterfeit miracles. We cannot deny but
that it is an ordinary thing, on S[t]. Anthonies day in Padua,
to bring divers mad men and dæmoniacal persons to be cured:
yet we make a doubt whether such parties be so affected indeed, but prepared by their priests by certain oyntments and
drams, to cosen the commonalty, as [2] Hildesheim well saith.
The like is commonly practised in Bohemia, as Mathiolus
gives us to understand in his preface to his comment upon
Dioscorides. But we need not run so far for examples in this
kind: we have a just volume published at home to this purpose: [3] *A Declaration of egregious Popish Impostures, to
with-draw the hearts of religious men under pretence of casting out Devils, practised by Father Edmunds, alias Weston, a
Jesuit, and divers Romish Priests, his wicked associates,* with
the several parties names, confessions, examinations, &c. which
were pretended to be possessed. But these are ordinary
tricks, only to get opinion and money, meer impostures.
Æsculapius of old, that counterfeit God, did as many famous
cures: his temple (as [4] Strabo relates) was daily full of patients,
and as many several tables, inscriptions, pendants, donaries,
&c. to be seen in his church, as at this day at our Lady of
Lorettas in Italy. It was a custome, long since,

> Suspendisse potenti
> Vestimenta maris Deo—*Hor. lib.* 1. *od.* 5.

To do the like, in former times, they were seduced and deluded
as they are now. 'Tis the same devil still, called heretofore
Apollo, Mars, Neptune, Venus, Æsculapius, &c. as [5] Lactan-

---

[1] Em Acosta, com. rerum in Oriente gest. a societat. Jesu, anno 1568. Epist.
Gonsalvi Fernandis. An. 1560, e Japoniâ.   [2] Spicil. de morbis dæmoniacis.
Sic a sacrificulis parati unguentis magicis corpori illitis, ut stultæ plebeculæ per-
suadeant tales curari a Sancto Antonio.   [3] Printed at London, 4to. by J. Ro-
binson, 1605.   [4] Greg. l. 8. Cujus fanum ægrotantium multitudine refertum
undiquaque, et tabellis pendentibus, in quibus sanati languores erant inscripti.
[5] Mali angeli sumserunt olim nomen Jovis, Junonis, Apollinis, &c. quos Gentiles
Deos credebant: nunc S. Sebastiani, Barbaræ, &c. nomen habent, et aliorum.

Mem. 4. Subs. 1.]   *Patient.*   465

tius (*lib. 2. de orig. erroris, c.* 17) observes. The same Jupiter,
and those bad angels, are now worshipped and adored by the
name of S[t]. Sebastian, Barbara, &c. Christopher and George
are come in their places. Our Lady succeeds Venus (as they
use her in many offices); the rest are otherwise supplyed (as
[1]*Lavater* writes); and so they are deluded: [2]*and God often
winks at these impostures, because they forsake his word, and
betake themselves to the devil, as they do that seek after holy
water, crosses, &c.* (Wierus, *lib. 4. cap.* 3). What can these
men plead for themselves more than those heathen gods? the
same cures done by both, the same spirit that seduceth: but
read more of the pagan gods effects in Austin, *de Civitate Dei,
l.* 10. *cap.* 6; and of Æsculapius, especially, in Cicogna, *l. 3.
cap.* 8; or put case they could help, why should we rather
seek to them, than to Christ himself? since that he so [3]kindly
invites us unto him: *Come unto me all ye that are heavy laden,
and I will ease you* (Matt. 11); and we know that there is one
God, *one Mediator betwixt God and man, Jesus Christ,* (1 Tim.
2. 5), *who gave himself a ransome for all men. We know that
we have an advocate with the Father Jesus Christ,* (1 John, 2.
1), that there is no [4]*other name under heaven, by which we can
be saved, but by his,* who is alwayes ready to hear us, and sits
at the right hand of God, and from [5]whom we can have no repulse: *solus vult, solus potest: curat universos tanquam singulos, et* [6] *unumquemque nostrûm ut solum ;* we are all as one
to him; he cares for us all as one; and why should we then
seek to any other but to him?

MEMB. IV.   SUBSECT. I.

Physician, Patient, Physick.

OF those divers gifts which, our apostle Paul saith, God
hath bestowed on man, this of physick is not the least, but most
necessary, and especially conducing to the good of mankind.
Next therefore to God, in all our extremities (*for of the Most
High cometh healing,* Ecclus. 38. 2) we must seek to, and rely
upon the physician, [7] who is *manus Dei* (saith Hierophilus), and
to whom he hath given knowledge, that he might be glorified in

---

[1] Part. 2. cap. 9. de spect. Veneri substituunt virginem Mariam.   [2] Ad hæc
ludibria Deus connivet frequenter, ubi, relicto verbo Dei, ad Satanam curritur ;
quales hi sunt, qui aquam lustralem, crucem, &c. lubricæ fidei hominibus offerunt.
[3] Carior est ipsis homo, quam sibi.   [4] Paul.   [5] Bernard.   [6] Austin.
[7] Ecclus. 38.   In the sight of great men, he shall be in admiration.

VOL. I.   H H

466 *Cure of Melancholy.* [Part. 2. Sec. 1.

his wondrous works. *With such doth he heal men, and taketh away their pains* (Ecclus. 38. 6. 7): *when thou hast need of him, let him not go from thee. The hour may come that their enterprises may have good success* (ver. 13). It is not therefore to be doubted, that, if we seek a physician as we ought, we may be eased of our infirmities—such a one, I mean, as is sufficient, and worthily so called; for there be many mountebanks, quacksalvers, empiricks, in every street almost, and in every village, that take upon them this name, make this noble and profitable art to be evil spoken of and contemned, by reason of these base and illiterate artificers : but such a physician I speak of, as is approved, learned, skilful, honest, &c. of whose duty Wecker, (*Antid. cap. 2. et Syntax. med.*) Crato, Julius Alexandrinus, (*medic.*) Heurnius, (*prax. med. lib. 3. cap.* 1) &c. treat at large. For this particular disease, him that shall take upon him to cure it, [1] Paracelsus will have to be a magician, a chymist, a philosopher, an astrologer; Thurnesserus, Severinus the Dane, and some other of his followers, require as much : *many of them cannot be cured but by magick.* [2] Paracelsus is so stiff for those chymical medicines, that, in his cures, he will admit almost of no other physick, deriding in the mean time Hippocrates, Galen, and all their followers. But magick, and all such remedies, I have already censured, and shall speak of chymistry [3] elsewhere. Astrology is required by many famous physicians, by Ficinus, Crato, Fernelius, [4] doubted of, and exploded by others. I will not take upon me to decide the controversie my self: Johannes Hossurtus, Thomas Boderius, and Maginus in the preface to his Mathematical physick, shall determine for me. Many physicians explode astrology in physick, (saith he) there is no use of it: *unam artem ac quasi temerariam insectantur, ac gloriam sibi ab ejus imperitiâ aucupari;* but I will reprove physicians by physicians, that defend and profess it, Hippocrates, Galen, Avicen, &c. that count them butchers without it, *homicidas medicos astrologiæ ignaros, &c.* Paracelsus goes farther, and will have his physician [5] predestinated to this mans cure, this malady, and time of cure, the scheme of each geniture inspected, gathering of herbs, of administering, astrologically observed ; in which Thurnesserus, and some iatromathematical professors, are too superstitious in my judgement. [6] *Hellebor will help, but not alway, not given by every*

---

[1] Tom. 4. Tract. 3. de morbis amentium. Horum multi non nisi a magis curandi et astrologis, quoniam origo ejus a cœlis petenda est.   [2] Lib. de Podagrâ. [3] Sect. 5.   [4] Langius. J. Cæsar Claudinus, consult.   [5] Prædestinatum ad hunc curandum.   [6] Helleborus curat; sed quod ab omni datus medico, vanum est.

physician, &c. But these men are too peremptory and self-conceited, as I think. But what do I do, interposing in that which is beyond my reach? A blind man cannot judge of colours, nor I peradventure of these things. Only thus much I would require, honesty in every physician, that he be not over-careless or covetous, Harpy-like to make a prey of his patient; *carnificis namque est* (as [1] Wecker notes) *inter ipsos cruciatus ingens pretium exposcere,* as an hungry chyrurgion often doth produce and wier-draw his cure, so long as there is any hope of pay,

> Non missura cutem, nisi plena cruoris, hirudo.

Many of them, to get a fee, will give physick to every one that comes, when there is no cause; and they do so *irritare silentem morbum,* as [2] Heurnius complains, stir up a silent disease, as it often falleth out, which, by good counsel, good advice alone, might have been happily composed, or, by rectification of those six non-natural things, otherwise cured. This is *naturæ bellum inferre,* to oppugn nature, and to make a strong body weak. Arnoldus in his eighth and eleventh Aphorisms, gives cautions against, and expressly forbiddeth it. [3] *A wise physician will not give physick, but upon necessity, and first try medicinal dyet, before he proceed to medicinal cure.* [4] In another place he laughs those men to scorn, that think *longis syrupis expugnare dæmones et animi phantasmata,* they can purge phantastical imaginations, and the devil, by physick. Another caution is, that they proceed upon good grounds, if so be there be need of physick, and not mistake the disease. They are often deceived by the [5] similitude of symptoms, saith Heurnius; and I could give instance in many consultations, wherein they have prescribed opposite physick. Sometimes they go too perfunctorily to work, in not prescribing a just [6] course of physick. To stir up the humour, and not to purge it, doth often more harm than good. Montanus (*consil.* 30) inveighs against such perturbations, *that purge to the halves, tire nature, and molest the body to no purpose.* 'Tis a crabbed humour to purge—and, as Laurentius calls this disease, the reproach of physicians; Bessardus, *flagellum medicorum,* their lash—and, for that cause, more carefully to be respected. Though the

---

[1] Antid. gen. lib. 3. cap. 2.   [2] Quod sæpe evenit, (lib. 3. cap. 1) cum non sit necessitas. Frustra fatigant remediis ægros, qui victûs ratione curari possunt. Heurnius.   [3] Modestus et sapiens medicus nunquam properabit ad pharmacum, nisi cogente necessitate. 41. Aphor. Prudens et pius medicus cibis prius medicinalibus, quam medicinis puris morbum expellere satagat.   [4] Brev. 1. c. 18.   [5] Similitudo sæpe bonis medicis imponit.   [6] Qui melancholicis præbent remedia non satis valida. Longiores morbi imprimis solertiam medici postulant, et fidelitatem: qui enim tumultuario hos tractant, vires absque ullo commodo lædunt et frangunt, &c.

468   *Cure of Melancholy.*   [Part. 2. Sec. 1.

patient be averse, saith Laurentius, desire help, and refuse it
again, though he neglect his own health, it behoves a good physician not to leave him helpless.   But, most part, they offend
in that other extream ; they prescribe too much physick, and
tire out their bodies with continual potions, to no purpose.
Aëtius (*tetrabib. 2. 2. ser. cap.* 90) will have them by all means
therefore [1] *to give some respite to nature*, to leave off now and
then ; and Lælius à Fonte Eugubinus, in his consultations,
found it (as he there witnesseth) often verified by experience,
[2] *that after a deal of physick to no purpose, left to themselves,
they have recovered.* 'Tis that which Nic. Piso, Donatus Altomarus, still inculcate—*dare requiem naturæ*, to give nature rest.

SUBSECT. II.

Concerning the Patient.

WHEN these precedent cautions are accurately kept, and
that we have now got a skilful, an honest physician to our
mind, if his patient will not be comformable, and content to
be ruled by him, all his endeavours will come to no good end.
Many things are necessarily to be observed and continued on
the patients behalf: first, that he be not too niggardly miserable of his purse, or think it too much he bestows upon himself, and, to save charges, endanger his health.   The Abderites, when they sent for Hippocrates, promised him what
reward he would—[3] *all the gold they had; if all the city were
gold, he should have it.*   Naaman the Syrian, when he went
into Israel to Elisha to be cured of his leprosie, took with him
ten talents of silver, six thousand pieces of gold, and ten
change of rayments (2 Kings, 5. 5).   Another thing is, that out
of bashfulness he do not conceal his grief: if ought trouble his
minde, let him freely disclose it.

> Stultorum incurata pudor malus ulcera celat.

By that means he procures to himself much mischief, and runs
into a greater inconvenience : he must be willing to be cured,
and earnestly desire it.   *Pars sanitatis velle sanari fuit.* (Seneca).   'Tis a part of his cure to wish his own health ; and not
to defer it too long.

> [4] Qui blandiendo dulce nutrivit malum,
>   Sero recusat ferre quod subiit jugum.   Et

---

[1] Naturæ remissionem dare oportet.   [2] Plerique hoc morbo medicinâ nihil
profecisse visi sunt, et sibi demissi invaluerunt.   [3] Abderitani, ep. Hippoc.
Quidquid auri apud nos est, libenter persolvemus, etiamsi tota urbs nostra aurum
esset.   [4] Seneca.

[Mem. 4. Subs. 2.] *Patient.* 469

> [1] Helleborum frustra, cum jam cutis ægra tumebit,
> Poscentes videas : venienti occurrite morbo.

He that by cherishing a mischief doth provoke,
Too late, at last refuseth, to cast off his yoke.

When the skin swels, to seek it to appease
With hellebor, is vain ; meet your disease.

By this means many times, or through their ignorance in not taking notice of their grievance and danger of it, contempt, supine negligence, extenuation, wretchedness, and peevishness, they undo themselves. The citizens I know not of what city now, when rumour was brought their enemies were coming, could not abide to hear it; and when the plague begins in many places, and they certainly know it, they command silence, and hush it up; but, after they see their foes now marching to their gates, and ready to surprise them, they begin to fortifie and resist when 'tis too late ; when the sickness breaks out, and can be no longer concealed, then they lament their supine negligence : 'tis no otherwise with these men. And often out of a prejudice, a loathing and distaste of physick, they had rather dye, or do worse, than take any of it. *Barbarous immanity* ([2] Melancthon terms it), *and folly to be deplored, so to contemn the precepts of health, good remedies, and voluntarily to pull death, and many maladies, upon their own heads :* though many again are in that other extreme, too profuse, suspicious, and jealous of their health, too apt to take physick on every small occasion, to aggravate every slender passion, imperfection, impediment ; if their finger do but ake, run, ride, send for a physician, as many gentlewomen do, that are sick without a cause, even when they will themselves, upon every toy or small discontent ; and when he comes, they make it worse than it is, by amplifying that which is not. [3] Hier. Capivaccius sets it down as a common fault of all *melancholy persons, to say their symptomes are greater than they are, to help themselves ;* and (which Mercurialis notes, *consil.* 53) *to be* [4] *more troublesome to their physicians, than other ordinary patients, that they may have change of physick.*

A third thing to be required in a patient, is confidence, to be of good chear, and have sure hope that his physician can help him. [5] Damascen the Arabian requires likewise in the

---

[1] Per. 3. Sat.   [2] De animâ. Barbarâ tamen immanitate, et deplorandâ inscitiâ, contemnunt præcepta sanitatis ; mortem et morbos ultro accersunt.   [3] Consul. 173. e Scoltziò, Melanch. Ægrorum hoc fere proprium est, ut graviora dicant esse symptomata, quam reverà sunt.   [4] Melancholici plerumque medicis sunt molesti, ut alia aliis adjungant.   [5] Oportet infirmo imprimere salutem, utcunque promittere, etsi ipse desperet. Nullum medicamentum efficax, nisi medicus etiam fuerit fortis imaginationis.

470   *Cure of Melancholy.*   [Part. 2. Sec. 1.

physician himself, that he be confident he can cure him, otherwise his physick will not be effectuall, and promise withall that he will certainly help him, make him beleeve so at least.   [1] Galeottus gives this reason, because the forme of health is contained in the physicians minde, and, as Galen holds, [2] *confidence and hope do more good than physick;* he cures most, in whom most are confident.   Axiochus, sick almost to death, at the very sight of Socrates recovered his former health.   Paracelsus assigns it for an only cause why Hippocrates was so fortunate in his cures, not for any extraordinary skill he had, [3] but *because the common people had a most strong conceipt of his worth.*   To this of confidence we may adde perseverance, obedience, and constancie, not to change his physician, or dislike him upon every toy; for he that so doth, (saith [4] Janus Damascen) *or consults with many, falls into many errours; or that useth many medicines.*   It was a chief caveat of [5] Seneca to his friend Lucilius, that he should not alter his physician, or prescribed physick: *nothing hinders health more: a wound can never be cured, that hath severall plasters.*   Crato (*consil.* 186) taxeth all melancholy persons of this fault: [6] *tis proper to them, if things fall not out to their minde, and that they have not present ease, to seek another and another; (as they do commonly that have sore eyes) twenty, one after another; and they still promise all to cure them, try a thousand remedies; and by this means they increase their malady, make it most dangerous, and difficil to be cured.*   They try many (saith [7] Montanus) *and profit by none:* and for this cause (*consil.* 24) he injoyns his patient, before he take him in hand, [8] *perseverance and sufferance; for in such a small time, no great matter can be effected; and upon that condition he will administer physick; otherwise all his endevour and counsell would be to small purpose.*   And in his 31 counsell for a notable matron, he tels her, [9] *if she will be cured, she must be of a most abiding patience, faithfull obedience and singular perseverance: if she remit or despair, she can expect or hope for no good success.*   *Consil.* 230, for an Italian abbot, he makes it one of the greatest reasons why this disease is

---

[1] De promisc. doct. cap. 15. Quoniam sanitatis formam animi medici continent.
[2] Spes et confidentia plus valent quam medicina.   [3] Felicior in medicinâ ob fidem ethnicorum.   [4] Aphoris. 89. Æger, qui plurimos consulit medicos, plerumque in errorem singulorum cadit.   [5] Nihil ita sanitatem impedit, ac remediorum crebra mutatio ; nec venit vulnus ad cicatricem, in quo diversa medicamenta tentantur.   [6] Melancholicorum proprium, quum ex eorum arbitrio non fit subita mutatio in melius, alterare medicos, qui quidvis, &c.   [7] Consil. 31. Dum ad varia se conferunt, nullo prosunt.   [8] Imprimis hoc statuere oportet, requiri perseverantiam, et tolerantiam.   Exiguo enim tempore nihil ex, &c.   [9] Si curari vult, opus est pertinaci perseverantiâ, fideli obedientiâ, et patientiâ singulari: si tædet aut desperet, nullum habebit effectum.

Mem. 4. Subs. 2.]   *Patient.*   471

so incurable, [1] *because the parties are so restless and impatient, and will therefore have him that intends to be eased,* [2] *to take physick, not for moneth, a year, but to apply himself to their prescriptions all the dayes of his life.* Last of all, it is required that the patient be not too bold to practise upon himself, without an approved physicians consent, or to try conclusions, if he read a receipt in a book; for, so, many grosly mistake, and do themselves more harme than good. That which is conducing to one man, in one case, the same time is opposite to another. [3] An asse and a mule went laden over a brook, the one with salt, the other with wooll; the mules packe was wet by chance; the salt melted; his burden the lighter, and he thereby much eased; he told the asse, who, thinking to speed as well, wet his packe likewise at the next water; but it was much the heavier; he quite tired. So one thing may be good and bad to severall parties, upon divers occasions. *Many things* (saith [4] *Penottus*) *are written in our books, which seem to the reader to be excellent remedies; but they that make use of them, are often deceived, and take, for physick, poyson.* I remember, in Valleriolas observations, a story of one John Baptist, a Neapolitan, that, finding by chance a pamphlet in Italian, written in praise of hellebor, would needs adventure on himself, and tooke one dram for one scruple: and, had not he been sent for, the poor fellow had poysoned himself. From whence he concludes (out of Damascenus, 2. et 3. *Aphoris.*) [5] *that, without exquisite knowledge, to work out of bookes is most dangerous: how unsavorie a thing it is to beleeve writers, and take upon trust, as this patient perceived by his own perill.* I could recite such another example, of mine own knowledge, of a friend of mine, that finding a receipt in Brassivola, would needs take hellebor in substance, and try it on his own person: but had not some of his familiars come to visit him by chance, he had by his indiscretion hazarded himself. Many such I have observed. These are those ordinary cautions, which I should thinke fit to be noted; and he that shall keep them, as [6] Montanus saith, shall surely be much eased, if not throughly cured.

---

[1] Ægritudine amittunt patientiam; et inde morbi incurabiles.   [2] Non ad mensem aut annum, sed oportet toto vitæ curriculo curationi operam dare.   [3] Camerarius, emb. 55. cent 2.   [4] Præfat. de nar. med. In libellis qui vulgo versantur apud literatos, incautiores multa legunt, a quibus decipiuntur, eximia illis: sed portentosum hauriunt venenum.   [5] Operari ex libris, absque cognitione et solerti ingenio, periculosum est. Unde monemur, quam insipidum scriptis auctoribus credere, quod hic suo didicit periculo.   [6] Consil. 23. Hæc omnia si, quo ordine decet, egerit, vel curabitur, vel certe minus afficietur.

472   *Cure of Melancholy.*   [Part. 2. Sec. 1.

SUBSECT. III.

Concerning Physick.

Physick itself in the last place is to be considered ; *for the Lord hath created medicines of the earth ; and he that is wise will not abhorre them*, Ecclus. 38. 4. and ver. 8. *of such doth the apothecary make a confection, &c.* Of these medicines there be divers and infinite kindes, plants, metals, animals, &c. and those of several natures, some good for one, hurtfull to another: some noxious in themselves, corrected by art, very wholesome and good, simples, mixt, &c. and therefore left to be managed by discreet and skillfull physicians, and thence applyed to mans use. To this purpose they have invented method, and severall rules of art, to put these remedies in order, for their particular ends. Physick (as Hippocrates defines it) is naught else but [1] addition and substraction ; and, as it is required in all other diseases, so in this of melancholy it ought to be most accurate ; it being (as [2] Mercurialis acknowledgeth) so common an affection in these our times, and therefore fit to be understood. Severall prescripts and methods I find in several men: some take upon them to cure all maladies with one medicine severally applyed, as that *panacea, aurum potabile,* so much controverted in these dayes, *herba solis, &c.* Paracelsus reduceth all diseases to four principall heads, to whom Severinus, Ravelascus, Leo Suavius, and others, adhere and imitate : those are leprosie, gout, dropsie, falling-sicknesse : to which they reduce the rest; as to leprosie, ulcers, itches, furfures, scabs, &c. to gout, stone, cholick, tooth-ach, head-ach, &c. to dropsie, agues, jaundies, cachexia, &c. To the falling-sicknesse, belong palsy, vertigo, cramps, convulsions, incubus, apoplexie, &c. [3] *If any of these four principall be cured,* (saith Ravelascus) *all the inferior are cured;* and the same remedies commonly serve : but this is too generall, and by some contradicted. For this peculiar disease of melancholy, of which I am now to speak, I find severall cures, severall methods and prescripts. They that intend the practick cure of melancholy, saith Duretus in his notes to Hollerius, set down nine peculiar scopes or ends ; Savanarola prescribes seven especiall canons. Ælianus Montaltus, *cap.* 26. Faventinus, in his Emperieks, Hercules de Saxoniâ, &c. have their severall injunctions and rules, all tending to one end. The ordinary is threefold, which I mean to fol-

---

[1] Fuchsius, cap. 2. lib. 1.   [2] In pract. med. Hæc affectio nostris temporibus frequentissima ; ergo maxime pertinet ad nos hujus curationem intelligere.   [3] Si aliquis horum morborum summus sanatur, sanantur omnes inferiores.

low,—Διαιτητικη, *Pharmaceutica,* and *Chirurgica,* diet or living, apothecary, chirurgery, which Wecker, Crato, Guianerius, &c. and most prescribe ; of which I will insist, and speak in their order.

SECT. II.

MEMB. I. SUBSECT. I.

Dyet rectified in substance.

DIET, διαιτητικη, *victus* or living, according to [1] Fuchsius and others, comprehends those six non-natural things, which, I have before specified, are especiall causes, and, being rectified, a sole, or chief part of the cure. [2] Johannes Arculanus (*cap.* 16. *in* 9 *Rhasis*) accounts the rectifying of these six a sufficient cure. Guianerius (*Tract.* 15. *cap.* 9) calls them, *propriam et primam curam,* the principall cure : so doth Montanus, Crato, Mercurialis, Altomarus, &c. first to be tried. Lemnius (*instit. cap.* 22) names them the hinges of our health ; [3] no hope of recovery without them. Reinerus Solenander, in his seventh consultation for a Spanish young gentlewoman, that was so melancholy she abhorred all company, and would not sit at table with her familiar friends, prescribes this physick above the rest ; [4] no good to be done without it. [5] Aretæus, (*lib.* 1. *cap.* 7) an old physician, is of opinion, that this is enough of it self, if the party be not too far gone in sicknesse. [6] Crato, in a consultation of his for a noble patient, tells him plainly, that, if his highness will keep but a good diet, he will warrant him his former health. [7] Montanus, *consil.* 27, for a nobleman of France, admonisheth his lordship to be most circumspect in his diet, or else all his other physick will [8] be to small purpose. The same injunction I finde verbatim in J. Cæsar Claudinus, *Respon.* 34. Scoltzii *consil.* 183. Trallianus, *cap.* 16. *lib.* 1. Lælius à Fonte Eugubinus often brags that he hath done more cures in this kinde by rectification of diet, than all other physick besides. So that, in a word, I may say to most me-

---

[1] Instit. cap. 8. sect. 1. Victûs nomine non tam cibus et potus, sed aër, exercitatio, somnus, vigilia, et reliquæ res sex non-naturales, continentur. [2] Sufficit plerumque regimen rerum sex non-naturalium. [3] Et in his potissima sanitas consistit. [4] Nihil hîc agendum sine exquisitâ vivendi ratione, &c. [5] Si recens malum sit, ad pristinum habitum recuperandum, aliâ medelâ non est opus. [6] Consil. 99. lib. 2. Si celsitudo tua rectam victûs rationem, &c. [7] Moneo, domine, ut sis prudens ad victum, sine quo cætera remedia frustra adhibentur. [8] Omnia remedia irrita et vana sine his. Novistis me plerosque, ita laborantes, victu potius quam medicamentis curâsse.

474   *Cure of Melancholy.*   [Part. 2. Sec. 2.

lancholy men, as the fox said to the wesell, that could not get
out of the garner, *Macra cavum repetas, quem macra sub-
isti;* the six non-naturall things caused it ; and they must cure
it.   Which howsoever I treat of, as proper to the meridian of
melancholy, yet nevertheless, that which is here said, with him
in [1] Tully, though writ especially for the good of his friends at
Tarentum and Sicily, yet it will generally serve [2] most other
diseases, and help·them likewise, if it be observed.

Of these six non-naturall things, the first is diet, properly so
called, which consists in meat and drink, in which we must
consider substance, quantity, quality, and that opposite to the
precedent. In substance, such meats are generally commended,
which are [3] *moist, easie of digestion, and not apt to engender
winde, not fryed, nor rosted, but sod,* (saith Valescus, Altomarus, Piso, &c.) *hot and moist, and of good nourishment.*
Crato (*Consil.* 21. *lib* 2) admits rost meat, [4] if the burned and
scorched superficies, the brown we call it, be pared off. Salvianus (*lib. 2. cap.* 1) cries out on cold and dry meats ; [5] young
flesh and tender is approved, as of kid, rabbets, chickens,
veale, mutton, capons, hens, partridge, phesant, quailes,
and all mountain birds, which are so familiar in some parts of
Africa, and in Italy, and (as [6] Dublinius reports) the common
food of boores and clownes in Palæstina.   Galen takes exception at mutton ; but without question he means that rammy
mutton, which is in Turkie and Asia Minor, which have those
great fleshie tailes, of 48 pound weight, as Vertomannus witnesseth, *navig. lib. 2. cap.* 5. The lean of fat meat is best ;
and all manner of brothes, and pottage, with borage, lettuce,
and such wholesome hearbs, are excellent good, specially of a
cock boyled; all spoon meat. Arabians commend braines ; but
[7] Laurentius (*c.* 8) excepts against them ; and so do many others;
[8] egges are justified, as a nutritive wholsome meat : butter and
oyle may passe, but with some limitation : so [9] Crato confines
it, and *to some men sparingly, at set times, or in sauce ;* and
so sugar and hony are approved. [10] All sharp and sowre sauces
must be avoided, and spices, or at least seldom used : and so
saffron, sometimes, in broth, may be tolerated ; but these things
may be more freely used, as the temperature of the party is hot

---

[1] 1. de finibus Tarentinis et Siculis.   [2] Modo non multum elongentur.
[3] Lib. 1. de melan. cap. 7.   Calidus et humidus cibus concoctu facilis, flatûs exsortes, elixi, non assi, neque cibi frixi sint.   [4] Si interna tantum pulpa devo-
retur, non superficies torrida ab igne.   [5] Bene nutrientes cibi; tenella ætas
multum valet; carnes non virosæ, nec pingues.   [6] Hodœpor. peregr. Hierosol.
[7] Inimico stomacho.   [8] Not fryed, or buttered, but potched.   [9] Consil. 16.
Non improbatur butyrum et oleum, si tamen plus quam par sit non profundatur :
sacchari et mellis usus utiliter ad ciborum condimenta comprobatur.   [10] Mercurialis, consil. 88. Acerba omnia evitentur.

Mem. 1. Subs. 1.]   *Dyet rectified.*   475

or cold, or as he shall finde inconvenience by them. The thinnest, whitest, smallest wine is best, not thick, nor strong; and so of beer, the midling is fittest. Bread of good wheat, pure, well purged from the bran is preferred; Laurentius (*cap.* 8) would have it kneaded with rain water, if it may be gotten.

Water.] Pure, thin, light water by all means use, of good smell and taste; like to the ayr in sight, such as is soon hot, soon cold, and which Hippocrates so much approves, if at least it may be had. Rain water is purest, so that it fall not down in great drops, and be used forthwith; for it quickly putrefies. Next to it fountain water, that riseth in the east, and runneth eastward, from a quick running spring, from flinty, chalky, gravelly, grounds: and the longer a river runneth, it is commonly the purest; though many springs do yeeld the best water at their fountains. The waters in hotter countries, as in Turkie, Persia, India, within the tropicks, are frequently purer than ours in the north, more subtile, thin, and lighter (as our merchants observe) by four ounces in a pound, pleasanter to drink, as good as our beer, and some of them, as Choaspis in Persia, preferred by the Persian kings, before wine it self.

[1] Clitorio quicunque sitim de fonte levârit,
Vina fugit, gaudetque meris abstemius undis.

Many rivers, I deny not, are muddy still, white, thick, like those in China, Nilus in Ægypt, Tibris at Rome, but after they be setled two or three dayes, defecate and clear, very commodious, usefull and good. Many make use of deep wels, as of old in the Holy Land, lakes, cisterns, when they cannot be better provided; to fetch it in carts or gundilos, as in Venice, or camels backs, as at Cairo in Ægypt: [2] Radzivilius observed 8000 camels daily there, employed about that business. Some keep it in trunks, as in the East Indies, made four square, with descending steps: and 'tis not amiss: for I would not have any one so nice as that Græcian Calis, sister to Nicephorus emperour of Constantinople, and [3] married to Dominicus Silvius Duke of Venice, that, out of incredible wantonness, *communi aquâ uti nolebat,* would use no vulgar water; but she died *tantâ* (saith mine author) *fœtidissimi puris copiâ,* of so fulsome a disease, that no water could wash her clean. [4] Plato would not have a traveller lodge in a city, that is not governed by laws, or hath not a quick stream running by it; *illud enim animum, hoc corrumpit valetudinem;* one corrupts the body, the other the minde. But this is more than needs; too much curiosity is

[1] Ovid. Met. lib. 15.   [2] Peregr. Hier.   [3] The dukes of Venice were then
permitted to marry.   [4] De Legibus.

476 *Cure of Melancholy.* [Part. 2. Sec. 2.

naught ; in time of necessity any water is allowed. Howsoever, pure water is best, and which (as Pindarus holds) is better than gold: an especiall ornament it is, and *very commodious to a city* (according to [1] Vegetius) *when fresh springs are included within the wals ;* as at Corinth, in the midst of the town almost, there was *arx altissima scatens fontibus,* a goodly mount full of fresh-water-springs : *if nature afford them not, they must be had by art.* It is a wonder to read of those [2] stupend aqueducts ; and infinite cost hath been bestowed, in Rome of old, Constantinople, Carthage, Alexandria, and such populous cities, to conveigh good and wholsome waters: read [3] Frontinus, Lipsius, *de admir.* [4] Plinius, *lib. 3. cap.* 11. Strabo, in his Geogr. That aqueduct of Claudius was most eminent, fetched upon arches 15 miles, every arch 109 foot high : they had 14 such other aqueducts, besides lakes and cisterns, 700, as I take it; [5] every house had private pipes and chanels to serve them for their use. Peter Gillius, in his accurate description of Constantinople, speaks of an old cistern which he went down to see, 336 foot long, 180 foot broad, built of marble, covered over with arch-work, and sustained by 336 pillars, twelve foot asunder, and in 11 rowes, to contain sweet water. Infinite cost in chanels and cisterns, from Nilus to Alexandria, hath been formerly bestowed, to the admiration of these times ; [6] their cisterns so curiously cemented and composed, that a beholder would take them to be all of one stone : when the foundation is laid, and cistern made, their house is half built. That Segovian aqueduct in Spain is much wondred at in these dayes, [7] upon three rows of pillars, one above another, conveying sweet water to every house: but each city almost is full of such aqueducts. Amongst the rest, [8] he is eternally to be commended, that brought that new stream to the north side of London at his own charge ; and Mr. Otho Nicholson, founder of our water-works and elegant conduit in Oxford. So much have all times attributed to this element, to be conveniently provided of it. Although Galen hath taken exceptions at such waters which run through leaden pipes, *ob cerussam quæ in iis generatur,* for that unctuous ceruse, which causeth dysenteries and fluxes ; [9] yet, as Alsarius Crucius of Genua well answers, it is opposite to common experience.

---

[1] Lib. 4. cap. 10. Magna urbis utilitas, cum perennes fontes muris includuntur ; quod si natura non præstat, effodiendi, &c.   [2] Opera gigantum dicit aliquis. [3] De aquæduct.   [4] Curtius fons à quadragesimo lapide in urbem opere arcuato perductus. Plin. lib. 36. 15.   [5] Quæque domus Romæ fistulas habebat et canales, &c.   [6] Lib. 2. cap. 20. Jod. a Meggen. cap. 15. pereg. Hier. Bellonius. [7] Cypr. Echovius, delic. Hisp. Aqua profluens inde in omnes fere domos ducitur ; in puteis quoque æstivo tempore frigidissima conservatur.   [8] Sir Hugh Middleton, baronet.   [9] De quæsitis med. cent. fol. 354.

Mem. 1. Subs. 1.] *Dyet rectified.*

If that were true, most of our Italian cities, Montpelier in France, with infinite others, would finde this inconvenience; but there is no such matter. For private families, in what sort they should furnish themselves, let them consult with P. Crescentius, *de Agric. l.* 1. *c.* 4. Pamphilus Hirelacus, and the rest.

Amongst fishes, those are most allowed of, that live in graveily or sandy waters, pikes, pearch, trout, gudgeon, smelts, flounders, &c. Hippolytus Salvianus takes exception at carp; but I dare boldly say, with [1] Dubravius, it is an excellent meat, if it come not from [2] muddy pooles, that it retain not an unsavory tast. *Erinaceus marinus* is much commended by Oribasius, Aëtius, and most of our late writers.

[3] Crato (*consil.* 21. *lib.* 2) censures all manner of fruits, as subject to putrefaction, yet tolerable at some times; after meales, at second course, they keep down vapours, and have their use. Sweet fruits are best, as sweet cherries, plums, sweet apples, peare-maines, and pippins, which Laurentius extols, as having a peculiar property against this disease, and Plater magnifies: *omnibus modis appropriata conveniunt;* but they must be corrected for their windiness : ripe grapes are good, and raysins of the sun, musk-millions well corrected, and sparingly used. Figs are allowed, and almonds blanched. Trallianus discommends figs. [4] Salvianus olives and capers, which [5] others especially like of, and so of pistick nuts. Montanus and Mercurialis (out of Avenzoar) admit peaches, [6] peares, and apples baked after meales, only corrected with sugar, and aniseed, or fennel-seed ; and so they may be profitably taken, because they strengthen the stomack, and keep down vapors. The like may be said of preserved cherries, plums, marmalit of plums, quinces, &c. but not to drink after them. [7] Pomegranates, lemons, oranges are tolerated, if they be not too sharp.

[8] Crato will admit of no herbs, but borage, bugloss, endive, fennell, aniseed, bawme : Calenus and Arnoldus tolerate lettuce, spinage, beets, &c. The same Crato will allow no roots at all to be eaten. Some approve of potatoes, parsnips, but all corrected for winde. No raw sallets ; but, as Lauren-

---

[1] De piscibus lib. Habent omnes in lautitiis, modo non sint e cœnoso loco. [2] De pisc. c. 2. l. 7. Plurimum præstat ad utilitatem et jucunditatem. Idem Trallianus, lib. 1. c. 16. Pisces petrosi, et molles carne. [3] Etsi omnes putredini sunt obnoxii, ubi secundis mensis, incepto jam priore, devorentur, commodi succi prosunt, qui dulcedine sunt præditi, ut dulcia cerasa, poma, &c. [4] Lib. 2. cap. 1. [5] Montanus, consil. 24. [6] Pyra quæ grato sunt sapore, cocta mala, poma tosta, et saccharo vel anisi semine conspersa, utiliter statim a prandio vel a cœnâ sumi possunt, eo quod ventriculum roborent, et vapores caput petentes reprimant. Mont. [7] Punica mala commodè permittuntur, modo non sint austera et acida. [8] Olera omnia, præter boraginem, buglossum, intybum, feniculum, anisum, melissum, vitari debent.

478   *Cure of Melancholy.*   [Part. 2. Sec. 2.

tius prescribes, in broths; and so Crato commends many of
them: or to use borage, hops, bawme, steeped in their ordinary
drink. [1] Avenzoar magnifies the juice of a pomegranate, if
it be sweet, and especially rose-water, which he would have
to be used in every dish; which they put in practice in those
hot countries about Damascus, where (if we may beleeve the
relations of Vertomannus) many hogsheads of rose-water are
to be sold in the market at once, it is in so great request
with them.

SUBSECT. II.

Dyet rectified in quantity.

MAN alone saith [2] Cardan, eates and drinks without appetite
and useth all his pleasure without necessity, *animæ vitio;* and
thence come many inconveniences unto him; for there is no
meat whatsoever, though otherwise wholsome and good, but,
if unseasonably taken, or immoderately used, more than the
stomack can well beare, it will ingender cruditie, and do much
harme. Therefore [3] Crato adviseth his patient to eat but twice
a day, and that at his set meales, by no means to eat without an appetite, or upon a full stomach, and to put seven
houres difference betwixt dinner and supper: which rule if we
did observe in our colleges, it would be much better for our
healths: but custome, that tyrant, so prevails, that, contrary
to all good order and rules of physick, we scarce admit of five.
If, after seven houres tarrying, he shall have no stomach, let
him defer his meal, or eat very little at his ordinary time of
repast. This very counsell was given by Prosper Calenus to
Cardinall Cæsius, labouring of this disease; and [4] Platerus prescribes it to a patient of his, to be most severely kept. Guianerius admits of three meals a day; but Montanus, *consil. 23.
pro Ab. Italo,* ties him precisely to two. And, as he must not
eat overmuch, so he may not absolutely fast; for, as Celsus contends (*lib.* 1), Jacchinus (15. *in* 9 *Rhasis*), [5] repletion and in-
anition may both do harm in too contrary extreams. Moreover,
that which he doth eat, must be well [6] chewed, and not hastily
gobled; for that causeth crudity and winde; and by all means

[1] Mercurialis, pract. med.   [2] Lib. 2. de com.   Solus homo edit bibitque, &c.
[3] Consil. 21. 18.   Si plus ingeratur quam par est, et ventriculus tolerare possit,
nocet, et cruditates generat, &c.   [4] Observat. lib. 1.   Assuescat bis in die
cibos sumere, certâ semper horâ.   [5] Ne plus ingerat, cavendum, quam ventriculus ferre potest; semperque surgat à mensâ non satur.   [6] Siquidem qui semi-
mansum velociter ingerunt cibum, ventriculo laborem inferunt, et flatus maximos
promovent.   Crato.

Mem. 1. Subs. 2.] *Dyet rectified.* 479

to eat no more than he can well digest. *Some think* (saith [1] Trincavellius, *lib.* 11. *cap.* 29. *de curand. part. hum.*) *the more they eat, the more they nourish themselves:* eat and live, as the proverb is, *not knowing that onely repairs man which is well concocted, not that which is devoured.* Melancholy men most part have good [2] appetites, but ill digestion; and for that cause they must be sure to rise with an appetite: and that which Socrates and Disarius the physicians, in [3] Macrobius, so much require, St. Hierom injoines Rusticus, to eat and drink no more than will [4] satisfie hunger and thirst. [5] Lessius the Jesuite holds 12, 13, or 14 ounces, or in our northern countries 16 at most, (for all students, weaklings, and such as lead an idle sedentary life) *of meat, bread, &c. a fit proportion for a whole day, and as much or little more of drink.* Nothing pesters the body and minde sooner than to be still fed, to eat and ingurgitate beyond all measure, as many do. [6] *By overmuch eating and continual feasts, they stifle nature, and choke up themselves; which, had they lived coursly, or, like galley-slaves been tyed to an oare, might have happily prolonged many fair years.*

A great inconvenience comes by variety of dishes, which causeth the precedent distemperature, [7] *than which* (saith Avicenna) *nothing is worse; to feed on diversity of meats, or overmuch,* Sertorius-like *in lucem cœnare,* and, as commonly they do in Muscovie and Island, to prolong their meals all day long, or all night. Our northern countries offend especially in this: and we in this island (*ampliter viventes in prandiis et cœnis,* as [8] Polydore notes) are most liberal feeders, but to our own hurt. [9] *Persicos odi, puer, apparatus: excess of meat breedeth sickness: and gluttony causeth cholerick diseases; by surfeiting, many perish: but he that dieteth himself, prolongeth his life,* Ecclus. 37. 29, 30. We account it a great glory for a man to have his table daily furnished with variety of meats: but hear the physician: he puls thee by the ear as thou sittest, and telleth thee, [10] *that nothing can be more noxious to thy health, than such variety and plenty.* Temperance is a bridle of gold;

---

[2] Quidam maxime comedere nituntur, putantes eâ ratione se vires refecturos; ignorantes, non ea quæ ingerunt posse vires reficere, sed quæ probe concoquunt. [2] Multa appetunt; pauca digerunt. [3] Saturnal. lib. 7. cap. 4. [4] Modicus et temperatus cibus et carni et animæ utilis est. [5] Hygiasticon, reg. 14. 16 unciæ per diem sufficiant, computato pane, carne, ovis, vel aliis opsoniis, et totidem vel paulo plures unciæ potûs. [6] Idem, reg. 27. Plures in domibus suis brevi tempore pascentes extinguuntur, qui, si triremibus vincti fuissent, aut gregario pane pasti, sani et incolumes in longam ætatem vitam prorogâssent. [7] Nihil deterius quam diversa nutrientia simul adjungere, et comedendi tempus prorogare. [8] Lib. 1. hist. [9] Hor. ad lib. 5. ode ult. [10] Ciborum varietate et copiâ in eâdem mensâ nihil nocentius homini ad salutem. Fr. Valeriola, observ. l. 2. cap. 6.

480   *Cure of Melancholy.*   [Part. 2. Sec. 2.

and he that can use it aright, [1] *ego non summis viris comparo, sed simillimum Deo judico,* is liker a God than a man : for, as it will transform a beast to a man again, so will it make a man a God. To preserve thine honour, health, and to avoid therefore all those inflations, torments, obstructions, crudities, and diseases, that come by a full diet, the best way is to [2] feed sparingly of one or two dishes at most, to have *ventrem bene moratum,* as Seneca calls it ; [3] *to choose one of many, and to feed on that alone,* as Crato adviseth his patient. The same counsell [4] Prosper Calenus gives to Cardinall Cæsius, to use a moderate and simple diet : and, though his table be jovially furnished by reason of his state and guests, yet, for his own part, to single out some one savoury dish, and feed on it. The same is inculcated by [5] Crato (*consil. 9. l. 2*) to a noble personage affected with this grievance : he would have his highness to dine or sup alone, without all his honourable attendance and courtly company, with a private friend or so, [6] a dish or two, a cup of Rhenish wine, &c. Montanus, *consil. 24.* for a noble matron, injoyns her one dish, and by no means to drink betwixt meals : the like, *consil. 229.* or not to eat till he be an hungry ; which rule Berengarius did most strictly observe, as Hilbertus Cenomecensis Episc. writes in his life.

> ————————cui non fuit unquam
> Ante sitim potus, nec cibus ante famem ;

and which all temperate men do constantly keep. It is a frequent solemnity still used with us, when friends meet, to go to the ale-house or tavern ; they are not sociable otherwise : and if they visit one anothers houses, they must both eat and drink. I reprehend it not, moderately used : but to some men nothing can be more offensive : they had better (I speak it with Saint [7] Ambrose) pour so much water in their shooes.

It much availes likewise to keep good order in our diet, [8] *to eat liquid things first, broaths, fish, and such meats as are sooner corrupted in the stomack ; harder meats of digestion, must come last.* Crato *would have the supper less than the dinner,* which Cardan (*contradict. lib. 1. Tract. 5. contra-*

---

[1] Tul. orat. pro M. Marcel.   [2] Nullus cibum sumere debet, nisi stomachus sit vacuus. Gordon. lib. med. 1. l. c. 11.   [3] E multis eduliis unum elige, relictisque cæteris, ex eo comede.   [4] L. de atrâ bile. Simplex sit cibus, et non varius : quod licet dignitati tuæ ob convivas difficile videatur, &c.   [5] Celsitudo tua prandeat sola, absque apparatu aulico, contentus sit illustrissimus princeps duobus tantum ferculis, vinoque Rhenano solum in mensâ utatur.   [6] Semper intra satietatem a mensâ recedat, uno ferculo contentus.   [7] Lib. de Hel. et Jejunio. Multo melius in terram vina fudisses.   [8] Crato. Multum refert non ignorare qui cibi priores, &c. liquida præcedant carnium jura, pisces, fructus, &c. Cœna brevior sit prandio.

Mem. 1. Subs. 2.] *Dyet rectified.* 481

dict. 18) disallowes, and that by the authority of Galen, 7. *art. curat. cap.* 6 ; and for four reasons he will have the supper biggest. I have read many treatises to this purpose ; I know not how it may concern some few sick men ; but, for my part, generally for all, I should subscribe to that custome of the Romans, to make a sparing dinner, and a liberal supper ; all their preparation and invitation was still at supper ; no mention of dinner. Many reasons I could give ; but when all is said *pro* and *con,* [1] Cardans rule is best, to keep that we are accustomed unto, though it be naught : and to follow our disposition and appetite in some things is not amiss ; to eat sometimes of a dish which is hurtful, if we have an extraordinary liking to it. Alexander Severus loved hares and apples above all other meats, as [2] Lampridius relates in his life : one pope pork, another peacock, &c. what harm came of it ? I conclude, our own experience is the best physician : that dyet which is most propitious to one, is often pernicious to another ; such is the variety of palats, humours, and temperatures, let every man observe, and be a law unto himself. Tiberius, in [3] Tacitus, did laugh at all such, that after 30 years of age would ask counsell of others concerning matters of diet : I say the same.

These few rules of diet he that keeps, shall surely finde great ease and speedy remedy by it. It is a wonder to relate that prodigious temperance of some hermites, anachorites, and fathers of the church. He that shall but read their lives, written by Hierom, Athanasius, &c. how abstemious heathens have bin in this kind, those Curii and Fabricii, those old philosophers, as Pliny records (*lib.* 11), Xenophon (*lib.* 1 *de vit. Socrat.*) emperours and kings, as Nicephorus relates (*Eccles. hist. lib.* 18. *cap.* 8), of Mauritius, Lodovicus Pius, &c. and that admirable [4] example of Lodovicus Cornarus, a patritian of Venice, cannot but admire them. This have they done voluntarily, and in health ; what shall these private men do, that are visited with sickness, and necessarily [5] injoyned to recover and continue their health ? It is a hard thing to observe a strict dyet ; *et qui medice vivit misere vivit,* as the saying is ; *quale hoc ipsum erit vivere, his si privatus fueris ?* as good be buried, as so much debarred of his appetite ; *excessit medicina malum,* the physick is more troublesome than the disease ; so he complained in the poet, so thou thinkest : yet he that loves himself, will easily endure this little misery, to avoid a greater inconvenience ;

---

[1] Tract. 6. contradict. 1. lib. 1.   [2] Super omnia quotidianum leporem habuit, et pomis indulsit.   [3] Annal. 6. Ridere solebat eos, qui post 30 ætatis annum, ad cognoscenda corpori suo noxia vel utilia, alicujus consilii indigerent.   [4] A Lessio edit. 1614.   [5] Ægyptii olim omnes morbos curabant vomitu et jejunio. Bohemus, lib. 1. cap. 5.

VOL. I.   I I

482   *Cure of Melancholy.*   [Part. 2. Sec. 2.

e malis minimum, better do this than do worse. And, as [1] Tully holds, *better be a temperate old man, than a lascivious youth.* 'Tis the only sweet thing, (which he adviseth) so to moderate our selves, that we may have *senectutem in juventute, et in senectute juventutem*, be youthful in our old age, staid in our youth, discreet and temperate in both.

MEMB. II.

Retention and Evacuation rectified.

I HAVE declared, in the Causes, what harm costiveness hath done in procuring this disease : if it be so noxious, the opposite must needs be good, or mean at least, as indeed it is, and to this cure necessarily required ; *maxime conducit*, saith Montaltus, *cap.* 27 ; it very much availes. [2] Altomarus (*cap.* 7) *commends walking in a morning, into some fair green pleasant fields ; but by all means first, by art or nature, he will have these ordinary excrements evacuated.* Piso calls it *beneficium ventris*, the benefit, help, or pleasure of the belly : for it doth much ease it. Laurentius (*cap.* 8), Crato (*consil.* 21. *l.* 2) prescribes it once a day at least : where nature is defective, art must supply, by those lenitive electuaries, suppositories, condite prunes, turpentine, clisters, as shall be shewed. Prosper Calenus (*lib. de atrâ bile*) commends clisters, in hypochondriacall melancholy, still to be used as occasion serves. [3] Peter Cnemander, in a consultation of his *pro hypochondriaco,* will have his patient continually loose, and to that end sets down there many forms of potions and clisters. Mercurialis (*consil.* 88), if this benefit come not of its own accord, prescribes [4] clisters in the first place : so doth Montanus, *consil.* 24. *consil.* 31. *et* 229 : he commends turpentine to that purpose : the same he ingeminates, *consil.* 230, for an Italian abbot. 'Tis very good to wash his hands and face often, to shift his clothes, to have fair linen about him, to be decently and comely attired ; for *sordes vitiant*, nastiness defiles, and dejects any man that is so voluntarily, or compelled by want; it dulleth the spirits.

Bathes are either artificiall or naturall ; both have their spe-

[1] Cat. Major. Melior conditio senis viventis ex præscripto artis medicæ, quam adolescentis luxuriosi. [2] Debet per amœna exerceri, et loca viridia, excretis prius arte vel naturâ alvi excrementis. [3] Hildesheim, spicil. 2. de mel. Primum omnium operam dabis ut singulis diebus habeas beneficium ventris, semper cavendo ne alvus sit diutius astricta. [4] Si non sponte, clysteribus purgetur.

Mem. 2.] *Retention and Evacuation rectified.* 483

cial uses in this malady, and (as [1] Alexander supposeth, *lib.* 1.
cap. 16) yeeld as speedy a remedy, as any other physick whatsoever. Aëtius would have them daily used, *assidua balnea*,
Tetra. 2. *sec.* 2. *c.* 9. Galen crakes how many severall cures he
hath performed in this kinde by use of bathes alone, and Rufus
pills, moistning them which are otherwise dry. Rhasis makes
it a principall cure (*tota cura sit in humectando*) to bathe
and afterwards anoint with oyle. Jason Pratensis, Laurentius,
cap. 8, and Montanus, set down their peculiar formes of artificiall
bathes. Crato (*consil.* 17. *lib.* 2) commends mallowes, camomile, violets, borage, to be boyled in it, and sometimes faire
water alone ; and in his following counsell, *balneum aquæ
dulcis solum sæpissime profuisse compertum habemus.* So
doth Fuchsius, *lib.* 1. *cap.* 33. Frisimelica, 2. *consil.* 42. *in*
Trincavellius. Some, beside hearbs, prescribe a rammes head
and other things to be boyled. [2] Fernelius (*consil.* 44.) *will
have them used* 10 or 12 dayes together ; to which he must
enter fasting, and so continue in a temperate heat, and, after
that, frictions all over the body. Lælius Eugubinus, *consil.*
142, and Christoph. Ærerus in a consultation of his, hold
once or twice a week sufficient to bathe, the [3] *water to be
warme, not hot, for fear of sweating.* Felix Plater (*observ.
lib.* 1. for a melancholy lawyer) [4] *will have lotions of the head
still joyned to these bathes, with a lee wherein capitall hearbs
have been boyled.* [5] Laurentius speaks of bathes of milk, which
I finde approved by many others. And still, after bath, the
body to be anointed with oyl of bitter almonds, of violets, new
or fresh butter, [6] capons grease, especially the back bone, and
then lotions of the head, embrocations, &c. These kinde of
bathes have been in former times much frequented, and diversly varied, and are still in generall use in those eastern countries. The Romanes had their publick baths very sumptuous
and stupend, as those of Antoninus and Dioclesian. Plin. 36.
saith there were an infinite number of them in Rome, and
mightily frequented. Some bathed seven times a day, as Commodus the emperour is reported to have done : usually twice a
day ; and they were after anointed with most costly oyntments ;
rich women bathed themselves in milke, some in the milke of
500 she asses at once. We have many ruines of such bathes
found in this iland, among those parietines and rubbish of

---

[1] Balneorum usus dulcium, siquid aliud, ipsis opitulatur. Credo hæc dici cum
aliquâ jactantiâ, inquit Montanus, consil. 26.   [2] In quibus jejunus diu sedeat
eo tempore, ne sudorem excitent aut manifestum teporem, sed quâdam refrigera-
tione humectent.   [3] Aqua non sit calida, sed tepida, ne sudor sequatur.
[4] Lotiones capitis ex lixivio, in quo herbas capitales coxerint.   [5] Cap. 8. de mel.
[6] Aut axungiâ pulli. Piso.

484   *Cure of Melancholy.*   [Part. 2. Sec. 2.

old Romane townes. Lipsius (*de mag. Urb. Rom. l. 3. c.* 8), Rosinus, Scot of Antwerp, and other antiquaries, tell strange stories of their baths. Gillius (*l.* 4. *cap. ult. Topogr. Constant.*) reckons up 155 publicke [1] baths in Constantinople, of faire building: they are still [2] frequented in that citie by the Turkes of all sorts, men and women, and all over Greece and those hot countries ; to absterge, belike, that fulsomeness of sweat, to which they are there subject. [3] Busbequius, in his epistles, is very copious in describing the manner of them, how their women go covered, a maid following with a box of oyntment to rub them. The richer sort have private baths in their houses: the poorer goe to the common, and are generally so curious in this behalf, that they will not eat nor drink until they have bathed; before and after meals some, [4] *and will not make water (but they will wash their hands) or go to stool.* Leo Afer (*l.* 3) makes mention of 100 severall baths at Fez in Africke, most sumptuous, and such as have great revenues belonging to them. Buxtorf (*cap.* 14. *Synagog. Jud.*) speakes of many ceremonies amongst the Jews in this kind; they are very superstitious in their bathes, especially women.

Naturall bathes are praised by some, discommended by others; but it is in a divers respect. [5] Marcus de Oddis, *in Hyp. affect.* consulted about baths, condemns them for the heat of the liver, because they dry too fast; and yet by and by, [6] in another counsell for the same disease, he approves them because they cleanse by reason of the sulphur, and would have their water to be drunk. Aretæus (*c.* 7) commends allome baths above the rest; and [7] Mercurialis (*consil.* 88) those of Luca in that hypochondriacall passion. *He would have his patient tarry there 15 days together, and drink the water of them, and to be bucketed, or have the water powred on his head.* John Baptista Silvaticus (*cont.* 64) commends all the baths in Italy, and drinking of their water, whether they be iron, allome, sulphur ; so doth [8] Hercules de Saxoniâ. But, in that they cause sweat, and dry so much, he confines himself to hypochondriacall melancholy alone, excepting that of the head, and the other. Trincavellius (*consil.* 14. *lib.* 1.) prefers those [9] Porrectan baths before the rest, because of the mixture

---

[1] Thermæ. Nymphea.   [2] Sandes, lib. 1. saith that women go twice a week to the baths at least.   [3] Epist. 3.   [4] Nec alvum excernunt, quin aquam secum portent, quâ partes obscœnas lavent. Busbequius, ep. 3. Leg. Turciæ. [5] Hildesheim spicil. 2. de mel. Hypochon. si non adesset jecoris caliditas, thermas laudarem, et si non nimia humoris exsiccatio esset metuenda.   [6] Fol. 141. [7] Thermas Lucenses adeat, ibique aquas ejus per 15 dies potet: et calidarum aquarum stillicidiis tum caput tum ventriculum de more subjiciat.   [8] In panth. [9] Aquæ Porrectanæ.

Mem. 2.] *Retention and Evacuation rectified.* 485

of brasse, iron, allome; and, *consil. 35. l. 3,* for a melancholy lawyer, and *consil.* 36, in that hypochondriacall passion, the [1] baths of Aquaria, and *consil.* 36, the drinking of them. Frisimelica, consulted among the rest (in Trincavellius, *consil.* 42. *lib.* 2) preferres the waters of [2] Apona before all artificiall baths whatsoever in this disease, and would have one nine years affected with hypochondriacall passions, flie to them, as to an holy anchor. Of the same minde is Trincavellius himself there; and yet both put a hot liver in the same party for a cause, and send him to the waters of [3] S. Helen, which are much hotter. Montanus (*consil.* 230) magnifies the [4] Chalderinian Baths; and (*consil.* 237 et 239) he exhorteth to the same, but with this caution, [5] *that the liver be outwardly anointed with some coolers, that it be not overheated.* But these baths must be warily frequented by melancholy persons, or if used to such as are very cold of themselves; for, as Gabelius concludes of all Dutch baths, and especially those of Baden, *they are good for all cold diseases,* [6] *naught for cholerick, hot and dry, and all infirmities proceeding of choler, inflammations of the spleen and liver.* Our English baths, as they are hot, must needs incur the same censure: but D. Turner of old, and D. Jones, have written at large of them. Of cold baths I find little or no mention in any physician: some speak against them: [7] Cardan alone (out of Agathinus) commends *bathing in fresh rivers, and cold waters, and adviseth all such as mean to live long to use it; for it agrees with all ages and complexions, and is most profitable for hot temperatures.* As for sweating, urine, bloud-letting by hæmrods, or otherwise, I shall elsewhere more opportunely speak of them.

Immoderate Venus, in excess, as it is a cause, or in defect; so, moderately used, to some parties an only help, a present remedy. Peter Forestus calls it, *aptissimum remedium,* a most apposite *remedy,* [8] *remitting anger, and reason, that was otherwise bound.* Avicenna (*Fen.* 3. 20), Oribasius (*med. collect. lib.* 6. *cap.* 37), contend, out of Ruffus and others, [9] *that many mad men, melancholy, and labouring of the falling sickness, have been cured by this alone.* Montaltus (*cap.* 27.

---

[1] Aquæ Aquariæ.   [2] Ad aquas Aponenses, velut ad sacram anchoram, confugiat.   [3] John Beauhinus (li. 3. ca. 14. hist. admir. fontis Bollensis in ducat. Wittemberg) laudat aquas Bollenses ad melancholicos morbos, mœrorem, fascinationem, aliaque animi pathemata.   [4] Balnea Chalderina.   [5] Hepar externe ungatur, ne calefiat.   [6] Nocent calidis et siccis, cholericis, et omnibus morbis ex cholerâ, hepatis, splenisque affectionibus.   [7] Lib. de aquâ. Qui breve hoc vitæ curriculum cupiunt sani transigere, frigidis aquis sæpe lavare debent, nulli ætati cum sit incongrua, calidis imprimis utilis.   [8] Solvit Venus rationis vim impeditam, ingentes iras remittit, &c.   [9] Multi comitiales, melancholici, insani, hujus usu solo sanati.

486   *Cure of Melancholy.*   [Part. 2. Sec. 2.

de melan.) will have it drive away sorrow, and all illusions of
the brain, to purge the heart and brain from ill smoakes and
vapours that offend them; [1] *and if it be omitted, as Valescus
supposeth, it makes the mind sad, the body dull and heavy.*
Many other inconveniences are reckoned up by Mercatus,
and by Rodericus a Castro, in their tracts *de melancholiá virginum et monialium: ob seminis retentionem, sæviunt sæpe
moniales et virgines;* but, as Platerus addes, *si nubant, sanantur;* they rave single, and pine away; much discontent; but
marriage mends all. Marcellus Donatus (*lib. 2. med. hist.
cap. 1.*) tells a storie to confirm this, out of Alexander Benedictus, of a maid that was mad, *ob menses inhibitos: cum in
officinam meritoriam incidisset, a quindecim viris eâdem nocte
compressa, mensium largo profluvio, quod pluribus annis ante
constiterat, non sine magno pudore, mane, menti restituta,
discessit.* But this must be warily understood; for as Arnoldus objects, *lib. 1. breviar. 18. cap. quid coitus ad melancholicum succum?* What affinity have these two? [2] *except it
be manifest that superabundance of seed or fulness of blood
be a cause, or that love, or an extraordinary desire of Venus,
have gone before,* or that, as Lod. Mercatus excepts, they be
very flatuous, and have been otherwise accustomed unto it.
Montaltus (*cap. 27*) will not allow of moderate Venus to such
as have the gout, palsie, epilepsie, melancholy, except they
be very lusty, and full of blood. [3] Lodovicus Antonius, *lib.
med. miscel.* in his chapter of Venus, forbids it utterly to all
wrestlers, ditchers, labouring men, &c. [4] Ficinus and [5] Marsilius Cognatus put Venus one of the five mortall enemies of a
student: *it consumes the spirits, and weakneth the brain.*
Halyabbas the Arabian (5 *Theor. cap.* 36), and Jason Pratensis, make it the fountain of most diseases, [6] *but most pernicious
to them who are cold and dry;* a melancholy man must not
meddle with it, but in some cases. Plutarch, in his book *de
san. tuend.* accounts of it as one of the three principall signs
and preservers of health, temperance in this kinde: [7] *to rise with
an appetite, to be ready to work, and abstain from venery, tria
saluberrima,* are three most healthful things. We see their
opposites, how pernicious they are to mankinde, as to all other
creatures: they bring death, and many ferall diseases:

---

[1] Si omittatur coitus, contristat et plurimum gravat corpus et animum.   [2] Nisi
certo constet nimium semen aut sanguinem caussam esse, aut amor præcesserit,
aut, &c.   [3] Athletis, arthriticis, podagricis nocet; nec opportuna prodest,
nisi fortibus, et qui multo sanguine abundant. Idem Scaliger, exerc. 269. Turcis
ideo luctatoribus prohibitum.   [4] De sanit. tuend. lib. 1.   [5] Lib. 1. ca. 7.
Exhaurit enim spiritus, animumque debilitat.   [6] Frigidis et siccis corporibus
inimicissima.   [7] Vesci intra satietatem, impigrum esse ad laborem, vitale semen conservare.

Mem. 3.] *Digression of Ayre.* **487**

Immodicis brevis est ætas et rara senectus.

Aristotle gives instance in sparrows, which are *parum vivaces ob salacitatem*,[1] short lived because of their salacity, which is very frequent, as Scoppius, *in Priapeis*, will better inform you. The extremes being both bad, [2] the *medium* is to be kept, which cannot easily be determined. Some are better able to sustain, such as are hot and moist, phlegmatick, as Hippocrates insinuateth, some strong and lustie, well fed like [3] Hercules, [4] Proculus the emperour, lusty Laurence, [5] *prostibulum feminæ*, Messalina the empress, that by philtres, and such kinde of lascivious meats, use all means to [6] inable themselves, and brag of it in the end; *confodi multas enim, occidi vero paucas per ventrem vidisti*, as that Spanish [7] Celestina merrily said: others impotent, of a cold and dry constitution, cannot sustain those gymnicks without great hurt done to their own bodies; of which number (though they be very prone to it) are melancholy men for the most part.

MEMB. III.

Ayr rectified.   With a digression of the Ayr.

As a long-winged hawk, when he is first whistled off the fist, mounts aloft, and for his pleasure fetcheth many a circuit in the ayr, still soaring higher and higher, till he be come to his full pitch, and in the end, when the game is sprung, comes down amain, and stoopes upon a sudden; so will I, having now come at last into these ample fields of ayre, wherein I may freely expatiate and exercise myself for my recreation, a while rove, wander round about the world, mount aloft to those æthereall orbs and celestiall spheres, and so descend to my former elements again: in which progress, I will first see whether that relation of the [8] Frier of Oxford be true, concerning those northern parts under the pole, (if I meet *obiter* with the wandring Jew, Elias Artifex, or Lucians Icaromenippus, they shall be my guides) whether there be such 4 Euripes,

---

[1] Nequitia est, quæ te non sinit esse senem.   [2] Vide Montanum, Pet. Godefridum, Amorum lib. 2. cap. 6. Curiosum de his, nam et numerum definite Talmudistis, unicuique sciatis assignari suum tempus, &c.   [3] Thespiadas genuit. [4] Vide Lampridium, vit. ejus 4.   [5] Et lassata viris, &c.   [6] Vid. Mizald. cent. 8. 11.   Lemnium, lib. 2. cap. 16.   Catullum ad Hypsithillam, &c.   Ovid. Eleg. lib. 3. et 6, &c. Quot itinera unâ nocte confecissent, tot coronas ludicro Deo puta Triphallo, Marsiæ, Hermæ, Priapo, donarent.   Cingemus tibi mentulam coronis, &c.   [7] Pornoboscodid. Gasp. Barthii.   [8] Nich. de Lynna, cited by Mercator in his Map.

488   *Cure of Melancholy.*   [Part. 2. Sec. 2.

and a great rock of loadstones, which may cause the needle
in the compass still to bend that way, and what should be the
true cause of the variation of the compass, [1] is it a magneticall
rock, or the pole-star, as Cardan will; or some other star in the
bear, as Marsilius Ficinus; or a magneticall meridian, as
Maurolicus; *vel situs in venâ terræ*, as Agricola; or the near-
ness of the next continent, as Cabeus will; or some other
cause, as Scaliger, Cortesius, Conimbricenses, Peregrinus, contend; why at the Azores it looks directly north, otherwise
not? In the Mediterranean or Levant (as some observe) it
varies 7 grad., by and by 12, and then 22. In the Baltick
Seas, near Rasceburgh in Finland, the needle runs round, if
any ships come that way, though [2] Martin Ridley write otherwise, that the needle near the pole will hardly be forced
from his direction. 'Tis fit to be enquired whether certain
rules may be made of it, as 11 *grad. Lond. variat. alibi* 36,
&c. and, that which is more prodigious, the variation varies in
the same place: now taken accurately, 'tis so much; after a
few years, quite altered from that it was: till we have better
intelligence, let our D. Gilbert and Nicholas [3] Cabeus the Jesuite, that have both written great volumes of this subject,
satisfie these inquisitors. Whether the sea be open and navigable by the pole arctick, and which is the likeliest way, that of
Bartison the Hollander, under the pole itself, which for some
reasons I hold best; or by *fretum* Davies, or Nova Zembla.
Whether [4] Hudsons discovery be true of a new found ocean,
any likelihood of Buttons bay in 50 degrees, Hubberds hope
in 60; that of *ut ultra* near Sir Thomas Roes welcome in
north-west Fox, being that the sea ebbs and flows constantly
there 15 foot in 12 hours; as our [5] new cards inform us
that California is not a cape, but an iland, and the west-
windes make the nepe tides equall to the spring, or that there
be any probability to pass by the straights of Anian to China,
by the promontory of Tabin. If there be, I shall soon perceive whether [6] Marcus Polus the Venetians narration be true
or false, of that great city of Quinsay and Cambalu; whether
there be any such places, or that, as [7] Matth. Riccius the Jesuite
hath written, China and Cataia be all one, the great Cham
of Tartary and the king of China be the same: Xuntain
and Quinsay, and the city of Cambalu be that new Paquin,
or such a wall 400 leagues long to part China from Tartary;

---

[1] Mons. Sloto. Some call it the highest hill in the world, next Teneriffe in the
Canaries, Lat. 81.   [2] Cap. 26. in his Treatise of magneticke bodies.   [3] Lege
lib. 1. cap. 23. et 24. de magneticâ philosophiâ, et lib. 3. cap. 4.   [4] 1612.
[5] M. Brigs, his Map, and Northwest Fox.   [6] Lib. 2. ca. 64. de nob. civitat.
Quinsay, et cap. 10. de Cambalu.   [7] Lib. 4. exped. ad Sinas, ca. 3. et lib. 5.
c. 16.

whether [1] Presbyter John be in Asia or Africk; M. Polus Venetus puts him in Asia; [2] the most received opinion is, that he is emperour of the Abissines, which of old was Æthiopia, now Nubia, under the Æquator in Africk. Whether [3] Guinea be an iland or part of the continent, or that hungry [4] Spaniards discovery of Terra Australis Incognita, or Magellanica, be as true as that of Mercurius Britannicus, or his of Utopia, or his of Lucinia. And yet in likelihood it may be so; for, without all question, it being extended from the tropick of Capricorn to the circle Antarctick, and lying as it doth in the temperate Zone, cannot chuse but yeeld in time some flourishing kingdomes to succeding ages, as America did unto the Spaniards. Shouten and Le Meir have done well in the discovery of the streights of Magellan, in finding a more convenient passage to *Mare Pacificum:* me thinks some of our modern Argonautes should prosequute the rest. As I go by Madagascar, I would see that great bird [5] Rucke, that can carry a man and horse or an elephant, with that Arabian Phœnix described by [6] Adrichomius; see the pellicanes of Ægypt, those Scythian gryphes in Asia: and afterwards in Africk examine the fountains of Nilus, whether Herodotus, [7] Seneca, Plin. *lib.* 5. *cap.* 9. Strabo, *lib.* 5. give a true cause of his annuall flowing, [8] Pagaphetta discourse rightly of it, or of Niger and Senega: examine Cardan, [9] Scaligers reasons, and the rest. Is it from those Etesian winds, or melting of snow in the mountains under the Æquator, (for Jordan yearly overflows when the snow melts in mount Libanus) or from those great dropping perpetual showres, which are so frequent to the inhabitants within the tropicks, when the sun is verticall, and cause such vast inundations in Senega, Maragnan, Orenoque, and the rest of those great rivers in *Zona Torrida,* which have all commonly the same passions at set times; and by good husbandry and policy, hereafter no doubt may come to be as populous, as well tilled, as fruitfull as Ægypt it self, or Cauchinchina? I would observe all those motions of the sea, and from what cause they proceed; from the moon (as the vulgar hold) or earths motion, which Galileus, in the fourth dialogue of his systeme of the world, so eagerly proves, and firmly demonstrates; or winds, as [10] some will. Why in that quiet ocean of Zur, *in mari pacifico,* it is

---

[1] M. Polus, in Asiâ, Presb. Joh. meminit. lib. 2. cap. 30. [2] Alluaresius et alii. [3] Lat. 10. gr. Aust. [4] Ferdinando de Quir. anno 1612. [5] Alarum pennæ continent in longitudine 12 passus: elephantem in sublime tollere potest. Polus, l. 3. c. 40. [6] Lib. 2. Descript. terræ sanctæ. [7] Natur. quæst. lib. 4. cap. 2. [8] Lib. de reg. Congo. [9] Exercit. 47. [10] See M. Carpenters Geography, lib. 2. cap. 6. et Bern. Telesius, lib. de mari.

490   *Cure of Melancholy.*   [Part. 2. Sec. 2.

scarce perceived, in our British seas most violent, in the Mediterranean and Red Sea so vehement and irregular, and diverse? Why the current in that Atlantick ocean should still be in some places from, in some again towards the north, and why they come sooner than go : and so from Moabar to Madagascar in that Indian ocean, the merchants come in three weeks, as [1] Scaliger discusseth, they return scarce in three moneths, with the same or like windes : the continuall current is from east to west. Whether Mount Athos, Pelion, Olympus, Ossa, Caucasus, Atlas, be so high as Pliny, Solinus, Mela relate, above clouds, meteors, *ubi nec auræ nec venti spirant*, (insomuch that they that ascend dy suddenly very often, the aire is so subtile) 1250 paces high, according to that measure of Dicæarchus, or 78 miles perpendicularly high, as Jacobus Mazonius, *sec. 3. et 4.* expounding that place of Aristotle about Mount Caucasus; and as [2] Blancanus the Jesuite contends out of Clavius and Nonius demonstrations *de Crepusculis :* or rather 32 stadiums, as the most received opinion is; or 4 miles, which the height of no mountain doth perpendicularly exceed, and is equal to the greatest depths of the sea, which is, as Scaliger holds, 1580 paces (*Exer.* 38), others 100 paces. I would see those inner parts of America, whether there be any such great city of Mannoa or Eldorado in that golden empire, where the high ways are as much beaten (one reports) as between Madrit and Valedolit in Spain ; or any such Amazones as he relates, or gigantical Patagones in Chica ; with that miraculous mountain, [3] Ybouyapab, in the northern Brasile, *cujus jugum sternitur in amœnissimam planitiem,* &c. or that of Pariacacca, so high elevated in Peru. [4] The pike of Teneriff how high is it? 79 miles, or 52, as Patricius holds, or 9 as Snellius demonstrates in his Eratosthenes : see that strange [5] Cirknickzerksey lake in Carniola, whose waters gush so fast out of the ground, that they will overtake a swift horseman, and by and by, with as incredible celerity, are supped up: which Lazius and Warnerus make an argument of the Argonautes sayling under ground. And that vast den or hole called [6] Esmellen in Muscovia, *quæ visitur horrendo hiatu,* &c. which, if any thing casually fall in, makes such a roaring noise, that no thunder, or ordnance, or warlike engine, can make the like. Such another is Gilberts

---

[1] Exercit. 52. de maris motu caussæ investigandæ : prima reciprocationis, secunda varietatis, tertia celeritatis, quarta cessationis, quinta privationis, sexta contrarietatis.   [2] Lib. de explicatione locorum Mathem. Aristot.   [3] Laët. lib. 17. cap. 18. descrip. occid. Ind.   [4] Patritius saith 52 miles in heighth. [5] Luge alii vocant. Geor. Wernerus. Aquæ tantâ celeritate erumpunt et absorbentur, ut expedito equiti aditum intercludant.   [6] Boissardus, de Magis, cap. de Pilapiis.

8

Mem. 3.]   *Digression of Ayre.*   491

cave in Lapland, with many the like. I would examine the
Caspian sea, and see where and how it exonerates it self, after
it hath taken in Volga, Iaxares, Oxus, and those great rivers ;
at the mouth of Oby, or where ? What vent the Mexican lake
hath, the Titicacan in Peru, or that circular pool in the vale
of Terapeia, (of which Acosta, *l. 3. c.* 16) hot in a cold country, the spring of which boils up in the middle twenty foot
square, and hath no vent but exhalation : and that of *Mare
mortuum* in Palestina, of Thrasumene, at Perusium in Italy :
the Mediterranean it self : for, from the ocean, at the straights
of Gibraltar, there is a perpetuall current into the Levant, and
so likewise by the Thracian Bosphorus out of the Euxine or
Black sea, besides all those great rivers of Nilus, Padus, Rhodanus, &c. : how is this water consumed ? by the sun, or otherwise ? I would find out, with Trajan, the fountains of Danubius, of Ganges, Oxus, see those Egyptian pyramids, Trajans
bridge, Grotta de Sibyllâ, Lucullus fish-ponds, the temple of
Nidrose, &c. and, if I could, observe what becomes of swallowes, storkes, cranes, cuckowes, nightingales, redstarts, and
many other kinde of singing birds, water-fowls, hawks, &c.
some of them are onely seen in summer, some in winter ;
some are observed in the [1] snow, and at no other times : each
have their seasons. In winter, not a bird is in Muscovie to be
found ; but, at the spring, in an instant the woods and
hedges are full of them, saith [2] Herbastein : how comes it to
pass ? do they sleep in winter, like Gesners Alpine mice ? or
do they lye hid (as [3] Olaus affirmes) *in the bottome of lakes
and rivers,* spiritum continentes ? *often so found by fisher-
men in Poland and Scandia, two together, mouth to mouth,
wing to wing ; and, when the spring comes, they revive
again, or if they be brought into a stove, or to the fire side.*
Or do they follow the sun, as Peter Martyr (*legat. Baby-
lonica, l.* 2) manifestly convicts, out of his own knowledge ?
for, when he was embassadour in Egypt, he saw swallowes,
Spanish kites, [4] and many other such European birds, in De-
cember and January very familiarly flying, and in great abundance, about Alexandria, *ubi floridæ tunc arbores ac viridaria,*
or lye they hid in caves, rocks, and hollow trees, as most think,
in deep tin-mines or sea-cliffes, as [5] Mr Carew gives out ? I con-

---

[1] In campis Lovicen. solum visuntur in nive ; et ubinam vere, æstate, autumno
se occultant ? Hermes, Polit. l. 1. Jul. Bellius.   [2] Statim ineunte vere
sylvæ strepunt eorum cantilenis. Muscovit. comment   [3] Immergunt se
fluminibus, lacubusque per hyemem totam, &c.   [4] Cæterasque volucres
Pontum hyeme adveniente e nostris regionibus Europæis transvolantes.   [5] Survey of Cornwall.

492   *Cure of Melancholy.*   [Part. 2. Sec. 2.

clude of them all, for my part, as [1] Munster doth of cranes and storks: whence they come, whither they goe, *incompertum adhuc*, as yet we know not. We see them here, some in summer, some in winter: *their coming and going is sure in the night: in the plains of Asia* (saith he) *the storkes meet on such a set day, he that comes last is torn in pieces ; and so they get them gon.* Many strange places, Isthmi, Euripi, Chersonnesi, creekes, havens, promontories, straights, lakes, bathes, rocks, mountaines, places, and fields, where cities have bin ruined or swallowed, battels fought, creatures, sea-monsters, remora, &c. minerals, vegetals. Zoöphites were fit to be considered in such an expedition, and, amongst the rest, that of [2] Herbastein his Tartar lambe, [3] Hector Boëthius goos-bearing tree in the Orchades, to which Cardan (*lib.* 7. *cap.* 36. *de rerum varietat.*) subscribes: [4] Vertomannus wonderfull palme, that [5] fly in Hispaniola, that shines like a torch in the night, that one may well see to write; those sphericall stones in Cuba which nature hath so made, and those like birds, beasts, fishes, crowns, swords, saws, pots, &c. usually found in the metall mines in Saxony about Mansfield, and in Poland neer Nokow and Pallukie, as [6] Munster and others relate. Many rare creatures and novelties each part of the world affords: amongst the rest I would know for a certain whether there be any such men, as Leo Suavius in his comment on Paracelsus *de sanit. tuend.* and [7] Gaguinus records in his description of Muscovie, *that, in Lucomoria, a province in Russia, lye fast asleep as dead all winter, from the* 27 *November, like frogges and swallowes, benumbed with cold, but about the* 24 *of April in the spring they revive again, and goe about their business.* I would examine that demonstration of Alexander Picolomineus, whether the earths superficies be bigger than the seas; or that of Archimedes be true, the superficies of all water is even. Search the depth and see that variety of sea-monsters and fishes, mare-maids, sea-men, horses,

---

[1] Porro ciconiæ quonam e loco veniant, quo se conferant, incompertum adhuc ; agmen venientium, descendentium, ut gruum, venisse cernimus, nocturnis opinor temporibus. In patentibus Asiæ campis certo die congregant se, eam quæ novissime advenit lacerant, inde avolant. Cosmog. l. 4. c. 126.   [2] Comment. Muscov.   [3] Hist. Scot. l. 1.   [4] Vertomannus, l. 5. c. 16. mentioneth a tree that bears fruits to eat, wood to burn, bark to make ropes, wine and water to drink, oyl and sugar, and leaves as tiles to cover houses, flowers for clothes, &c.   [5] Animal insectum Cusino, ut quis legere vel scribere possit sine alterius ope luminis.   [6] Cosmog. lib. 1. cap. 435. et lib. 3. cap. 1. Habent ollas a naturâ formatas, e terrâ extractas, similes illis a figulis factis, coronas, pisces, aves, et omnes animantium species.   [7] Ut solent hirundines et ranæ præ frigoris magnitudine mori, et postea, redeunte vere, 24 Aprilis reviviscere.

Mem. 3.] *Digression of Ayre.* 493

&c. which it affords. Or whether that be true which Jordanus Brunus scoffes at, that, if God did not detain it, the sea would overflow the earth by reason of his higher site, and which Josephus Blancanus the Jesuite, in his interpretation on those mathematicall places of Aristotle, foolishly feares, and in a just tract proves by many circumstances, that in time the sea will waste away the land, and all the globe of the earth shall be covered with waters; *risum teneatis, amici?* what the sea takes away in one place, it addes in another. Mee thinks he might rather suspect the sea should in time be filled by land, trees grow up, carcasses, &c. that all-devouring fire, *omnia devorans et consumens*, will sooner cover and dry up the vast ocean with sands and ashes. I would examine the true seat of that terrestriall [1] Paradise, and where Ophir was, whence Solomon did fetch his gold; from Peruana, which some suppose, or that Aurea Chersonnesus, as Dominicus Niger, Arias Montanus, Goropius, and others, will. I would censure all Plinies, Solinus, Strabos, Sr John Mandevils, Olaus Magnus, Marcus Polus lyes, correct those errors in navigation, reforme cosmographicall chartes, and rectifie longitudes, if it were possible; not by the compass, as some dream, with Mark Ridley in his treatise of magneticall bodies, *cap.* 43: for, as Cabeus (*magnet. philos. lib. 3. cap.* 4.) fully resolves, there is no hope thence; yet I would observe some better meanes to find them out.

I would have a convenient place to go down with Orpheus, Ulysses, Hercules, [2] Lucians Menippus, at St. Patricks purgatory, at Trophonius den, Hecla in Island, Ætna in Sicily, to descend and see what is done in the bowels of the earth; do stones and metalls grow there still? how come firre trees to be [3] digged out from tops of hills, as in our mosses and marishes all over Europe? How come they to dig up fish bones, shells, beams, iron-works, many fathomes under ground, and anchors in mountains, far remote from all seas? [4] Anno 1460, at Berna in Switzerland, 50 fathom deep, a ship was dig'd out of a mountain, where they got metall ore, in which were 48 carcasses of men, with other merchandise. That such things are ordinarily found in tops of hils, Aristotle insinuates in his meteors, [5] Pomponius Mela in his first book, *c. de Numidiâ;* and familiarly in the Alpes, saith [6] Blancanus the Jesuite, the like is to be seen. Came this from earth-quakes, or from Noahs floud, as Christians suppose? or is there a

---

[1] Vid. Pererium, in Gen. Cor. a Lapide, et alios.   [2] In Necyomantiâ, Tom. 2.   [3] Fracastorius, lib. de simp. Georgius Merula, lib. de mem. Julius Billius, &c.   [4] Simlerus, Ortelius. Brachiis centum sub terrâ reperta est, in quâ quadraginta octo cadavera inerant, anchoræ, &c.   [5] Pisces et conchæ in montibus reperiuntur.   [6] Lib. de locis Mathemat. Aristot.

494   *Cure of Melancholy.*   [Part. 2. Sec. 2.

vicissitude of sea and land? as Anaximenes held of old, the
mountaines of Thessaly would become seas, and seas again
mountaines. The whole world, belike, should be new moulded,
when it seemed good to those all-commanding powers, and
turned inside out, as we do hay-cocks in harvest, top to bottom, or bottom to top; or, as we turn apples to the fire, move
the world upon his center; that which is under the Poles
now, should be translated to the Æquinoctiall, and that which
is under the torrid zone, to the circle Arctique and Antarctique another while, and so be reciprocally warmed by the
sun; or if the worlds be infinite, and every fixed star a sun,
with his compassing planets (as Brunus and Campanella conclude), cast three or four worlds into one; or else of one old
world make three or four new, as it shall seem to them best.
To proceed, if the earth be 21500 miles in [1] compass, its diameter is 7000 from us to our antipodes; and what shall be
comprehended in all that space? What is the center of the
earth? is it pure element onely, as Aristotle decrees, inhabited (as [2] Paracelsus thinks) with creatures, whose chaos is
the earth: or with fairies, as the woods and waters (according
to him) are with nymphes, or as the aire with spirits? Diony-
siodorus, a mathematician in [3] Pliny, that sent a letter *ad
superos* after he was dead, from the center of the earth, to signifie what distance the same center was from the *superficies* of
the same, viz. 42000 *stadiums*, might have done well to have
satisfied all these doubts. Or is it the place of hell, as Virgil
in his Æneïdes, Plato, Lucian, Dante, and others, poetically
describe it, and as many of our divines think? In good earnest,
Anthony Rusca, one of the society of that Ambrosian college
in Millan, in his great volume *de Inferno, lib.* 1. *cap.* 47, is
stiffe in this tenent: 'tis a corporeall fire tow, *cap.* 5. *l.* 2. as
he there disputes. *Whatsoever philosophers write,* (saith
'Surius) *there be certain mouthes of hell, and places appointed
for the punishment of mens souls, as at Hecla in Island,
where the ghosts of dead men are familiarly seen, and sometimes talk with the living. God would have such visible
places, that mortal men might be certainly informed, that
there be such punishments after death, and learn hence to
fear God.* Kranzius (*Dan. hist. lib.* 2. *cap.* 24) subscribes
to this opinion of Surius; so doth Colerus, *cap.* 12. *lib. de
immortal. animæ,* (out of the authority, belike, of S[t]. Gregory,

---

[1] Or plain, as Patricius holds, which Austin, Lactantius, and some others, held
of old, as round as a trencher.   [2] Lib. de Zilphia et Pygmæis. They penetrate
the earth, as we do the aire.   [3] Lib. 2. c. 112.   [4] Commentar. ad annum
1537.   Quidquid dicunt philosophi, quædam sunt Tartari ostia, et loca puniendis
animis destinata, ut Hecla mons, &c. ubi mortuorum spiritus visuntur, &c. voluit
Deus exstare talia loca, ut discant mortales.

Durand, and the rest of the schoolmen, who derive as much from Ætna in Sicily, Lipara, Hiera, and those sulphureous Vulcanian islands) making Terra del Fuego, and those frequent vulcanes in America, of which Acosta, *lib. 3. cap. 24.* that fearfull mount Hecklebirg in Norway, an especiall argument to prove it, [1] *where lamentable screeches and howlings are continually heard, which strike a terrour to the auditors: fiery chariots are commonly seen to bring in the souls of men in the likeness of crows, and divels ordinarily goe in and out.* Such another proofe is that place neer the pyramids in Egypt, by Cairo, as well to confirm this as the resurrection, mentioned by [2] Kornmannus, *mirac. mort. lib. 1. cap. 38.* Camerarius *oper. suc. cap. 37.* Bredenbachius, *pereg. ter. sanct.* and some others, *where once a yeere dead bodies arise about March, and walk, and after a while hide themselves again: thousands of people come yearly to see them.* But these and such like testimonies others reject, as fables, illusions of spirits; and they will have no such locall known place, more than Styx or Phlegeton, Plutos court, or that poeticall *infernus*, where Homers soul was seen hanging on a tree, &c. to which they ferried over in Charons boat, or went down at Hermione in Greece, *compendiaria ad inferos via*, which is the shortest cut *quia nullum a mortuis naulum eo loci exposcunt*, (saith [3] Gerbelius) and besides there were no fees to be paid. Well then, is it hell, or purgatory, as Bellarmine; or *Limbus patrum*, as Gallucius will, and as Rusca will (for they have made maps of it), [4] or Ignatius parler? Virgil, sometimes bishop of Saltburg (as Aventinus, anno 745, relates) by Bonifacius bishop of Mentz was therefore called in question, because he held *antipodes* (which they made a doubt whether Christ died for), and so by that means took away the seat of hell, or so contracted it, that it could bear no proportion to heaven, and contradicted that opinion of Austin, Basil, Lactantius, that held the earth round as a trencher (whom Acosta and common experience more largely confute), but not as a ball; and Jerusalem, where Christ died, the middle of it ; or Delos, as the fabulous Greeks fained ; because, when Jupiter let two eagles loose, to fly from the worlds ends east and west, they met at Delos. But that scruple of Bonifacius is now quite taken away by our latter divines : Franciscus Ribera (*in cap. 14. Apocalyps.*) will have hell a materiall and locall fire in the center of the earth, 200 Italian miles in diameter, as he defines it out of those words *Exivit sanguis de terrâ* . . . . . . *per stadia mille*

---

[1] Ubi miserabiles ejulantium voces audiuntur, quæ auditoribus horrorem incutiunt haud vulgarem, &c. [2] Ex sepulcris apparent mense Martio, et rursus sub terram se abscondunt, &c. [3] Descript. Græc. lib. 6. de Pelop. [4] Conclave Ignatii.

496   *Cure of Melancholy.*   [Part. 2. Sec. 2.

sexcenta, &c. But Lessius (*lib.* 13. *de moribus divinis, cap.* 24)
will have this locall hell far less, one Dutch mile in diameter, all filled with fire and brimstone; because, as he there
demonstrates, that space, cubically multiplied, will make a
sphere able to hold eight hundred thousand millions of damned
bodies (allowing each body six foot square); which will
abundantly suffice, *cum certum sit, inquit, factâ subductione,
non futuros centies mille milliones damnandorum.* But, if it
be no materiall fire (as Sco-Thomas, Bonaventure, Soncinas,
Vossius, and others argue) it may be there or elsewhere, as
Keckerman disputes, *System. Theol.* for sure somewhere it
is: *certum est alicubi, etsi definitus circulus non assignetur.*
I will end the controversie in [1] Austins words, *better doubt of
things concealed, than to contend about uncertainties: where
Abrahams bosome is, and hell fire,* [2] *vix a mansuetis, a con-
tentiosis nunquam, invenitur;* scarce the meek, the contentious shall never finde. If it be solid earth, 'tis the fountain of
metals, waters, which by his innate temper turns aire into
water, which springs up in several chinks, to moisten the
earths *superficies,* and that in a tenfold proportion (as Aristotle
holds); or else these fountains come directly from the sea, by
[3] secret passages, and so made fresh again, by running through
the bowels of the earth; and are either thick, thin, hot, cold,
as the matter or minerals are by which they pass; or, as Peter
Martyr (*Ocean. Decad. lib.* 9) and some others hold, from
[4] abundance of rain that fals, or from that ambient heat and
cold, which alters that inward heat, and so *per consequens* the
generation of waters. Or else it may be full of winde, or sulphureous innate fire, as our meteorologists enform us, which,
sometimes breaking out, causeth those horrible earth-quakes,
which are so frequent in these dayes in Japan, China, and
oftentimes swallow up whole cities. Let Lucians Menippus
consult with or aske of Tiresias, if you will not beleeve philosophers: he shall cleare all your doubts when he makes a
second voiage.

In the mean time let us consider of that which is *sub dio,*
and finde out a true cause, if it be possible, of such accidents,
meteors, alterations, as happen above the ground. Whence
proceed that variety of manners, and a distinct character (as
it were) to severall nations? Some are wise, subtil, witty; others
dull, sad, and heavy; some big, some little, as Tully *de Fato,*

---

[1] Melius dubitare de occultis, quam litigare de incertis, ubi flamma inferni, &c.
[2] See Dr. Raynolds prælect. 55. in Apoc.   [3] As they come from the sea, so
they return to the sea again by secret passages, as in all likelihood the Caspian
sea vents itself into the Euxine or Ocean.   [4] Seneca, quæst. lib. cap. 3, 4, 5,
6, 7, 8, 9, 10, 11, 12. de caussis aquarum perpetuis.

Mem. 3.] *Digression of Ayre.* 497

Plato in Timæo, Vegetius, and Bodine proves at large, *method. cap.* 5; some soft, and some hardy, barbarous, civill, black, dun, white: is it from the aire, from the soyle, influence of stars, or some other secret cause? Why doth Africa breed so many venemous beasts, Ireland none? Athens owles, Creet none? [1] Why hath Daulis and Thebes no swallowes (so Pausanias informeth us) as well as the rest of Greece? [2] Ithaca no hares, Pontus asses, Scythia swine? whence come this variety of complections, colours, plants, birds, beasts, [3] metals, peculiar almost to every place? Why so many thousand strange birds and beasts proper to America alone, as Acosta demands, *lib.* 4. *cap.* 36? were they created in the six dayes, or ever in Noahs Arke? if there, why are they not dispersed and found in other countries? It is a thing (saith he) hath long held me in suspence; no Greek, Latine, Hebrew, ever heard of them before, and yet as differing from our European animals, as an egg and a chesnut: and, which is more, kine, horses, sheep, &c. till the Spaniards brought them, were never heard of in those parts. How comes it to pass, that, in the same site, in one latitude, to such as are *periœci*, there should be such difference of soyle, complexion, colour, metall, aire, &c. The Spaniards are white, and so are Italians, when as the inhabitants about [4] *Caput bonæ Spei* are blackemores, and yet both alike distant from the æquator: nay, they that dwell in the same parallel line with these Negros, as about the straights of Magellan, are white coloured, and yet some in Presbyter Johns country in Æthiopia are dun; they in Zeilan and Malabar, parallel with them, again black: Manamotapa in Africk, and St. Thomas isle are extreme hot, both under the line, cole black their inhabitants, whereas in Peru they are quite opposite in colour, very temperate, or rather cold, and yet both alike elevated. Mosco, in 53 degrees of latitude, extreme cold, as those northern countries usually are, having one perpetuall hard frost all winter long: and in 52 deg. lat. sometimes hard frost and snow all summer, as in Buttons bay, &c. or by fits; and yet [5] England neere the same latitude, and Ire-

---

[1] In iis nec pullos hirundines excludunt, neque, &c. [2] Th. Ravennas, lib. de vit. hom. prorog. ca. ult. [3] At Quito in Peru, plus auri quam terræ foditur in aurifodinis. [4] Ad Caput bonæ Spei incolæ sunt nigerrimi. Si sol caussa, cur non Hispani et Itali æque nigri, in eâdem latitudine, æque distantes ab Æquatore, hi ad Austrum, illi ad Boream? qui sub Presbytero Johan habitant, subfusci sunt, in Zeilan et Malabar nigri, æque distantes ab Æquatore, eodemque cœli parallelo: sed hoc magis mirari quis possit, in totâ Americâ nusquam nigros inveniri, præter paucos in loco Quareno illis dicto: quæ hujus coloris caussa efficiens, cœlive an terræ qualitas, an soli proprietas, aut ipsorum hominum innata ratio, aut omnia? Ortelius, in Africâ, Theat. [5] Regio quocunque anni tempore temperatissima. Ortel. Multas Galliæ et Italiæ regiones, molli tepore, et benignâ quâdam temperie, prorsus antecellit Jovius.

VOL. I. K K

498 *Cure of Melancholy.* [Part. 2. Sec. 2.

land, very moist, warme, and more temperate in winter than Spain, Italy, or France. Is it the sea that causeth this difference, and the aire that comes from it? Why then is [1] Ister so cold neere the Euxine, Pontus, Bithynia, and all Thrace? *frigidas regiones* Maginus calls them; and yet their latitude is but 42, which should be hot. [2] Quevira, or Nova Albion in America, bordering on the sea, was so cold in July, that our [3] Englishmen could hardly endure it. At Noremberga, in 45 lat. all the sea is frozen ice, and yet in a more southern latitude than ours. New England, and the island of Cambriall Colchos, which that noble gentleman M[r]. Vaughan, or Orpheus Junior, describes in his Golden Fleece, is in the same latitude with little Britaine in France; and yet their winter begins not till January, their spring till May; which search he accounts worthy of an astrologer: is this from the easterly winds, or melting of ice and snow dissolved within the circle arctick; or that the aire, being thick, is longer before it be warm by the sun beams, and, once heated, like an oven, will keep it self from cold? Our climes breed lice: [4] Hungary and Ireland *male audiunt* in this kinde; come to the Azores, by a secret vertue of that aire they are instantly consumed, and all our European vermine almost, saith Ortelius. Egypt is watred with Nilus not far from the sea; and yet there it seldome or never raines: Rhodes, an iland of the same nature, yeelds not a cloud; and yet our iland's ever dropping and inclining to rain. The Atlantick ocean is still subject to storms, but in Del Zur, or *Mari pacifico*, seldome or never any. Is it from topick stars, *apertio portarum*, in the dodecatemories or constellations, the moons mansions, such aspects of planets, such winds, or dissolving ayre, or thick ayre, which causeth this and the like differences of heat and cold? Bodin relates of a Portugal embassadour, that, coming from [5] Lisbon to [6] Dantzick in Spruce, found greater heat there than at any time at home. Don Garcia de Sylva, legat to Philip 3 king of Spain, residing at Spahan in Persia, 1619, in his letter to the marquess of Bedmar, makes mention of greater cold in Spahan, whose lat. is 31 gr. than ever he felt in Spain, or any part of Europe. The torrid zone was by our predecessors held to be uninhabitable, but by our modern travelers found to be most temperate, bedewed with frequent rains, and moistening showers; the brise and cooling blasts in some parts, as [7] Acosta describes, most pleasant and fertile. Arica in Chili is by report one of the sweetest places that ever the sun shined on, *Olympus terræ*, an heaven on earth:

---

[1] Lat. 45 Danubii.　　　[2] Quevira, lat. 40.　　　[3] In Sir Fra. Drakes voiage.
[4] Lansius, orat. contra Hungaros.　　　[5] Lisbon, lat. 38.　　　[6] Dantzick, lat. 54.
[7] De nat. novi orbis, lib. 1. cap. 9. Suavissimus omnium locus, &c.

Mem. 3.] *Digression of Ayre.* 499

how incomparably do some extoll Mexico in Nova Hispania, Peru, Brasile, &c.? in some again hard, dry, sandy, barren, a very desert, and still in the same latitude. Many times we finde great diversity of aire in the same [1] country, by reason of the site to seas, hills, or dales, want of water, nature of soil, and the like; as, in Spain Arragan is *aspera et sicca*, harsh and evill inhabited; Estramadura is dry, sandy, barren most part, extreme hot by reason of his plains; Andaluzia another paradise, Valence a most pleasant aire, and continually green; so is it about [2] Granado, on the one side fertile plains, on the other, continuall snow to be seen all summer long on the hill tops. That their houses in the Alpes are three quarters of the yeer covered with snow, who knows not? That Tenariffa is so cold at the top, extreme hot at the bottome: Mons Atlas in Africk, Libanus in Palæstina, with many such, *tantos inter ardores fidos nivibus*, [3] Tacitus calls them, and Radzivilius (*epist. 2. fol. 27*) yeelds it to be far hotter there than in any part of Italy : 'tis true ; but they are highly elevated, near the middle region, and therefore cold, *ob paucam solarium radiorum refractionem*, as Serrarius answers, *com. in 3. cap. Josua, quæst. 5.* Abulensis, *quæst. 37.* In the heat of summer, in the kings palace in Escuriall, the aire is most temperate, by reason of a cold blast which comes from the snowie mountains of Sierra de Cadarama hard by, when as in Toledo it is very hot: so in all other countries. The causes of these alterations are commonly by reason of their neerness (I say) to the middle region : but this diversity of aire, in places equally site elevated, and distant from the pole, can hardly be satisfied with that diversity of plants, birds, beasts, which is so familiar with us. With Indians, every where, the sun is equally distant, the same verticall stars, the same irradiations of planets, aspects alike, the same neerness of seas, the same superficies, the same soyl, or not much different. Under the Æquator it self, amongst the Sierras, Andes, Lanes, as Herrera, Laët. and [4] Acosta contend, there is *tam mirabilis et inopinata varietas*, such variety of weather, *ut merito exerceat ingenia*, that no philosophy can yet finde out the true cause of it. When I consider how temperate it is in one place, saith [5] Acosta, within the tropick of Capricorn, as about La-Plate, and yet hard by at Potosa, in that same altitude, mountainous alike, extreme cold; extreme hot in Brasile, &c. *hîc ego*, saith Acosta, *philosophiam Aristotelis meteorologicam vehementer irrisi, cum, &c.* when the sun comes neerest to

---

[1] The same variety of weather Lod. Guicciardine observes betwixt Liege and Aix not far distant. Descript. Belg.   [2] Magin. Quadus.   [3] Hist. lib. 5. [4] Lib. 11. cap. 7.   [5] Lib. 2. cap. 9. Cur Potosa et Plata, urbes in tam tenui intervallo, utraque montosa, &c.

500   *Cure of Melancholy.*   [Part. 2. Sec. 2.

them, they have great tempests, storms, thunder and lightning, great store of rain, snow, and the foulest weather; when the sun is verticall, their rivers over-flow, the morning fair and hot, noon day cold and moist: all which is opposite to us. How comes it to pass? Scaliger (*poëtices l. 3. c.* 16) discourseth thus of this subject. How comes, or wherefore is this *temeraria siderum dispositio*, this rash placing of stars, or, as Epicurus will, *fortuita*, or accidentall? Why are some big, some little? why are they so confusedly, unequally site in the heavens, and set so much out of order? In all other things, Nature is equall, proportionable, and constant: there be *justæ dimensiones, et prudens partium dispositio*, as in the fabrick of man, his eyes, ears, nose, face, members are correspondent; *cur non idem cœlo, opere omnium pulcherrimo?* Why are the heavens so irregular, *neque paribus molibus, neque paribus intervallis?* whence is this difference? *Diversos* (he concludes) *efficere locorum Genios*, to make diversity of countries, soils, maners, customs, characters and constitutions among us, *ut quantum vicinia ad charitatem addat, sidera distrahant ad perniciem;* and so by this means *fluvio vel monte distincti sunt dissimiles*, the same places almost shall be distinguished in maners. But this reason is weak, and most unsufficient. The fixed stars are removed, since Ptolomies time, 26 gr. from the first of Aries; and if the earth be immovable, as their site varies, so should countries vary, and divers alterations would follow. But this we perceive not; as, in Tullies time, with us in Britain, *cœlum visu fœdum, et in quo facile generantur nubes, &c.* 'tis so still. Wherefore Bodine (*Theat. nat. lib.* 2) and some others will have all these alterations and effects immediately to proceed from those genii, spirits, angels, which rule and domineer in several places; they cause storms, thunder, lightning, earthquakes, ruins, tempests, great winds, floods, &c. The philosophers of Conimbra will refer this diversity to the influence of that *empyrean* heaven: for some say the *excentricity* of the sun is come neerer to the earth than in Ptolomies time; the vertue therefore of all the vegetals is decayed; [1] men grow less, &c. There are that observe new motions of the heavens, new stars, *palantia sidera*, comets, clouds, (call them what you will) like those Medicean, Burbonian, Austrian planets lately detected, which do not decay, but come and go, rise higher and lower, hide and shew themselves amongst the fixed stars, amongst the planets, above and beneath the moon, at set times, now neerer, now farther off, together, asunder; as he that plaies upon a sagbut, by pulling it up and down, alters

---

[1] Terra malos homines nunc educat, atque pusillos.

Mem. 3.] *Digression of Ayre.* 501

his tones and tunes, do they their stations and places, though
to us undiscerned; and from those motions proceed (as they
conceive) divers alterations. Clavius conjectures otherwise:
but they be but conjectures. About Damascus in Cœle-Syria
is a [1] paradise, by reason of the plenty of waters; *in promptu
caussa est ;* and the desarts of Arabia barren, because of rockes,
rolling seas of sands, and dry mountaines ; *quod inaquosa,*
(saith Adricomius) *montes habens asperos, saxosos, præcipites,
horroris et mortis speciem præ se ferentes,* uninhabitable therefore of men, birds, beasts, void of all greene trees, plants and
fruits, a vast rocky horrid wilderness, which by no art can be
manured; 'tis evident. Bohemia is cold, for that it lyes all
along to the north. But why should it be so hot in Egypt, or
there never rain ? Why should those [2] Etesian and north-east-
ern winds blow continually and constantly so long together, in
some places, at set times, one way still, in the dog-dayes only:
here perpetual draught, there dropping showres; here foggy
mists, there a pleasant aire; here [3] terrible thunder and lightning
at such set seasons, here frozen seas all the yeare, there open in
the same latitude, to the rest no such thing, nay quite opposite
is to be found ? Sometimes (as in [4] Peru) on the one side of
the mountaines it is hot, on the other cold, here snow, there
winde, with infinite such. Fromundus, in his Meteors, will
excuse or salve all this by the suns motion : but when there is
such diversity to such as *periœci,* or very neare site, how can
that position hold?

Who can give a reason of this diversity of meteors ? that it
should rain [5] stones, frogs, mice, &c. rats, which they call
lemmer in Norway, and are manifestly observed (as [6] Munster
writes) by the inhabitants, to descend and fall with some fæculent showres, and, like so many locusts, consume all that is
green. Leo Afer speaks as much of locusts ; about Fez in Barbary there be infinite swarmes in their fields upon a sudden : so
at Arles in France, 1553, the like happened by the same mischief; all their grass and fruits were devoured ; *magná incolarum admiratione et consternatione* (as Valleriola, *obser. med.
lib.* 1. *obser.* 1. relates) *cœlum subito obumbrabant, &c.* he
concludes, [7] it could not be from natural causes; they cannot
imagine whence they come, but from heaven. Are these and
such creatures, corn, wood, stones, worms, wooll, blood, &c.

---

[1] Nav. l. 1. c. 5.   [2] Strabo.   [3] As under the æquator in many
parts, showres here at such a time, windes at such a time, the brise they call it.
[4] Ferd. Cortesius, lib. Novus orbis inscript.   [5] Lapidatum est. Livie.
[6] Cosmog. lib. 4. ca. 22. Hæ tempestatibus decidunt e nubibus fæculentis, de-
pascunturque more locustarum omnia virentia.   [7] Hort. Genial. An a
terrâ sursum rapiuntur a solo, iterumque cum pluviis præcipitantur ? &c.

502 *Cure of Melancholy.* [Part. 2. Sec. 2.

lifted up into the middle region by the sun beams, as [1] Paracelsus the physician disputes, and thence let fall with showres, or there ingendred? [2] Cornelius Gemma is of that opinion, they are there conceived by celestiall influences : others suppose they are immediately from God, or prodigies raised by art and illusions of spirits, which are princes of the ayre; to whom Bodin (*lib. 2. Theat. Nat.*) subscribes. In fine, of meteors in generall, Aristotles reasons are exploded by Bernardinus Telesius, by Paracelsus, his principles confuted, and other causes assigned, sal, sulphur, mercury, in which his disciples are so expert, that they can alter elements, and separate at their pleasure, make perpetuall motions, not as Cardan, Tasneir, Peregrinus, by some magneticall vertue, but by mixture of elements; imitate thunder, like Salmoneus, snow, hail, the seas ebbing and flowing, give life to creatures (as they say) without generation, and what not? P. Nonius Saluciensis, and Kepler, take upon them to demonstrate that no meteors, cloudes, fogges, [3] vapours, arise higher than 50 or 80 miles, and all the rest to be purer aire or element of fire : which [4] Carden, [5] Tycho, and [6] John Pena manifestly confute by refractions, and many other arguments, there is no such element of fire at all. If, as Tycho proves, the moon be distant from us 50 and 60 semidiameters of the earth : and as Peter Nonius will have it, the aire be so angust, what proportion is there betwixt the other three elements and it? to what use serves it? Is it full of spirits which inhabit it, as the Paracelsians and Platonists hold, the higher the more noble, [7] full of birds, or a meer *vacuum* to no purpose? It is much controverted betwixt Tycho Brahe and Christopher Rotman the Lantsgrave of Hessias mathematician, in their Astronomicall Epistles, whether it be the same *diaphanum*, cleerness, matter of aire and heavens, or two distinct essences? Christopher Rotman, John Pena, Jordanus Brunus, with many other mathematicians, contend it is the same, and one matter throughout, saving that the higher still, the purer it is, and more subtile; as they finde by experience in the top of some hills in [8] America : if a man ascend, he faints instantly for want of thicker ayre to refrigerate the heart. Acosta (*l. 3. c.* 9) calls this mountain Periacaca in Peru : it makes men cast and vomit, he saith, that climb it, as some other of those Andes do in the desarts of Chila for 500 miles together, and, for extre-

---

[1] Tam ominosus proventus in naturales caussas referri vix potest. [2] Cosmog. c. 6. [3] Cardan saith vapours rise 288 miles from the earth, Eratosthenes 48 miles. [4] De subtil. l. 2. [5] In progymnas. [6] Præfat. ad Euclid. Catop. [7] Manucodiatæ, birds that live continually in the ayre, and are never seen on ground but dead. See Ulysses Aldrovand. Ornithol. Scal. exerc. cap. 229. [8] Laët. descrip. Amer.

Mem. 3.] *Digression of Ayre.* 503

mity of cold, to lose their fingers and toes. Tycho will have
two distinct matters of heaven and ayre : but to say truth,
with some small qualification, they have one and the self same
opinion about the essence and matter of heavens ; that it is
not hard and impenetrable, as Peripateticks hold, transparent,
of a *quinta essentia,* [1] *but that it is penetrable and soft as the
ayre it self is, and that the planets move in it, as birds in the
ayre, fishes in the sea.* This they prove by motion of comets,
and otherwise (though Claremontius in his Antitycho stiffly
opposes) which are not generated, as Aristotle teacheth, in the
aeriall region, of an hot and dry exhalation, and so consumed :
but, as Anaxagoras and Democritus held of old, of a celestiall
matter : and as [2] Tycho, [3] Helisæus Rœslin, Thaddeus Haggesius, Pena, Rotman, Fracastorius, demonstrate by their progress, parallaxes, refractions, motions of the planets, (which
enterfeire and cut one anothers orbes, now higher, and then
lower, as ♂, amongst the rest, which sometimes, as [4] Kepler
confirms by his own and Tychos accurate observations, comes
nearer the earth than the ☉, and is again eftsoons aloft in Jupiters orbe) and [5] other sufficient reasons, far above the moon :
exploding in the mean time that element of fire, those fictitious
first watry movers, those heavens I mean above the firmament, which Delrio, Lodovicus Imola, Patricius, and many
of the fathers, affirm ; those monstrous orbes of eccentricks,
and *eccentre epicycles deserentes;* which howsoever Ptolo-
my, Alhasen, Vitellio, Purbachius, Maginus Clavius, and
many of their associates stiffly maintain to be reall orbes, ex-
centrick, concentrick, circles æquant, &c. are absurd and ridiculous. For who is so mad to think, that there should be so
many circles, like subordinate wheels in a clock, all impenetrable and hard, as they fain, adde and substract at their pleasure ?
[6] Maginus makes eleven heavens, subdivided into their orbes and
circles, and all too little to serve those particular appearances :
Fracastorius, 72 homocentricks : Tycho Brahe, Nicholas Ramerus, Helisæus Rœslin, have peculiar hypotheses of their own
inventions ; and they be but inventions, as most of them acknowledge, as we admit of æquators, tropicks, colures, circles, arctique and antarctique, for doctrines sake (though Ra-

---

[1] Epist. lib. 1. p. 83. Ex quibus constat nec diversa aëris et ætheris diaphana
esse, nec refractiones aliunde quam a crasso aëre caussari.—Non dura aut im-
pervia, sed liquida, subtilis, motuique planetarum facile cedens. [2] In Pro-
gymn. lib. 2. exemplis quinque. [3] In Theoriâ novâ Met. cœlestium, 1578.
[4] Epit. Astron. lib. 4. [5] Multa sane hinc consequuntur absurda, et si
nihil aliud, tot cometæ in æthere animadversi, qui nullius orbis ductum comitantur, id ipsum sufficienter refellunt. Tycho, astr. epist. pag. 107. [6] In
Theoricis planetarum, three above the firmament, which all wise men reject.

504   *Cure of Melancholy.*   [Part. 2. Sec. 2.

mus thinks them all unnecessary) they will have them supposed
onely for method and order.   Tycho hath fained I know not
how many subdivisions of epicycles in epicycles, &c. to calculate and express the moons motion; but, when all is done, as a
supposition, and no otherwise; not (as he holds) hard, impenetrable, subtile, transparent, &c. or making musick, as Pythagoras maintained of old, and Robert Constantine of late, but
still quiet, liquid, open, &c.

If the heavens then be penetrable, as these men deliver, and
no lets, it were not amiss, in this aereall progress, to make
wings, and fly up; which that Turk, in Busbequius, made his
fellow-citizens in Constantinople beleeve he would perform,
and some new-fangled wits, methinks, should some time or
other finde out: or if that may not be, yet with a Galilies
glass, or Icaromenippus wings in Lucian, command the
spheres and heavens, and see what is done amongst them: whether there be generation and corruption, as some think, by
reason of æthereall comets, that in Cassiopea 1572, that in
Cygno 1600, that in Sagittarius 1604, and many like, which
by no means Jul. Cæsar la Galla, that Italian philosopher, (in
his physicall disputation with Galileus, *de phænomenis in orbe
Lunæ, cap.* 9) will admit: or that they were created *ab initio*,
and shew themselves at set times; and, as [1] Helisæus Rœslin
contends, have poles, axeltrees, circles of their own, and
regular motions.   For *non pereunt, sed minuuntur et dispa-
rent,* [2] Blancanus holds; they come and go by fits, casting
their tailes still from the sun: some of them, as a burning glass
projects the sun beams from it; though not alwaies neither;
for sometimes a comet casts his taile from Venus, as Tycho observes; and, as [3] Helisæus Rœslin of some others, from the
moon, with little stars about them, *ad stuporem astronomo-
rum; cum multis aliis in cœlo miraculis,* all which argue,
with those Medicean, Austrian, and Burbonian stars, that
the heaven of the planets is indistinct, pure and open, in
which the planets move *certis legibus ac metis.*   Examine
likewise, *an cœlum sit coloratum?*   Whether the stars be of
that bigness, distance, as astronomers relate, so many in
' number, 1026, or 1725, as J. Bayerus; or, as some Rabbins,
29000 myriades; or, as Galilie discovers by his glasses, infinite, and that *via lactea*, a confused light of small stars,
like so many nailes in a door: or all in a row, like those
12000 iles of the Maldives, in the Indie ocean? whether
the least visible star in the eighth sphere be 18 times bigger

---

[1] Theor. nova cœlest. Meteor.   [2] Lib. de fabricâ mundi.   [3] Lib. de
Cometis.   [4] An sit crux et nubecula in cœlis ad Polum Antarcticum, quod
ex Corsalio refert Patritius.

Mem. 3.] *Digression of Ayre.* 505

than the earth ; and, as Tycho calculates, 14000 semidiameters
distant from it ? Whether they be thicker parts of the orbes, as
Aristotle delivers ; or so many habitable worlds, as Democritus?
whether they have light of their own, or from the sun, or
give light round, as Patritius discourseth ? *An æque distent a
centro mundi ?* Whether light be of their essence ; and that
light be a substance or an accident ? whether they be hot by
themselves or by accident cause heat? whether there be such
a precision of the æquinoxes, as Copernicus holds, or that the
eighth sphere move ? *An bene philosophentur R. Bacon, et
J. Dee, Aphorism. de multiplicatione specierum?* Whether
there be any such images ascending with each degree of
the Zodiack in the east, as Aliacensis feignes? *An aqua super
cœlum?* as Patritius and the schoolmen will, a crystalline
[1] watry heaven, which is [2] certainly to be understood of that in
the middle region? for otherwise, if at Noahs floud the water
came from thence, it must be above an hundred yeeres falling
down to us, as [3] some calculate. Besides, *an terra sit animata?* which some so confidently beleeve, with Orpheus,
Hermes, Averroes, from which all other souls of men, beasts,
divels, plants, fishes, &c. are derived, and into which again,
after some revolutions, as Plato in his Timæus, Plotinus in his
Enneades, more largely discusse, they return (See Chalcidius
and Bennius, Platos commentators) as all philosophicall
matter, *in materiam primam.* Keplerus, Patritius, and some
other neotericks have in part revived this opinion : and
that every star in heaven hath a soul, angel, or intelligence
to animate or move it, &c. or to omit all smaller controversies,
as matters of less moment, and examine that main paradox,
of the earths motion, now so much in question : Aristarchus Samius, Pythagoras maintained it of old, Democritus,
and many of their scholars. Didacus Astunica, Anthony Fas-
carinus a Carmelite, and some other commentators, will have
Job to insinuate as much, *cap. 9. ver. 4. Qui commovet
terram de loco suo, &c.* and that this one place of Scripture
makes more for the earths motion, than all the other prove
against it ; whom Pineda confutes, most contradict. Howsoever,
it is revived since by Copernicus, not as a truth, but a supposition, as he confesseth himself in the Preface to Pope Nicholas,
but now maintained in good earnest by [4]Calcagninus, Telesius, Kepler, Rotman, Gilbert, Digges, Galileus, Campanella, and especially by [5] Lansbergius, *naturæ rationi, et*

[1] Gilbertus Origanus.   [2] See this discussed in Sir Walter Raleighs history,
in Zanch. ad Casman.   [3] Vid. Fromundum, de Meteoris, lib. 5. artic. 5. et
Lansbergium.   [4] Peculiari libello.   [5] Comment. in motum terræ
Middlebergi, 1630. 4.

506   *Cure of Melancholy.*   [Part. 2. Sec. 2.

veritati consentaneum, by Origanus, and some [1] others of his
followers.   For, if the earth be the center of the world, stand
still, and the heavens move, as the most received opinion is,
which they call *inordinatam cœli dispositionem,* though stifly
maintained by Tycho, Ptolomæus, and their adherents, *quis
ille furor?* &c. what fury is that, saith [2] Dr. Gilbert, *satis
animose,* as Cabeus notes, that shall drive the heavens
about with such incomprehensible celerity in 24 houres, when
as every point of the firmament, and in the æquator, must
needs move (so [3] Clavius calculates) 176660 in one 246th part
of an houre : and an arrow out of a bow must goe seven times
about the earth, whilest a man can say an *Ave Maria,* if it
keep the same space, or compass the earth 1884 times in an
houre ; which is *supra humanam cogitationem,* beyond human
conceit : *Ocyor et jaculo, et ventos æquante sagittâ.*   A
man could not ride so much ground, going 40 miles. a day,
in 2904 yeeres, as the firmament goes in 24 houres : or so much
in 203 yeeres, as the said firmament in one minute ; *quod incredibile videtur :* and the [4] pole star, which to our thinking
scarce moveth out of his place, goeth a bigger circuit than the
sun, whose diameter is much larger than the diameter of the
heaven of the sun, and 20000 semidiameters of the earth from
us, with the rest of the fixed stars, as Tycho proves.   To avoid
therefore these impossibilities, they ascribe a triple motion to
the earth, the sun immovable in the centre of the whole world,
the earth center of the moon, alone, above ♀ and ☿, beneath
♄, ♃, ♂, (or, as [5] Origanus and others wil, one single motion
to the earth, still placed in the center of the world, which is
more probable) a single motion to the firmament, which moves
in 30 or 26 thousand yeeres ; and so the planets, Saturne in 30
yeeres absolves his sole and proper motion, Jupiter in 12,
Mars in 3, &c. and so salve all apparances better than any way
whatsoever : calculate all motions, be they in *longum* or *latum,*
direct, stationary, retrograde, ascent or descent, without epicycles, intricate, eccentricks, &c. *rectius commodiusque per
unicum motum terræ,* saith Lansbergius, much more certain
than by those Alphonsine, or any such tables, which are
grounded from those other suppositions.   And 'tis true, they
say, according to optick principles, the visible apparances of the
planets do so indeed answer to their magnitudes and orbes, and
come neerest to mathematicall observations, and precedent cal-
culations ; there is no repugnancy to physicall axiomes, because

[1] Peculiari libello.   [2] See M. Carpenters Geogr. cap. 4. lib. 1. Campanella
et Origanus præf. Ephemer. where Scripture places are answered. [3] De Magnete.
Comment. in 2. cap. sphær. Jo. de Sacr. Bosc.   [4] Dist. 3. gr. 1. a Polo.
[5] Præf. Ephem.

Mem. 3.]   *Digression of Ayre.*   **507**

no penetration of orbes: but then, between the sphere of Saturne and the firmament, there is such an incredible and vast
[1] space or distance (7000000 semidiameters of the earth, as Tycho
calculates) void of stars: and besides, they do so inhance the
bigness of the stars, enlarge their circuit, to salve those ordinary objections of parallaxes and retrogradations of the fixed
stars, that alteration of the poles, elevation in severall places or
latitude of cities here on earth (for, say they, if a mans eye were
in the firmament, he should not at all discern that great annuall
motion of the earth, but it would still appear *punctum indivi-
sibile*, and seem to be fixed in one place, of the same bigness)
that it is quite opposite to reason, to naturall philosophy, and
all out as absurd as disproportionall (so some will), as prodigious, as that of the Suns swift motion of heavens. But *hoc
posito*, to grant this their tenent of the earths motion; if the
earth move, it is a planet and shines to them in the moon, and
to the other planetary inhabitants, as the moon and they do to
us upon the earth: but shine she doth, as Galilie, [2] Kepler, and
others prove; and then *per consequens*, the rest of the planets
are inhabited, as well as the moon; which he grants in his dis-
sertation with Galilies Nuncius Sidereus, [3] *that there be Joviall
and Saturnine inhabitants*, &c. and those severall planets have
their severall moons about them, as the earth hath hers, as
Galileus hath already evinced by his glasses; [4] four about Jupiter, two about Saturne (though Sitius the Florentine, For-
tunius Licetus, and Jul. Cæsar le Galla cavill at it): yet Kepler, the emperours mathematician, confirmes out of his experience, that he saw as much by the same help, and more about
Mars, Venus; and the rest they hope to find out, peradventure
even amongst the fixed stars, which Brunus and Brutius
have already averred. Then (I say) the earth and they be
planets alike, inhabited alike, moved about the sun, the common center of the world alike: and it may be, those two green
children, which [5] Nubrigensis speaks of in his time, that fell
from heaven, came from thence; and that famous stone that
fell from heaven, in Aristotles time, olymp. 84, *anno tertio, ad
Capuæ Fluenta*, recorded by Laërtius and others, or Ancile

---

[1] Which may be full of planets, perhaps, to us unseen, as those about Jupiter,
&c.   [2] Luna circumterrestris planeta quum sit, consentaneum est esse in
lunâ viventes creaturas; et singulis planetarum globis sui serviunt circulatores;
ex quâ consideratione de eorum incolis summâ probabilitate concludimus, quod et
Tychoni Braheo, e solâ consideratione vastitatis eorum, visum fuit. Kepl. dissert.
cum nun. sid. f. 29.   [3] Temperare non possum quin ex inventis tuis hoc
moneam, veri non absimile, non tam in Lunâ, sed etiam in Jove, et reliquis pla-
netis incolas esse. Kepl. fo. 26. Si non sint accolæ in Jovis globo, qui notent
admirandam hanc varietatem oculis, cui bono quatuor illi planetæ Jovem circum-
cursitant?   [4] Some of those about Jupiter I have seen myself by the help of
a glass 8 foot long.   [5] Rerum Angl. l. 1. c. 27. de viridibus pueris.

508   *Cure of Melancholy.*   [Part. 2. Sec. 2.

or buckler in Numas time, recorded by Festus. We may
likewise insert with Campanella and Brunus, that which Pythagoras, Aristarchus Samius, Heraclitus, Epicurus, Melissus,
Democritus, Leucippus, maintained in their ages, there be
[1] *infinite worlds*, and infinite earths or systemes, *in infinito
æthere ;* which [2] Eusebius collects out of their tenents, because
infinite stars and planets like unto this of ours, which some
stick not still to maintain and publikely defend; *sperabundus
exspecto innumerabilium mundorum in æternitate perambu-
lationem, &c.* (Nic. Hill Londinensis *philos. Epicur.*) For if
the firmament be of such an incomparable bigness, as these
Copernicall giants will have it, *infinitum, aut infinito proximum,*
so vast and full of innumerable stars, as being infinite in
extent, one above another, some higher, some lower, some
neerer, some farther off, and so far asunder, and those so huge
and great ; insomuch that, if the whole sphere of Saturn, and
all that is included in it, *totum aggregatum* (as Fromundus of
Lovain in his tract *de immobilitate terræ* argues) *evehatur
inter stellas, videri a nobis non poterit, tam immanis est di-
stantia inter tellurem et fixas; sed instar puncti, &c.* If our
world be small in respect, why may we not suppose a plurality
of worlds, those infinite stars visible in the firmament to be so
many suns, with particular fixt centers ; to have likewise their
subordinate planets, as the sun hath his dancing still round
him ? which cardinall Cusanus, Walkarinus, Brunus, and some
others, have held, and some still maintain. *Animæ Aristo-
telismo innutritæ, et minutis speculationibus assuetæ, secus
forsan, &c.* Though they seem close to us, they are infinitely
distant, and so *per consequens,* there are infinite habitable
worlds: what hinders?   Why should not an infinite cause
(as God is) produce infinite effects? as Nic. Hill (*Democrit.
philos.*) disputes : Kepler (I confess) will by no means admit
of Brunus infinite worlds, or that the fixed stars should be so
many suns, with their compassing planets; yet the said [3] Kepler,
betwixt jest and earnest, in his Perspectives, Lunar Geography,
[4] *et Somnio suo, Dissertat. cum nunc. sider.* seems in part to
agree with this, and partly to contradict. For the planets, he
yeelds them to be inhabited ; he doubts of the stars: and so
doth Tycho in his Astronomicall Epistles, out of a consideration
of their vastity and greatness, break out into some such like
speeches, that he will never beleeve those great and huge bodies
were made to no other use than this that we perceive, to illu-

---

[1] Infiniti alii mundi, vel, ut Brunus, terræ, huic nostræ similes.   [2] Libro
cont. philos. cap. 29.   [3] Kepler, fol. 2. dissert. Quid impedit quin credamus
ex his initiis, plures alios mundos detegendos, vel (ut Democrito placuit) infinitos?
[4] Lege somnium Kepleri, edit. 1635.

Mem. 3.] *Digression of Ayre.* 509

minate the earth, a point insensible, in respect of the whole. But who shall dwell in these vast bodies, earths, worlds, [1] *if they be inhabited? rationall creatures?* as Kepler demands; *or have they souls to be saved? or do they inhabit a better part of the world than we do? are we or they lords of the world? and how are all things made for man? Difficile est nodum hunc expedire, eo quod nondum omnia, quæ huc pertinent, explorata habemus;* 'tis hard to determin; this only he proves, that we are in *præcipuo mundi sinu,* in the best place, best world, neerest the heart of the sun. [2] Thomas Campanella, a Calabrian monk, (in his second book *de sensu rerum, cap.* 4) subscribes to this of Keplerus; that they are inhabited he certainly supposeth, but with what kind of creatures, he cannot say; he labours to prove it by all means: and that there are infinite worlds, having made an apologie for Galileus, and dedicates this tenet of his to Cardinall Cajetanus. Others freely speak, mutter, and would perswade the world (as [3] Marinus Marcenus complaines) that our modern divines are too severe and rigid against mathematicians; ignorant and peevish, in not admitting their true demonstrations and certain observations, that they tyrannize over art, science, and all philosophy, in suppressing their labours, (saith Pomponatius) forbidding them to write, to speak a truth, all to maintain their superstition, and for their profits sake. As for those places of Scripture which oppugne it, they will have spoken *ad captum vulgi,* and if rightly understood, and favorably interpreted, not at all against it: and as Otho Casman (*Astrol. cap.* 1. *part.* 1) notes, many great divines, besides Porphyrius, Proclus, Simplicius, and those heathen philosophers, *doctrinâ et ætate venerandi, Mosis Genesin mundanam popularis nescio cujus ruditatis, quæ longe absit a verâ philosophorum eruditione, insimulant:* for Moses makes mention but of two planets, ☉ and ☾. no 4 elements, &c. Reade more in him, in [4] Grossius and Junius. But to proceed, these and such like insolent and bold attempts, prodigious paradoxes, inferences must needs follow, if it once be granted, which Rotman, Kepler, Gilbert, Diggeus, Origanus, Galileus, and others maintain of the earths motion, that 'tis a planet, and shines as the moon doth,

---

[1] Quid igitur inquies, si sint in cœlo plures globi, similes nostræ telluris? an cum illis certabimus, quis meliorem mundi plagam teneat? Si nobiliores illorum globi, nos non sumus creaturarum rationalium nobilissimi: quomodo igitur omnia propter hominem? quomodo nos domini operum Dei? Kepler. fol. 29.   [2] Francofurt. quarto, 1620. ibid. quarto, 1622.   [3] Præfat. in Comment. in Genesin. Modo suadent theologos summâ ignoratione versari, veras scientias admittere nolle, et tyrannidem exercere, ut eos falsis dogmatibus, superstitionibus, et religione catholicâ detineant.   [4] Theat. Biblico.

510   *Cure of Melancholy.*   [Part. 2. Sec. 2.

which containes in it [1] *both land and sea as the moon doth:*
for so they find by their glasses that *maculæ in facie Lunæ,
the brighter parts are earth, the duskie sea,* which Thales,
Plutarch, and Pythagoras, formerly taught; and manifestly
discern hills and dales, and such like concavities, if we may
subscribe to and beleeve Galilies observations. But to avoid
these paradoxes of the earths motion (which the church of
Rome hath lately [2] condemned as hereticall, as appeares by
Blancanus and Fromundus writings), our latter mathematicians
have rolled all the stones that may be stirred; and, to salve all
appearances and objections, have invented new hypotheses,
and fabricated new systems of the world, out of their own
Dædalean heads. Fracastorius will have the earth stand still,
as before; and to avoid that supposition of eccentricks and
epicycles, he has coined 72 homocentricks, to salve all appearances. Nicholas Ramerus will have the earth the center
of the world, but moveable, and the eighth sphere immoveable, the five upper planets to move above the sun, the sun
and moon about the earth. Of which orbes, [3] Tycho Brahe
puts the earth the center immoveable, the stars immoveable,
the rest with Ramerus, the planets without orbes to wander in
the aire, keep time and distance, true motion, according to
that vertue which God hath given them. [4] Helisæus Rœslin
censureth both, with Copernicus (whose hypothesis *de terræ
motu,* Philippus Lansbergius hath lately vindicated, and de-
monstrated with solid arguments in a just volume, Jansonius
Cæsius hath illustrated in a sphere). The said Johannes Lansbergius, 1633, hath since defended his assertion against all the
cavills and calumnies of Fromundus his Anti-Aristarchus, Baptista Morinus, and Petrus Bartholinus: Fromundus, 1634,
hath written against him again, J. Rosseus of Aberdine, &c.
(sound drummes and trumpets) whilest Rœslin (I say) censures
all, and Ptolomæus himself as unsufficient: one offends against
naturall philosophy, another against optick principles, a third
against mathematicall, as not answering to astronomicall observations: one puts a great space betwixt Saturnus orbe and
the eighth sphere, another too narrow. In his own hypothesis
he makes the earth, as before, the universall center, the sun to
the five upper planets: to the eighth sphere he ascribes di-
urnall motion, eccentricks and epicycles to the seven planets,
which hath been formerly exploded; and so,

(Dum vitant stulti vitia, in contraria currunt)

---

[1] His argumentis plane satisfecisti; do maculas in lunâ esse maria; do lucidas
partes esse terram. Kepler. fol. 16.   [2] Anno 1616.   [3] In Hypothes. de
mundo, Edit. 1597.   [4] Lugduni 1633.

8

Mem. 3.] *Digression of Ayre.* 511

as a tinker stops one hole and makes two, he corrects them, and doth worse himself; reformes some, and marres all. In the mean time, the world is tossed in a blanket amongst them; they hoyse the earth up and down like a ball, make it stand and goe at their pleasures. One saith the sun stands; another, he moves: a third comes in, taking them all at rebound; and, lest there should any paradox be wanting, he [1] findes certain spots and cloudes in the sun, by the help of glasses, which multiply (saith Keplerus) a thing seen a thousand times bigger *in plano*, and make it come 32 times nearer to the eye of the beholder: but see the demonstration of this glass in [2] Tarde, by means of which, the sun must turn round upon his own center, or they about the sun. Fabricius puts only three, and those in the sun: Apelles, 15, and those without the sun, floating like the Cyanean isles in the Euxine sea. [3] Tarde the Frenchman hath observed 33, and those neither spots nor clouds, as Galileus (*Epist. ad Velserum*) supposeth, but planets concentrick with the sun, and not far from him, with regular motions. [4] Christopher Schemer a German Suisser Jesuit, Ursica Rosa, divides them *in maculas et faculas*, and will have them to be fixed *in solis superficie*, and to absolve their periodicall and regular motion in 27 or 28 dayes; holding withall the rotation of the sun upon his center: and are all so confident, that they have made skemes and tables of their motions. The [5] Hollander, in his *dissertatiuncula cum Apelle*, censures all; and thus they disagree amongst themselves, old and new, irreconcileable in their opinions; thus Aristarchus, thus Hipparchus, thus Ptolomæus, thus Albateginus, thus Alfraganus, thus Tycho, thus Ramerus, thus Rœslinus, thus Fracastorius, thus Copernicus and his adherents, thus Clavius and Maginus, &c. with their followers, vary and determine of these celestiall orbs and bodies; and so, whilest these men contend about the sun and moon, like the philosophers in Lucian, it is to be feared the sun and moon will hide themselves, and be as much offended as [6] shee was with those, and send another message to Jupiter, by some new fangled Icaromenippus, to make an end of all those curious controversies, and scatter them abroad.

But why should the sun and moon be angry, or take exceptions at mathematicians and philosophers, when as the like measure is offered unto God himself, by a company of theolo-

---

[1] Jo. Fabricius, de maculis in sole, Witeb. 1611.   [2] In Burboniis sideribus.
[3] Lib. de Burboniis sid. Stellæ sunt erraticæ, quæ propriis orbibus feruntur, non longe a sole dissitis, sed juxta solem.   [4] Braccini, fol. 1630. lib. 4. cap. 52, 55, 59, &c.   [5] Lugdun. Bat. An. 1612.   [6] Ne se subducant, et relictâ statione decessum parent, ut curiositatis finem faciant.

512   *Cure of Melancholy.*   [Part. 2. Sec. 2.

gasters? They are not contented to see the sun and moon, measure their site and biggest distance in a glass, calculate their
motions, or visit the moon in a poeticall fiction, or a dream, as
he saith: [1] *audax facinus et memorabile nunc incipiam, neque
hoc sæculo usurpatum prius: quid in Lunæ regno hac nocte
gestum sit, exponam, et quo nemo unquam nisi somniando per-
venit,* but he and Menippus: or as [2] Peter Cuneus, *bonâ fide
agam: nihil eorum, quæ scripturus sum, verum esse scitote,
&c. quæ nec facta, nec futura sunt, dicam,* [3] *styli tantum et
ingenii caussâ:* not in jest, but in good earnest, these gygan-
ticall Cyclopes will transcend spheres, heaven, stars, into that
empyrean heaven; soare higher yet, and see what God himself doth.   The Jewish Thalmudists take upon them to determine how God spends his whole time, sometimes playing with
Leviathan, sometime over-seeing the world, &c. like Lucians
Jupiter, that spent much of the year in painting butter-flies
wings, and seeing who offered sacrifice; telling the houres
when it should rain, how much snow should fall in such a place,
which way the winde should stand in Greece, which way in
Africk.   In the Turks Alcoran, Mahomet is taken up to
heaven, upon a Pegasus sent a purpose for him, as he lay in
bed with his wife, and, after some conference with God, is set
on ground again.   The pagans paint him and mangle him after
a thousand fashions; our hereticks, schismaticks, and some
schoolmen, come not far behind: some paint him in the habit
of an old man, and make maps of heaven, number the angels,
tell their several [4] names, offices: some deny God and his providence; some take his office out of his hand, will [5] binde and
loose in heaven, release, pardon, forgive, and be quarter-master
with him; some call his godhead in question, his power and
attributes, his mercy, justice, providence; they will know with
[6] Cæcilius, why good and bad are punished together, wars, fires,
plagues, infest all alike, why wicked men flourish, good are
poor, in prison, sick, and ill at ease.   Why doth he suffer so
much mischief and evill to be done, if he be [7] able to help? why
doth he not assist good, or resist bad, reform our wills, if he be
not the author of sin, and let such enormities be committed,
unworthy of his knowledge, wisdome, government, mercy, and
providence? why lets he all things be done by fortune and
chance? Others as prodigiously enquire after his omnipotency,

---

[1] Hercules, tuam fidem! Satyra Menip. edit. 1608.   [2] Sardi venales. Satyr.
Menip. an. 1612.   [3] Puteani Comus sic incipit, or as Lipsius Satyre in a
dream.   [4] Trithemius, l. de 7. secundis.   [5] They have fetched Trajanus
soul out of hell, and canonize for saints whom they list.   [6] In Minutius. Sine
delectu tempestates tangunt loca sacra et profana; bonorum et malorum fata
juxta; nullo ordine res fiunt: soluta legibus fortuna dominatur.   [7] Vel malus
vel impotens, qui peccatum permittit, &c. unde hæc superstitio?

Mem. 3.]   *Digression of Ayre.*   513

*an possit plures similes creare Deos? an ex scarabæo Deum?
&c. et quo demum ruetis, sacrificuli?* Some, by visions and revelations, take upon them to be familiar with God, and to be
of privie counsell with him; they will tell how many, and who,
shall be saved, when the world shall come to an end, what year,
what moneth, and whatsoever else God hath reserved unto himself, and to his angels. Some again, curious phantasticks, will
know more than this, and enquire, with [1] Epicurus, what God
did before the world was made? was he idle? where did he
bide? what did he make the world of? why did he then make
it, and not before? If he made it new, or to have an end, how
is he unchangeable, infinite? &c. Some will dispute, cavill,
and object, as Julian did of old, whom Cyrill confutes, as Simon Magus is fained to do, in that [2] dialogue betwixt him and
Peter: and Ammonius the philosopher, in that dialogicall disputation with Zacharias the Christian. If God be infinitely and
only good, why should he alter or destroy the world? if he
confound that which is good, how shall himself continue good?
if he pull it down because evill, how shall he be free from the
evill, that made it evill? &c. with many such absurd and brain-
sick questions, intricacies, froth of humane wit, and excrements of curiosity, &c. which, as our Saviour told his inquisitive disciples, are not fit for them to know. But hoo! I am
now gone quite out of sight: I am almost giddy with roving
about: I could have ranged farther yet; but I am an infant,
and not [3] able to dive into these profundities, or sound these
depths; not able to understand, much less to discuss. I leave
the contemplation of these things to stronger wits, that have
better ability, and happier leisure, to wade into such philosophicall mysteries: for put case I were as able as willing, yet
what can one man do? I will conclude with [4] Scaliger, *Nequa-
quam nos homines sumus, sed partes hominis: ex omnibus aliquid fieri potest, idque non magnum; ex singulis fere nihil.*
Besides (as Nazianzen hath it) *Deus latere nos multa voluit:*
and with Seneca, (*cap. 35. de Cometis*) *Quid miramur tam
rara mundi spectacula non teneri certis legibus, nondum intelligi? multæ sunt gentes, quæ tantum de facie sciunt cœlum: veniet tempus fortasse, quo ista, quæ nunc latent, in
lucem dies extrahat longioris ævi diligentiâ: una ætas non
sufficit: posteri, &c.* when God sees his time, he will reveal
these mysteries to mortall men, and show that to some few at

---

[1] Quid fecit Deus ante mundum creatum? ubi vixit otiosus a suo subjecto, &c.
[2] Lib. 3. recog. Pet. cap. 3. Peter answers by the simile of an egge-shell, which
is cunningly made, yet of necessity to be broken; so is the world, &c. that the excellent state of heaven might be made manifest.   [3] Ut me pluma levat, sic
grave mergit onus.   [4] Exercit. 184.

VOL. I.   L L

514   *Cure of Melancholy.*   [Part. 2. Sec. 2.

last, which he hath concealed so long. For I am of [1] his mind, that Columbus did not find out America by chance, but God directed him at that time to discover it: it was contingent to him, but necessary to God; he reveals and conceals, to whom and when he will: and, which [2] one said of history and records of former times, *God in his providence, to check our presumptuous inquisition, wraps up all things in uncertainty, bars us from long antiquity, and bounds our search within the compass of some few ages.* Many good things are lost, which our predecessors made use of, as Pancirolla will better enform you; many new things are daily invented, to the public good; so kingdomes, men, and knowledge, ebbe and flow, are hid and revealed: and, when you have all done, as the preacher concluded, *Nihil est sub sole novum.* But my melancholy spaniels quest, my game is sprung, and I must suddenly come down and follow.

Jason Pratensis, in his book *de morbis capitis,* and chapter of Melancholy, hath these words out of Galen, [3] *Let them come to me to know what meat and drink they shall use; and, besides that, I will teach them what temper of ambient aire they shall make choice of, what wind, what countries they shall chuse, and what avoid.* Out of which lines of his, thus much we may gather, that, to this cure of melancholy, amongst other things, the rectification of aire is necessarily required. This is performed, either in reforming naturall or artificiall aire. Naturall is that which is in our election to chuse or avoid: and 'tis either generall, to countries, provinces; particular, to cities, towns, villages, or private houses. What harm those extremities of heat or cold do in this malady, I have formerly shewed: the *medium* must needs be good, where the aire is temperate, serene, quiet, free from bogs, fens, mists, all manner of putrefaction, contagious and filthy noisom smels. The [4] Egyptians by all geographers are commended to be *hilares,* a conceited and merry nation: which I can ascribe to no other cause than the serenity of their aire. They that live in the Orchades are registred by [5] Hector Boëthius and [6] Cardan to be fair of complexion, long-lived, most healthfull, free from all manner of infirmities of body and mind, by reason of a sharp purifying aire, which comes from the sea. The Bœotians in Greece were dull and heavy, *crassi Bœoti,* by reason of a foggy aire in which they lived,

---

[1] Laët. descrip. occid. Indiæ.   [2] Daniel, principio historiæ.   [3] Veniant ad me, audituri quo esculento, quo item poculento uti debeant, et præter alimentum ipsum, potumque, ventos ipsos docebo, item aëris ambientis temperiem, insuper regiones quas eligere, quas vitare, ex usu sit.   [4] Leo Afer, Maginus, &c.   [5] Lib. 1. Scot. Hist.   [6] Lib. 1. de rer. var.

Mem. 3.]   *Ayre rectified.*   515

(¹ Bœotûm in crasso jurares aëre natum.)

Attica most acute, pleasant, and refined.   The clime changeth
not so much customes, manners, wits, (as Aristotle, *Polit.
lib. 6. cap. 4.* Vegetius, Plato, Bodine, *method. hist. cap. 5.*
hath proved at large) as constitutions of their bodies, and temperature it self. In all particular provinces we see it confirmed
by experience; as the aire is, so are the inhabitants, dull, heavy, witty, subtle, neat, cleanly, clownish, sick, and sound.   In
² Perigort in France, the aire is subtile, healthfull, seldome any
plague or contagious disease, but hilly and barren: the men,
sound, nimble, and lusty; but in some parts of Quienne full of
moores and marishes, the people dull, heavy, and subject to
many infirmities.   Who sees not a great difference betwixt
Surry, Sussex, and Rumny marsh, the wolds in Lincolnshire,
and the fens? He, therefore, that loves his health, if his ability
will give him leave, must often shift places, and make choice of
such as are wholsome, pleasant, and convenient: there is nothing better than change of aire in this malady, and, generally for health, to wander up and down, as those ³ Tartari
Zamolhenses, that live in hordes, and take opportunity of times,
places, seasons.   The kings of Persia had their summer and
winter houses; in winter at Sardis, in summer at Susa; now
at Persepolis, then at Pasargada.   Cyrus lived seven cold months
at Babylon, three at Susa, two at Ecbatana, saith ⁴ Xenophon,
and had by that means a perpetual spring.   The Great Turk
sojourns sometimes at Constantinople, sometimes at Adrianople, &c.   The kings of Spain have their Escuriall in heat of
summer, ⁵ Madritte for an wholsome seat, Villadolitte a pleasant site, &c. variety of *secessus*, as all princes and great men
have, and their severall progresses to this purpose.   Lucullus
the Roman had his house at Rome, at Baiæ, &c.   ⁶ When
Cn. Pompeius, Marcus Cicero, (saith Plutarch) and many noble men, in the summer came to see him, at supper Pompeius
jested with him, that it was an elegant and pleasant village, full
of windows, galleries, and all offices fit for a summer house:
but, in his judgment, very unfit for winter; Lucullus made answer, that the lord of the house had wit like a crane, that
changeth her country with the season; he had other houses
furnished and built for that purpose, all out as commodious as
this.   So Tully had his Tusculane, Plinius his Lauretan vil-

---

¹ Horat.   ² Maginus.   ³ Hatonus, de Tartaris.   ⁴ Cyropæd. lib. 8.
Perpetuum inde ver.   ⁵ The aire so clear, it never breeds the plague.   ⁶ Leander Albertus, in Campaniâ, e Plutarcho, vitâ Luculli. Cum Cn. Pompeius, Marcus Cicero, multique nobiles viri L. Lucullum æstivo tempore convenissent, Pompeius inter cœnandum familiariter jocatus est, eam villam imprimis sibi sumptuo-
sam et elegantem videri, fenestris, porticibus, &c.

L L 2

516 *Cure of Melancholy.* [Part. 2. Sec.

lage, and every gentleman of any fashion in our times hath the like. The [1] bishop of Exeter had 14 severall houses all furnished, in times past. In Italy, though they bide in cities in winter, which is more gentleman-like, all the summer they come abroad to their country-houses, to recreate themselves. Our gentry in England live most part in the country (except it be some few castles), building still in bottoms (saith [2] Jovius) or neer woods, *coronâ arborum virentium :* you shall know a village by a tuft of trees at or about it, to avoid those strong winds wherewith the island is infested, and cold winter blasts. Some discommend moted houses, as unwholesome, (so Camden saith of [3] Ew-elme, that it was therefore unfrequented, *ob stagni vicini halitus*) and all such places as be neer lakes or rivers. But I am of opinion, that these inconveniences will be mitigated, or easily corrected, by good fires, as [4] one reports of Venice, that *graveolentia* and fog of the moors is sufficiently qualified by those innumerable smoaks. Nay more, [5] Thomas Philol. Ravennas, a great physician, contends that the Venetians are generally longer lived than any city in Europe, and live, many of them, 120 years. But it is not water simply that so much offends, as the slime and noisome smels that accompany such overflowed places, which is but at some few seasons after a floud, and is sufficiently recompensed with sweet smels and aspects in summer, (*Ver pingit vario gemmantia prata colore*) and many other commodities of pleasure and profit; or else may be corrected by the site, if it be somewhat remote from the water, as Lindly, [6] Orton *super montem*, [7] Drayton, or a little more elevated, though neerer, as [8] Caucut, as [9] Amington, [10] Polesworth, [11] Weddington, (to insist in such places best to me known) upon the river of Anker in Warwickshire, [12] Swarston, and [13] Drakesly upon Trent. Or, howsoever they be unseasonable in winter, or at some times, they have their good use in summer. If so be that their means be so slender, as they may not admit of any such variety, but must determine once for all, and make one house serve each season, I know no men that have given better rules in this behalf, than our husbandry writers. [14] Cato and Columella prescribe a good house to stand by a navigable river, good high-waies, neer some city and in a good soile; but that is more for commodity than health.

[1] Godwin, vita Jo. Voysye al. Harman.   [2] Descript. Brit.   [3] In Oxfordshire.   [4] Leander Albertus.   [5] Cap. 21. de vit. hom prorog. [6] The possession of Robert Bradshaw, Esq.   [7] Of George Purefey, Esq. [8] The possession of William Purefey, Esq.   [9] The seat of Sir John Reppington, Kt.   [10] Sir Henry Goodieres, lately deceased.   [11] The dwelling house of Hum. Adderly, Esq.   [12] Sir John Harpars, lately deceased.   [13] Sir George Greselies, Kt.   [14] Lib. 1. cap. 2.

Mem. 3.] *Ayre rectified.* 517

The best soile commonly yeelds the worst aire: a dry sandy plat is fittest to build upon, and such as is rather hilly than plain, full of downes, a cotswold country, as being most commodious for hawking, hunting, wood, waters, and all manner of pleasures. Perigot in France is barren, yet, by reason of the excellency of the aire, and such pleasures that it affords, much inhabited by the nobility; as Noremberg in Germany, Toledo in Spain. Our countryman Tusser will tell us so much, that the fieldone is for profit, the woodland for pleasure and health, the one commonly a deep clay, therefore noisome in winter, and subject to bad high-waies: the other a dry sand. Provision may be had elsewhere, and our towns are generally bigger in the woodland than the fieldone, more frequent and populous, and gentlemen more delight to dwell in such places. Sutton Coldfield in Warwickshire (where I was once a grammar schollar) may be a sufficient witness, which stands, as Camden notes, *loco ingrato et sterili*, but in an excellent aire, and full of all maner of pleasures. [1] Wadley in Barkshire is situate in a vale, though not so fertil a soile as some vales afford, yet a most commodious site, wholsome, in a delicious aire, a rich and pleasant seat. So Segrave in Leicestershire (which towne [2] I am now bound to remember) is sited in a champian, at the edge of the wolds, and more barren than the villages about it: yet no place likely yeelds a better aire. And he that built that faire house, [3] Wollerton in Nottinghamshire, is much to be commended, (though the tract be sandy and barren about it) for making choice of such a place. Constantine (*lib. 2. cap. de agricult.*) praiseth mountaines, hilly, steep places, above the rest by the sea side, and such as look toward the [4] north upon some great river, as [5] Farmack in Darbishire on the Trent, environed with hills, open only to the north, like Mount Edgemond in Cornwall, which M[r] [6] Carew so much admires for an excellent seat: such as is the generall site of Bohemia: *serenat Boreas;* the north wind clarifies; [7] *but neer lakes or marishes, in holes, obscure places, or to the south and west, he utterly disproves:* those winds are unwholsome, putrifying, and make men subject to diseases. The best building for health, according to him, is in [8] *high places, and in an excellent prospect,* like that of Cuddeston

---

[1] The seat of G. Purefey, Esq. [2] For I am now incumbent of that rectory, presented thereto by my right honorable patron, the Lord Berkly. [3] Sir Francis Willoughby. [4] Montani et maritimi salubriores, acclives, et ad Boream vergentes. [5] The dwelling of Sir To. Burdet, Knight Baronet. [6] In his Survay of Cornwall, book 2. [7] Prope paludes, stagna, et loca concava, vel ad Austrum, vel ad Occidentem inclinatæ, domus sunt morbosæ. [8] Oportet igitur ad sanitatem domus in altioribus ædificare, et ad speculationem.

518   *Cure of Melancholy.*   [Part. 2. Sec. 2.

in Oxfordshire (which place I must, *honoris ergo,* mention) is
lately and fairly [1] built in a good aire, good prospect, good
soile, both for profit and pleasure, not so easily to be matched.
P. Crescentius (in his *lib.* 1. *de Agric. cap.* 5) is very copious
in this subject, how a house should be wholsomely sited, in a
good coast, good aire, wind, &c. Varro (*de re rust. lib.* 1.
cap. 12) [2] forbids lakes and rivers, marish and manured
grounds : they cause a bad aire, gross diseases, hard to be
cured : [3] *if it be so that he cannot help it, better, as he adviseth,
sell thy house and land, than lose thine health.* He that respects not this in chusing of his seat, or building his house, is
mente captus, mad, [4] Cato saith, *and his dwelling next to hell
it self,* according to Columella ; he commends, in conclusion,
the middle of a hill, upon a descent. Baptista Porta (*Villæ,
lib.* 1. *cap.* 22) censures Varro, Cato, Collumella, and those
ancient rusticks, approving many things, disallowing some,
and will by all means have the front of an house stand to the
south, which how it may be good in Italy and hotter climes,
I know not ; in our northern countries I am sure it is best.
Stephanus a Frenchman (*prædio rustic. lib.* 1. *cap.* 4) subscribes to this, approving especially the descent of an hill south
or south east, with trees to the north, so that it be well wa-
tered ; a condition, in all sites, which must not be omitted, as
Herbastein inculcates, *lib.* 1. : Julius Cæsar Claudinus, a physician, *consult.* 24 for a nobleman in Poland, melancholy given,
adviseth him to dwell in a house inclining to the [5] east, and [6] by
all means to provide the aire be cleer and sweet ; which Montanus (*consil.* 229) counselleth the earle of Monfort his patient—to inhabit a pleasant house, and in a good aire. If it be
so the naturall site may not be altered of our city, town, village, yet by artificiall means it may be helped. In hot countries, therefore, they make the streets of their cities very
narrow, all over Spain, Africk, Italy, Greece, and many cities
of France, in Languedock especially, and Provence, those
southern parts : Montpelier, the habitation and university of
physicians, is so built, with high houses, narrow streets, to divert the sun's scalding rayes, which Tacitus commends, (*lib.* 15.
Annal.) as most agreeing to their health, [7] *because the height*

---

[1] By John Bancroft, Dr. of Divinity, my quondam tutor in Christ-Church,
Oxon, now the Right Reverend Lord Bishop of Oxon, who built this house for
himself and his successors.   [2] Hyeme erit vehementer frigida, et æstate non
salubris : paludes enim faciunt crassum aërem, et difficiles morbos.   [3] Vendas
quot assibus possis, et, si nequeas, relinquas.   [4] Lib. 1. cap. 2. In Orco habi-
tat.   [5] Aurora Musis amica. Vitruv.   [6] Ædes Orientem spectantes vir
nobilissimus inhabitet, et curet ut sit aër clarus, lucidus, odoriferus. Eligat ha-
bitationem optimo aëre jucundam.   [7] Quoniam angustiæ itinerum et altitudo
tectorum non perinde solis calorem admittunt.

of buildings, and narrowness of streets, keep away the sun beams. Some cities use galleries, or arched cloysters towards the street, as Damascus, Bologna, Padua, Berna in Switzerland, Westchester with us, as well to avoid tempests, as the suns scorching heat. They build on high hills in hot countries, for more aire : or to the sea side, as Baiæ, Naples, &c. In our northern coasts we are opposite; we commend straight, broad, open, fair streets, as most befitting and agreeing to our clime. We build in bottomes for warmth : and that site of Mitylene in the island of Lesbos, in the Ægæan sea, (which Vitruvius so much discommends, magnificently built with fair houses, *sed imprudenter positam,* unadvisedly sited, because it lay along to the south, and when the south wind blew, the people were all sick) would make an excellent site in our northern climes.

Of that artificiall site of houses I have sufficiently discoursed: if the site of the dwelling may not be altered, yet there is much in choice of such a chamber or room, in opportune opening and shutting of windowes, excluding forrain aire and winds, and walking abroad at convenient times. [1] Crato, a German, commends east and south site (disallowing cold aire and northern winds in this case, rainy weather and misty dayes) free from putrefaction, fens, bogs, and muckhills. If the aire be such, open no windowes: come not abroad. Montanus will have his patient not to [2] stir at all, if the wind be big or tempestuous, as most part in March it is with us ; or in cloudy, louring, dark dayes, as in November, which we commonly call the black moneth ; or stormy, let the wind stand how it will : *consil.* 27. and 30 he must not [3] *open a casement in bad weather,* or in a boisterous season ; *consil.* 299, he especially forbids us to open windowes to a south wind. The best site for chamber windowes, in my judgement, are north, east, south; and which is the worst, west. Levinus Lemnius (*lib. 3. cap. 3. de occult. nat. mir.*) attributes so much to aire, and rectifying of wind and windowes, that he holds it alone sufficient to make a man sick or well; to alter body and minde. [4] *A cleer aire cheares up the spirits, exhilarates the minde; a thick, black, misty, tempestuous, contracts, overthrows.* Great heed is therefore to be taken at what times we walke, how we place our windowes, lights, and houses, how we let in or exclude this ambient aire. The Egyp-

---

[1] Consil. 21. li. 2. Frigidus aër, nubilosus, densus, vitandus, æque ac venti septemtrionales, &c. [2] Consil. 24. [3] Fenestram non aperiat. [4] Discutit sol horrorem crassi spiritûs, mentem exhilarat ; non enim tam corpora, quam et animi, mutationem inde subeunt, pro cœli et ventorum ratione, et sani aliter affecti sunt cœlo nubilo, aliter sereno. De naturâ ventorum, see Pliny, lib. 2. cap. 26, 27, 28. Strabo, lib. 7. &c.

520   *Cure of Melancholy.*   [Part. 2. Sec. 2.

tians, to avoid immoderate heat, make their windows on the
top of the house, like chimnies, with two tunnells to draw a
through aire.   In Spain they commonly make great opposite
windows without glass, still shutting those which are next to
the sun.   So likewise in Turkey and Italy (Venice excepted,
which brags of her stately glazed palaces) they use paper windows to like purpose; and lye *sub dio*, in the top of their flat-
roofed houses, so sleeping under the canopy of heaven.   In
some parts of [1] Italy they have windmills, to draw a cooling
aire out of hollow caves, and disperse the same through all the
chambers of their palaces, to refresh them; as at Costoza the
house of Cæsareo Trento, a gentleman of Vicenza, and elsewhere.   Many excellent means are invented to correct nature
by art.   If none of these courses help, the best way is to make
artificial aire, which howsoever is profitable and good, still to
be made hot and moist, and to be seasoned with sweet perfumes, [2] pleasant and lightsome as may be; to have roses,
violets, and sweet smelling flowers ever in their windows, po-
sies in their hand.   Laurentius commends water-lillies, a ves-
sell of warm water to evaporate in the room, which will make
a more delightsome perfume, if there be added orange flowers,
pils of citrons, rosemary, cloves, bayes, rose-water, rose-
vinegar, belzoin, ladanum, styrax, and such like gums, which
make a pleasant and acceptable perfume.   [3] Bessardus Bisanti-
nus prefers the smoak of juniper to melancholy persons, which
is in great request with us at Oxford, to sweeten our chambers,
[4] Guianerius prescribes the aire to be moistened with water,
and sweet herbs boiled in it, vine and sallow leaves, &c. [5] to
besprinkle the ground and posts with rose-water, rose-vinegar,
which Avicenna much approves.   Of colours it is good to behold green, red, yellow, and white, and by all means to have
light enough with windows in the day, wax candles in the night,
neat chambers, good fires in winter, merry companions; for,
though melancholy persons love to be darke and alone, yet
darkness is a great encreaser of the humour.

Although our ordinary aire be good by nature or art, yet it is
not amiss, as I have said, still to alter it; no better physick for
a melancholy man than change of aire and variety of places, to
travel abroad and see fashions.   [6] Leo Afer speaks of many of
his countrymen so cured, without all other physick: amongst

---

[1] Fines Morison, part. 1. c. 4.   [2] Altomarus, cap. 7. Bruel. Aër sit lucidus,
bene olens, humidus. Montaltus idem. ca. 26. Olfactus rerum suavium. Laurentius, c. 8.   [3] Ant. Philos. cap. de melanc.   [4] Tract. 15. c. 9. Ex redolen-
tibus herbis et foliis vitis viniferæ, salicis, &c.   [5] Pavimentum aceto et aquâ
rosaceâ irrorare. Laurent. c. 8.   [6] Lib. 1. cap. de morb. Afrorum. In Nigri-
tarum regione tanta aëris temperies, ut siquis alibi morbosus eo advehatur, optimæ
statim sanitati restituatur; quod multis accidisse ipse meis oculis vidi.

Mem. 3.] *Ayre rectified.* 521

the Negroes, *there is such an excellent aire, that if any of them be sick elsewhere, and brought thither, he is instantly recovered; of which he was often an eye-witness.* [1] Lipsius, Zuinger, and some other, adde as much of ordinary travell. No man, saith Lipsius, in an epistle to Phil. Lanoius, a noble friend of his, now ready to make a voyage, [2] *can be such a stock or stone, whom that pleasant speculation of countries, cities, towns, rivers, will not affect.* [3] Seneca the philosopher was infinitely taken with the sight of Scipio Africanus house, near Linternum, to view those old buildings, cisterns, bathes, tombs, &c. And how was [4] Tully pleased with the sight of Athens, to behold those ancient and faire buildings, with a remembrance of their worthy inhabitants. Paulus Æmilius, that renowned Roman captain, after he had conquered Perseus, the last king of Macedonia, and now made an end of his tedious wars, though he had been long absent from Rome, and much there desired, about the beginning of autumne (as [5] Livy describes it) made a pleasant peregrination all over Greece, accompanied with his son Scipio, and Athenæus the brother of king Eumenes, leaving the charge of his army with Sulpitius Gallus. By Thessaly he went to Delphos, thence to Megaris, Aulis, Athens, Argos, Lacedæmon, Megalopolis, &c. He took great content, exceeding delight, in that his voyage; as who doth not that shall attempt the like, though his travell be *ad jactationem magis quam ad usum reipub.* (as [6] one well observes) to cracke, gaze, see fine sights and fashions, spend time, rather than for his own or publike good? (as it is to many gallants that travel out their best daies, together with their means, manners, honesty, religion) yet it availeth howsoever. For peregrination charmes our senses with such unspeakable and sweet variety, [7] that some count him unhappy that never travelled, a kinde of prisoner, and pity his case, that from his cradle to his old age beholds the same still; still, still the same, the same : insomuch that [8] Rhasis (*cont. lib.* 1. *Tract.* 2) doth not only commend but enjoyn travell, and such variety of objects, to a melancholy man, *and to lye in diverse innes, to be drawn into severall companies.* Montaltus (*cap.* 36) and many neotericks are of the same minde. Celsus adviseth him, therefore, that will continue his health, to have *varium vitæ genus,* diversity of callings, occupations, to be busied about, [9] *sometimes to live in*

---

[1] Lib. de peregrinat. [2] Epist. 2. cen. 1. Nec quisquam tam lapis aut frutex, quem non titillat amœna illa, variaque spectio locorum, urbium, gentium, &c. [3] Epist. 86. [4] Lib. 2. de legibus. [5] Lib. 45. [6] Keckerman, præfat. polit. [7] Fines Morison, c. 3. part. 1. [8] Mutatio de loco in locum, itinera et viagia longa et indeterminata, et hospitare in diversis diversoriis. [9] Modo ruri esse, modo in urbe, sæpius in agro venari, &c.

522   *Cure of Melancholy.*   [Part. 2. Sec. 2.

*the city, sometimes in the countrey ; now to study or work, to be
intent, then again to hawk or hunt, swim, run, ride, or exercise
himself.* A good prospect alone will ease melancholy, as
Gomesius contends, *lib. 2. c. 7. de Sale.* The citizens of [1] Bar-
cino, saith he, otherwise penned in, melancholy, and stirring
little abroad, are much delighted with that pleasant prospect
their city hath into the sea, which, like that of old Athens, besides Ægina, Salamina, and many pleasant islands, had all the
variety of delicious objects: so are those Neapolitanes, and inhabitants of Genua, to see the ships, boats and passengers,
go by, out of their windowes, their whole cities being sited on
the side of an hill, like Pera by Constantinople, so that each
house almost hath a free prospect to the sea, as some part of
London to the Thames: or to have a free prospect all over the
city at once, as at Granado in Spain, and Fez in Africk, the
river running betwixt two declining hills, the steepness causeth
each house almost as well to oversee, as to be overseen of the
rest. Every country is full of such [2] delightsome prospects as
well within land as by sea, as Hermon and [3] Rama in Palæstina,
Colalto in Italy, the top of Täygetus, or Acrocorinthus, that old
decayed castle in Corinth, from which Peloponnesus, Greece,
the Ionian and Ægæan seas, were *semel et simul*, at one view
to be taken. In Egypt the square top of the great Pyramis 300
yards in height, and so the sultans palace in Grand Cairo the
country being plain, hath a marveilous faire prospect, as well
over Nilus, as that great city, five Italian miles long, and two
broad, by the river side: from mount Sion in Jerusalem the holy
land is of all sides to be seen. Such high places are infinite :
with us, those of the best note are Glassenbury tower, Bever
castle, Rodway Grange, [4] Walsby in Lincolnshire, where I
lately received a real kindness by the munificence of the right
honourable my noble lady and patroness, the Lady Frances
countess dowager of Exeter ; and two amongst the rest, which
I may not omit for vicinities sake, Oldbury in the confines of
Warwickshire, where I have often looked about me with
great delight, at the foot of which hill [5] I was born ; and Hanbury in Staffordshire, contiguous to which is Falde a pleasant
village, and an ancient patrimony belonging to our family,
now in the possession of mine elder brother William Burton,
esquire. [6] Barclay the Scot commends that of Greenwich
tower for one of the best prospects in Europe, to see London
on the one side, the Thames, ships, and pleasant meadows, on

---

[1] In Catalonia in Spaine.   [2] Laudaturque domus, longos quæ prospicit
agros.   [3] Many towns there are of that name, saith Adricomius, all high-sited.
[4] Lately resigned for some speciall reasons.   [5] At Lindley in Leicestershire,
the possession and dwelling place of Ralph Burton, Esquire, my late deceased
father.   [6] In Icon animorum.

Mem. 4.]   *Exercise rectified.*   523

the other.   There be those that say as much and more of S^t.
Marks steeple in Venice.   Yet these are at too great a distance;
some are especially affected with such objects as be near, to see
passengers go by in some great rode way, or boats in a river,
in subjectum forum despicere, to oversee a fair, a market-
place, or out of a pleasant window into some thorough-fare
street to behold a continual concourse, a promiscuous route,
coming and going, or a multitude of spectators at a theater,
a maske, or some such like shew.   But I rove: the sum is this,
that variety of actions, objects, aire, places, are excellent good
in this infirmity and all others, good for man, good for beast.
[1] Constantine the emperour (*lib.* 18. *cap.* 13. *ex Leontio*) *holds
it an only cure for rotten sheep, and any manner of sicke cattel.*
Lælius a Fonte Æugubinus, that great doctor, at the latter end
of many of his consultations, (as commonly he doth set down
what success his physik had) in melancholy most especially
approves of this above all other remedies whatsoever, as appears,
consult. 69. *consult.* 229, &c.   [2] *Many other things helped; but
change of aire was that which wrought the cure, and did most
good.*

MEMB. IV.

Exercise rectified of Body and Minde.

To that great inconvenience, which comes on the one side
by immoderate and unseasonable exercise, too much solitariness and idleness on the other, must be opposed, as an antidote, a moderate and seasonable use of it, and that both of
body and minde, as a most materiall circumstance, much conducing to this cure, and to the generall preservation of our health.
The heavens themselves run continually round; the sun riseth
and sets; the moon increaseth and decreaseth; stars and planets
keep their constant motions; the aire is still tossed by the winds;
the waters eb and flow, to their conservation no doubt, to teach
us that we should ever be in action.   For which cause Hierom
prescribes Rusticus the monk, that he be alwayes occupied about
some business or other, [3] *that the devil do not find him idle.*
[4] Seneca would have a man do something, though it be to no
purpose.   [5] Xenophon wisheth one rather to play at tables,

---

[1] Ægrotantes oves in alium locum transportandæ sunt, ut alium aërem et aquam
participantes, coalescant et corroborentur.   [2] Alia utilia; sed ex mutatione
aëris potissimum curatus.   [3] Ne te dæmon otiosum inveniat.   [4] Præstat
aliud agere quam nihil.   [5] Lib. 3. de dictis Socratis.   Qui tesseris et risus
excitando vacant, aliquid faciunt, etsi liceret his meliora agere.

524   *Cure of Melancholy.*   [Part. 2. Sec. 2.

dice, or make a jester of himself (though he might be far
better imployed) than do nothing. The [1] Ægyptians of old, and
many flourishing commonwealths since, have enjoyned labour
and exercise to all sorts of men, to be of some vocation and
calling, and to give an account of their time, to prevent those
grievous mischiefs that come by idleness ; *for, as fodder, whip,
and burthen, belong to the asse, so meat, correction, and worke,
unto the servant.* Ecclus. 33. 23. The Turks injoyn all men
whatsoever, of what degree, to be of some trade or other : the
grand Signior himself is not excused. [2] *In our memory*
(saith Sabellicus) *Mahomet the Turke, he that conquered
Greece, at that very time when he heard ambassadours of other
princes, did either carve or cut wooden spoones, or frame something upon a table.* [3] This present sultan makes notches for
bows. The Jews are most severe in this examination of time.
All well-governed places, towns, families, and every discreet
person, will be a law unto himself. But, amongst us, the badge
of gentry is idleness : to be of no calling, not to labour (for
that's derogatory to their birth), to be a meer spectator, a drone,
fruges consumere natus, to have no necessary employment to
busie himself about in church and commonwealth (some few
governors exempted), *but to rise to eat, &c.* to spend his
dayes in hawking, hunting, &c. and such like disports and recreations ([4] which our casuists tax), are the sole exercise almost
and ordinary actions of our nobility, and in which they are
too immoderate. And thence it comes to pass, that in city and
country so many grievances of body and mind, and this ferall
disease of melancholy so frequently rageth, and now domineers
almost all over Europe amongst our great ones. They know
not how to spend their times (disports excepted, which are all
their business), what to do, or otherwise how to bestow
themselves ; like our modern Frenchmen, that had rather lose
a pound of blood in a single combate, than a drop of sweat in
any honest labour. Every man almost hath something or
other to employ himself about, some vocation, some trade : but
they do all by ministers and servants ; *ad otia duntaxat se natos
existimant, imo ad sui ipsius plerumque et aliorum perniciem,*
[5] as one freely taxeth such kinde of men : they are all for pastimes ; 'tis all their study : all their invention tends to this alone,
to drive away time, as if they were born, some of them, to no
other ends. Therefore to correct and avoid these errors and

---

[1] Amasis compelled every man once a year to tell how he lived.   [2] Nostrâ memoriâ Mahometes Othomanus, qui Græciæ imperium subvertit, cum
oratorum postulata audiret externarum gentium, cochlearia lignea assidue cæla-
bat, aut aliquid in tabulâ affingebat.   [3] Sands, fol. 37. of his voyage to Jerusalem.   [4] Perkins cases of conscience, l. 3. c. 4. q. 3.   [5] Lusci-
nius Grunnio.

Mem. 4.] *Exercise rectified.* 525

inconveniences, our divines, physicians, and politicians, so much labour, and so seriously exhort : and for this disease in particular, [1] *there can be no better cure than continuall business,* as Rhasis holds, *to have some employment or other, which may set their mind aworke, and distract their cogitations.* Riches may not easily be had without labour and industry, nor learning without study ; neither can our health be preserved without bodily exercise. If it be of the body, Guianerius allowes that exercise which is gentle, [2] *and still after those ordinary frications,* which must be used every morning. Montaltus (*cap.* 26) and Jason Pratensis use almost the same words, highly commending exercise, if it be moderate : *a wonderful help, so used,* Crato calls it, *and a great means to preserve our health, as adding strength to the whole body, increasing naturall heat, by means of which, the nutriment is well concocted in the stomacke, liver, and veins, few or no crudities left, is happily distributed over all the body.* Besides, it expells excrements by sweat, and other insensible vapours ; in so much that [3] Galen prefers exercise before all physick, rectification of diet, or any regimen in what kinde soever ; 'tis Natures physician. [4] Fulgentius (out of Gordonius, *de conserv. vit. hom. lib.* 1. *cap.* 7) tearms exercise *a spur of a dull sleepy nature, the comforter of the members, cure of infirmity, death of diseases, destruction of all mischiefes and vices.* The fittest time for exercise is a little before dinner, a little before supper, [5] or at any time when the body is empty. Montanus (*consil.* 31) prescribes it every morning to his patient, and that, as [6] Calenus addes, *after he hath done his ordinary needs, rubbed his body, washed his hands and face, combed his head, and gargarized.* What kinde of exercise he should use, Galen tells us, *lib.* 2. *et* 3. *de sanit. tuend.* and in what measure, [7] *till the body be ready to sweat,* and roused up, *ad ruborem,* some say, *non ad sudorem,* lest it should dry the body too much ; others injoyn those wholesome businesses, as to dig so long in his garden, to hold the plough, and the like. Some prescribe frequent and violent labour and exercises, as sawing

---

[1] Non est cura melior quam injungere iis necessaria, et opportuna ; operum administratio illis magnum sanitatis incrementum, et quæ repleant animos eorum, et incutiant iis diversas cogitationes. Cont. 1. tract. 9.   [2] Ante exercitium, leves toto corpore fricationes conveniunt Ad hunc morbum exercitationes, quum recte et suo tempore fiunt, mirifice conducunt, et sanitatem tuentur, &c.   [3] Lib. 1. de san. tuend.   [4] Exercitium naturæ dormientis stimulatio, membrorum solatium, morborum medela, fuga vitiorum, medicina languorum, destructio omnium malorum. Crato.   [5] Alimentis in ventriculo probe concoctis.   [6] Jejuno ventre, vesicâ et alvo ab excrementis purgato, fricatis membris, lotis manibus et oculis, &c. Lib. de atrâ bile.   [7] Quousque corpus universum intumescat, et floridum appareat, sudoremque, &c.

526 *Cure of Melancholy.* [Part. 2. Sec. 2.

every day, so long together, (*epid.* 6. Hippocrates confounds them) but that is in some cases, to some peculiar men; [1] the most forbid, and by no means will have it go farther than a beginning sweat, as being [2] perilous if it exceed.

Of these labours, exercises, and recreations, which are likewise included, some properly belong to the body, some to the mind, some more easie, some hard, some with delight, some without, some within doors, some naturall, some are artificiall. Amongst bodily exercises, Galen commends *ludum parvæ pilæ,* to play at ball: be it with the hand or racket, in tennis courts, or otherwise, it exerciseth each part of the body, and doth much good, so that they sweat not too much. It was in great request of old amongst the Greeks, Romanes, Barbarians, mentioned by Homer, Herodotus, and Plinius. Some write, that Aganella, a fair maide of Corcyra, was the inventer of it; for she presented the first ball that ever was made, to Nausica, the daughter of king Alcinoüs, and taught her how to use it.

The ordinary sports which are used abroad, are hawking, hunting : *hilares venandi labores,* [3] one calls them, because they recreate body and minde; [4] another, [5] *the best exercise that is, by which alone many have been* [6] *freed from all ferall diseases.* Hegesippus (*lib.* 1. *cap.* 37) relates of Herod, that he was eased of a grievous melancholy by that means. Plato (7 *de leg.*) highly magnifies it, dividing it into three parts, by land, water, ayre. Xenophon (in *Cyropæd.*) graces it with a great name, *Deorum munus,* the gift of the Gods, a princely sport, which they have ever used, saith Langius, (*epist.* 59. *lib.* 2) as well for health as pleasure, and do at this day, it being the sole almost and ordinary sport of our noblemen in Europe, and elsewhere all over the world. Bohemus (*de mor. gent. lib.* 3. *cap.* 12) stiles it therefore *studium nobilium; communiter venantur, quod sibi solis licere contendunt;* 'tis all their study, their exercise, ordinary business, all their talk : and indeed some dote too much after it; they can do nothing else, discourse of naught else. Paulus Jovius (*descr. Brit.*) doth in some sort tax our [7] *English nobility for it, for living in the country so much, and too frequent use of it, as if they had no other means but hawking and hunting to approve themselves gentlemen with.*

---

[1] Omnino sudorem vitent. cap. 7. lib. 1. Valescus de Tar. [2] Exercitium si excedat, valde periculosum. Sallust. Salvianus, de remed. lib. 2. cap. 1. [3] Camden in Staffordshire. [4] Fridevallius, lib. 1. cap. 2. Optima omnium exercitationum : multi ab hac solummodo morbis liberati. [5] Josephus Quercetanus, dial. polit. sect. 2. cap. 11. Inter omnia exercitia præstantiæ laudem meretur. [6] Chiron in monte Pelio, præceptor heroum, eos a morbis animi venationibus et puris cibis tuebatur. M. Tyrius. [7] Nobilitas omnis fere urbes fastidit, castellis et liberiore cœlo gaudet, generisque dignitatem unâ maxime venatione et falconum aucupiis tuetur.

Mem. 4.]   *Exercise rectified.*   527

Hawking comes neer to hunting, the one in the aire, as the other on the earth, a sport as much affected as the other, by some preferred. [1] It was never heard of amongst the Romans, invented some 1200 years since, and first mentioned by Firmicus, *lib. 5. cap. 8.* The Greek emperours began it, and now nothing so frequent: he is nobody, that in the season hath not a hawke on his fist: a great art, and many [2] books written of it. It is a wonder to hear [3] what is related of the Turkes officers in this behalf, how many thousand men are employed about it, how many hawks of all sorts, how much revenewes consumed on that only disport, how much time is spent at Adrianople alone every year to that purpose. The [4] Persian kings hawk after butterflies with sparrows, made to that use, and starrs; lesser hawks for lesser games they have, and bigger for the rest, that they may produce their sport to all seasons. The Muscovian emperours reclaime eagles to fly at hindes, foxes, &c. and such a one was sent for a present to [5] Queen Elizabeth: some reclaime ravens, castrils, pies, &c. and man them for their pleasures.

Fowling is more troublesome, but all out as delightsome to some sorts of men, be it with guns, lime, nets, glades, ginnes, strings, baits, pitfalls, pipes, calls, stawking-horses, setting-doggs, coy-ducks, &c. or otherwise. Some much delight to take larks with day-nets, small birds with chaffe-nets, plovers, partridge, herons, snite, &c. Henry the third, king of Castile, (as Mariana the Jesuite reports of him, *lib. 3. cap. 7.*) was much affected [6] *with catching of quailes:* and many gentlemen take a singular pleasure at morning and evening to go abroad with their quaile-pipes, and will take any paines to satisfie their delight in that kinde. The [7] Italians have gardens fitted to such use, with nets, bushes, glades, sparing no cost or industry, and are very much affected with the sport. Tycho Brahe, that great astronomer, in the Chorography of his Isle of Huena, and castle of Uraniburge, puts down his nets, and manner of catching small birds as an ornament, and a recreation, wherein he himself was sometimes employed.

Fishing is a kinde of hunting by water, be it with nets, weeles, baits, angling or otherwise, and yeelds all out as much pleasure to some men, as dogs, or hawks, [8] *when they draw*

---

[1] Jos. Scaliger, comment. in Cirin. fol. 344. Salmuth, 23 de Nov. repert. com. in Pancir.   [2] Demetrius Constantinop. de re accipitrariâ liber, a P. Gillar Latine redditus. Ælius, epist. Aquilæ, Symmachi, et Theodotionis ad Ptolemæum, &c.   [3] Lonicerus, Getfreus, Jovius.   [4] S. Antony Sherlies relations.   [5] Hacluit.   [6] Coturnicum aucupio.   [7] Fines Morison, part. 3. c. 8.   [8] Non majorem voluptatem animo capiunt, quam qui feras insectantur, aut missis canibus comprehendunt, quum retia trahentes, squamosas pecudes in ripas adducunt.

528   *Cure of Melancholy.*   [Part. 2. Sec. 2.

their fish upon the bank, saith Nic. Henselius, *Silesiographiæ cap.* 3, speaking of that extraordinary delight his countrymen took in fishing, and in making of pooles.   James Dubravius, that Moravian, in his book *de pisc.* telleth, how travelling by the highway side in Silesia, he found a nobleman [1] *booted up to the groins*, wading himself, pulling the nets, and labouring as much as any fisherman of them all: and when some belike objected to him the baseness of his office, he excused himself, [2] *that if other men might hunt hares, why should not he hunt carpes ?*   Many gentlemen in like sort, with us, will wade up to the arm-holes, upon such occasions, and voluntarily undertake that to satisfie their pleasure, which a poor man for a good stipend would scarce be hired to undergo. Plutarch, in his book *de soler. animal.* speaks against all fishing, [3] *as a filthy, base, illiberall imployment, having neither wit nor perspicacity in it, nor worth the labour.*   But he that shall consider the variety of baits, for all seasons, and pretty devices which our anglers have invented, peculiar lines, false flies, severall sleights, &c. will say, that it deserves like commendation, requires as much study and perspicacity as the rest, and is to be preferred before many of them ; because hawking and hunting are very laborious, much riding, and many dangers accompany them ; but this is still and quiet : and if so be the angler catch no fish, yet he hath a wholesome walk to the brook side, pleasant shade, by the sweet silver streams ; he hath good aire, and sweet smels of fine fresh meadow flowers ; he hears the melodious harmony of birds ; he sees the swans, herns, ducks, water-hens, cootes, &c. and many other fowle, with their brood, which he thinketh better than the noise of hounds, or blast of hornes, and all the sport that they can make.

Many other sports and recreations there be, much in use, as ringing, bowling, shooting, which Askam commends in a just volume, and hath in former times been injoyned by statute, as a defensive exercise, and an [4] honour to our land, as well may witness our victories in France ; keelpins, tronks, coits, pitching bars, hurling, wrestling, leaping, running, fencing, mustring, swimming, wasters, foiles, foot-ball, balown, quintans, &c. and many such, which are the common recreations of the country folks ; riding of great horses, running at rings, tilts and turnaments, horse-races, wilde-goose chases, which are the

---

[1] More piscatorum cruribus ocreatus.   [2] Si principibus venatio leporis non sit inhonesta, nescio quomodo piscatio cyprinorum videri debeat pudenda. [3] Omnino turpis piscatio, nullo studio digna, illiberalis credita est, quod nullum habet ingenium, nullam perspicaciam.   [4] Præcipua hinc Anglis gloria, crebræ victoriæ partæ. Jovius.

Mem. 4.]   *Exercise rectified.*   529

disports of greater men, and good in themselves, though many gentlemen, by that means, gallop quite out of their fortunes.

But the most pleasant of all outward pastimes is that of [1] Aretæus, *deambulatio per amœna loca,* to make a petty progress, a merry journey now and then with some good companions, to visit friends, see cities, castles, towns,

> [2] Visere sæpe amnes nitidos, peramœnaque Tempe,
> Et placidas summis sectari in montibus auras :

> To see the pleasant fields, the crystall fountains,
> And take the gentle aire amongst the mountains :

[3] to walk amongst orchards, gardens, bowers, mounts, and arbours, artificiall wildernesses, green thickets, arches, groves, lawns, rivulets, fountains and such like pleasant places, like that Antiochian Daphne, brooks, pooles, fishponds, betwixt wood and water, in a fair meadow, by a river side, [4] *ubi variæ avium cantationes, florum colores, pratorum frutices, &c.* to disport in some pleasant plain, park, run up a steep hill sometimes, or sit in a shady seat, must needs be a delectable recreation. *Hortus principis et domus ad delectationem facta, cum sylvâ, monte, et piscinâ, vulgo La Montagna :* the princes garden at Ferrara, [5] Schottus highly magnifies, with the groves, mountaines, ponds, for a delectable prospect : he was much affected with it : a Persian paradise, or pleasant parke, could not be more delectable in his sight. S. Bernard, in the description of his monastery, is almost ravished with the pleasures of it. *A sick* [6] *man* (saith he) *sits upon a green bank : and when the dog-star parcheth the plaines, and dries up rivers, he lies in a shadie bowre ;*

> Fronde sub arboreâ ferventia temperat astra,

and feeds his eyes with variety of objects, hearbs, trees ; and to comfort his misery, he receives many delightsome smels, and fils his ears with that sweet and various harmony of birdes. Good God ! (saith he) *what a company of pleasures hast thou made for man !* He that should be admitted on a sudden to the sight of such a palace as that of Escuriall in Spain, or to that which the Moores built at Granado, Fountenblewe in France, the Turkes gardens in his seraglio, wherein all manner of birds and beasts are kept for pleasure, wolves, bears, lynces, tygers, lyons, elephants, &c. or upon the

---

[1] Cap. 7.   [2] Fracastorius.   [3] Ambulationes subdiales, quas hortenses auræ ministrant, sub fornice viridi, pampinis virentibus concameratâ.   [4] Theophylact.   [5] Itinerar. Ital.   [6] Sedet ægrotus cæspite viridi ; et cum inclementia canicularis terras excoquit, et siccat flumina, ipse securus sedet sub arboreâ fronde, et, ad doloris sui solatium, naribus suis gramineas redolet species ; pascit oculos herbarum amœna viriditas ; aures suavi modulamine demulcet pictarum concentus avium, &c.   Deus bone ! quanta pauperibus procuras solatia !

VOL. I.   M M

530   *Cure of Melancholy.*   [Part. 2. Sec. 2.

banks of that Thracian Bosphorus: the popes Belvedere in
Rome [1] as pleasing as those *horti pensiles* in Babylon, or that
Indian kings delightsome garden in [2] Ælian; or [3] those famous
gardens of the Lord Cantelow in France, could not choose,
though he were never so ill apaid, but be much recreated for
the time; or many of our noblemens gardens at home. To
take a boat in a pleasant evening, and with musick [4] to row
upon the waters, which Plutarch so much applaudes, Ælian
admires, upon the river Peneus, in those Thessalian fields beset
with green bayes, where birds so sweetly sing, that passengers,
enchanted as it were with their heavenly musick, *omnium laborum et curarum obliviscantur,* forget forthwith all labours,
care and grief; or in a gundilo through the grand canale in
Venice, to see those goodly palaces, must needs refresh and
give content to a melancholy dull spirit. Or to see the inner
roomes of a fair-built and sumptuous ædifice, as that of the
Persian kings so much renowned by Diodorus and Curtius, in
which all was almost beaten gold, [5] chaires, stooles, thrones,
tabernacles, and pillars of gold, plane trees, and vines of gold,
grapes of precious stones, all the other ornaments of pure gold,

> ([6] Fulget gemma toris, et iaspide fulva supellex;
> Strata micant Tyrio——)

with sweet odours and perfumes, generous wines, opiparous
fare, &c. besides the gallantest young men, the fairest [7] virgins, *puellæ scitulæ ministrantes,* the rarest beauties the world
could afford, and those set out with costly and curious attires,
ad stuporem usque spectantium, with exquisite musick, as in
[8] Trimalchions house, in every chamber, sweet voices ever
sounding day and night, *incomparabilis luxus,* all delights
and pleasures in each kinde which to please the senses could
possibly be devised or had, *convivæ coronati, deliciis ebrii, &c.*
Telemachus in Homer is brought in as one ravished almost, at
the sight of that magnificent palace, and rich furniture of
Menelaus, when he beheld

> [9] Æris fulgorem, et resonantia tecta corusco
> Auro, atque electro nitido, sectoque elephanto,
> Argentoque simul. Talis Jovis ardua sedes,
> Aulaque Cœlicolûm stellans splendescit Olympo.

---

[1] Diod. Siculus, lib. 2.   [2] Lib. 13. de animal. cap. 13.   [3] Pet. Gillius.
Paul. Hentzerus, Itinerar. Italiæ, 1617. Jod. Sincerus, Itinerar. Galliæ, 1617.
Simp. lib. 1. quæst. 4.   [4] Jucundissima deambulatio juxta mare, et navigatio
prope terram.—In utrâque fluminis ripâ.   [5] Aurei panes, aurea opsonia, vis
margaritarum aceto subacta, &c.   [6] Lucan.   [7] 300 pellices, pocillatores,
et pincernæ innumeri, pueri loti purpurâ induti, &c. ex omnium pulchritudine
delecti.   [8] Ubi omnia cantu strepunt.   [9] Odyss. 8.

Mem. 4.] *Exercise rectified.* 531

> Such glittering of gold and brightest brass to shine,
> Cleer amber, silver pure, and ivory so fine :
> Jupiters lofty palace, where the gods do dwell,
> Was even such a one, and did it not excell.

It will *laxare animos*, refresh the soule of man, to see fair-built cities, streets, theatres, temples, obelisks, &c. The temple of Jerusalem was so fairly built of white marble, with so many pyramids covered with gold; *tectumque templi, fulvo coruscans auro, nimio suo fulgore obcæcabat oculos itinerantium*, was so glorious and so glistered afar off, that the spectators might not well abide the sight of it. But the inner parts were all so curiously set out with cedar, gold, jewels, &c. (as he said of Cleopatras palace in Egypt,

> ———[1] Crassumque trabes absconderat aurum)

that the beholders were amazed. What so pleasant as to see some pageant or sight go by, as at coronations, weddings, and such like solemnities;—to see an embassadour or a prince met, received, entertained with masks, shewes, fireworks, &c.—to see two kings fight in single combat, as Porus and Alexander, Canutus and Edmond Ironside, Scanderbeg and Ferat Bassa the Turke, when not honour alone but life it self is at stake, (as the [2] poet of Hector,

> ——————nec enim pro tergore tauri,
> Pro bove nec certamen erat, quæ præmia cursûs
> Esse solent, sed pro magni vitâque animâque
> Hectoris) ;——

to behold a battle fought, like that of Cressy, or Agencourt, or Poictiers, *quâ nescio* (saith Froissard) *an vetustas ullam proferre possit clariorem;*—to see one of Cæsars triumphs in old Rome revived, or the like ;—to be present at an interview, [3] as that famous of Henry the 8th, and Francis the first, so much renowed all over Europe ; *ubi tanto apparatu* (saith Hubertus Vellius) *tamque triumphali pompâ ambo reges cum eorum conjugibus coiêre, ut nulla unquam ætas tam celebria festa viderit aut audierit*, no age ever saw the like. So infinitely pleasant are such shewes, to the sight of which often times they will come hundreds of miles, give any money for a place, and remember many years after with singular delight. Bodine, when he was embassadour in England, said he saw the noblemen go in their robes to the parliament house, *summâ cum jucunditate vidimus;* he was much affected with the sight of it. Pomponius Columna, saith Jovius in his life, saw

---

[1] Lucan. l. 8.   [2] Iliad. 10.   [3] Betwixt Ardes and Guines, 1519.

M M 2

532   *Cure of Melancholy.*   [Part. 2. Sec. 2.

13 Frenchmen, and so many Italians, once fight for a whole
army : *quod jucundissimun spectaculum in vitâ dicit suâ*, the
pleasantest sight that ever he saw in his life. Who would not
have been affected with such a spectacle ? Or that single combat of [1] Breaute the Frenchman, and Anthony Schets a Dutch-
man, before the walls of Sylvaducis in Brabant, anno 1600.
They were 22 horse on the one side, as many on the other,
which, like Livies Horatii, Torquati, and Corvini, fought for
their own glory and countries honour, in the sight and view of
their whole city and army. [2] When Julius Cæsar warred
about the bankes of Rhene, there came a barbarian prince
to see him and the Roman army ; and when he had beheld
Cæsar a good while, [3] *I see the gods now*, (saith he) *which before I heard of, nec feliciorem ullam vitæ meæ aut optavi aut
sensi diem :* it was the happiest day that ever he had in his life.
Such a sight alone were able of it self to drive away melancholy ; if not for ever, yet it must needs expell it for a time.
Radzivilius was much taken with the bassas palace in Cairo ;
and, amongst many other objects which that place afforded,
with that solemnity of cutting the bankes of Nilus, by Im-
bram Bassa, when it overflowed, besides two or three hundred
guilded gallies on the water, he saw two millions of men gathered together on the land, with turbants as white as snow ;
and twas a goodly sight. The very reading of feasts, triumphs,
interviews, nuptials, tilts, turnaments, combats, and monomachies, is most acceptable and pleasant. [4] Franciscus Modius
hath made a large collection of such solemnities in two great
tomes, which who so will may peruse. The inspection alone
of those curious iconographies of temples and palaces, as that
of the Lateran church in Albertus Durer, that of the temple
of Jerusalem in [5] Josephus, Adricomius, and Villalpandus: that
of the Escuriall in Guadas, of Diana at Ephesus in Pliny,
Neros golden palace in Rome, [6] Justinians in Constantinople,
that Peruvian Ingos in [7] Cusco, *ut non ab hominibus, sed a
dæmoniis, constructum videatur ;* S. Marks in Venice by Ignatius, with many such : *priscorum artificum opera* (saith that
[8] interpreter of Pausanias) the rare workmanship of those ancient Greeks, in theaters, obelisks, temples, statues, gold,
silver, ivory, marble images, *non minore ferme, quum leguntur,
quam quum cernuntur, animum delectatione complent,* affect
one as much by reading almost, as by sight.

---

[1] Senertius, in deliciis, fol. 487. Veteri Horatiorum exemplo, virtute et successu
admirabili, cæsis hostibus 17 in conspectu patriæ, &c.   [2] Paterculus, vol. post.
[3] Quos antea audivi, inquit, hodie vidi Deos.   [4] Pandectæ Triumph. fol.
[5] Lib. 6. cap. 14. de bello Jud.   [6] Procopius.   [7] Laët. lib. 10. Amer.
descript.   [8] Romulus Amaseus, præfat. Pausan.

The country hath his recreations, the city his severall gymnicks and exercises, May-games, feasts, wakes, and merry meetings, to solace themselves. The very being in the country, that life it self, is a sufficient recreation to some men, to enjoy such pleasures, as those old patriarks did. Dioclesian the emperour was so much affected with it, that he gave over his scepter, and turned gardiner. Constantine wrote 20 books of husbandry, Lysander, when embassadours came to see him, bragged of nothing more than of his orchard: *hi sunt ordines mei.* What shall I say of Cincinnatus, Cato, Tully, and many such? how have they been pleased with it, to prune, plant, inoculate, and graft, to shew so many severall kindes of pears, apples, plums, peaches, &c.

> [1] Nunc captare feras laqueo, nunc fallere visco,
> Atque etiam magnos canibus circumdare saltus,
> Insidias avibus moliri, incendere vepres.

> Sometimes with traps deceive, with line and string
> To catch wild birds and beasts, encompassing
> The grove with dogs, and out of bushes firing.

> ———— et nidos avium scrutari, &c.

Jucundus, in his preface to Cato, Varro, Columella, &c. put out by him, confesseth of himself, that he was mightily delighted with these husbandry studies, and took extraordinary pleasure in them. If the theorick or speculation can so much affect, what shall the place and exercise it self, the practick part, do? The same confession I find in Herbastein, Porta, Camerarius, and many others, which have written of that subject. If my testimony were ought worth, I could say as much of myself; I am *verè Saturninus;* no man ever took more delight in springs, woods, groves, gardens, walks, fishponds, rivers, &c. But

> Tantalus a labris sitiens fugientia captat
> Flumina;

and so do I; *velle licet; potiri non licet.*

Every palace, every city almost, hath his peculiar walkes, cloysters, tarraces, groves, theaters, pageants, games, and severall recreations; every country, some professed gymnicks, to exhilarate their minds, and exercise their bodyes. The [2] Greeks had their Olympian, Pythian, Isthmian, Nemean games, in honour of Neptune, Jupiter, Apollo; Athens, hers; some for honour, garlands, crowns; for [3] beauty, dancing, running,

---

[1] Virg. l. Geor. [2] Boterus, lib. 3. polit. cap. l. [3] See Athenæus, dipnoso.

534   *Cure of Melancholy.*   [Part. 2. Sec. 2.

leaping, like our silver games. The [1] Romanes had their feasts
(as the Athenians and Lacedæmonians held their publike ban-
quets *in Prytanæo, Panathenæis, Thesmophoriis, Phiditiis*),
playes, naumachies, places for sea-fights, [2] theaters, amphi-
theaters able to contain 70000 men, wherein they had severall
delightsome shews to exhilarate the people; [3] gladiators, combats of men with themselves, with wild beasts, and wild beasts
one with another, like our bull-baitings, or bear-baitings (in
which many countrymen and citizens amongst us so much delight and so frequently use), dancers on ropes, juglers, wrestlers,
comedies, tragedies, publikely exhibited at the emperours and
cities charge, and that with incredible cost and magnificence.
In the Low-countries, (as [4] Meteran relates) before these wars,
they had many solemn feasts, playes, challenges, artillery
gardens, colleges of rimers, rhetoricians, poets; and to this
day, such places are curiously maintained in Amsterdam, as
appears by that description of Isaacus Pontanus, *rerum Am-
stelrod. lib. 2. cap. 25.* So likewise not long since at Friburg
in Germany, as is evident by that relation of [5] Neander, they
had *ludos septennales,* solemn playes every seven years, which
Bocerus one of their own poets hath elegantly described:

> At nunc magnifico spectacula structa paratu
> Quid memorem, veteri non concessura Quirino
> Ludorum pompâ, &c.

In Italy they have solemn declamations of certain select young
gentlemen in Florence (like those reciters in old Rome), and
publike theaters in most of their cities for stage-players and
others, to exercise and recreate themselves. All seasons almost, all places, have their severall pastimes; some in som-
mer, some in winter; some abroad, some within; some of
the body, some of the minde; and divers men have divers recreations, and exercises. Domitian the emperour was much
delighted with catching flies; Augustus to play with nuts
amongst children; [6] Alexander Severus was often pleased to
play with whelps and young pigs. [7] Adrian was so wholly enamoured with dogs and horses, that he bestowed monuments
and tombes on them, and buried them in graves. In fowle

---

[1] Ludi votivi, sacri, ludicri, Megalenses, Cereales, Florales, Martiales, &c.
Rosinus, 5. 12.   [2] See Lipsius, Amphitheatrum. Rosinus, lib. 5. Meursius
de ludis Græcorum.   [3] 1500 men at once, tigers, lions, elephants, horses, dogs,
beares, &c.   [4] Lib. ult. et l. 1. ad finem. Consuetudine non minus laudabili,
quam veteri, contubernia rhetorum, rhythmicorum in urbibus et municipiis; cer-
tisque diebus exercebant se sagittarii, gladiatores, &c.   Alia ingenii, animique
exercitia, quorum præcipuum studium, principem populum tragœdiis, comœdiis,
fabulis scenicis, aliisque id genus ludis recreare.   [5] Orbis terræ descript.
part. 3.   [6] Lampridius.   [7] Spartian.

Mem. 4.]   *Exercise rectified.*   535

weather, or when they can use no other convenient sports, by
reason of the time, as we do cock-fighting to avoide idleness
I think, (though some be more seriously taken with it, spend
much time, cost and charges, and are too solicitous about it.)
[1] Severus used partridges and quailes, as many Frenchmen
do still, and to keep birds in cages, with which he was much
pleased, when at any time he had leasure from publike cares
and businesses.   He had (saith Lampridius) tame pheasants,
ducks, partridges, peacocks, and some 20000 ringdoves and
pigeons.   Busbequius, the emperors orator, when he lay in
Constantinople, and could not stir much abroad, kept for his
recreation, busying himself to see them fed, almost all manner
of strange birds and beasts; this was something, though not to
exercise his body, yet to refresh his minde.   Conradus Gesner,
at Zurick in Switzerland, kept so likewise for his pleasure a
great company of wilde beasts, and (as he saith) took great
delight to see them eat their meat.   Turkie gentlewomen, that
are perpetuall prisoners, still mewed up according to the custome of the place, have little else besides their houshold business, or to play with their children, to drive away time, but to
dally with their cats, which they have *in deliciis*, as many of
our ladies and gentlewomen use monkies and little doggs.
The ordinary recreations which we have in winter, and in
most solitary times busie our minds with, are cardes, tables
and dice, shovelboard, chesse-play, the philosophers game,
small trunks, shuttle-cock, balliards, musick, masks, singing, dancing, ulegames, frolicks, jests, riddles, catches, pur-
poses, questions and commands, [2] merry tales of errant knights,
queens, lovers, lords, ladies, giants, dwarfes, theeves, cheaters,
witches, fayries, goblins, friers, &c. such as the old women
told Psyche in [3] Apuleius, Bocace novels, and the rest,
quarum auditione pueri delectantur, senes narratione, which
some delight to hear, some to tell; all are well pleased with.
Amaranthus the philosopher met Hermocles, Diophantus, and
Philolaus, his companions, one day busily discoursing about
Epicurus and Democritus tenents, very solicitous which was
most probable and came nearest to truth.   To put them
out of that surly controversie, and to refresh their spirits,
he told them a pleasant tale of Stratocles the physicians
wedding, and of all the particulars, the company, the chear,
the musick, &c. for he was new come from it; with which
relation they were so much delighted, that Philolaus wished

---

[1] Delectatus lusu catulorum, porcellorum, ut perdices inter se pugnarent, aut ut
aves parvulæ sursum et deorsum volitarent, his maxime delectatus, ut solicitudines publicas sublevaret.   [2] Brumales læte ut possint producere noctes.
[3] Miles. 4.

a blessing to his heart, and many a good wedding, [1]many such merry meetings might he be at, *to please himself with the sight, and others with the narration of it.* Newes are generally welcome to all our ears: *avide audimus; aures enim hominum novitate lætantur* ([2] as Pliny observes), we long after rumour, to hear and listen to it; [3]*densum humeris bibit aure vulgus.* We are most part too inquisitive and apt to hearken after newes; which Cæsar in his [4]Commentaries observes of the old Gaules; they would be enquiring of every carrier and passenger, what they had heard or seen, what newes abroad ?

> ———————— quid toto fiat in orbe,
> Quid Seres, quid Thraces agant, secreta novercæ,
> Et pueri, quis amet, &c.

as at an ordinary with us, bakehouse, or barbers shop. When that great Gonsalva was upon some displeasure confined by king Ferdinand to the city of Loxa in Andalusia, the onely comfort (saith [5]Jovius) he had to ease his melancholy thoughts, was to hear newes, and to listen after those ordinary occurrents, which were brought him, *cum primis,* by letters or otherwise out of the remotest parts of Europe. Some mens whole delight is to take tobacco, and drink all day long in a tavern or alehouse, to discourse, sing, jest, roare, talk of a cock and bull over a pot, &c. or, when three or four good companions meet, tell old stories by the fire side, or in the sun, as old folkes usually do, *quæ aprici meminére senes,* remembring afresh and with pleasure ancient matters, and such like accidents, which happened in their younger yeares. Others best pastime is to game : nothing to them so pleasant.

> [6] Hic Veneri indulget, hunc decoquit alea.———

Many too nicely take exceptions at cardes, [7]tables, and dice, and such mixt lusorious lots (whom Gataker well confutes), which, though they be honest recreations in themselves, yet may justly be otherwise excepted at, as they are often abused, and forbidden as things most pernicious; *insanam rem et damnosam,* [8]Lemnius calls it: *for, most part, in these kind of*

---

[1] O Dii! similibus sæpe conviviis date ut ipse videndo delectetur, et postmodum narrando delectet. Theod. prodromus Amorum, dial. interpret. Gilberto Gaulinio. [2] Epist. lib. 8. Ruffino. [3] Hor. [4] Lib. 4. Gallicæ consuetudinis est, ut viatores etiam invitos consistere cogant, et quid quisque eorum de quâque re audierit aut cognôrit, quærant. [5] Vitæ ejus, lib. ult. [6] Juven. [7] They account them unlawful, because sortilegious. [8] Instit. c. 44. In his ludis plerumque non ars aut peritia viget, sed fraus, fallacia, dolus, astutia, casus, fortuna, temeritas, locum habent, non ratio, consilium, sapientia, &c.

Mem. 4.] *Exercise rectified.*

disports, 'tis not art or skill, but subtilty, cunnycatching, knavery, chance and fortune, carries all away: 'tis *ambulatoria pecunia,*

———————————— puncto mobilis horæ
Permutat dominos, et cedit in altera jura.

They labour, most part, not to pass their time in honest disport, but for filthy lucre, and covetousness of money. *In fœdissimum lucrum et avaritiam hominum convertitur,* as Daneus observes. *Fons fraudum et maleficiorum,* 'tis the fountain of cosenage and villany: [1] *a thing so common all over Europe at this day, and so generally abused, that many men are utterly undone by it,* their means spent, patrimonies consumed, they and their posterity beggered; besides swearing, wrangling, drinking, loss of time, and such inconveniences, which are ordinary concomitants; [2] *for, when once they have got a haunt of such companies, and habit of gaming, they can hardly be drawn from it; but, as an itch, it will tickle them; and, as it is with whoremasters, once entered, they cannot easily leave it off: vexat mentes insana cupido,* they are mad upon their sport. And in conclusion (which Charles the Seventh, that good French king, published in an edict against gamesters) *unde piæ et hilaris vitæ suffugium sibi suisque liberis, totique familiæ, &c.* that which was once their livelihood, should have maintained wife, children, family, is now spent and gone; *mœror et egestas,* &c. sorrow and beggery succeeds. So good things may be abused; and that which was first invented to [3] refresh mens weary spirits when they come from other labours and studies, to exhilarate the minde, to entertain time and company, tedious otherwise in those long solitary winter nights, and keep them from worse matters, an honest exercise, is contrarily perverted.

Chesse-play is a good and witty exercise of the mind, for some kinde of men, and fit for such melancholy (Rhasis holds) as are idle, and have extravagant impertinent thoughts, or troubled with cares; nothing better to distract their mind, and alter their meditations; invented (some say) by the [4] generall of an army in a famine, to keep souldiers from mutiny: but

---

[1] Abusus tam frequens hodie in Europâ, ut plerique crebro harum usu patrimonium profundant, exhaustisque facultatibus, ad inopiam redigantur. [2] Ubi semel prurigo ista animum occupat, ægre discuti potest; solicitantibus undique ejusdem farinæ hominibus, damnosas illas voluptates repetunt; quod et scortatoribus insitum, &c. [3] Instituitur ista exercitatio, non lucri, sed valetudinis et oblectamenti ratione, et quo animus defatigatus respiret, novasque vires ad subeundos labores denuo concipiat. [4] Latrunculorum ludus inventus est a duce, ut, cum miles intolerabili fame laboraret, altero die edens, altero ludens, famis oblivisceretur. Bellonius. See more of this game in Daniel Souters Palamedes, vel de variis ludis, l. 3.

538   *Cure of Melancholy.*   [Part. 2. Sec. 2.

if it proceed from over much study, in such a case it may do
more harm than good; it is a game too troublesome for some
mens braines, too full of anxiety, all out as bad as study; besides, it is a testy cholerick game, and very offensive to him
that loseth the mate. [1] William the Conqueror, in his younger
yeares, playing at chesse with the prince of France, (Dauphine
was not annexed to that crown in those dayes) losing a mate,
knocked the chesse-board about his pate, which was a cause
afterward of much enmity betwixt them.   For some such reason it is, belike, that Patritius (in his 3. book, *Tit.* 12. *de reg.
instit.*) forbids his prince to play at chesse : hawking and hunting, riding, &c. he will allow; and this to other men, but by
no means to him.   In Muscovy, where they live in stoves and
hot houses all winter long, come seldome or little abroad, it is
again very necessary, and therefore in those parts (saith [2] Herbastein) much used.   At Fessa in Africk, where the like inconvenience of keeping within doors is through heat, it is very
laudable; and (as [3] Leo Afer relates) as much frequented : a
sport fit for idle gentlemen, souldiers in garrison, and courtiers
that have nought but love matters to busie themselves about,
but not altogether so convenient for such as are students.
The like I may say of Cl. Bruxers philosophy game, D. Fulkes
Metromachia and his *Ouranomachia*, with the rest of those
intricate astrologicall and geometricall fictions, for such especially as are mathematically given : and the rest of those curious games.

Dancing, singing, masking, mumming, stage-plaies, howsoever they be heavily censured by some severe Catoes, yet, if
opportunely and soberly used, may justly be approved. *Melius
est fodere, quam saltare,* saith Austin : but what is that, if
they delight in it? [4] *Nemo saltat sobrius.*   But in what kinde
of dance?   I know these sports have many oppugners, whole
volumes writ against them; when as all they say (if duly considered) is but *ignoratio elenchi;* and some again, because
they are now cold and wayward, past themselves, cavel at all
such youthfull sports in others, as he did in the comedy ; they
think them, *illico nasci senes, &c.*   Some, out of præposterous
zeal, object many times triviall arguments, and, because of some
abuse, will quite take away the good use, as if they should
forbid wine, because it makes men drunk; but, in my judgement, they are too stern : there *is a time for all things, a
time to mourne, a time to dance* (Eccles. 3. 4); *a time to
embrace, a time not to embrace* (vers. 5); *and nothing better
than that a man should rejoyce in his own works* (vers. 22).

---

[1] D. Hayward, in vitâ ejus.   [2] Muscovit. commentarium.   [3] Inter cives
Fessanos latrunculorum ludus est usitatissimus. lib. 3. de Africâ.   [4] Tullius.

Mem. 4.]   *Exercise rectified.*   539

For my part, I will subscribe to the *kings declaration*, and
was ever of that mind, those May-games, wakes, and Whit-
sonales, &c. if they be not at unseasonable hours, may justly
be permitted. Let them freely feast, sing, and dance, have their
poppet-playes, hobby-horses, tabers, crouds, bag-pipes, &c.
play at ball, and barley-breaks, and what sports and recreations they like best. In Franconia, a province of Germany,
(saith [1] Aubanus Bohemus) the old folks, after evening prayer,
went to the ale-house, the younger sort to dance : and, to say
truth with [2] Sarisburiensis, *satius fuerat sic otiari, quam turpius
occupari*, better do so than worse, as without question otherwise (such is the corruption of mans nature) many of them
will do. For that cause, playes, masks, jesters, gladiators,
tumblers, juglers, &c. and all that crew is admitted and winked
at : [3] *tota jocularium scena procedit, et ideo spectacula admissa
sunt, et infinita tyrocinia vanitatum, ut his occupentur, qui per-
niciosius otiari solent :* that they might be busied about such
toyes, that would otherwise more perniciously be idle. So that,
as [4] Tacitus said of the astrologers in Rome, we may say of
them, *genus hominum est, quod in civitate nostrâ et vitabitur
semper et retinebitur;* they are a deboshed company, most
part, still spoken against, as well they deserve some of them,
(for I so relish and distinguish them as fidlers, and musicians)
and yet ever retained. *Evil is not to be done* (I confess), that
good may come of it : but this is evil *per accidens*, and, in a
qualified sense, to avoide a greater inconvenience, may justly be
tolerated. S[r] Thomas More, in his Utopian Commonwealth,
[5] *as he will have none idle, so will he have no man labour over
hard, to be toiled out like an horse : 'tis more than slavish
infelicity, the life of most of our hired servants, and tradesmen
elsewhere* (excepting his Utopians): *but half the day allotted for
work, and half for honest recreation, or whatsover imployment
they shall think fit themselves.* If one half-day in a week were
allowed to our household servants for their merry meetings, by
their hard masters, or in a year some feasts, like those Roman
Saturnals, I think they would labour harder all the rest of their
time, and both parties be better pleased: but this needs not
(you will say); for some of them do nought but loyter all the
week long.

This, which I aim at, is for such as are *fracti animis*,
troubled in mind, to ease them, over-toiled on the one part,

---

[1] De mor. gent.   [2] Polycrat. l. 1. cap. 8.   [3] Idem Sarisburiensis.
[4] Hist. lib. 1.   [5] Nemo desidet otiosus; ita nemo asinino more ad seram noctem
laborat; nam ea plusquam servilis ærumna, quæ opificum vita est, exceptis Uto-
piensibus, qui diem in 24 horas dividunt, 12 duntaxat operi deputant, reliquum
somno et cibo cujusque arbitrio permittitur.

8

540   *Cure of Melancholy.*   [Part. 2. Sec. 2.

to refresh : over idle on the other, to keep themselves busied.
And to this purpose, as any labour or imployment will serve
to the one, any honest recreation will conduce to the other, so
that it be moderate and sparing, as the use of meat and drink ;
not to spend all their life in gaming, playing, and pastimes, as
too many gentlemen do ; but to revive our bodies and recreate
our souls with honest sports : of which as there be divers sorts,
and peculiar to severall callings, ages, sexes, conditions, so
there be proper for severall seasons, and those of distinct natures, to fit that variety of humors which is amongst them, that
if one will not, another may : some in summer, some in winter ;
some gentle, some more violent ; some for the mind alone,
some for the body and mind : (as, to some it is both business
and a pleasant recreation to oversee workmen of all sorts,
husbandry, cattle, horse, &c. to build, plot, project, to make
models, cast up accompts, &c.) some without, some within
doors : new, old, &c. as the season serveth, and as men are
inclined. It is reported of Philippus Bonus, that good duke of
Burgundy, (by Lodovicus Vives, in *Epist.* and Pont. [1] Heuter
in his history) that the said duke, at the marriage of Eleonora,
sister to the king of Portugal, at Bruges in Flanders, which
was solemnized in the deep of winter, when as by reason of
unseasonable weather he could neither hawk nor hunt, and
was now tired with cards, dice, &c. and such other domestical
sports, or to see ladies dance, with some of his courtiers, he
would in the evening walk disguised all about the town. It so
fortuned as he was walking late one night, he found a country
fellow dead drunk, snorting on a bulk : [2] he caused his followers to bring him to his palace, and there stripping him of
his old cloaths, and attiring him after the court fashion, when
he waked, he and they were all ready to attend upon his excellency, perswading him he was some great duke. The poor
fellow, admiring how he came there, was served in state all
the day long ; after supper he saw them dance, heard musick,
and the rest of those court-like pleasures : but late at night,
when he was well tipled, and again fast asleep, they put on his
old robes, and so conveighed him to the place where they first
found him. Now the fellow had not made them so good sport
the day before, as he did when he returned to himself: all the
jest was, to see how he [3] looked upon it. In conclusion, after
some little admiration, the poor man told his friends he had
seen a vision, constantly believed it, would not otherwise be

---

[1] Rerum Burgund. lib. 4.   [2] Jussit hominem deferri ad palatium, et lecto
ducali collocari, &c. Mirari homo, ubi se eo loci videt.   [3] Quid interest, inquit Lodovicus Vives, (epist. ad Francisc. Barducem) inter diem illius et nostros
aliquot annos ? nihil penitus, nisi quod, &c.

persuaded; and so the jest ended. [1] Antiochus Epiphanes would often disguise himself, steal from his court, and go into merchants, goldsmiths, and other tradesmens shops, sit and talk with them, and sometimes ride or walk alone, and fall aboord with any tinker, clowne, serving man, carrier, or whomsover he met first. Sometimes he did *ex insperato* give a poor fellow money, to see how he would look, or on set purpose lose his purse as he went, to watch who found it, and withall how he would be affected; and with such objects he was much delighted. Many such tricks are ordinarily put in practice by great men, to exhilarate themselves and others; all which are harmless jests, and have their good uses.

But, amongst those exercises, or recreations of the minde within doors, there is none so generall, so aptly to be applyed to all sorts of men, so fit and proper to expell idleness and melancholy, as that of study. *Studia senectutem oblectant, adolescentiam alunt, secundas res ornant, adversis perfugium et solatium præbent, domi delectant, &c.* find the rest in Tully *pro Archiâ Poëtâ.* What so full of content, as to read, walke, and see mappes, pictures, statues, jewels, marbles, which some so much magnifie, as those that Phidias made of old, so exquisite and pleasing to be beheld, that (as [2] Chrysostome thinketh) *if any man be sickly, troubled in minde, or that cannot sleep for griefe, and shall but stand over against one of Phidias images, he will forget all care, or whatsoever else may molest him, in an instant?* There be those as much taken with Michael Angelos, Raphael d'Urbinos, Francesco Francias pieces, and many of those Italian and Dutch painters, which were excellent in their ages; and esteem of it as a most pleasing sight, to view those neat architectures, devices, scutchions, coats of armes, read such bookes, to peruse old coynes of severall sorts in a fair gallery; artificiall works, perspective glasses, old reliques, Roman antiquities, variety of colours. A good picture is *falsa veritas, et muta poësis:* and though (as [3] Vives saith) *artificialia delectant, sed mox fastidimus,* artificiall toyes please but for a time: yet who is he that will not be moved with them for the present? When Achilles was tormented and sad for the loss of his dear friend Patroclus, his mother Thetis brought him a most elaborate and curious buckler made by Vulcan, in which were engraven sun, moon, stars, planets, sea, land, men fighting, running, riding, women scolding, hils, dales, townes, castles, brooks, rivers, trees,

[1] Hen. Stephan. præfat. Herodoti. [2] Orat. 12. Siquis animo fuerit afflictus aut æger, nec somnum admittens, is mihi videtur, e regione stans talis imaginis, oblivisci omnium posse, quæ humanæ vitæ atrocia et difficilia accidere solent. [3] 3. De animâ.

542   *Cure of Melancholy.*   [Part. 2. Sec. 2.

&c. with many pretty landskips, and perspective pieces; with sight of which he was infinitely delighted, and much eased of his grief.

> [1] Continuo eo spectaculo captus, delenito mœrore,
> Oblectabatur, in manibus tenens Dei splendida dona.

Who will not be affected so in like case, or to see those wel-furnished cloisters and galleries of the Roman cardinals, so richly stored with all modern pictures, old statues and antiquities? *Cum se spectando recreet simul et legendo,* to see their pictures alone, and read the description, as [2] Boissardus well addes, whom will it not affect? which Bozius, Pomponius Lætus, Marlianus, Schottus, Cavelerius, Ligorius, &c. and he himself hath well performed of late. Or in some princes cabinets, like that of the great dukes in Florence, of Felix Platerus in Brasil, or noblemens houses, to see such variety of attires, faces, so many, so rare, and such exquisite peeces, of men, birds, beasts, &c. to see those excellent landskips, Dutch-works, and curious cuts of Sadlier of Prague, Albertus Durer, Goltzius, Urintes, &c. such pleasant peeces of perspective, Indian pictures made of feathers, China works, frames, thaumaturgical motions, exotick toyes, &c. Who is he that is now wholly overcome with idleness, or otherwise involved in a labyrinth of worldly cares, troubles, and discontents, that will not be much lightned in his mind by reading of some inticing story, true or fained, where, as in a glass, he shall observe what our forefathers have done, the beginnings, ruins, fals, periods of common-wealths, private mens actions displayed to the life, &c.? [3] Plutarch therefore cals them *secundas mensas et bellaria,* the second course and junkets, because they were usually read at noblemens feasts. Who is not earnestly affected with a passionate speech, well penned, an elegant poem, or some pleasant betwitching discourse, like that of [4] Heliodorus, *ubi oblectatio quædam placide fluit, cum hilaritate conjuncta?* Julian the Apostate was so taken with an oration of Libanius the sophister, that, as he confesseth, he could not be quiet till he had read it all out. *Legi orationem tuam magná ex parte, hesterná die ante prandium: pransus vero sine ullá intermissione totam absolvi. O argumenta! O compositionem!* I may say the same of this or that pleasing tract, which will draw his attention along with it. To most kind of men it is an extraordinary delight to study. For what a world of books offers itself, in all subjects, arts, and

[1] Iliad. 19.   [2] Topogr. Rom. part. 1.   [3] Quod heroum conviviis legi solitæ.   [4] Melancthon, de Heliodoro.

Mem. 4.] *Exercise rectified.* 543

sciences, to the sweet content and capacity of the reader? In arithmetick, geometry, perspective, optick, astronomy, architecture, *sculpturâ, picturâ*, of which so many and such elaborate treatises are of late written : in mechanicks and their mysteries, military matters, navigation, [1] riding of horses, [2] fencing, swimming, gardening, planting, great tomes of husbandry, cookery, faulconry, hunting, fishing, fowling, &c. with exquisite pictures of all sports, games, and what not? In musick, metaphysicks, natural and moral philosophy, philologie, in policy, heraldry, genealogy, chronology, &c. they afford great tomes, or those studies of [3] antiquity, &c. *et* [4] *quid subtilius arithmeticis inventionibus? quid jucundius musicis rationibus? quid divinius astronomicis? quid rectius geometricis demonstrationibus?* What so sure, what so pleasant? He that shall but see that geometrical tower of Garezenda at Bologne in Italy, the steeple and clock at Strasborough, will admire the effects of art, or that engine of Archimedes to remove the earth itself, if he had but a place to fasten his instrument; *Archimedis cochlea*, and rare devises to corrivate waters, musick instruments, and trisyllable echoes again, again, and again repeated, with miriades of such. What vast tomes are extant in law, physick, and divinity, for profit, pleasure, practice, speculation, in verse or prose, &c.? their names alone are the subject of whole volumes : we have thousands of authors of all sorts, many great libraries full well furnished, like so many dishes of meat, served out for several palates ; and he is a very block that is affected with none of them. Some take an infinite delight to study the very languages wherein these books are written, Hebrew, Greek, Syriack, Chalde, Arabick, &c. Me thinks it would well please any man to look upon a geographical map, ([5] *suavi animum delectatione allicere, ob incredibilem rerum varietatem et jucunditatem, et ad pleniorem sui cognitionem excitare*) chorographical, topographical delineations; to behold, as it were, all the remote provinces, townes, cities of the world, and never to go forth of the limits of his study ; to measure, by the scale and compasse, their extent, distance, examine their site. Charles the great (as Platina writes) had three faire silver tables, in one of which superficies was a large map of Constantinople, in the second Rome neatly engraved, in the third an exquisite description of the whole world ; and much delight he took in them. What greater pleasure can there now be,

---

[1] Pluvines. [2] Thibault. [3] As, in travelling, the rest go forward and look before them, an antiquary alone looks round about him, seeing things past, &c. hath a compleat horizon, Janus Bifrons. [4] Cardan. [5] Hondius, præfat. Mercatoris.

544   *Cure of Melancholy.*   [Part. 2. Sec. 2.

than to view those elaborate maps of Ortelius, [1] Mercator,
Hondius, &c. to peruse those books of cities, put out by
Braunus, and Hogenbergius? to read those exquisite descrip-
tions of Maginus, Munster, Herrera, Laet, Merula, Boterus,
Leander Albertus, Camden, Leo Afer, Adricomius, Nic. Gerbelius, &c.? those famous expeditions of Christoph. Columbus, Americus Vesputius, Marcus Polus the Venetian, Lod.
Vertomannus, Aloysius Cadamustus, &c.? those accurate
diaries of Portugals, Hollanders, of Bartison, Oliver a Nort,
&c. Hacluits voyages, Pet. Martyrs Decades, Benzo, Lerius,
Linschotens relations, those Hodœporicons of Jod. a Meggen,
Brocarde the monke, Bredenbachius, Jo. Dublinius, Sands,
&c. to Jerusalem, Egypt, and other remote places of the
world? those pleasant itineraries of Paulus Hentzerus, Jodocus Sincerus, Dux Polonus, &c. to read Bellonius observations, P. Gillius his survayes; those parts of America, set out,
and curiously cut in pictures, by Fratres a Bry. To see a well
cut herbal, hearbs, trees, flowers, plants, all vegetals, expressed in their proper colours to the life, as that of Matthiolus
upon Dioscorides, Delacampius, Lobel, Bauhinus, and that
last voluminous and mighty herbal of Besler of Noremberge,
wherein almost every plant is to his own bignesse. To see
birds, beasts, and fishes of the sea, spiders, gnats, serpents,
flies, &c. all creatures set out by the same art, and truly expressed in lively colours, with an exact description of their
natures, vertues, qualities, &c. as hath been accurately performed by Ælian, Gesner, Ulysses Aldrovandus, Bellonius,
Rondoletius, Hippolytus Salvianus, &c. [2] *Arcana cœli, naturæ secreta, ordinem universi scire, majoris felicitatis et
dulcedinis est, quam cogitatione quis assequi possit, aut mortalis sperare.* What more pleasing studies can there be, than
the mathematicks, theorick, or practick parts? as to survay
land, make maps, models, dials, &c. with which I was ever
much delighted my self. *Talis est mathematum pulchritudo,*
saith [3] Plutarch) *ut his indignum sit divitiarum phaleras
istas et bullas et puellaria spectacula comparari;* such is the
excellency of these studies, that all those ornaments and
childish bubbles of wealth are not worthy to be compared to
them: *crede mihi,* ([4] saith one) *exstingui dulce erit mathema-
ticarum artium studio;* I could even live and die with such
meditations, [5] and take more delight, true content of mind in
them, than thou hast in all thy wealth and sport, how rich
soever thou art. And, as [6] Cardan well seconds me, *honorificum*

---

[1] Atlas Geog.   [2] Cardan.   [3] Lib. de cupid. divitiarum.   [4] Leon.
Diggs, præfat. ad perpet. prognost.   [5] Plus capio voluptatis, &c.   [6] In
Hyperchen. divis. 3.

Mem. 4.]   *Exercise rectified.*   545

*magis est et gloriosum hæc intelligere, quam provinciis præ-
esse, formosum aut ditem juvenem esse.* The like pleasure
there is in all other studies, to such as are truly addicted to
them: [1]*ea suavitas,* (one holds) *ut, cum quis ea degusta-
verit, quasi poculis Circeis captus, non possit unquam ab illis
divelli;* the like sweetnesse, which, as Circes cup, bewitcheth
a student, he cannot leave off, as well may witnesse those
many laborious houres, dayes, and nights, spent in the voluminous treatises written by them; the same content. [2] Julius
Scaliger was so much affected with poetry, that he brake out
into a pathetical protestation, he had rather be the author of
12 verses in Lucian, or such an ode in [3] Horace, than emperour of Germany. [4] Nicholas Gerbelius, that good old man,
was so much ravished with a few Greek authors restored
to light, with hope and desire of enjoying the rest, that he
exclaims forthwith, *Arabibus atque Indis omnibus erimus
ditiores,* we shall be richer than all the Arabick or Indian
princes ; of such [5] esteem they were with him, incomparable
worth and value.   Seneca prefers Zeno and Chrysippus, two
doting Stoicks, (he was so much enamoured on their works)
before any prince or general of an army ; and Orontius the
mathematician so far admires Archimedes, that he cals him,
divinum et homine majorem, a petty god, more than a man ;
and well he might, for ought I see, if you respect fame or
worth.   Pindarus of Thebes is as much renowned for his
poems, as Epaminondas, Pelopidas, Hercules, or Bacchus, his
fellow citizens, for their warlike actions: *et si famam respi-
cias, non pauciores Aristotelis quam Alexandri meminerunt :*
(as Cardan notes) Aristotle is more known than Alexander ;
for we have a bare relation of Alexanders deeds; but Aristotle
totus vivit in monumentis, is whole in his works: yet I
stand not upon this; the delight is it, which I aim at; so
great pleasure, such sweet content there is in study. [6] King
James, 1605, when he came to see our university of Oxford,
and, amongst other ædifices, now went to view that famous library, renewed by S[r]. Thomas Bodley, in imitation of Alexander, at his departure brake out into that noble speech, If I
were not a king, I would be a university man: [7] *and if it were
so that I must be a prisoner, if I might have my wish, I would
desire to have no other prison than that library, and to be
chained together with so many good authors, et mortuis ma-*

---

[1] Cardan. præfat. rerum variet.   [2] Poëtices lib.   [3] Lib. 3. Ode 9.
Donec gratus eram tibi, &c.   [4] De Peloponnes. lib. 6. descrip. Græc.   [5] Quos
si integros haberemus, Dii boni ! quas opes, quos thesauros teneremus !   [6] Isaack
Wake, musæ regnantes.   [7] Si unquam mihi in fatis sit, ut captivus ducar, si
mihi daretur optio, hoc cuperem carcere concludi, his catenis illigari, cum hisce
captivis concatenatus ætatem agere.

VOL. I.   N N

546 *Cure of Melancholy.* [Part. 2. Sec. 2.

gistris. So sweet is the delight of study, the more learning they have, (as he that hath a dropsie, the more he drinks, the thirstier he is) the more they covet to learn; and the last day is *prioris discipulus;* harsh at first learning is; *radices amaræ,* but *fructus dulces,* according to that of Isocrates, pleasant at last; the longer they live, the more they are enamoured with the Muses. Heinsius, the keeper of the library at Leiden in Holland, was mewed up in it all the year long; and that which to thy thinking should have bred a loathing, caused in him a greater liking. [1] *I no sooner* (saith he) *come into the library, but I bolt the door to me, excluding lust, ambition, avarice, and all such vices, whose nurse is Idlenesse the mother of Ignorance, and Melancholy her self; and in the very lap of eternity, amongst so many divine souls, I take my seat, with so lofty a spirit and sweet content, that I pitty all our great ones, and rich men, that know not this happinesse.* I am not ignorant in the mean time (notwithstanding this which I have said) how barbarously and basely for the most part our ruder gentry esteem of libraries and books, how they neglect and contemn so great a treasure, so inestimable a benefit, as Æsops cock did the jewel he found in the dunghil; and all through error, ignorance, and want of education. And 'tis a wonder withal to observe how much they will vainly cast away in unnecessary expences, *quot modis pereant* (saith [2] Erasmus) *magnatibus pecuniæ, quantum absumant alea, scorta, compotationes, profectiones non necessariæ, pompæ, bella quæsita, ambitio, colax, morio, ludio, &c.* what in hawkes, hounds, lawsuits, vain building, gurmundizing, drinking, sports, playes, pastimes, &c. If a well-minded man to the Muses would sue to some of them for an exhibition, to the farther maintenance or inlargement of such a work, be it college, lecture, library, or whatsoever else may tend to the advancement of learning, they are so unwilling, so averse, they had rather see these which are already with such cost and care erected, utterly ruined, demolished, or otherwise employed; for they repine, many, and grudge at such gifts and revenews so bestowed: and therefore it were in vain, as Erasmus well notes, *vel ab his, vel a negotiatoribus qui se Mammonæ dediderunt, improbum fortasse tale officium exigere,* to solicite or aske any thing of such men (that are, likely, damn'd to riches) to this purpose. For my part, I pity these men; *stultos jubeo esse libenter;* let

---

[1] Epist. Primiero. Plerumque in quâ simul ac pedem posui, foribus pessulum abdo; ambitionem autem, amorem, libidinem, &c. excludo, quorum parens est ignavia, imperitia nutrix; et in ipso æternitatis gremio, inter tot illustres animas sedem mihi sumo, cum ingenti quidem animo, ut subinde magnatum me misereat, qui felicitatem hanc ignorant.   [2] Chil. 2. Cent. 1. adag. 1.

Mem. 4.]   *Exercise rectified.*   547

them go as they are, in the catalogue of Ignoramus. How
much, on the other side, are we all bound, that are schollers,
to those munificent Ptolemies, bountifull Mæcenates, heroi-
call patrons, divine spirits, ———— [1] *qui nobis hæc otia fe-*
cerunt: namque erit ille mihi semper Deus ———— that have
provided for us so many well furnished libraries, as well in
our publike academies in most cities, as in our private colleges?
How shall I remember [2] S[r]. Thomas Bodley, amongst the rest,
[3] Otho Nicholson, and the right reverend John Williams lord
bishop of Lincolne, (with many other pious acts) who, besides
that at S[t]. Johns college in Cambridge, that in Westminster,
is now likewise in *fieri* with a library at Lincolne (a noble
president for all corporate towns and cities to imitate) *O quam*
te memorem, vir illustrissime? quibus elogiis? but to my taske
again.

Whosoever he is, therefore, that is overrun with solitariness,
or carried away with pleasing melancholy and vain conceits,
and for want of imployment knows not how to spend his
time, or crucified with worldly care, I can prescribe him no
better remedy than this of study, to compose himself to the
learning of some art or science; provided alwayes that his
malady proceed not from overmuch study; for in such cases
he addes fuell to the fire; and nothing can be more pernicious.
Let him take heed he do not overstretch his wits, and make a
skeleton of himself; or such inamoratoes as read nothing but
play-books, idle poems, jests, Amadis de Gaul, the Knight of
the Sun, the Seven Champions, Palmerin de Oliva, Huon of
Burdeaux, &c. Such many times prove in the end as mad
as Don Quixot. Study is only prescribed to those that are
otherwise idle, troubled in minde, or carried headlong with vain
thoughts and imaginations, to distract their cogitations, (although variety of study, or some serious subject, would do
the former no harm) and divert their continuall meditations
another way. Nothing in this case better than study; *semper*
aliquid memoriter ediscant, saith Piso; let them learn something without book, transcribe, translate, &c. read the scriptures, which Hyperius (*lib.* 1. *de quotid. script. lec. fol.* 77)
holds available of it self: [4] *the mind is erected thereby from*
all worldly cares, and hath much quiet and tranquillity: for,
as [5] Austin well hath it, 'tis *scientia scientiarum, omni melle*
dulcior, omni pane suavior, omni vino hilarior: 'tis the best
nepenthes, surest cordiall, sweetest alterative, present'st di-

---

[1] Virg. eclog. 1.   [2] Founder of our publike library in Oxon.   [3] Ours
in Christ-church, Oxon.   [4] Animus levatur inde a curis, multâ quiete et
tranquillitate fruens.   [5] Ser. 38. ad Fratres Erem.

548   *Cure of Melancholy.*   [Part. 2. Sec. 2.

verter: for neither, as [1] Chrysostome well adds, *those boughs and leaves of trees which are plashed for cattle to stand under, in the heat of the day, in summer, so much refresh them with their acceptable shade, as the reading of the scripture doth recreate and comfort a distressed soul, in sorrow and affliction.* Paul bids *pray continually; quod cibus corpori, lectio animæ facit,* saith Seneca; as meat is to the body, such is reading to the soul. [2] *To be at leasure without books is another hell, and to be buried alive.* [3] Cardan cals a library the physick of the soul; [4] *divine authors fortifie the mind, make men bold and constant; and* (as Hyperius adds) *godly conference will not permit the mind to be tortured with absurd cogitations.* Rhasis injoynes continuall conference to such melancholy men, perpetuall discourse of some history, tale, poem, news, &c. *alternos sermones edere ac bibere, æque jucundum quam cibus, sive potus,* which feeds the minde, as meat and drink doth the body, and pleaseth as much: and therefore the said Rhasis, not without good cause, would have some body still talke seriously, or dispute with them, and sometimes [5] *to cavil and wrangle* (so that it break not out to a violent perturbation); *for such altercation is like stirring of a dead fire, to make it burn afresh;* it whets a dull spirit, *and will not suffer the minde to be drowned in those profound cogitations, which melancholy men are commonly troubled with.* [6] Ferdinand and Alphonsus, kings of Arragon and Sicily, were both cured by reading the history, one of Curtius, the other of Livy, when no prescribed physick would take place. [7] Camerarius relates as much of Laurence Medices. Heathen philosophers are so full of divine precepts in this kind, that, as some think, they alone are able to settle a distressed mind—

     [8] Sunt verba et voces, quibus hunc lenire dolorem, &c.

Epictetus, Plutarch, and Seneca. *Qualis ille! quæ tela,* saith Lipsius, *adversus omnes animi casus, administrat, et ipsam mortem! quomodo vitia eripit, infert virtutes!* when I read Seneca, [9] *me thinks I am beyond all humane fortunes, on the top of an hill above mortalitie.* Plutarch saith as much of

---

[1] Hom. 4. de pœnitentiâ. Nam neque arborum comæ, pro pecorum tuguriis fractæ, meridie per æstatem optabilem exhibentes umbram, oves ita reficiunt, ac scripturarum lectio afflictas angore animas solatur et recreat. [2] Otium sine literis mors est, et vivi hominis sepultura. Seneca. [3] Cap. 99. l. 57. de rer. var. [4] Fortem reddunt animum et constantem; et pium colloquium non permittit animum absurdâ cogitatione torqueri. [5] Altercationibus utantur, quæ non permittunt animum submergi profundis cogitationibus, de quibus otiose cogitat, et tristatur in iis. [6] Bodin. præfat. ad meth. hist. [7] Operum subcis. cap. 15. [8] Hor. [9] Fatendum est, cacumine Olympi constitutus mihi videor, supra ventos et procellas, et omnes res humanas.

Homer; for which cause, belike, Niceratus, in Xenophon, was made by his parents to con Homers Iliads and Odysses without book, *ut in virum bonum evaderet,* as well to make him a good and honest man, as to avoid idleness. If this comfort may be got by philosophy, what shall be had from divinity? What shall Austin, Cyprian, Gregory, Bernards divine meditations, afford us?

> Qui, quid sit pulchrum, quid turpe, quid utile, quid non,
> Plenius et melius Chrysippo et Crantore dicunt.

Nay what shall the scripture it self, which is like an apothecaries shop, wherein are all remedies for all infirmities of minde, purgatives, cordials, alteratives, corroboratives, lenitives, &c.? *Every disease of the soul,* saith [1] Austin, *hath a peculiar medicine in the scripture; this onely is required, that the sick man take the potion which God hath already tempered.* [2] Gregory calls it *a glass wherein we may see all our infirmities; ignitum colloquium,* Psalm 119, 140; [3] Origen, a charme. And therefore Hierome prescribes Rusticus the monke, [4] *continually to read the scripture, and to meditate on that which he hath read; for, as mastication is to meat, so is meditation on that which we read.* I would, for these causes, wish him that is melancholy, to use both humane and divine authors, voluntarily to impose some taske upon himself, to divert his melancholy thoughts; to study the art of memory, Cosmus Rosselius, Pet. Ravennas, Scenkelius detectus, or practise brachygraphy, &c. that will ask a great deale of attention: or let him demonstrate a proposition in Euclide in his five last books, extract a square root, or studie algebra; than which, as [5] Clavius holds, *in all humane disciplines, nothing can be more excellent and pleasant, so abstruse and recondite, so bewitching, so miraculous, so ravishing, so easie withall, and full of delight, omnem humanum captum superare videtur.* By this means you may define *ex ungue leonem,* as the diverbe is, by his thumb alone the bigness of Hercules, or the true dimensions of the great [6] Colossus, Solomons temple, and Domitians amphitheater, out of a little part. By this art you may contemplate the variation of the 23 letters, which may be so infinitely varied, that the words complicated and deduced thence will not be contained within the compass of the firma-

---

[1] In Ps. 36. Omnis morbus animi in scripturâ habet medicinam; tantum opus est, ut qui sit æger, non recuset potionem quam Deus temperavit. [2] In moral. speculum quo nos intueri possimus. [3] Hom. 28. Ut incantatione virus fugatur, ita lectione malum. [4] Iterum atque iterum moneo, ut animam sacræ scripturæ lectione occupes. Masticat divinum pabulum meditatio. [5] Ad. 2. definit. 2. elem. In disciplinis humanis nihil præstantius reperitur: quippe miracula quædam numerorum eruit tam abstrusa et recondita, tantâ nihilominus facilitate et voluptate, ut, &c. [6] Which contained 1080000 weight of brass.

550   *Cure of Melancholy.*   [Part. 2. Sec. 2.

ment; ten words may be varied 40320 severall wayes: by this art you may examine how many men may stand one by another in the whole superficies of the earth: some say 148456800000000, *assignando singulis passum quadratum;* how many men, supposing all the world as habitable as France, as fruitfull, and so long lived, may be born in 60000 years; and so may you demonstrate, with [1] Archimedes, how many sands the mass of the whole world might contain, if all sandy, if you did but first know how much a small cube as big as a mustard-seed might hold; with infinite such. But, in all nature, what is there so stupend as to examine and calculate the motion of the planets, their magnitudes, apogeums, perigeums, excentricities, how far distant from the earth, the bigness, thickness, compass of the firmament, each star, with their diameters and circumference, apparent *area, superficies,* by those curious helps of glasses, astrolabes, sextants, quadrants, of which Tycho Brahe in his mechanicks, opticks ([2] divine opticks), arithmetick, geometry, and such like arts and instruments? What so intricate, and pleasing withall, as to peruse and practise Heron Alexandrinus works, *de spiritalibus, de machinis bellicis, de machinâ se movente, Jordani Nemorarii de ponderibus proposit.* 13. that pleasant tract of Machometes Bragdedinus *de superficierum divisionibus,* Apollonius Conicks, or Commandinus labours in that kinde, *de centro gravitatis,* with many such geometricall theorems, and problems? Those rare instruments and mechanical inventions of Jac. Bessonus, and Cardan to this purpose, with many such experiments intimated long since by Roger Bacon in his tract *de* [3] *Secretis artis et naturæ,* as to make a chariot to move *sine animali,* diving boats, to walk on the water by art, and to fly in the air, to make several cranes and pullies, *quibus homo trahat ad se mille homines,* lift up and remove great weights, mils to move themselves, Archytas dove, Albertus brasen head, and such thaumaturgical works; but especially to do strange miracles by glasses, of which Proclus and Bacon writ of old, burning glasses, multiplying glasses, perspectives, *ut unus homo appareat exercitus,* to see afar off, to represent solid bodies, by cylinders and concaves, to walk in the air, *ut veraciter videant* (saith Bacon) *aurum et argentum, et quicquid aliud volunt, et, quum veniant ad locum visionis, nihil inveniant,* which glasses are much perfected of late by Baptista Porta and Galileus, and much more is promised by Maginus and Midorgius, to be performed in this kinde. Otacousticons some speak of, to intend hearing, as the other do sight; Marcellus Vrencken, an Hollander, in his epistle to Burgravius, makes mention of a friend of his that is about an

---

[1] Vide Clavium, in com. de Sacrobosco.   [2] Distantias cœlorum sola optica dijudicat.   [3] Cap. 4 et 5.

Mem. 4.] *Exercise rectified.* 551

instrument, *quo videbit quæ in altero horizonte sint.* But our alchymists, methinks, and Rosie-cross men afford most rarities, and are fuller of experiments: they can make gold, separate and alter metals, extract oyls, salts, lees, and do more strange works than Geber, Lullius, Bacon, or any of those ancients. Crollius hath made, after his master Paracelsus, *aurum fulminans,* or *aurum volatile,* which shall imitate thunder and lightning, and crack lowder than any gunpowder; Cornelius Drible a perpetual motion, inextinguible lights, *linum non ardens,* with many such feats: see his book *de naturâ elementorum,* besides hail, wind, snow, thunder, lightning, &c. those strange fire-works, devilish petards, and such like warlike machinations derived hence, of which read Tartalea and others. Ernestus Burgravius, a disciple of Paracelsus, hath published a discourse, in which he specifies a lamp to be made of mans blood, *lucerna vitæ et mortis index,* so he terms it, which, chymically prepared 40 dayes, and afterward kept in a glass, shall shew all the accidents of this life; *si lampas hic clarus, tunc homo hilaris et sanus corpore et animo; si nebulosus et depressus, male afficitur; et sic pro statu hominis variatur, unde sumptus sanguis;* and, which is most wonderful, it dies with the party; *cum homine perit, et evanescit;* the lamp, and the man whence the blood was taken, are extinguished together. The same author hath another tract of Mumia (all out as vain and prodigious as the first) by which he will cure most diseases, and transfer them from a man to a beast, by drawing blood from one, and applying it to the other, *vel in plantam derivare,* and an *alexipharmacum* (of which Roger Bacon of old, in his *Tract. de retardandâ senectute*) to make a man young again, live three or foure hundred years: besides panaceas, martial amulets, *unguentum armarium,* balsomes, strange extracts, elixars, and such like magico-magnetical cures. Now what so pleasing can there be as the speculation of these things, to read and examine such experiments; or, if a man be more mathematically given, to calculate, or peruse Napiers Logarithmes, or those tables of artificiall [1] sines and tangents, not long since set out by mine old collegiate good friend, and late fellow student of Christ-church in Oxford, [2] M[r]. Edmund Gunter, which will perform that by addition and subtraction only, which heretofore Regiomontanus tables did by multiplication and division, or those elaborate conclusions of his [3] sector, quadrant, and crossestaffe? Or let him that is melancholy calculate spherical triangles, square a circle, cast a nativity, which howsoever some taxe, I say with [4] Garcæus, *dabimus hoc petulantibus ingeniis,* we will in some cases allow: or let

---

[1] Printed at London, anno 1620.   [2] Late astronomy-reader at Gresham college.   [3] Printed at London by William Jones, 1623.   [4] Præfat. Meth. Astrol.

552   *Cure of Melancholy.*   [Part. 2. Sec. 2.

him make an ephemerides, read Suisset the calculators works, Scaliger *de emendatione temporum,* and Petavius his adversary, till he understand them, peruse subtile Scotus and Suarez metaphysicks, or school divinity, Occam, Thomas, Entisberus, Durand, &c. If those other do not affect him, and his means be great, to imploy his purse and fill his head, he may go find the philosophers stone; he may apply his mind, I say, to heraldry, antiquity, invent impresses, emblems; make epithalamiums, epitaphs, elegies, epigrams, *palindroma epigrammata,* anagrams, chronograms, acrosticks upon his friends names; or write a comment on Martianus Capella, Tertullian *de pallio,* the Nubian geography, or upon *Ælia Lælia Crispis,* as many idle fellowes have assayed; and rather than do nothing, vary a [1]verse a thousand waies with Putean, so torturing his wits, or as Rainnerus of Luneburge, [2]2150 times in his *Proteus Poëticus,* or Scaliger, Chrysolithus, Cleppisius, and others have in like sort done. If such voluntary tasks, pleasure and delight, or crabbednesse of these studies, will not yet divert their idle thoughts, and alienate their imaginations, they must be compelled, saith Christophorus a Vega, *cogi debent, l. 5. c. 14.* upon some mulct, if they perform it not, *quod ex officio incumbat,* loss of credit or disgrace, such as are our publike university exercises. For, as he that playes for nothing, will not heed his game: no more will voluntary imployment so thoroughly affect a student, except he be very intent of himself, and take an extraordinary delight in the study about which he is conversant. It should be of that nature his business, which *volens nolens* he must necessarily undergo, and without great loss, mulct, shame, or hindrance, he may not omit.

Now for women, instead of laborious studies, they have curious needle-works, cut works, spinning, bone-lace, and many pretty devices of their own making, to adorn their houses, cushions, carpets, chaires, stools, (*for she eats not the bread of idleness,* Prov. 31. 27. *quæsivit lanam et linum*) confections, conserves, distillations, &c. which they shew to strangers.

> [3]Ipsa comes præsesque operis venientibus ultro
> Hospitibus monstrare solet, non segniter horas
> Contestata suas, sed nec sibi deperiisse.

> Which to her guests she shews, with all her pelfe:
> "Thus far my maids : but this I did my selfe."

This they have to busie themselves about, houshold offices, &c. [4]neat gardens, full of exotick, versicolour, diversly varied, sweet

---

[1] Tot tibi sunt dotes, virgo, quot sidera cœlo.   [2] Da, pie Christe, urbi bona sit pax tempore nostro.   [3] Chalonerus, Lib. 9. de Rep. Ang.   [4] Hortus coronarius, medicus, et culinarius, &c.

Mem. 4.] *Exercise rectified.* 553

smelling flowers, and plants in all kinds, which they are most ambitious to get, curious to preserve and keep, proud to possess, and much many times brag of. Their merry meetings and frequent visitations, mutual invitations in good towns, I voluntarily omit, which are so much in use, gossiping among the meaner sort, &c. Old folks have their beads; an excellent invention to keep them from idleness, that are by nature melancholy, and past all affairs, to say so many *paternosters, ave-maries, creeds,* if it were not prophane and superstitious. In a word, body and mind must be exercised, not one, but both, and that in a mediocrity : otherwise it will cause a great inconvenience. If the body be overtired, it tires the mind. The mind oppresseth the body, as with students it oftentimes fals out, who (as [1] Plutarch observes) have no care of the body, *but compel that which is mortal, to do as much as that which is immortal; that which is earthly, as that which is ethereall. But as the oxe, tyred, told the camel (both serving one master) that refused to carry some part of his burden, before it were long, he should be compelled to carry all his pack, and skin to boot (which by and by, the oxe being dead, fell out), the body may say to the soul, that will give him no respite or remission: a little after, an ague, vertigo, consumption seiseth on them both; all his study is omitted, and they must be compelled to be sick together.* He that tenders his own good estate and health, must let them draw with equal yoke both alike, [2] *that so they may happily enjoy their wished health.*

---

[1] Tom. 1. de sanit. tuend. Qui rationem corporis non habent, sed cogunt mortalem immortali, terrestrem æthereæ æqualem præstare industriam. Cæterum ut camelo usu venit, quod ei bos prædixerat, cum eidem servirent domino, et parte oneris levare illum camelus recusâsset, paulo post et ipsius cutem, et totum onus cogeretur gestare (quod mortuo bove impletum), ita animo quoque contingit, dum defatigato corpori, &c.   [2] Ut pulchram illam et amabilem sanitatem præstemus.

554   *Cure of Melancholy.*   [Part. 2. Sec. 2.

MEMB. V.

Waking and terrible dreams rectified.

As waking, that hurts, by all means, must be avoided, so
sleep, which so much helps, by like waies, [1] *must be procured,
by nature or art, inward or outward medicines, and be pro-
tracted longer than ordinary, if it may be, as being an especiall
help.* It moystens and fattens the body, concocts, and helps
digestion, as we see in dormice, and those Alpine mice that
sleep all winter, (which Gesner speaks of) when they are so
found sleeping under the snow in the dead of winter, as fat as
butter. It expels cares, pacifies the minde, refresheth the
weary limbs after long work.

> [2] Somne, quies rerum, placidissime, Somne, Deorum,
> Pax animi, quem cura fugit, qui corpora, duris
> Fessa ministeriis, mulces, reparasque labori.

> Sleep, rest of things, O pleasing deity,
> Peace of the soul, which cares dost crucifie,
> Weary bodies refresh and mollifie.

The chiefest thing in all physick [3] Paracelsus calls it, *omnia
arcana gemmarum superans et metallorum.* The fittest time is
[4] *two or three hours after supper, when as the meat is now settled
at the bottome of the stomack; and 'tis good to lie on the right
side first, because at that site the liver doth rest under the stomach, not molesting any way, but heating him, as a fire doth a
kettle, that is put to it. After the first sleep, 'tis not amiss to lie
on the left side, that the meat may the better descend,* and sometimes again on the belly, but never on the back. Seven or eight
hours is a competent time for a melancholy man to rest, as
Crato thinks; but, as some do, to lie in bed, and not sleep, a
day, or half a day together, to give assent to pleasing conceits
and vain imaginations, is many wayes pernicious. To procure
this sweet moistning sleep, it's best to take away the occasions
(if it be possible) that hinder it, and then to use such inward
or outward remedies, which may cause it. *Constat hodie* (saith
Boissardus, in his Tract *de magiâ, cap. 4*) *multos ita fascinari,*

---

[1] Interdicendæ vigiliæ; somni paullo longiores conciliandi. Altomarus, cap. 7.
Somnus supra modum prodest, quovis modo conciliandus. Piso.   [2] Ovid.
[3] In Hippoc. Aphoris.   [4] Crato, cons. 21. lib. 2. Duabus aut tribus horis post
cœnam, quum jam cibus ad fundum ventriculi resederit, primum super latere dex-
tro quiescendum, quod in tali decubitu jecur sub ventriculo quiescat, non gravans,
sed cibum calefaciens, perinde ac ignis lebetem qui illi admovetur; post primum
somnum, quiescendum latere sinistro, &c.

8

Mem. 5.]   *Waking and Dreams rectified.*   555

ut noctes integras exigant insomnes, summâ inquietudine ani-morum et corporum: many cannot sleep for witches and fasci-nations, which are too familiar in some places: they call it, *dare alicui malam noctem.* But the ordinary causes are heat and dryness, which must first be removed. [1] A hot and dry brain never sleeps well: grief, fears, cares, expectations, anxie-ties, great businesses, ([2] *in aurem utramque otiose ut dormias*) and all violent perturbations of the mind, must in some sort be qualified, before we can hope for any good repose. He that sleeps in the day time, or is in suspense, fear, any way troubled in minde, or goes to bed upon a full [3] stomack, may never hope for quiet rest in the night. *Nec enim meritoria somnos admit-tunt,* as the [4] poet saith: innes, and such like troublesome places, are not for sleep; one calls ostler, another tapster; one cryes and shouts, another sings, whoupes, hollows,

—— [5] absentem cantat amicam,
Multâ prolutus vappâ, nauta atque viator.

Who, not accustomed to such noyses, can sleep amongst them? He that will intend to take his rest, must go to bed *animo securo, quieto, et libero,* with a [6] secure and composed minde, in a quiet place;

(Omnia noctis erunt placidâ compôsta quiete)

and if that will not serve, or may not be obtained, to seek then such means as are requisite: to lye in clean linnen and sweet: before he goes to bed, or in bed, to hear [7] *sweet musick,* (which Ficinus commends, *lib.* 1. *cap.* 24) or (as Jobertus, *med. pract. lib. 3. cap.* 10) [8] *to read some pleasant author till he be asleep, to have a bason of water still dropping by his bed side,* or to lie near that pleasant murmure, [9] *lene sonantis aquæ,* some floud-gates, arches, falls of water, like London bridge, or some continuate noise which may benum the senses. *Lenis motus, silentium, et tenebræ, tum et ipsa voluntas, somnos fa-ciunt;* as a gentle noyse to some procures sleep, so, which Ber-nardius Tilesius (*lib. de somno*) well observes, silence, in a darke roome, and the will it self, is most available to others. Piso commends frications, Andrew Borde a good draught of strong drink before one goes to bed; I say, a nutmeg and ale, or a good draught of muscadine, with a tost and a nutmeg, or a posset of the same, which many use in a morning, but, me

---

[1] Sæpius accidit melancholicis, ut, nimium exsiccato cerebro vigiliis, attenuen-tur. Ficinus, lib. 1. cap. 29.   [2] Ter.   [3] Ut sis nocte levis, sit tibi cœna brevis.   [4] Juven. Sat. 3.   [5] Hor. Ser. lib. 1. Sat. 5.   [6] Sepositis curis omnibus, quantum fieri potest, una cum vestibus, &c. Kirkst.   [7] Ad horam somni, aures suavibus cantibus et sonis delenire.   [8] Lectio jucunda, aut sermo, ad quem attentior animus convertitur; aut aqua ab alto in subjectam pel-vim dela batur, &c.   [9] Ovid.

556   *Cure of Melancholy.*   [Part. 2. Sec. 2.

thinks, for such as have dry brains, are much more proper at
night.   Some prescribe a [1] sup of vinegar as they go to bed, a
spoonfull, saith Aëtius, *Tetrabib. lib. 3. ser. 2. cap.* 10. *lib.* 6.
cap. 10.   Ægineta, *lib. 3. cap.* 14.   Piso, *a little after meat,*
[2] *because it rarifies melancholy, and procures an appetite to*
sleep. Donat. ab Altomar. *cap.* 7, and Mercurialis, approve
of it, if the malady proceed from the [3] spleen. Sallust. Salvian.
(*lib. 2. cap.* 1. *de remed.*)   Hercules de Saxoniâ, (*in Pan.*)
Ælianus Montaltus, (*de morb. capitis, cap.* 28. *de Melan.*) are
altogether against it. Lod. Mercatus (*de inter. morb. cau. lib.* 1.
cap. 17) in some cases doth allow it.   [4] Rhasis seems to deliberate of it : though Simeon commend it (in sawce peradventure) he makes a question of it: as for baths, fomentations,
oyls, potions, simples or compounds, inwardly taken to this
purpose, [5] I shall speak of them elsewhere.   If in the midst of
the night they lie awake, which is usuall, to toss and tumble,
and not sleep, [6] Ranzovius would have them, if it bee in warme
weather, to rise and walk three or four turnes (till they be
cold) about the chamber, and then go to bed again.

Against fearful and troublesome dreams, *incubus,* and such
inconveniences, wherewith melancholy men are molested, the
best remedy is to eat a light supper, and of such meats as are
easie of digestion, no hare, venison, beef, &c. not to lie on
his back, not to meditate or think in the day time of any terrible
objects, or especially talke of them before he goes to bed. For,
as he said in Lucian, after such conference, *Hecatas somniare*
mihi videor, I can think of nothing but hobgoblins : and, as
Tully notes, [7] *for the most part our speeches in the day time*
cause our phantasy to work upon the like in our sleep ; which
Ennius writes of Homer :

> Et canis in somnis leporis vestigia latrat :

as a dog dreams of an hare, so do men, on such subjects they
thought on last.

> Somnia, quæ mentes ludunt volitantibus umbris,
> Nec delubra Deum, nec ab æthere Numina mittunt,
> Sed sibi quisque facit, &c.

For that cause, when [8] Ptolemy king of Egypt had posed the
70 interpreters in order, and asked the nineteenth man, what
would make one sleep quietly in the night, he told him,

---

[1] Aceti sorbitio.   [2] Attenuat melancholiam, et ad conciliandum somnum
juvat.   [3] Quod lieni acetum conveniat.   [4] Cont. 1. tract. 9. meditandum
de aceto.   [5] Sect. 5. memb. 1. subsect. 6.   [6] Lib. de sanit. tuendâ.
[7] In Som. Scip.   Fit enim fere ut cogitationes nostræ et sermones pariant aliquid
in somno,quale de Homero scribit Ennius, de quo videlicet sæpissime vigilans
solebat cogitare et loqui.   [8] Aristeæ hist.

Mem. 6. Subs. 1.]   *Passions rectified.*   557

[1] *The best way was to have divine and celestiall meditations, and to use honest actions in the day time.* [2] Lod. Vives *wonders how schoolemen could sleep quietly, and were not terrified in the night, or walke in the darke, they had such monstrous questions, and thought of such terrible matters all day long.* They had need, amongst the rest, to sacrifice to God Morpheus, whom [3] Philostratus paints in a white and black coat, with a horn and ivory box full of dreams, of the same colours, to signify good and bad. If you will know how to interpret them, read Artemidorus, Sambucus, and Cardan : but how to help them, [4] I must refer you to a more convenient place.

MEMB. VI. SUBSECT. I.

Perturbations of the minde rectified. From himself, by resisting to the utmost, confessing his grief to a friend, &c.

WHOSOEVER he is, that shall hope to cure this malady in himself or any other, must first rectifie these passions and perturbations of the minde ; the chiefest cure consists in them. A quiet mind is that *voluptas,* or *summum bonum* of Epicurus; *non dolere, curis vacare, animo tranquillo esse,* not to grieve, but to want cares, and have a quiet soul, is the only pleasure of the world, as Seneca truly recites his opinion, not that of eating and drinking, which injurious Aristotle maliciously puts upon him, and for which he is still mistaken, *male audit et vapulat,* slandered without a cause, and lashed by all posterity. [5] *Fear and sorrow therefore are especially to be avoided, and the minde to be mitigated with mirth, constancy, good hope : vain terror, bad objects, are to bee removed, and all such persons in whose companies they be not well pleased.* Gualter Bruel, Fernelius, *consil.* 43. Mercurialis, *consil.* 6. Piso, Jacchinus, *cap.* 15. *in* 9 Rhasis, Capivaccius, Hildesheim, &c. all inculcate this as an especiall meanes of their cure, that their [6] *minds be quietly pacified, vain conceits diverted, if it be possible, with terrors, cares,* [7] *fixed studies, cogitations, and whatsoever it is that shall*

---

[1] Optimum de cœlestibus et honestis meditari, et ea facere.   [2] Lib. 3. de caussis corr. art. Tam. mira monstra quæstionum sæpe nascuntur inter eos, ut mirer eos interdum in somniis non terreri, aut de illis in tenebris audere verba facere, adeo res sunt monstrosæ.   [3] Icon. lib. 1.   [4] Sect. 5. memb. 1. subs 6.   [5] Animi perturbationes summe fugiendæ, metus potissimum et tristitia ; eorumque loco, animus demulcendus hilaritate, animi constantiâ, bonâ spe ; removendi terrores, et eorum consortium quos non probant.   [6] Phantasiæ eorum placide subvertendæ, terrores ab animo removendi.   [7] Ab omni fixâ cogitatione quovis modo avertantur.

558   *Cure of Melancholy.*   [Part. 2. Sec. 2.

any way molest or trouble the soul, because that otherwise there
is no good to be done. [1] *The bodies mischiefes*, as Plato proves,
*proceed from the soul: and if the mind be not first satisfied, the
body can never be cured.* Alcibiades raves (saith [2] Maximus
Tyrius), and is sick; his furious desires carry him from Lyceus
to the pleading place, thence to the sea, so into Sicily, thence
to Lacedæmon, thence to Persia, thence to Samos, then again
to Athens; Critias tyrannizeth over all the city; Sardanapalus
is love-sick; these men are ill-affected all, and can never be
cured, till their minds be otherwise qualified. Crato therefore,
in that often cited counsell of his for a noble man his patient,
when he had sufficiently informed him in diet, air, exercise,
Venus, sleep, concludes with these as matters of greatest moment : *quod reliquum est, animæ accidentia corrigantur*, from
which alone proceeds melancholy ; they are the fountain, the
subject, the hinges whereon it turns, and must necessarily be
reformed.   [3] *For anger stirs choler, heats the blood and vital
spirits: sorrow on the other side refrigerates the body, and extinguisheth natural heat, overthrows appetite, hinders concoction, dries up the temperature, and perverts the understanding:*
fear dissolves the spirits, infects the heart, attenuates the soul:
and for these causes all passions and perturbations must, to
the uttermost of our power, and most seriously, be removed.
Ælianus Montaltus attributes so much to them, [4] *that he holds
the rectification of them alone to be sufficient to the cure of
melancholy in most patients.* Many are fully cured when they
have seen or heard, &c. enjoy their desires, or be secured and
satisfied in their minds.   Galen, the common master of them
all, from whose fountain they fetch water, brags (*lib*. 1. *de san.
tuend.*) that he for his part hath cured divers of this infirmity,
solum animis ad rectum institutis, by right settling alone of
their minds.

   Yea, but you will here infer, that this is excellent good indeed, if it could be done ; but how shall it be effected, by
whom, what art, what means ? *hic labor, hoc opus est.* 'Tis a
natural infirmity, a most powerful adversary: all men are subject to passions, and melancholy above all others, as being distempered by their innate humors, abundance of choler adust,

---

   [1] Cuncta mala corporis ab animo procedunt, quæ nisi curentur, corpus curari
minime potest. Charmid.   [2] Disputat, an morbi graviores corporis an animi.
Renoldo interpret. Ut parum absit a furore, rapitur a Lyceo in concionem, a con-
cione ad mare, a mari in Siciliam, &c.   [3] Ira bilem movet, sanguinem
adurit, vitales spiritus accendit; mœstitia universum corpus infrigidat, calorem
innatum exstinguit, appetitum destruit, concoctionem impedit, corpus exsiccat,
intellectum pervertit. Quamobrem hæc omnia prorsus vitanda sunt, et pro virili
fugienda.   [4] De mel. c. 26. Ex illis solum remedium ; multi ex visis, auditis,
&c. sanati sunt.

Mem. 6. Subs. 1.] *Passions rectified.* **559**

weakness of parts, outward occurrences; and how shall they be . avoided? The wisest men, greatest philosophers, of most excellent wit, reason, judgment, divine spirits, cannot moderate themselves in this behalf: such as are sound in body and mind, stoicks, heroes, Homers gods, all are passionate, and furiously carryed sometimes; and how shall we that are already crased, *fracti animis,* sick in body, sick in mind, resist? we cannot perform it. You may advise and give good precepts, as who cannot? But, how shall they be put in practice? I may not deny but our passions are violent, and tyrannize over us; yet there be means to curb them; though they be headstrong, they may be tamed, they may be qualified, if he himself or his friends will but use their honest endeavours, or make use of such ordinary helps as are commonly prescribed.

He himself (I say); from the patient himself the first and chiefest remedy must be had; for, if he be averse, peevish, waspish, give way wholly to his passion, will not seek to be helped, or be ruled by his friends, how is it possible he should be cured? But if he be willing at least, gentle, tractable, and desire his own good, no doubt but he may *magnam morbi deponere partem,* be eased at least, if not cured. He himself must do his utmost endeavour to resist and withstand the beginnings. *Principiis obsta : Give not water passage,* no not *a little,* Eccles. 25. 27. If they open a little, they will make a greater breach at length. Whatsoever it is that runneth in his mind, vain conceit, be it pleasing or displeasing, which so much affects or troubleth him, [1] *by all possible means he must withstand it, expel those vain, false, frivolous imaginations, absurd conceits, fained fears and sorrowes (from which,* saith Piso, *this disease primarily proceeds, and takes his first occasion or beginning) by doing something or other that shall be opposite unto them, thinking of something else, perswading by reason, or howsoever, to make a sudden alteration of them.* Though he have hitherto run in a full career, and precipitated himself, following his passions, giving reins to his appetite, let him now stop upon a sudden, curb himself in, and, as [2] Lemnius adviseth, *strive against with all his power, to the utmost of his endeavour, and not cherish those fond imaginations, which so covertly creep into his mind, most pleasing and*

---

[1] Pro viribus annitendum in prædictis, tum in aliis, a quibus malum, velut a primariâ caussâ, occasionem nactum est ; imaginationes absurdæ falsæque et mœstitia quæcunque subierit, propulsetur, aut aliud agendo, aut ratione persuadendo earum mutationem subito facere. [2] Lib. 2. c. 16. de occult. nat. Quisquis huic malo obnoxius est, acriter obsistat, et summâ curâ obluctetur, nec ullo modo foveat imaginationes tacite obrepentes animo, blandas ab initio et amabiles, sed quæ adeo convalescunt, ut nullâ ratione excuti queant.

560   *Cure of Melancholy.*   [Part. 2. Sec. 2.

*amiable at first, but bitter as gall at last, and so head-strong,
that, by no reason, art, counsel, or perswasion, they may be
shaken off.* Though he be far gone, and habituated unto such
phantastical imaginations, yet (as [1] Tully and Plutarch advise)
let him oppose, fortifie, or prepare himself against them, by
premeditation, reason, or (as we do by a crooked staffe) bend
himself another way.

> [2] Tu tamen interea effugito quæ tristia mentem
> Solicitant; procul esse jube curasque metumque
> Pallentem, ultrices iras ; sint omnia læta.

> In the mean time expel them from thy mind,
> Pale fears, sad cares, and griefs, which do it grind,
> Revengeful anger, pain and discontent :
> Let all thy soule be set on merriment.

> Curas tolle graves : irasci crede profanum.

If it be idleness hath caused this infirmity, or that he perceive
himself given to solitariness, to walk alone and please his
mind with fond imaginations, let him by all means avoid it ;
'tis a bosome enemy ; 'tis delightsome melancholy, a friend in
shew, but a secret devil, a sweet poyson ; it will in the end be
his undoing ; let him go presently, task or set himself a work,
get some good company. If he proceed, as a gnat flies about
a candle so long till at length he burn his body, so in the end
he will undo himself : if it be any harsh object, ill company,
let him presently go from it. If by his own default through ill
diet, bad aire, want of exercise, &c. let him now begin to reform himself. *It would be a perfect remedy against all corruption, if* (as [3] Roger Bacon hath it) *we could but moderate
our selves in those six non-natural things.* [4] *If it be any
disgrace, abuse, temporal loss, calumny, death of friends, imprisonment, banishment, be not troubled with it ; do not fear, be
not angry, grieve not at it, but with all courage sustain it.*
(Gordonius, *lib.* 1. c. 13. *de conser. vit.*) *Tu contra audentior
ito.* [5] If it be sickness, ill success, or any adversity, that hath
caused it, oppose an invincible courage ; *fortify thy self by
Gods word ; or otherwise, mala bonis persuadenda,* set pro-

---

[1] Tusc. ad Apollonium.   [2] Fracastorius.   [3] Epist. de secretis artis et
naturæ, cap. 7. de retard. sen. Remedium esset contra corruptionem propriam, si
quilibet exerceret regimen sanitatis, quod consistat in rebus sex non naturabilus.
[4] Pro aliquo vituperio non indigneris, nec pro amissione alicujus rei, pro morte
alicujus, nec pro carcere, nec pro exilio, nec pro aliâ re, nec irascaris, nec timeas,
nec doleas, sed cum summâ præsentiâ hæc sustineas.   [5] Quod si incommoda
adversitatis infortunia hoc malum invexerint, his infractum animum opponas :
Dei verbo ejusque fiduciâ te suffulcias, &c. Lemnius, lib. 1. c. 16.

Mem. 6. Subs. 1.] *Passions rectified.* 561

sperity against adversity: as we refresh our eyes by seeing some pleasant meadow, fountain, picture, or the like, recreate thy mind by some contrary object, with some more pleasing meditation divert thy thoughts.

Yea, but you infer again, *facile consilium damus aliis,* we can easily give counsel to others; every man, as the saying is, can tame a shrew, but he that hath her: *si hic esses, aliter sentires;* if you were in our misery, you would find it otherwise; 'tis not so easily performed. We know this to be true; we should moderate our selves; but we are furiously carryed; we cannot make use of such precepts; we are overcome, sick, *male sani,* distempered, and habituated in these courses; we can make no resistance; you may as well bid him that is diseased, not to feel pain, as a melancholy man not to fear, not to be sad: 'tis within his blood, his brains, his whole temperature: it cannot be removed. But he may chuse whether he will give way too far unto it; he may in some sort correct himself. A philosopher was bitten with a mad dog; and, as the nature of that disease is to abhor all waters, and liquid things, and to think still they see the picture of a dog before them, he went, for all this, *reluctante se,* to the bath, and seeing there (as he thought) in the water the picture of a dog, with reason overcame this conceit: *quid cani cum balneo?* what should a dog do in a bath? a meer conceit. Thou thinkest thou hearest and seest devils, black men, &c. 'tis not so; 'tis thy corrupt phantasie; settle thine imagination; thou art well. Thou thinkest thou hast a great nose, thou art sick, every man observes thee, laughs thee to scorn: perswade thy self 'tis no such matter: this is fear only, and vain suspicion. Thou art discontent, thou art sad and heavy, but why? upon what ground? consider of it: thou art jealous, timorous, suspicious; for what cause? examine it throughly; thou shalt find none at all, or such as is to be contemned, such as thou wilt surely deride, and contemn in thy self, when it is past. Rule thy self then with reason; satisfie thy self; accustom thy self; wean thy self from such fond conceits, vain fears, strong imaginations, restless thoughts. Thou mayest do it: *est in nobis assuescere* (as Plutarch saith): we may frame our selves as we will. As he that useth an upright shooe, may correct the obliquity or crookedness by wearing it on the other side; we may overcome passions if we will. *Quicquid sibi imperavit animus, obtinuit* (as [1] Seneca saith): *nulli tam feri affectus, ut non disciplinâ perdomentur:* whatsoever the will desires, she may command: no such cruel affections, but by discipline they may be tamed. Voluntarily thou

---

[1] Lib. 2. de irâ.

VOL. I. O O

562   *Cure of Melancholy.*   [Part. 2. Sec. 2.

wilt not do this or that, which thou oughtest to do, or refrain,
&c. but when thou art lashed like a dull jade, thou wilt reform
it; fear of a whip will make thee do, or not do. Do that
voluntarily then which thou canst do, and must do by compulsion: thou maist refrain if thou wilt, and master thine
affections. [1] *As, in a city,* (saith Melancthon) *they do by stubborn rebellious rogues, that will not submit themselves to political judgement, compel them by force; so must we do by our
affections. If the heart will not lay aside those vicious motions,
and the phantasie those fond imaginations, we have another
form of government to enforce and refrain our outward members, that they be not led by our passions.* If appetite will not
obey, let the moving faculty over-rule her; let her resist and
compel her to do otherwise. In an ague, the appetite would
drink; sore eyes that itch, would be rubbed; but reason saith
no; and therefore the moving faculty will not do it. Our
phantasie would intrude a thousand fears, suspicions, chimeras
upon us; but we have reason to resist; yet we let it be overborne by our appetite. [2] *Imagination enforceth spirits, which
by an admirable league of nature compel the nerves to obey,
and they our several limbs:* we give too much way to our passions. And as, to him that is sick of an ague, all things are
distastful and unpleasant, *non ex cibi vitio,* saith Plutarch,
not in the meat, but in our taste: so many things are offensive
to us, not of themselves, but out of our corrupt judgement,
jealousie, suspicion, and the like; we pull these mischiefs upon
our own heads.

If then our judgement be so depraved, our reason over-ruled,
will precipitated, that we cannot seek our own good, or moderate our selves, as in this disease commonly it is, the best way
for ease is to impart our misery to some friend, not to smother
it up in our own breast; *alitur vitium, crescitque, tegendo, &c.*
and that which was most offensive to us, a cause of fear and
grief, *quod nunc te coquit,* another hell; for

[3] Strangulat inclusus dolor, atque exæstuat intus,

grief concealed strangles the soul; but when as we shall but
impart it to some discreet, trusty, loving friend, it is [4]instantly
removed by his counsel happily, wisdome, perswasion, advice,

---

[1] Cap. 3. de affect. anim. Ut in civitatibus contumaces, qui non cedunt politico
imperio, vi coërcendi sunt; ita Deus nobis indidit alteram imperii formam; si cor
non deponit vitiosum affectum, membra foras coërcenda sunt, ne ruant in quod
affectus impellat; et locomotiva, quæ herili imperio obtemperat, alteri resistat.
[2] Imaginatio impellit spiritus, et inde nervi moventur, &c. et obtemperant imaginationi et appetitui mirabili fœdere, ad exsequendum quod jubent.   [3] Ovid.
Trist. lib. 5.   [4] Participes inde calamitatis nostræ sunt; et, velut exoneratâ
in eos sarcinâ, onere levamur. Arist. Eth. lib. 9.

his good means, which we could not otherwise apply unto our selves. A friends counsel is a charm; like mandrake wine, *curas sopit;* and as a [1] bull that is tyed to a fig-tree, becomes gentle on a sudden (which some, saith [2] Plutarch, interpret of good words), so is a savage, obdurate heart mollified by faire speeches. *All adversity finds ease in complaining* (as [3] Isidore holds); *and 'tis a solace to relate it:*

[4] Αγαθη δε παραιφασις εστιν έταιρου,

friends confabulations are comfortable at all times, as fire in winter, shade in summer; *quale sopor fessis in gramine,* meat and drink to him that is hungry or athirst. Democritus colly-rium is not so soveraign to the eyes, as this is to the heart; good words are cheerful and powerful of themselves, but much more from friends, as so many props, mutually sustaining each other, like ivie and a wal, which [5] Camerarius hath well illus-trated in an embleme. *Lenit animum vel simplex sæpe nar-ratio,* the simple narration many times easeth our distressed mind; and in the midst of greatest extremities, so divers have been relieved, by [6] exonerating themselves to a faithful friend: he sees that which we cannot see for passion and discontent; he pacifies our minds; he will ease our pain, asswage our anger. *Quanta inde voluptas! quanta securitas!* Chrysostome addes: what pleasure! what security by that means! [7] *Nothing so available, or that so much refresheth the soul of man.* Tully, as I remember, in an epistle to his dear friend Atticus, much condoles the defect of such a friend. [8] *I live here* (saith he) *in a great citie, where I have a multitude of acquaintance, but not a man of all that companie, with whom I dare familiarly breath, or freely jest. Wherefore I expect thee, I desire thee, I send for thee; for there be many things which trouble and molest me, which, had I but thee in presence, I could quickly disburden myself of in a walking discourse.* The like perad-venture may he and he say with that old man in the comedy,

Nemo est meorum amicorum hodie,
Apud quem expromere occulta mea audeam:

and much inconvenience may both he and he suffer in the mean time by it. He or he, or whosoever then labours of this malady, by all means let him get some trusty friend,

[9] Semper habens Pyladen aliquem, qui curet Oresten,

---

[1] Camerarius, Embl. 26. Cen. 2. [2] Sympos. lib. 6. cap. 10. [3] Epist. 8. lib. 3. Adversa fortuna habet in querelis levamentum; et malorum relatio, &c. [4] Alloquium cari juvat, et solamen, amici. [5] Emblem. 54. cent. 1. [6] As David did to Jonathan, 1 Sam. 20. [7] Seneca, Epist. 67. [8] Hîc in civitate magnâ et turbâ magnâ neminem reperire possumus, quocum suspirare familiariter, aut jocari libere, possimus. Quare te exspectamus, te desideramus, te arcessimus. Multa sunt enim, quæ me solicitant et angunt, quæ mihi videor, aures tuas nactus, unius ambulationis sermone exhaurire posse. [9] Ovid.

564 *Cure of Melancholy.* [Part. 2. Sec. 2.

a Pylades, to whom freely and securely he may open himself. For, as in all other occurrences, so it is in this—*si quis in cœlum ascendisset, &c.* as he said in [1] Tully, if a man had gone to heaven, *seen the beauty of the skies*, stars errant, fixed, &c. *insuavis erit admiratio*, it will do him no pleasure, except he have some body to impart what he hath seen. It is the best thing in the world, as [2] Seneca therefore adviseth in such a case, *to get a trusty friend, to whom we may freely and sincerely pour out our secrets. Nothing so delighteth and easeth the minde, as when we have a prepared bosome, to which our secrets may descend, of whose conscience we are assured as our own, whose speech may ease our succourless estate, counsell relieve, mirth expell our mourning, and whose very sight may be acceptable unto us.* It was the counsell which that politick [3] Commineus gave to all princes, and others distressed in mind, by occasion of Charles duke of Burgundy, that was much perplexed, *first to pray to God, and lay himself open to him, and then to some speciall friend, whom we hold most dear, to tell all our grievances to him. Nothing so forcible to strengthen, recreate, and heal the wounded soul of a miserable man.*

SUBSECT. II.

Help from Friends by Counsell, Comfort, fair and foul Means, witty Devices, Satisfaction, Alteration of his Course of Life, removing Objects, &c.

WHEN the patient of himself is not able to resist or overcome these heart-eating passions, his friends or physician must be ready to supply that which is wanting. *Suæ erit humanitatis et sapientiæ,* (which [4] Tully injoyneth in like case) *siquid erratum, curare, aut improvisum, suâ diligentiâ corrigere.* They must all joyn; *nec satis medico,* saith [5] Hippocrates, *suum fecisse officium, nisi suum quoque ægrotus, suum astantes, &c.* First they must especially beware, a melancholy discontented person (be it in what kinde of melancholy soever) never be left alone or idle: but, as physicians prescribe physick, *cum custodiâ,* let them not be left unto themselves, but with some company or other, lest by that means they aggra-

---

[1] De amicitiâ.   [2] De tranquil. c. 7. Optimum est amicum fidelem nancisci, in quem secreta nostra infundamus. Nihil æque oblectat animum, quam ubi sint præparata pectora, in quæ tuto secreta descendant, quorum conscientia æque ac tua; quorum sermo solitudinem leniat, sententia consilium expediat, hilaritas tristitiam dissipet, conspectusque ipse delectet.   [3] Comment. l. 7. Ad Deum confugiamus, et peccatis veniam precemur, inde ad amicos, et cui plurimum tribuimus, nos patefaciamus totos, et animi vulnus quo affligimur: nihil ad reficiendum animum efficacius.   [4] Ep. ad Q. frat.   [5] Aphor. prim.

Mem. 6. Subs. 2.]   *Mind rectified.*   565

vate and increase their disease. *Non oportet ægros hujusmodi
esse solos, vel inter ignotos, vel inter eos quos non amant aut
negligunt,* as Rod. a Fonseca, (*Tom.* 1. *consul.* 35) prescribes.
Lugentes custodire solemus, (saith [1] Seneca) *ne solitudine male
utantur;* we watch a sorrowfull person, lest he abuse his
solitariness: and so should we do a melancholy man; set
him about some business, exercise, or recreation, which may
divert his thoughts, and still keep him otherwise intent; for
his phantasie is so restless, operative and quick, that, if it be
not in perpetuall action, ever employed, it will work upon
it self, melancholize, and be carried away instantly with some
fear, jealousie, discontent, suspicion, some vain conceit or
other.   If his weakness be such, that he cannot discern what
is amiss, correct or satisfie, it behoves them, by counsel, comfort, or perswasion, by fair or foul means, to alienate his
mind by some artificial invention or some contrary passion,
to remove all objects, causes, companies, occasions, as may
any wayes molest him, to humour him, please him, divert
him, and, if it be possible, by altering his course of life, to
give him security and satisfaction.   If he conceal his grievances, and will not be known of them, [2] *they must observe, by
his looks, gestures, motions, phantasie, what it is that offends,*
and then to apply remedies unto him.   Many are instantly
cured when their minds are satisfied.   [3] Alexander makes
mention of a woman, *that, by reason of her husbands long
absence in travel, was exceeding peevish and melancholy; but,
when she heard her husband was returned, beyond all expectation, at the first sight of him, she was freed from all fear,
without help of any other physick restored to her former
health.* Trincavelius (*consil.* 12. *lib.* 1) hath such a story of
a Venetian, that, being much troubled with melancholy, [4] *and
ready to dye for grief, when he heard his wife was brought to
bed of a son, instantly recovered.* As Alexander concludes,
[5] *if our imaginations be not inveterate, by this art they may
be cured, especially if they proceed from such a cause.* No
better way to satisfy, than to remove the object, cause, occasion, if by any art or means possible we may finde it out.   If
he grieve, stand in fear, be in suspicion, suspence, or any way
molested, secure him; *solvitur malum:* give him satisfaction;
the cure is ended: alter his course of life, there needs no

---

[1] Epist. 10.   [2] Observando motus, gestus, manus, pedes, oculos, phantasiam.   Piso.   [3] Mulier, melancholiâ correpta ex longâ viri peregrinatione,
et iracunde omnibus respondens, quum maritus domum reversus præter spem, &c.
[4] Præ dolore moriturus, quum nuntiatum esset uxorem peperisse filium, subito
recuperavit.   [5] Nisi affectus longo tempore infestaverit, tali artificio imaginationes curare oportet, præsertim ubi malum ab his, velut a primariâ caussâ, occasionem habuerit.

566   *Cure of Melancholy.*   [Part. 2. Sec. 2.

other physick. If the party be sad, or otherwise affected, *consider* (saith [1] Trallianus) *the manner of it, all circumstances, and forthwith make a sudden alteration,* by removing the occasions; avoid all terrible objects, heard or seen, [2] *monstrous and prodigious aspects,* tales of devils, spirits, ghosts, tragicall stories: to such as are in fear, they strike a great impression, renew many times, and recal such chimeras and terrible fictions into their minds. [3] *Make not so much as mention of them in private talk, or a dumb shew tending to that purpose: such things* (saith Galateus) *are offensive to their imaginations.* And to those that are now in sorrow, [4] Seneca *forbids all sad companions, and such as lament: a groaning companion is an enemy to quietness.* [5] *Or if there be any such party, at whose presence the patient is not well pleased, he must be removed: gentle speeches and fair means must first be tryed; no harsh language used, or uncomfortable words; and not expel,* as some do, one madness with another; he that so doth is madder than the patient himself: all things must be quietly composed; *eversa non evertenda, sed erigenda,* things down must not be dejected, but reared, as Crato counselleth: [6] *he must be quietly and gently used;* and we should not do any thing against his mind, but by little and little effect it. As an horse that starts at a drum or trumpet, and will not endure the shooting of a piece, may be so manned by art, and animated, that he cannot only endure, but is much more generous at the hearing of such things, much more couragious than before, and much delighteth in it; they must not be reformed *ex abrupto,* but, by all art and insinuation, made to such companies, aspects, objects, they could not formerly away with. Many at first cannot endure the sight of a green wound, a sick man, which afterward become good chyrurgians, bold empericks. A horse starts at a rotten post afar off, which, coming neer, he quietly passeth. 'Tis much in the manner of making such kind of persons: be they never so averse from company, bashful, solitary, timorous, they may be made at last, with those Roman matrons, to desire nothing more than, in a publike shew, to see a full company of gladiators breath out their last.

[1] Lib. 1. cap. 16. Si ex tristitiâ aut alio affectu cœperit, speciem considera, aut aliud quid eorum, quæ subitam alterationem facere possunt.   [2] Evitandi monstrifici aspectus, &c.   [3] Neque enim tam actio aut recordatio rerum hujusmodi displicet, sed iis vel gestus alterius imaginationi adumbrare, vehementer molestum. Galat. de mor. cap. 7.   [4] Tranquil. Præcipue vitentur tristes, et omnia deplorantes: tranquillitati inimicus est comes perturbatus, omnia gemens.   [5] Illorum quoque hominum, a quorum consortio abhorrent, præsentia amovenda, nec sermonibus ingratis obtundendi. Si quis insaniam ab insaniâ sic curari æstimat, et proterve utitur, magis quam æger insanit. Crato, consil. 184. Scoltzii.   [6] Molliter ac suaviter æger tractetur, nec ad ea adigatur quæ non curat.

[Mem. 6. Subs. 2.] *Mind rectified.*

If they may not otherwise be accustomed to brook such distastful and displeasing objects, the best way then is generally to avoid them. Montanus, *consil.* 229, to the earl of Montfort a courtier, and his melancholy patient, adviseth him to leave the court, by reason of those continual discontents, crosses, abuses, [1] *cares, suspicions, emulations, ambition, anger, jealousie, which that place afforded, and which surely caused him to be so melancholy at the first :*

Maxima quæque domus servis est plena superbis :

a company of scoffers and proud Jacks, are commonly conversant and attendant in such places, and able to make any man that is of a soft quiet disposition (as many times they do), *ex stulto insanum*, if once they humour him, a very idiot, or starke mad : a thing too much practised in all common societies; and they have no better sport than to make themselves merry by abusing some silly fellow, or to take advantage of another mans weaknes. In such cases, as in a plague, the best remedy is *cito, longe, tarde,* (for to such a party, especially if he be apprehensive, there can be no greater misery) to get him quickly gone far enough off, and not to be over-hasty in his return. If he be so stupid, that he do not apprehend it, his friends should take some order, and by their discretion supply that which is wanting in him, as in all other cases they ought to do. If they see a man melancholy given, solitary, averse from company, please himself with such private and vain meditations, though he delight in it, they ought by all means to seek to divert him, to dehort him, to tell him of the event and danger that may come of it. If they see a man idle, that, by reason of his means otherwise, will betake himself to no course of life, they ought seriously to admonish him, he makes a noose to intangle himself, his want of employment will be his undoing. If he have sustained any great losse, suffered a repulse, disgrace, &c. if it be possible, relieve him. If he desire ought, let him be satisfied : if in suspence, fear, suspicion, let him be secured : and if it may conveniently be, give him his hearts content; for the body cannot be cured till the mind be satisfied. [2] Socrates, in Plato, would prescribe no physick for Charmides head-ach, *till first he had eased his troublesome mind; body and soul must be cured together, as head and eyes.*

[3] Oculum non curabis sine toto capite,
Nec caput sine toto corpore,
Nec totum corpus sine animâ.

[1] Ob suspiciones, curas, æmulationem, ambitionem, iras, &c. quas locas ille ministrat, et quæ fecissent melancholicum.   [2] Nisi prius animum turbatissimum curâsset; nec oculi sine capite, nec corpus sine animâ curari potest.
[3] E Græco.

568   *Cure of Melancholy.*   [Part. 2. Sec. 2.

If that may not be hoped or expected, yet ease him with comfort, chearful speeches, fair promises, and good words; perswade
him; advise him. *Many,* saith [1]Galen, *have been cured by good
counsel and perswasion alone.   Heaviness of the heart of man
doth bring it down; but a good word rejoiceth it* (Prov. 12. 25);
*and there is he that speaketh words like the pricking of a
sword; but the tongue of a wise man is health* (ver. 18): *oratio
namque saucii animi est remedium;* a gentle speech is the true
cure of a wounded soul, as [2]Plutarch contends out of Æschylus
and Euripides: *if it be wisely administered, it easeth grief and
pain, as divers remedies do many other diseases;* 'tis *incanta-
tionis instar,* a charm, *æstuantis animi refrigerium,* that true
nepenthes of Homer, which was no Indian plant or fained medicine, which Epidamna, Thonis wife, sent Helena for a token,
as Macrobius, 7. *Saturnal.* Goropius, *Hermet. lib.* 9. Greg.
Nazianzen, and others, suppose, but opportunity of speech:
for Helenus boule, Medeas unction, Venus girdle, Circes cup,
cannot so inchant, so forcibly move or alter, as it doth.   A
letter sent or read will do as much; *multum allevor, quum tuas
literas lego;* I am much eased, as [3]Tully writ to Pomponius
Atticus, when I read thy letters; and as Julianus the Apostate
once signified to Maximus the philosopher—as Alexander slept
with Homers works, so do I with thine epistles, *tamquam
Pæoniis medicamentis, easque assidue tanquam recentes et
novas iteramus: scribe ergo, et assidue scribe;* or else come
thy self; *amicus ad amicum venies.*   Assuredly a wise and
well spoken man may do what he will in such a case: a good
orator alone, as [4]Tully holds, can alter affections by power of
his eloquence, *comfort such as are afflicted, erect such as are
depressed, expel and mitigate fear, lust, anger, &c.*   And how
powerful is the charm of a discreet and dear friend!

Ille regit dictis animos, et temperat iras.

What may not he effect? as [5]Chremes told Menedemus,
*Fear not; conceal it not, O friend; but tell me what it is that
troubles thee; and I shall surely help thee by comfort, counsel,
or in the matter it self.* [6]Arnoldus (*lib.* 1. *breviar. cap.* 18)
speaks of an usurer in his time, that, upon a loss, much
melancholy and discontent, was so cured.   As imagination,
fear, grief, cause such passions, so conceipts alone, rectified

---

[1] Et nos non paucos sanavimus, animi motibus ad debitum revocatis. lib. 1. de
sanit. tueud.   [2] Consol. ad Apollonium.   Si quis sapienter et suo tempore
adhibeat, remedia morbis diversis diversa sunt : dolentem sermo benignus sublevat.
[3] Lib. 12. Epist.   [4] De nat. Deorum. Consolatur afflictos ; deducit perterri-
tos a timore ; cupiditates imprimis, et iracundias, comprimit.   [5] Heauton.
Act. I. Scen. I. Ne metue; ne verere ; crede, inquam, mihi ; aut consolando, aut
consilio, aut re, juvero.   [6] Novi fœneratorem avarum apud meos sic curatum,
qui multam pecuniam amiserat.

Mem. 6. Subs. 2.]   *Mind rectified.*   569

by good hope, counsel, &c. are able again to help : and 'tis incredible how much they can do in such a case, as [1] Trincavelius illustrates by an example of a patient of his.   Porphyrius the philosopher (in Plotinus life, written by him) relates, that, being in a discontented humor through unsufferable anguish of mind, he was going to make away himself : but, meeting by chance his master Plotinus, who perceiving by his distracted looks all was not wel, urged him to confess his grief; which when he had heard, he used such comfortable speeches, that he redeemed him *e faucibus Erebi*, pacified his unquiet mind, insomuch that he was easily reconciled to himself, and much abashed to think afterwards that he should ever entertain so vile a motion.   By all means, therefore, fair promises, good words, gentle perswasions, are to be used, not to be too rigorous at first, [2] *or to insult over them, not to deride, neglect, or contemn, but rather*, as Lemnius exhorteth, *to pity, and by all plausible means to seek to reduce them :* but if satisfaction may not be had, mild courses, promises, comfortable speeches, and good counsel will not take place ; then, as Christopherus a Vega determines, *lib. 3. cap.* 14. *de Mel.* to handle them more roughly, to threaten and chide, saith [3] Altomarus, terrifie sometimes, or, as Salvianus will have them, to be lashed and whipped, as we do by a starting horse, [4] that is affrighted without a cause, or, as [5] Rhasis adviseth, *one while to speak fair and flatter, another while to terrifie and chide*, as they shall see cause.

When none of these precedent remedies will avail, it will not be amiss, which Savanarola and Ælian Montaltus so much commend, *clavum clavo pellere*, [6] *to drive out one passion with another, or by some contrary passion*, as they do bleeding at nose by letting blood in the arm, to expel one fear with another, one grief with another.   [7] Christopherus a Vega accounts it rational physick, *non alienum a ratione :* and Lemnius much approves it, *to use an hard wedge to an hard knot*, to drive out one disease with another, to pull out a tooth, or wound him, to geld him, saith [8] Platerus, as they did epileptical patients of old, because it quite alters the temperature, that the pain of the one may mitigate the grief of

---

[1] Lib. 1. consil. 12.   Incredibile dictu quantum juvent.   [2] Nemo istiusmodi conditionis hominibus insultet, aut in illos sit severior; verum miseriæ potius indolescat, vicemque deploret. lib. 2. cap. 16.   [3] Cap. 7. Idem Piso Laurentius, cap. 8.   [4] Quod timet nihil est, ubi cogitur et videt.   [5] Unâ vice blandiantur, unâ vice iisdem terrorem incutiant.   [6] Si vero fuerit ex novo malo audito, vel ex animi accidente, aut de amissione mercium, aut morte amici, introducantur nova contraria his, quæ ipsum ad gaudia moveant; de hoc semper niti debemus, &c.   [7] Lib. 3. cap. 14.   [8] Cap. 3. Castratio olim a veteribus usa in morbis desperatis, &c.

570   *Cure of Melancholy.*   [Part. 2. Sec. 2.

the other : [1] *and I knew one that was so cured of a quartan ague, by the sudden comming of his enemies upon him.* If we may believe [2] Pliny, whom Scaliger cals *mendaciorum patrem,* the father of lies, Q. Fabius Maximus, that renowned consul of Rome, in a battle fought with the king of the Allobroges at the river Isaurus, was so rid of a quartan ague. Valesius, in his controversies, holds this an excellent remedy, and, if it be discreetly used in this malady, better than any physick.

Sometimes again, by some [3] fained lye, strange newes, witty device, artificial invention, it is not amiss to deceive them. [4] *As they hate those,* saith Alexander, *that neglect or deride, so they will give ear to such as will sooth them up. If they say they have swallowed froggs, or a snake, by all means grant it, and tell them you can easily cure it :* 'tis an ordinary thing. Philodotus the physician cured a melancholy king, that thought his head was off, by putting a leaden cap thereon; the weight made him perceive it, and freed him of his fond imagination. A woman, in the said Alexander, swallowed a serpent, as she thought : he gave her a vomit, and conveyed a serpent, such as she conceived, into the bason : upon the sight of it, she was amended. The pleasantest dotage that ever I read, saith [5] Laurentius, was of a gentleman at Senes in Italy, who was afraid to piss, lest all the town should be drowned; the physicians caused the bels to be rung backward, and told him the town was on fire; whereupon he made water, and was immediately cured. Another supposed his nose so big that he should dash it against the wall, if he stirred; his physician took a great peece of flesh, and holding it in his hand, pinched him by the nose, making him beleeve that flesh was cut from it. Forestus (*obs. lib.* 1) had a melancholy patient, who thought he was dead : [6] *he put a fellow in a chest, like a dead man, by his beds side, and made him reare himself a little, and eat : the melancholy man asked the counterfeit, whether dead men use to eat meat ? he told him yea; whereupon he did eat likewise, and was cured.* Lemnius (*lib.* 2. *cap.* 6. *de* 4. *complex.*) hath many such instances, and Jovianus Pontanus (*lib.* 4. *cap.* 2. *of Wisd.*) of the like : but amongst the rest I find one most memorable, registred in the [7] French Chronicles, of an advocate

---

[1] Lib. 1. cap. 5. Sic morbum morbo, ut clavum clavo, retundimus, et malo nodo malum cuneum adhibemus. Novi ego qui ex subito hostium incursu, et inopinato timore, quartanam depulerat.   [2] Lib. 7. cap. 50. In acie pugnans febre quartanâ liberatus est.   [3] Jacchinus, c. 15, in 9 Rhasis. Mont. cap. 26. [4] Lib. 1. cap. 16. Aversantur eos qui eorum affectus rident, contemnunt. Si ranas et viperas comedisse se putant, concedere debemus, et spem de curâ facere. [5] Cap. 8. de mel.   [6] Cistam posuit ex medicorum consilio prope eum, in quem alium se mortuum fingentem posuit ; hic in cistâ jacens, &c.   [7] Serres, 1550.

8

[Mem. 6. Subs. 3.] *Perturbation rectified.* 571

of Paris before mentioned, who beleeved verily he was dead, &c. I read a multitude of examples, of melancholy men cured by such artificial inventions.

SUBSECT. III.

Musick a remedy.

MANY and sundry are the means which philosophers and physicians have prescribed to exhilarate a sorrowful heart, to divert those fixed and intent cares and meditations, which in this malady so much offend; but, in my judgement, none so present, none so powerfull, none so apposite, as a cup of strong drink, mirth, musick, and merry company. Ecclus. 40. 20: *Wine and musick rejoyce the heart.* [1] Rhasis (*cont.* 9. *Tract.* 15), Altomarus (*cap.* 7), Ælianus Montaltus (*c.* 26), Ficinus, Bened. Victor. Faventinus, are almost immoderate in the commendation of it; a most forcible medicine [2] Jacchinus calls it: Jason Pratensis, *a most admirable thing, and worthy of consideration, that can so mollifie the minde, and stay those tempestuous affections of it. Musica est mentis medicina mœstæ,* a roaring-meg against melancholy, to rear and revive the languishing soul; [3] *affecting not onely the ears, but the very arteries, the vital and animal spirits, it erects the minde, and makes it nimble.* Lemnius, *instit. cap.* 44. This it will effect in the most dull, severe, and sorrowfull souls, [4] *expell griefe with mirth; and, if there be any cloudes, dust, or dregs of cares yet lurking in our thoughts, most powerfully it wipes them all away* (Salisbur. *polit. lib.* 1. *cap.* 6); and that which is more, it will perform all this in an instant— [5] *chear up the countenance, expell austerity, bring in hilarity,* (Girald. Camb. *cap.* 12. *Topogr. Hiber.*) *informe our manners, mitigate anger.* Athenæus (*Dipnosophist. lib.* 14. *cap.* 10) calleth it an infinite treasure to such as are endowed with it.

Dulcisonum reficit tristia corda melos. (Eobanus Hessus.)

Many other properties [6] Cassiodorus (*epist.* 4) reckons up of this our divine musick, not only to expell the greatest griefs, but *it doth extenuate fears and furies, appeaseth cruelty,*

---

[1] In 9 Rhasis. Magnam vim habet musica. [2] Cap. de Maniâ. Admiranda profecto res est, et digna expensione, quod sonorum concinnitas mentem emolliat, sistatque procellosas ipsius affectiones. [3] Languens animus inde erigitur et reviviscit; nec tam aures afficit, sed et sonitu per arterias undique diffuso, spiritus tum vitales tum animales excitat, mentem reddens agilem, &c. [4] Musica venustate suâ mentes severiores capit, &c. [5] Animos tristes subito exhilarat, nubilos vultus serenat, austeritatem reponit, jucunditatem exponit, barbariemque facit deponere gentes, mores instituit, iracundiam mitigat. [6] Cithara tristitiam jucundat, tumidos furores attenuat, cruentam sæviitam blande reficit, languorem, &c.

572   *Cure of Melancholy.*   [Part. 2. Sec. 2.

abateth heaviness; and, to such as are watchfull, it causeth quiet rest; it takes away spleen and hatred, bee it instrumentall, vocall, with strings, winde, [1] *quæ a spiritu, sine manuum dexteritate, gubernetur, &c.* it cures all irksomness and heaviness of the soul. [2] Labouring men, that sing to their work, can tell as much; and so can souldiers when they go to fight, whom terror of death cannot so much affright, as the sound of trumpet, drum, fife, and such like musick, animates; *metus enim mortis,* as [3] Censorinus enformeth us, *musicâ depellitur. It makes a childe quiet,* the nurses song; and many times the sound of a trumpet on a sudden, bells ringing, a carremans whistle, a boy singing some ballad tune early in the street, alters, revives, recreates a restless patient that cannot sleep in the night, &c. In a word, it is so powerfull a thing that it ravisheth the soul, *regina sensuum,* the queen of the senses, by sweet pleasure (which is an happy cure); and corporall tunes pacifie our incorporeall soul: *sine ore loquens, dominatum in animam exercet,* and carries it beyond it self, helps, elevates, extends it. Scaliger (*exercit.* 302) gives a reason of these effects, [4] *because the spirits about the heart take in that trembling and dancing air into the body, are moved together, and stirred up with it,* or else the minde, as some suppose, harmonically composed, is roused up at the tunes of musick.' And 'tis not onely men that are so affected, but almost all other creatures. You know the tale of Hercules, Gallus, Orpheus, and Amphion, (*felices animas* Ovid cals them) that could *saxa movere sono testudinis,* &c. make stocks and stones, as well as beasts, and other animals, dance after their pipes: the dog and hare, wolf and lamb,

> (Vicinumque lupo præbuit agna latus)

clamosus graculus, stridula cornix, et Jovis aquila, as Philostratus describes it in his images, stood all gaping upon Orpheus; and [5] trees, pulled up by the roots, came to hear him;

> Et comitem quercum pinus amica trahit.

Arion made fishes follow him, which, as common experience evinceth, [6] are much affected with musick. All singing birds are much pleased with it, especially nightingales, if we may beleeve Calcagninus; and bees among the rest, though they be flying away, when they hear any tingling sound, will tarry behinde. [7] *Harts, hindes, horses, dogs, bears, are exceedingly*

---

[1] Pet. Aretine.   [2] Castilio, de aulic. lib. 1. fol. 27.   [3] Lib. de Natali, cap. 12.   [4] Quod spiritus, qui in corde agitant, tremulum et subsaltantem recipiunt aërem in pectus, et inde excitantur, a spiritu musculi moventur, &c. [5] Arbores radicibus avulsæ, &c.   [6] M. Carew of Anthony, in descript. Cornwal, saith of whales. that they will come and show themselves dancing at the sound of a trumpet, fol. 35. 1. et fol. 154. 2. book.   [7] De cervo, equo, cane, urso, idem compertum; musicâ afficiuntur.

Mem. 6. Subs. 3.]   *Perturbation rectified.*   573

delighted with it, Scal. *exerc.* 302. Elephants, Agrippa addes, *lib. 2. cap.* 24. and in Lydia in the midst of a lake there be certain floating ilands, (if he will beleeve it) that, after musick, will dance.

But to leave all declamatory speeches in praise [1] of divine musick, I will confine my self to my proper subject: besides that excellent power it hath to expell many other diseases, it is a soveraigne remedy against [2] despair and melancholy, and will drive away the devil himself. Canus, a Rhodian fidler in [3] Philostratus, when Apollonius was inquisitive to know what he could do with his pipe, told him, *that he would make a melancholy man merry, and him that was merry much merrier than before, a lover more inamoured, a religious man more devout.* Ismenias the Theban, [4] Chiron the Centaure, is said to have cured this and many other diseases by musick alone: as now they do those, saith [5] Bodine, that are troubled with S. Vitus Bedlam dance. [6] Timotheus the musician compelled Alexander to skip up and down, and leave his dinner (like the tale of the frier and the boy); whom Austin (*de civ. Dei, lib.* 17. *cap.* 14.) so much commends for it. Who hath not heard how Davids harmony drove away the evill spirits from king Saul? (1 Sam. 16) and Elisha, when he was much troubled by importunate kings, called for a minstrel; *and, when he played, the hand of the Lord came upon him* (2 Kings, 3). Censorinus (*de natali, cap.* 12) reportes how Asclepiades the physician helped many frantike persons by this means, *phreneticorum mentes morbo turbatas.*—Jason Pratensis (*cap. de Mania*) hath many examples, how Clinias and Empedocles cured some desperately melancholy, and some mad, by this our musick; which because it hath such excellent virtues, belike, [7] Homer brings in Phemius playing, and the Muses singing at the banquet of the gods. Aristotle, *Polit. l.* 8. *c.* 5, Plato 2, *de legibus,* highly approve it, and so do all politicians. The Greekes, Romanes, have graced musick, and made it one of the liberall sciences, though it be now become mercenary. All civill commonwealths allow it: Cneius Manlius (as [8] Livius relates) A° *ab urb. cond.* 567, brought first out of Asia to Rome singing wenches, players, jesters, and all kinde of musick to their feasts.

---

[1] Numen inest numeris.   [2] Sæpe graves morbos modulatum carmen abegit, Et desperatis conciliavit opem.   [3] Lib. 5. cap. 7. Mœrentibus mœrorem adimam, lætantem vero scipso reddam hilariorem, amantem calidiorem, religiosum divino numine correptum, et ad Deos colendos paratiorem.   [4] Natalis Comes, Myth. lib. 4. cap. 12.   [5] Lib. 5. de rep. Curat musica furorem Sancti Viti. [6] Exsilire e convivio. Cardan, subtil. lib. 13.   [7] Iliad. 1   [8] Libro 9. cap. 1. Psaltrias, sambucistriasque, et convivialia ludorum oblectamenta addita epulis, ex Asiâ invexit in urbem.

574   *Cure of Melancholy.*   [Part. 2. Sec. 2.

Your princes, emperours, and persons of any quality, maintain it in their courts: no mirth without musick. Sr Thomas Moore, in his absolute Utopian common-wealth, allowes musick as an appendix to every meal, and that throughout, to all sorts. Epictetus cals *mensam mutam præsepe,* a table without musick a manger; for *the concert of musicians at a banquet is a carbuncle set in gold; and as the signet of an emerald well trimmed with gold, so is the melody of musick in a pleasant banquet.* Ecclus. 32, v. 5, 6. [1] Lewes the eleventh, when he invited Edward the fourth to come to Paris, told him, that, as a principall part of his entertainment, he should hear sweet voices of children, Ionicke and Lydian tunes, exquisite musick, he should have a . . . . , and the Cardinal of Burbon to be his confessor; which he used as a most plausible argument, as to a sensuall man indeed it is. [2] Lucian, in his book *de saltatione,* is not ashamed to confess that he took infinite delight in singing, dancing, musick, womens company, and such like pleasures; *and if thou* (saith he) *didst but hear them play and dance, I know thou wouldst be so well pleased with the object, that thou wouldst dance for company thy self: without doubt thou wilt bee taken with it:* So Scaliger ingenuously confesseth, *exercit.* 274. [3] *I am beyond all measure affected with musick; I do most willingly behold them dance: I am mightily detained and allured with that grace and comeliness of fair women; I am well pleased to bee idle amongst them.* And what young man is not? As it is acceptable and conducing to most, so especially to a melancholy man; provided alwaies, his disease proceed not originally from it, that he bee not some light *inamorato,* some idle phantastick, who capers in conceit all the day long, and thinks of nothing else, but how to make jigs, sonnets, madrigals, in commendation of his mistress. In such cases, musick is most pernicious, as a spur to a free horse will make him run himself blinde, or break his wind; *incitamentum enim amoris musica;* for musick enchants, as Menander holds; it will make such melancholy persons mad; and the sound of those jigs and horn-pipes will not bee removed out of the ears a week after. [4] Plato, for this reason, forbids musick and wine to all young men, because they are most part amorous, *ne ignis addatur igni,* lest one fire increase another. Many men are melancholy by hearing musick; but it is a pleasing melancholy that it causeth; and

---

[1] Commineus.   [2] Ista libenter et magnâ cum voluptate spectare soleo. Et scio te illecebris hisce captum iri, et insuper tripudiaturum: haud dubie demulcebere.   [3] In musicis supra omnem fidem capior et oblector; choreas libentissime aspicio; pulchrarum feminarum venustate detineor: otiari inter has solutus curis possum.   [4] 3 De legibus.

therefore to such as are discontent, in wo, fear, sorrow, or dejected, it is a most present remedy : it expels cares, alters their grieved minds, and easeth in an instant. Otherwise, saith [1] Plutarch, *musica magis dementat quam vinum:* musick makes some men mad as a tygre ; like Astolphos horn in Ariosto, or Mercuries golden wand in Homer, that made some wake, others sleep, it hath divers effects : and [2] Theophrastus right well prophesied, that diseases were either procured by musick, or mitigated.

SUBSECT. IV.

Mirth and merry company, fair objects, remedies.

MIRTH and merry company may not be separated from musick, both concerning and necessarily required in this business. Mirth (saith [3] Vives) *purgeth the blood, confirms health, causeth a fresh, pleasing, and fine colour,* prorogues life, whets the wit, makes the body young, lively, and fit for any manner of imployment. The merrier heart, the longer life: *a merry heart is the life of the flesh* (Prov. 14. 30) ; *Gladness prolongs his days* (Ecclus. 30. 22) ; and this is one of the three Salernitan doctors, D. Merryman, D. Diet, and D. Quiet, [4] which cure all diseases——*Mens hilaris, requies, moderata diæta.* [5] Gomesius (*præfat. lib. 3. de sal. gen.*) is a great magnifyer of honest mirth, by which (saith he) *we cure many passions of the minde, in our selves, and in our friends :* which [6] Galateus assignes for a cause why we love merry companions : and well they deserve it, being that (as [7] Magninus holds) a merry companion is better than musick, and, as the saying is, *comes jucundus in viâ pro vehiculo,* as a wagon to him that is wearied on the way. *Jucunda confabulatio, sales, joci,* pleasant discourse, jests, conceits, merry tales, *melliti verborum globuli,* (as Petronius, [8] Pliny, [9] Spondanus, [10] Cælius, and many good authors plead) are that sole *nepenthes* of Homer, Helenas

---

[1] Sympos. quæst. 5. Musica multos magis dementat quam vinum. [2] Animi morbi vel a musicâ curantur vel inferuntur. [3] Lib. 3. de animâ. Lætitia purgat sanguinem, valetudinem conservat, colorem inducit florentem, nitidum, gratum. [4] Spiritus temperat, calorem excitat, naturalem virtutem corroborat, juvenile corpus diu servat, vitam prorogat, ingenium acuit, et hominem negotiis quibuslibet aptiorem reddit. Schola Salern. [5] Dum contumeliâ vacant, et festivâ lenitate mordent, mediocres animi ægritudines sanari solent, &c. [6] De mor. fol. 57. Amamus ideo eos qui sunt faceti et jucundi. [7] Regim. sanit. part. 2. Nota quod amicus bonus et dilectus socius narrationibus suis jucundis superat omnem melodiam. [8] Lib. 21. cap. 27. [9] Comment. in 4. Odyss. [10] Lib. 26. c. 15.

576 *Cure of Melancholy.* [Part. 2. Sec. 2.

boule, Venus girdle, so renowned of old [1] to expell grief and care, to cause mirth and gladness of heart, if they be rightly understood, or seasonably applied. In a word,

[2] Amor, voluptas, Venus, gaudium,
Jocus, ludus, sermo suavis, suaviatio,

are the true *nepenthes.* For these causes our physicians generally prescribe this as a principal engine, to batter the walls of melancholy, a chief antidote, and a sufficient cure of it self. *By all means* (saith [3] Mesue) *procure mirth to these men, in such things as are heard, seen, tasted, or smelled, or any way perceived; and let them have all enticements, and fair promises, the sight of excellent beauties, attires, ornaments, delightsome passages, to distract their minds from fear and sorrow, and such things on which they are so fixed and intent.* [4] *Let them use hunting, sports, playes, jests, merry company,* as Rhasis prescribes, *which will not let the minde be molested, a cup of good drinke now and then, hear musick, and have such companions with whom they are especially delighted,* [5] *merry tales or toyes, drinking, singing, dancing, and whatsoever else may procure mirth:* and by no means, saith Guianerius, suffer them to be alone. Benedictus Victorius Faventinus, in his Empericks, accompts it an especial remedy against melancholy, [6] *to hear and see singing, dancing, maskers, mummers, to converse with such merry fellowes, and fair maids. For the beauty of a woman cheareth the countenance,* Ecclus. 36. 22. [7] Beauty alone is a soveraign remedy against fear, grief, and all melancholy fits; a charm, as Peter de la Seine and many other writers affirme, a banquet it self; he gives instance in discontented Menelaüs that was so often freed by Helenas fair face: and [8] Tully (3 *Tusc.*) cites Epicurus as a chief patron of this tenent. To expell grief, and procure pleasance, sweet smells, good diet, touch, taste, embracing, singing, dancing, sports, playes, and, above the rest, exquisite beauties, *quibus oculi jucunde moventur et animi,* are most powerfull means;

---

[1] Homericum illud nepenthes, quod mœrorem tollit, et euthymiam et hilaritatem parit. [2] Plaut. Bacch. [3] De ægritud. capitis. Omni modo generet lætitiam in iis, de iis quæ audiuntur et videntur, aut odorantur, aut gustantur, aut quocunque modo sentiri possunt, et aspectu formarum multi decoris et ornatûs, et negotiatione jucundâ, et blandientibus ludis, et promissis distrahantur eorum animi de re aliquâ quam timent et dolent. [4] Utantur venationibus, ludis, jocis, amicorum consortiis, quæ non sinunt animum turbari, vino, et cantu, et loci mutatione, et biberiâ, et gaudio, et quibus præcipue delectantur. [5] Piso: fabulis et ludis quærenda delectatio. His versetur qui maxime grati sunt: cantus et chorea ad lætitiam prosunt. [6] Præcipue valet ad expellendam melancholiam stare in cantibus, ludis, et sonis, et habitare cum familiaribus, et præcipue cum puellis jucundis. [7] Par. 5. de avocamentis. lib. de absolvendo luctu. [8] Corporum complexus, cantus, ludi, formæ, &c.

Mem. 6. Subs. 4.] *Mind rectified by Mirth.* 577

obvia forma, to meet, or see a fair maid pass by, or to be in company with her. He found it by experience, and made good use of it in his own person, if Plutarch bely him not; for he reckons up the names of some more elegant pieces, [1] Leontia, Boedina, Hedieia, Nicedia, that were frequently seen in Epicurus garden, and very familiar in his house. Neither did he try it himself alone; but, if we may give credit to [2] Athenæus, he practised it upon others: For, when a sad and sick patient was brought unto him to be cured, *he laid him on a down bed, crowned him with a garland of sweet-smelling flowers, in a fair perfumed closet delicately set out; and, after a potion or two of good drink which he administred, he brought in a beautiful yong [3] wench that could play upon a lute, sing and dance, &c.* Tully (3 *Tusc.*) scoffes at Epicurus for this his prophane physick (as well he deserved); and yet Phavorinus and Stobæus highly approve of it. Most of our looser physicians, in some cases, to such parties especially, allow of this; and all of them will have a melancholy, sad, and discontented person, make frequent use of honest sports, companies, and recreations, *et incitandos ad Venerem* (as [4] Rodericus a Fonseca will) *aspectu et contactu pulcherrimarum feminarum;* to be drawn to such consorts, whether they will or no; not to be an auditor only, or a spectator, but sometimes an actor himself. *Dulce est desipere in loco;* to play the fool now and then, is not amiss; there is a time for all things. Grave Socrates would be merry by fits, sing, dance, and take his liquor too, or else Theodoret belies him; so would old Cato; [5] Tully by his own confession, and the rest. Xenophon, in his Sympos. brings in Socrates as a principal actor; no man merrier then himself; and sometimes he would [6] *ride a cock horse with his children,*

——— equitare in arundine longâ

(though Alcibiades scoffed at him for it); and well he might; for now and then (saith Plutarch) the most vertuous, honest, and gravest men will use feasts, jests, and toys, as we do sauce to our meats. So did Scipio and Lælius,

[7] Quin, ubi se, a vulgo et scenâ, in secreta remôrant
Virtus Scipiadæ et mitis sapientia Lælì,

---

[1] Circa hortos Epicuri frequentes. [2] Dipnosoph. lib. 10. Coronavit florido serto incendens odores, in culcitâ plumeâ collocavit, dulciculam potionem propinans psaltriam adduxit, &c. [3] Ut reclinatâ suaviter in lectum puellâ, &c. [4] Tom. 2. consult. 85. [5] Epist. fam. lib. 7. 22. epist. Heri domum, bene potus, seroque redieram. [6] Valer. Max. cap. 8. lib. 8. Interpositâ arundine cruribus suis, cum filiis ludens, ab Alcibiade risus est. [7] Hor.

578   *Cure of Melancholy.*   [Part. 2. Sec. 2.

Nugari cum illo, et discincti ludere, donec
Decoqueretur olus, soliti——

Valorous Scipio and gentle Lælius,
Removed from the scene and rout so clamorous,
Were wont to recreate themselves, their robes laid by,
Whilst supper by the cook was making ready.

Machiavel, in the 8 book of his Florentine history, gives this
note of Cosmus Medices, the wisest and gravest man of his
time in Italy, that he would [1] *now and then play the most
egregious fool in his carriage, and was so much given to
jesters, players, and childish sports, to make himself merry,
that he that should but consider his gravity on the one part,
his folly and lightness on the other, would surely say, there
were two distinct persons in him.* Now, me thinks he did
well in it, though [2] Salisburiensis be of opinion that magistrates, senators, and grave men, should not descend to lighter
sports, *ne respublica ludere videatur;* but, as Themistocles,
still keep a stern and constant carriage. I commend Cosmus
Medices, and Castruccius Castrucanus, then whom Italy never
knew a worthier captain, another Alexander, if [3] Machiavel do
not deceive us in his life: *when a friend of his reprehended
him for dancing beside his dignity* (belike at some cushen
dance) he told him again, *qui sapit interdiu, vix unquam noctu
desipit;* he that is wise in the day, may dote a little in the
night. Paulus Jovius relates as much of Pope Leo Decimus,
that he was a grave, discreet, stay'd man, yet sometimes most
free, and too open in his sports. And 'tis not altogether
[4] unfit or mis-beseeming the gravity of such a man, if that
decorum of time, place, and such circumstances, be observed.
[5] *Misce stultitiam consiliis brevem :* and, as [6] he said in an epigram to his wife, I would have every man say to himself, or to
his friend,

Moll, once in pleasant company, by chance
I wisht that you for company would dance :
Which you refus'd, and said, your years require,
Now, matron-like, both manners and attire.
Well, Moll, if needs you will be matron-like,
Then trust to this, I will thee matron like :

---

[1] Hominibus facetis et ludis puerilibus ultra modum deditus, adeo ut, sicut in eo
tam gravitatem quam levitatem considerare liberet, duas personas distinctas in eo
esse diceret.   [2] De nugis curial. lib. 1. cap. 4. Magistratus et viri graves a
ludis levioribus arcendi.   [3] Machiavel. vitâ ejus. Ab amico reprehensus,
quod præter dignitatem tripudiis operam daret, respondet, &c.   [4] There is
a time for all things, to weep, laugh, mourn, dance. Eccles. 3. 4.   [5] Hor.
[6] Sir John Harrington, Epigr. 50.

Mem. 6. Subs. 4.]   *Mind rectified by Mirth.*   579

Yet so to you my love may never lessen,
As you, for church, house, bed, observe this lesson :
Sit in the church as solemn as a saint ;
No deed, word, thought, your due devotion taint :
Vaile, if you will, your head ; your soul reveal
To him that only wounded soules can heal.
Be in my house as busie as a bee,
Having a sting for every one but me ;
Buzzing in every corner, gath'ring hony :
Let nothing waste, that costs or yieldeth mony.
[1] And, when thou seest my heart to mirth incline,
Thy tongue, wit, blood, warm with good cheere and wine :
Then of sweet sports let no occasion scape,
But be as wanton, toying, as an ape.

Those old [2] Greeks had their *Lubentiam Deam,* goddess of
Pleasance, and the Lacedæmonians, instructed from Lycurgus,
did *Deo Risui sacrificare,* after their wars especially, and in
times of peace ; which was used in Thessaly, as it appears by
that of [3] Apuleius, who was made an instrument of their
laughter himself ; [4] *because laughter and merriment was to season their labours and modester life.*

[5] Risus enim Divûm atque hominum est æterna voluptas.

Princes use jesters, players, and have those masters of revels
in their courts. The Romans, at every supper, (for they had
no solemn dinner) used musick, gladiators, jesters, &c. as
[6] Suetonius relates of Tiberius, Dion of Commodus ; and so
did the Greeks. Besides musick, in Xenophons *Sympos.*
Philippus ridendi artifex, Philip, a jester, was brought to
make sport. Paulus Jovius, in the eleventh book of his
history, hath a pretty digression of our English customes,
which howsoever some may misconster, I, for my part, will interpret to the best. [7] *The whole nation, beyond all other mortal
men, is most given to banqueting and feasts ; for they prolong
them many houres together, with dainty cheere, exquisite
musick, and facete jesters ; and afterwards they fall a dancing
and courting their mistresses, till it be late in the night.*
Volaterran gives the same testimony of this island, commending our jovial manner of entertainment, and good mirth ; and
me thinks he saith well ; there is no harm in it ; long may
they use it, and all such modest sports. Ctesias reports of a
Persian king, that had 150 maids attending at his table, to

[1] Lucretia toto Sis licet usque die, Thaïda nocte volo.   [2] Lil. Giraldus, hist.
Deor. syntag. 1.   [3] Lib. 2. de aur. as.   [4] Eo quod risus esset laboris et
modesti victûs condimentum.   [5] Calcag. epig.   [6] Cap. 61. In deliciis
habuit scurras et adulatores.   [7] Universa gens supra mortales cæteros convi-
viorum studiosissima. Ea enim per varias et exquisitas dapes, interpositis musicis et joculatoribus, in multas sæpius horas extrahunt, ac subinde productis
choreis et amoribus fœminarum indulgent, &c.

P P 2

580   *Cure of Melancholy.*   [Part. 2. Sec. 2.

play, sing, and dance by turns; and [1] Lil. Giraldus of an Egyptian prince, that kept nine virgins still to wait upon him, and those of most excellent feature, and sweet voices, which afterwards gave occasion to the Greeks of that fiction of the nine muses. The king of Æthiopia in Africk, most of our Asiatick princes, have done so, and do; those Sophies, Mogors, Turkes, &c. solace themselves after supper amongst their queens and concubines, *quæ, jucundioris oblectamenti caussâ* ([2] saith mine author) *coram rege psallere et saltare consueverant;* taking great pleasure to see and hear them sing and dance. This and many such means, to exhilarate the heart of men, have been still practised in all ages, as knowing there is no better thing to the preservation of mans life. What shall I say then, but to every melancholy man,

> [3] Utere convivis non tristibus; utere amicis
> Quas nugæ et risus et joca salsa juvant.

> Feast often, and use friends not still so sad,
> Whose jests and merriments may make thee glad.

Use honest and chast sports, scenical shews, playes, games;

> [4] Accedant juvenumque chori, mixtæque puellæ.

And, as Marsilius Ficinus concludes an epistle to Bernard Canisianus and some other of his friends, will I this tract to all good students; [5] *Live merrily, O my friends, free from cares, perplexity, anguish, grief of mind; live merrily;* lætitiæ cœlum vos creavit: [6] *again and again I request you to be merry; if any thing trouble your hearts, or vex your souls, neglect and contemn it;* [7] *let it passe.* [8] *And this I enjoyn you, not as a divine alone, but as a physician; for, without this mirth, which is the life and quintessence of physick, medicines, and whatsoever is used and applyed to prolong the life of man, is dull, dead, and of no force.* Dum fata sinunt, vivite læti (Seneca): I say be merry:

> [9] Nec lusibus virentem
> Viduemus hanc juventam.

---

[1] Syntag. de Musis.   [2] Athenæus, lib. 12 et 14. Assiduis mulierum vocibus, cantuque symphoniæ palatium Persarum regis totum personabat. Jovius, hist. lib. 18.   [3] Eobanus Hessus.   [4] Fracastorius.   [5] Vivite ergo læti, O amici; procul ab angustiâ, vivite læti.   [6] Iterum precor et obtestor, vivite læti: illud, quod cor urit, negligite.   [7] Lætus in præsens animus quod ultra est oderit curare. Hor.   [8] He was both sacerdos et medicus. Hæc autem non tam ut sacerdos, amici, mando vobis, quam ut medicus; nam absque hac unâ tamquam medicinarum vitâ, medicinæ omnes ad vitam producendam adhibitæ moriuntur; vivite læti.   [9] Locheus. Anacreon.

15

Mem. 6. Subs. 4.] *Mind rectified.* 581

It was Tiresias the prophets counsel to [1] Menippus, that travelled all the world over, even down to hell it self, to seek content, and his last farewell to Menippus, to be merry. [2] *Contemn the world* (saith he) *and count all that is in it vanity and toyes: this only covet all thy life long; be not curious, or over solicitous in any thing, but with a well composed and contented estate to enjoy thy self, and above all things to be merry.*

> Si, Mimnermus uti censet, sine amore jocisque
> Nil est jucundum, vivas in amore jocisque.

Nothing better, (to conclude with Solomon Eccles. 3. 22.) *then that a man should rejoyce in his affairs.* 'Tis the same advice which every physician in this case rings to his patient, as [3] Capivaccius to his: *avoid over much study and perturbations of the minde, and, as much as in thee lies, live at hearts ease:* Prosper Calenus to that melancholy cardinal Cæsius, [4] *amidst thy serious studies and business, use jests and conceits, playes and toyes, and whatsoever else may recreate thy mind.* Nothing better then mirth and merry company in this malady. [5] *It begins with sorrow* (saith Montanus): *it must be expelled with hilarity.*

But see the mischief; many men, knowing that merry company is the only medicine against melancholy, will therefore neglect their business, and in another extreme, spend all their dayes among good fellowes in a tavern or an ale-house, and know not otherwise how to bestow their time but in drinking ; malt-worms, men-fishes, or water-snakes, [6] *qui bibunt solum ranarum more, nihil comedentes*, like so many frogs in a puddle. 'Tis their sole exercise to eat and drink: to sacrifice to Volupia, Rumina, Edulica, Potina, Mellona, is all their religion. They wish for Philoxenus neck, Jupiters trinoctium, and that the sun would stand still as in Joshuas time, to satisfy their lust, that they might *dies noctesque pergræcari et bibere.* Flourishing wits, and men of good parts, good fashion, and good worth, basely prostitute themselves to

---

[1] Lucian. Necyomantia, tom. 2.   [2] Omnia mundana nugas æstima. Hoc solum totâ vitâ persequere, ut, præsentibus bene compositis, minime curiosus, aut ullâ in re solicitus, quam plurimum potes vitam hilarem traducas.   [3] Hildesheim, spicil. 2. de Maniâ fol. 161. Studia literarum et animi perturbationes fugiat, et quantum potest, jucunde vivat.   [4] Lib. de atrâ bile. Gravioribus curis ludos et facetias aliquando interpone, jocos, et quæ solent animum relaxare. [5] Consil. 30. Mala valetudo aucta et contracta est tristitia, ac propterea exhilaratione animi removenda.   [6] Athen. dipnosoph. lib. 1.

582   *Cure of Melancholy.*   [Part. 2. Sec. 2.

every rogues company, to take tobacco and drink, to roare and sing scurrile songs in base places.

> [1] Invenies aliquem cum percussore jacentem,
> Permixtum nautis, aut furibus, aut fugitivis:

Which Thomas Erastus objects to Paracelsus, that he would lye drinking all day long with car-men and tapsters in a brothel-house, is too frequent amongst us, with men of better note : like Timocreon of Rhodes, *multa bibens, et multa vorans, &c.* they drown their wits, seeth their brains in ale, consume their fortunes, lose their time, weaken their temperatures, contract filthy diseases, rheumes, dropsies, calentures, tremor, get swoln juglars, pimpled red faces, sore eyes, &c. heat their livers, alter their complexions, spoil their stomacks, overthrow their bodies (for drink drowns more then the sea and all the rivers that fall into it)—meer funges and casks—confound their souls, suppress reason, go from Scylla to Charybdis, and use that which is an help, to their undoing.

> [2] Quid refert, morbo an ferro pereamve ruinâ ?

[3] When the Black Prince went to set the exil'd king of Castile into his kingdome, there was a terrible battel fought betwixt the English and the Spanish; at last the Spanish fled; the English followed them to the river side, *where some drowned themselves to avoid their enemies, the rest were killed.* Now tell me what difference is between drowning and killing? As good be melancholy still, as drunken beasts and beggars. Company, a sole comfort, and an only remedy to all kind of discontent, is their sole misery and cause of perdition. As Hermione lamented in Euripides, *malæ mulieres me fecerunt malam,* evil company marr'd her, may they justly complain bad companions have been their bane. For, [4] *malus malum vult, ut sit sui similis;* one drunkard in a company, one thief, one whoremaster, will, by his good will, make all the rest as bad as himself :

> ————[5] et si
> Nocturnos jures te formidare vapores,

be of what complexion you will, inclination, love or hate, be it good or bad, if you come amongst them, you must do as

---

[1] Juven. Sat. 8.   [2] Hor.   [3] Froissard. hist. lib. 1.   Hispani, cum Anglorum vires ferre non possent, in fugam se dederunt, &c. Præcipites in fluvium se dederunt, ne in hostium manus venirent.   [4] Ter.   [5] Hor.

Mem. 6. Subs. 4.]   *Mind rectified.*   583

they do; yea, [1] though it be to the prejudice of your health, you must drink *venenum pro vino*. And so, like grass-hoppers, whilst they sing over their cups all summer, they starve in winter; and, for a little vain merriment, shall find a sorrowful reckoning in the end.

[1] Η πιθι η απιθι.

END OF VOL. I.

LONDON:
GILBERT & RIVINGTON, PRINTERS,
St. John's Square.

CPSIA information can be obtained
at www.ICGtesting.com
Printed in the USA
LVHW041734241120
672596LV00004B/1020